THE DOCTORS BOOK
OF HOME REMEDIES

THE DOCTORS BOOK OF

HOME REMEDIES

THOUSANDS OF TIPS AND TECHNIQUES ANYONE CAN USE TO HEAL EVERYDAY HEALTH PROBLEMS

By the Editors of Prevention Magazine Health Books

Don Barone
Deborah Grandinetti
Marcia Holman
Lance Jacobs
William LeGro

Judith Lin
Claudia Allen Lowe
Jean Rogers
Don Wade
Russell Wild

Edited by Debora Tkac

Rodale Press, Emmaus, Pennsylvania

Printed in the United States of America on acid-free, recycled paper

Book Designer: Glen Burris
Cover Designer: Denise Mirabello
Copy Editor: Sally Schaffer

If you have any questions or comments concerning this book, please write:

Rodale Press
Book Reader Service
33 East Minor Street
Emmaus, PA 18098

Library of Congress Cataloging-in-Publication Data

The Doctors book of home remedies : thousands of tips and techniques anyone can
    use to heal everyday health problems / by the editors of Prevention Magazine Health
    Books ; edited by Debora Tkac.
        p.   cm.
    ISBN 0-87857-873-0   hardcover
    1. Medicine, Popular.   I. Tkac, Debora.   II. Prevention (Emmaus, Pa.)
RC81.D65   1990
610—dc20   89-38656
                                                                                  CIP

Distributed in the book trade by St. Martin's Press

    6 8 10 9 7 5   hardcover

Contents

Introduction
Your Healing Companion

You've probably seen the commercial: A rag-clad guy looking like a hybrid of Robinson Crusoe and Peter Jennings stands on a desert island. He tells you that most doctors would pick a certain brand of aspirin — the wonder drug — as their one healing companion if they were stranded on the island. Well, this introduction is a clone of that commercial, and here's the claim:

If you were stranded on a desert island and needed *one* self-help book — one medical companion that would let you effectively and safely treat almost any health problem — this would be the book.

What you're holding in your hands is the print equivalent of a wonder drug: a remarkably powerful, all-purpose product with enough extra strength to heal millions of people, including yourself. You're holding the distilled experience and wisdom of hundreds of doctors and health professionals — their very best curative techniques for dozens and dozens of conditions and diseases. And these techniques — like a wonder drug — are simple, accessible, and virtually risk-free.

How was this wonder drug formulated? The editors of Prevention Magazine Health Books spent months interviewing medical experts and asking them for home remedies — for ways that our readers could treat their annoyances and ills themselves. And those experts answered. They told us 27 ways to cut cholesterol. Eighteen remedies for hemorrhoids. Thirty-eight ways to relieve the pain of a sting. Fourteen tips to muffle a shingles infection. In all, they shared with us over 2,300 methods for relieving over 130 problems — a cornucopia of cures.

I've been in the health journalism business for 14 years. I've written and edited thousands of articles and chapters; I've read hundreds of how-to books. And never — never — have I come across a more complete, practical collection of healing tips and techniques. So if you take one book to that desert island — or just want one healing companion in the island of your home — choose this one. The doctors we talked to would agree; it's truly wonderful.

For better health,

William Gottlieb

William Gottlieb
Editor in Chief
Prevention Magazine Health Books

Acne

18 Remedies for Smoother Skin

As you wipe the steam off your bathroom mirror, you find yourself face-to-face with a huge pink dot on the end of your nose. This is not a good way to begin the week.

You give the mirror another wipe with your hand, then get up on your toes and lean over the sink to get a better look. It's there all right. But what's this? When you move your chin up to get a better view, you happen to glimpse a couple of whiteheads sprouting under your bottom lip.

You don't like this at all. You place one knee up on the sink and press your face close to the mirror, and there, in the gully between your nose and cheek, you find a lone blackhead staring back at you.

Stunned, you stumble back from the mirror. Sitting on the edge of the bathtub, you place your newly blemished face in your hands. Your thoughts drift back eons to a time of pimples and proms. Rocking back and forth, you wonder: What's going on here?

The answer is simple enough: You have acne. Acne may be the scourge of the adolescent years, but it can follow some people into middle age and beyond. "Women can have flare-ups at 25 or 35 years old and even older. In fact, my mother was still breaking out when she was 62," says dermatologist James E. Fulton, Jr., M.D., Ph.D., founder of the Acne Research Institute in Newport Beach, California.

Acne is really a catchall term for a variety of symptoms such as pimples, whiteheads, and blackheads, says Peter E. Pochi, M.D., professor of dermatology at Boston University School of Medicine. "It's a condition where the pores of the skin become clogged and the person gets inflamed and noninflamed lesions."

So what's the cause of all the clogging?

"Chocolate doesn't cause acne," says Dr. Fulton. "Dirty hair or skin doesn't cause it. Sex, either too much of it or a lack of it, doesn't cause it either."

MEDICAL ALERT

Accutane to the Rescue

A huge pimple on the end of a nose can seem like a serious problem to the person connected to that nose. It may even seem serious to the people who find themselves staring at it when they talk to him. But acne can get much more serious than a simple blemish.

Acne is classified in four grades, the first being a mild bout with a few whiteheads and blackheads. The fourth and most serious grade consists of many whiteheads, blackheads, pustules, nodules, and cysts. Grade four acne is often accompanied by severe inflammation that becomes red or purple. And it's a sign that you should see a dermatologist.

Severe acne can result in permanent scarring if it isn't treated properly, says Peter E. Pochi, M.D. "The prescription drug Accutane will take care of severe acne very well."

So what does? Heredity—at least for the most part.

"Acne is genetic; it tends to run in families," says Dr. Fulton. "It is an inherited defect of your pores."

If both of your parents had acne, three out of four of your brothers and sisters will get it, too. But if your sister is pimple-free while your face is a war zone, be aware that other factors *can* aggravate an acne outbreak. "Stress, sun exposure, seasonal changes, and climate can precipitate an acne attack," says Dr. Fulton. Certain types of makeup and taking birth control pills can also cause a breakout.

"Working women are especially vulnerable," adds Dr. Fulton. "They're prone to lots of stress, plus they tend to wear makeup a lot."

So here's some blemish-free advice, keeping in mind those who need it the most.

Change your makeup. In adult women, makeup is the major factor in acne outbreaks. "Oil-based makeup is the problem," says Dr. Fulton. "The pigments in foundation makeups, rouges, cleansing creams, or night moisturizers aren't the problem, and neither is the water in the products. It's just the oil. The oil is usually a derivative of fatty acids that are more potent than your own fatty acids. Use a non-oil-based makeup if you are prone to acne."

How Hollywood Hides Blemishes

You think that tiny, little pimple on your face is unsightly? Well, imagine how you would feel if that pimple were, say, the size of a 30-gallon garbage can.

That's the size it would appear to be if you were a star of the silver screen. Bette Davis's big, beautiful eyes would go unnoticed compared to the pimple on the tip of her nose if that pimple were allowed to remain in sight.

Ah, but we never see pimples, whiteheads, or blackheads on the faces of the stars. And why is that? Don't these folks break out? "You bet they do," says Hollywood makeup artist Maurice Stein. "The difference is, they can't let their pimples or any other blemish show."

Stein has been a makeup artist for over 25 years and he's touched up the famous faces in such movies as *M*A*S*H, Funny Girl,* and all five of the *Planet of the Apes* films.

Guerrilla warfare is the only way you can fight the pimple that always sprouts at the wrong time. So here are a few combat tips from the trenches in Hollywood. Stein says he's used these on "some of the most expensive faces in the world."

Go under cover. You can totally block out the discoloration, whether it's pink, red, or purple, according to Stein. To do that, "a person should look for a foundation makeup that has a high pigment level," he says. The more pigment per ounce, the better chance there is of putting the product on thin and still getting good coverage. "When I cover a pimple on an entertainer's face, I look for a pigment level of 50 to 70 percent. The normal range for most foundations is around 15 to 18 percent."

Do a swatch test. You can't really tell the pigment level by looking at a product, but you can tell by sampling it. "Take a drop of it and rub it on your skin," suggests Stein. "If it's so solid in color that you can't see your own skin underneath it, then you know it has a high pigment level and will do well in covering your blemish."

Read the labels. Cosmetic products that contain lanolins, isopropyl myristate, sodium lauryl sulfate, laureth-4, and D & C red dyes should also be avoided. Like oil, these ingredients are too rich for the skin.

Rinse that rouge. "Wash your makeup off thoroughly every night," says Dr. Fulton. "Use a mild soap twice a day and make sure you rinse the soap entirely off your face. Rinsing six or seven times with fresh water should do it."

Fishing for a Cause?

It may sound fishy, but if you are prone to acne, there is at least one doctor who believes that seafood and other foods containing iodine could bring on an attack.

"Iodine is a factor in some people who are prone to acne," says James E. Fulton, Jr., M.D., Ph.D. "Iodine enters the body and mixes into the bloodstream, with the excess excreted through the oil glands. As it is excreted, it irritates the pores and brings on an acne flare-up."

If you've been fishing around for a clue to the cause of your acne, here's a table of some foods and beverages and the amount, in parts per million, of iodides that they contain.

Dr. Fulton does not currently know at what level the iodides could bring on an acne attack, but he warns that "excessive *long-term* ingestion can induce acne attacks."

Food/Beverage	Iodides (ppm)	Food/Beverage	Iodides (ppm)
Dairy Products		Salt	
Cheddar cheese spread	27	Iodized	54
Butter	26	Seasoned	40
Homogenized milk	11	Seafood	
Sour cream	7	Kelp	1,020
Cottage cheese	5	Squid	39
Yogurt	3	Crab	33
Drinking water (U.S. average)	8	Sole	24
Meat and Poultry		Clams	20
Beef liver	325	Shrimp	17
Turkey	132	Lobster	9
Chicken	67	Oysters	8
Hamburger	44	Vegetables	
Miscellaneous		Asparagus	169
Tortilla chips	80	Broccoli	90
Wheat germ	46	Onions (white)	82
Potato chips	40	Corn	45
Pretzels	15	Brussels sprouts	23
White bread	8	Potato	9
Coca-Cola	3	Green beans	7
Sugar	2		

A Slick Test for Oil

Here's an easy test that you can do at home to find out just how oily your cosmetics really are.

Get a sheet of 25 percent cotton-bond typing paper and rub a thick streak of your makeup onto it. Wait 24 hours and then check for an oil ring. "Within a day the oil will spread out and you'll see a big grease ring," explains James E. Fulton, Jr., M.D., Ph.D. "The bigger the ring, the more oil there is in your makeup. Stay away from makeup that produces big oil slicks."

Go for the natural look. "Whatever makeup you use, the less you use of it, the better," says Dr. Fulton.

Blame it on the Pill. Research conducted by Dr. Fulton indicates that certain birth control pills such as Ovral, Loestrin, Norlestrin, and Norinyl can aggravate acne. If you're on the Pill and have an acne problem, discuss it with your doctor. He may be able to switch you to another pill or prescribe another birth control method.

Leave well enough alone. "You shouldn't squeeze pimples or whiteheads," says Dr. Pochi. "A pimple is an inflammation, and you could add to the inflammation by squeezing it. You may cause an infection." You can't do anything to a pimple to make it go away faster, he notes. "Normally a pimple will last from one to four weeks, but it will always go away."

A whitehead is a noninflamed plugged pore, notes Dr. Pochi. "The core of a whitehead is much smaller than the core of a blackhead. When you squeeze the whitehead, the wall of the pore could break and the contents could leak out into the skin and cause a pimple. A pimple naturally forms from the rupture of a whitehead pore wall."

Know when to squeeze. Although most pimples are best left alone, there is one kind that you can squeeze to help get rid of it. "Sometimes a pimple will have a little central yellow pus head in it," explains Dr. Pochi. "Gentle squeezing usually pops these open very nicely. Once the pus is out, the pimple will heal more quickly."

Attack blackheads. You can also get rid of a blackhead by squeezing it. "A blackhead is a very blocked pore. The material inside the blocked pore is solid, and the surface of the pore is widened," explains Dr.

Pochi. The black part of a blackhead is not dirt. In fact, dermatologists aren't really sure what it is, but whatever it is, it will not result in a pimple.

Use OTCs to KO acne. You can fight back an acne attack with over-the-counter products. "Use OTCs with benzoyl peroxide in them," says Dr. Fulton. "The benzoyl part pulls the peroxide into the pore and releases oxygen that kills the bacteria that aggravates acne. It's like two drugs in one. The benzoyl also suppresses the fatty acid cells that irritate the pores."

OTC acne products come in various forms, such as gels, liquids, lotions, or creams. Dr. Fulton suggests using a water-based gel. It is the least likely to irritate the skin.

He also suggests using it for an hour or so in the evening, then washing it off very thoroughly at bedtime, especially in the areas around the eyes and neck.

Don't be fooled by the numbers. Acne medications contain concentrations of benzoyl peroxide ranging from 2.5 percent to around 10 percent. The percentage, however, has little to do with the product's effectiveness. "In most tests that have been conducted, the lower-strength products were as effective as the upper-strength ones," says Thomas Gossel, Ph.D., R.Ph., a professor of pharmacology and toxicology at Ohio Northern University. "Five percent works as well as 10 percent."

Give dry skin extra care. Dry skin can be sensitive to benzoyl peroxide, so Dr. Gossel recommends you start with a lower-strength product first, then increase the concentration slowly. "You're going to get reddening of the skin when you put it on, but that is a normal reaction," he says.

Stay out of the sun. Acne medications may cause adverse reactions to the sun. "Minimize exposure to sunlight, infrared heat lamps, and sunscreens until you know how you will react," cautions Dr. Gossel, who advises a patch test for sunscreen sensitivity.

Scrub that skin. "Cleanse your skin thoroughly every time before applying any over-the-counter acne medication," says Dr. Gossel. A clean face is a happy face.

Use one treatment at a time. Don't mix treatments. If you are using an OTC acne product, you should stop using it if you are given prescription medication for your acne. "Benzoyl peroxide is a close cousin to Retin-A and other products containing vitamin A derivatives, such as Accutane," says Dr. Gossel. A person shouldn't use both of them together."

Stop the spread of acne. Apply acne medication about a half inch around the affected area, says Dr. Fulton, to help keep the acne from spreading. "The medication really doesn't fight the pimple you already have," he explains. "It acts more like a pimple preventive." Acne moves across the face from the nose out to the ear. You need to treat beyond the red inflammatory area. "When you buy an OTC product, it says to apply it to the affected area. To most people the affected area is where they see the pimples. But that's not the case at all."

PANEL OF ADVISERS

James E. Fulton, Jr., M.D., Ph.D., is a dermatologist and founder of the Acne Research Institute in Newport Beach, California. He is also coauthor of *Dr. Fulton's Step-by-Step Program for Clearing Acne* and codiscoverer of Retin-A (synthetic vitamin A), a prescription drug used to treat a variety of skin problems.

Thomas Gossel, Ph.D., R.Ph., is a professor of pharmacology and toxicology at Ohio Northern University in Ada and chairman of the university's Department of Pharmacology and Biomedical Sciences. He is an expert on over-the-counter products.

Peter E. Pochi, M.D., is a professor of dermatology at Boston University School of Medicine in Massachusetts.

Maurice Stein is a cosmetologist and Hollywood makeup artist. He is the owner of Cinema Secrets, a theatrical makeup house in Burbank, California.

Allergies

15 Ways to Alleviate the Symptoms

An allergy is what happens when your body detects a foreign substance it doesn't like. Your nose plugs up and starts dripping, your eyes itch and run, your lungs burn and wheeze.

Like people, allergies come in almost infinite variety. But most fit into three basic categories: contact, food, or inhalant allergies. Inhalant allergies—allergies we experience in response to material in the air we breathe—are the most common. The four biggest airborne troublemakers are house dust, pollen, pet dander, and mold.

"You find a bit of everything in house dust," says Thomas Platts-Mills, M.D., head of the University of Virginia Medical Center's Division of Allergy and Immunology. "Different people are allergic to different things—pieces of cockroach are pretty potent, actually— but the single biggest cause of problems is the dust mite."

For the record, the dust mite is an almost-microscopic relative of ticks and spiders. But the living mite is not the problem. It's the fecal material they expel in their wanderings about our carpets and furniture— their primary residences—and the bodies of dead mites that cause reactions.

As for the other common allergens, pollen blows in from outside, pet dander falls off Fido in a shower of dead skin, and mold grows wherever it's dark and humid—under your carpet, in the basement. But it doesn't matter which one you encounter. Inhale any one of them, and if you are allergic, you'll start sneezing.

Not every home can lay claim to all four of the Big Four, but every home that's not hermetically sealed can lay claim to one or more. So what to do? Is there ever any escape from these ubiquitous denizens of the modern home, or are the allergic masses condemned to a life of endless snuffling and eternal sniffling?

Rest easy—there's a lot you can do to minimize the misery your allergy brings to your life. The following doctor-tested and -recommended tips will plant you firmly on the path to easy breathing and dry eyes.

Treat your symptoms. A certain amount of exposure to whatever bothers you is unavoidable. Allergy shots available from your doctor are a great way to make sure your forays into the outside world are pleasant instead of painful. But you don't have to rely on them. Over-the-counter antihistamines, available from your local druggist, work wonders on drippy noses and red, itchy eyes.

"For the most part, they do a good job," says Richard Podell, M.D., clinical associate professor of family medicine at the University of Medicine and Dentistry of New Jersey, Robert Wood Johnson Medical School. "But if you have an allergy that persists for more than five to seven days, you should probably see your doctor."

Air-condition your house. This is probably the single most important thing you can do to alleviate pollen problems, and it can help with two other chief inhalants—molds and dust mites.

How the Home Became Dust-Mite Haven

Central heating and the vacuum cleaner: They were welcomed with enthusiasm—the vac about 50 years ago, central heating about 40. We can clean in half the time and stay warm in *every* room, not just in the kitchen, next to the stove.

But the same technology that makes our lives easier today has indirectly contributed heavily to one common medical problem—allergies to dust mites.

"The vacuum cleaner made carpeting attractive instead of throw rugs," says David Lang, M.D. Central heating meant that homes tended to stay at least 60° to 65°F year-round. Add very tight, well-insulated homes and cold-water washes to the package (courtesy of the energy crisis), and you end up with a perfect environment for dust mites.

"The basic idea is to create an oasis of sorts," says Dr. Podell. "You want your home to be a place of sanctuary, a place you can count on to provide escape."

Air-conditioning units can help in two ways. They keep humidity low, which discourages mites and molds, and they can filter the air in the course of cooling it—if you also install an air cleaner. But it's the sealing of the house that provides the real benefit, Dr. Podell says.

"If you've got the windows open, then hey, the inside of the house is essentially the same environment as the outside of the house—full of pollens."

Air-condition your car. If walking outside makes you start wheezing and sneezing, imagine what tearing through all those pollen clouds at 55 miles per hour is going to do! Be sensible, air-condition your automobile, too. And if the expense bothers you, remember—you're doing it for your health.

Install an air cleaner. When the experts say install an air cleaner, they don't mean the $14.95 special at the local hardware store. They mean one of the industrial-quality models that bolts into the air intake or outlet of your central heating and cooling unit.

"The room air cleaners certainly take particles out of the air, but they can also move it around," Dr. Platts-Mills says. "The cure can be worse than the condition." They're good, however, at removing pollen that's already in the air.

MEDICAL ALERT

Signs of Complications

If you have a known allergy, notice any of the following symptoms, and have never experienced them before during an allergy attack, you should see your doctor.

- A whistling sound when you breathe—otherwise known as wheezing.
- Congestion of the chest severe enough to make breathing difficult, often accompanied by wheezing—also known as asthma.
- An attack that doesn't respond to over-the-counter medications within a week.
- Welts that spring up in response to exposure to an allergen—also known as hives. They may indicate the onset of anaphylactic shock—an allergic reaction severe enough to kill.

Anaphylactic shock—a very severe allergic reaction—is most commonly associated with bee or fire ant stings, but it can occur in response to other allergens, too. If welts erupt following a sting, it could indicate a severe allergic reaction and should be viewed as a warning flag for prompt medical attention.

Buy a dehumidifier. Keeping the air clean in your home will bring relief from pollens, molds, and pet dander. Keeping it dry will help put a stop to dust mite problems, too.

"They really don't do very well at humidities below about 45 percent," Dr. Platts-Mills says. "Generally, the drier, the better."

If that creates a problem for a child or someone else sensitive to dry air, try putting a small room humidifier close to his bed.

Wipe down humid areas with fungicides. Clorox kills mold, and unlike some other exotic chemicals, you can get it in many grocery stores. Wipe down surfaces in your bathroom as needed to control problems. The Clorox label suggests you clean floors, vinyl, tile, woodwork, and appliances (Clorox will bleach fabrics) with a solution of ¾ cup Clorox bleach per gallon of water. Let stand 5 minutes and rinse. Use a regular fungicide for tough locations like the basement.

Isolate your pets. Pet dander is something many people are allergic to—cat dander usually causes the most problems. The simplest solution: Give your pets away. But for many people, that's not an option.

The alternative: Make your bedroom a haven, sealed off from the rest of the house and absolutely forbidden territory for Whiskers.

"One walk a week through a room is all it takes for a pet to keep a dander allergy going," Dr. Podell says.

Wear a face mask. Use one when doing anything that's likely to expose you to the material you're allergic to. A simple chore like vacuuming can throw huge quantities of dust and whatever else is in your home into the air, where it will hang for several minutes, says David Lang, M.D., a senior staff member in the Division of Allergy and Clinical Immunology at Henry Ford Hospital in Detroit, Michigan. And gardening can expose you to huge volumes of pollen. A small mask that covers nose and mouth, known professionally as a dust and mist respirator, can cut the allergen reaching your lungs. The 3M Company makes an inexpensive version that comes highly recommended and can be found in most hardware stores.

Hire help. If you're allergic to house dust or something else like pet dander that hides in your carpet, get someone else to take care of cleaning that carpet—a teenager or a professional cleaning service. The cost of a hired hand is a small price to pay for guaranteed escape from an allergic reaction.

Seal your bedding in plastic. A joint communiqué from Dr. Podell and Dr. Lang: If dust mites are the bane of your existence, encasing your mattress and pillows in plastic will help bring relief. The little bugs *love* bedding, but with the plastic in place, you breathe clean air instead of mite wastes.

Throw out your carpets. For an allergic person sensitive to house dust, pet dander, or mold, carpets are an absolute no-no. They make an almost perfect home for dust mites and molds, and the tightly woven modern carpet very effectively attracts and holds pollen and pet dander. Even steam cleaning may not help.

"It's not hot enough to kill the mites," Dr. Platts-Mills says. "About all it really does is make it warmer and wetter underneath—an ideal climate for both mites and mold."

Buy throw rugs. Replace your carpets with throw rugs and you'll achieve two major benefits. You'll eliminate that part of your home that captures and holds more dust, pollen, pet dander, and mold than any other, and you'll make keeping it allergen-free much easier. Rugs *can* be washed at temperatures hot enough to kill dust mites, and the floors underneath—courtesy of a rug's loose weave— stay cooler and drier, conditions distinctly hostile to mold and mites.

"Mites can't survive on a dry, polished floor," Dr. Platts-Mills says. "And that kind of floor dries in seconds versus weeks for a steam-cleaned carpet."

Buy synthetic pillows. Dust mites like synthetic (Hollofil or Dacron) pillows just as much as those made from down and foam, but synthetic pillows have one major advantage—you can wash them in hot water.

Wash mattress pads often and in hot water. Your pillows aren't the only problem. Mites love your mattress pads just as much. Run them through a hot-cycle wash weekly and you will kill the resident bugs.

Make at least one room a sanctuary. If you can't afford central air and don't want to rip the wall-to-wall carpeting out of every room in your house, there's still hope. Make just *one* room a sanctuary.

"Most people spend the largest part of their time at home in the bedroom," Dr. Platts-Mills says. "Making just that one room a mite-free area can do a great deal to alleviate the allergy."

Do it by air-conditioning the room in summer, sealing it from the rest of the house (keep the door closed), replacing carpets with throw rugs, and generally applying everything else you've read here.

PANEL OF ADVISERS

David Lang, M.D., is a senior staff member in the Division of Allergy and Clinical Immunology at Henry Ford Hospital in Detroit and a clinical assistant professor of medicine at the University of Michigan in Ann Arbor.

Thomas Platts-Mills, M.D., is a professor of medicine and head of the Division of Allergy and Immunology at the University of Virginia Medical Center in Charlottesville.

Richard Podell, M.D., is a clinical associate professor of family medicine at the University of Medicine and Dentistry of New Jersey, Robert Wood Johnson Medical School, in Piscataway.

Angina

17 Ways to Stop the Pain

Ollie slumps on the couch after gorging himself on Eula Mae's latest offering of his favorite meal: roast ham, baked potato with sour cream, hot, buttered corn on the cob, and apple pie à la mode. He lights up a cigarette. But he can't relax because he and Eula Mae are beginning their nightly postdinner argument — this time over who's going to shovel the snow. It's not long before an aggravated, red-faced Ollie rolls off the couch and waddles out into the frigid January night, vanquished once again.

Minutes later, Ollie is gasping and clenching his chest in pain as a heavy, squeezing pressure radiates from his heart. "Oh, Lord!" he cries. "Eula Mae! Eula Mae! This is The Big One! I'm a goner fer sure! I want to *live!*"

But it's not The Big One, and Ollie is not headed for that Big Greasy Spoon in the Sky. Five minutes later the pain has subsided and Ollie recalls what Dr. Hartebeest had told him just last week. His pain is not a heart attack, and it's not heartburn. It's angina. And it's a sign that the arteries in Ollie's heart are clogging up with fat. The blood can't get through to nourish his heart. That high-fat, high-salt feast, that argument with Eula Mae, going out into the cold, shoveling snow. Any one of those things can bring on angina.

"Here are some pills to take when you get the pain," Dr. Hartebeest had said. "But I'm warning you, Ollie. If you don't change your ways, you're asking for trouble."

What are poor Ollie and others like him to do? Here's what the experts advise.

Get a new outlook on life. Sidney C. Smith, Jr., M.D., director of cardiology at Sharp Memorial Hospital in San Diego, California, is tough and outspoken about the need for angina patients to see the light and make some lifelong lifestyle changes.

MEDICAL ALERT

The Signs of Trouble

You've been diagnosed as having angina—attacks of chest pain that result from a decrease in the supply of blood to your heart. You know what induces an attack and how to avoid it. You also know what to do when you feel one coming on. But do you know when your symptoms are saying something else, when something serious could be wrong? If not, here are a few signs that say "see your doctor—ASAP."

- You've been exercising to a certain level *without* getting angina, but now you're beginning to get angina at that level.
- You experience angina at a *lower* level of exercise than before.
- You've had stable angina (attacks that come on only with exertion), but now you've developed *unstable* angina (attacks that occur during rest).

These may all be signs that the arterial blockage that affects blood flow to your heart is getting worse, says Sidney C. Smith, Jr., M.D.

Another warning sign is angina pain that lasts for more than 15 to 20 minutes. "This could be a sign of heart attack or what we call coronary insufficiency, which is the most extreme form of unstable angina," says George Beller, M.D. "Coronary insufficiency causes prolonged pain but without the irreversible damage characteristic of a heart attack. But you can't tell the difference, so consider it a medical emergency."

"It's a source of major concern to me to see patients take expensive drugs and not make a commitment to modify their lifestyles," he says. "They're only going to get angina again. At times we look for quick answers to tough problems. That doesn't work with angina and heart disease.

"I spend a lot of time educating patients about their symptoms, what to do when they have them, the importance of clean living," he says. "But we don't feel we've done a complete job unless the patient is involved." With a good attitude and the desire to live a healthier life, the other necessary changes will come a whole lot easier.

Clear the air. For those of you who smoke, kicking the habit is the most important thing you can do. On a scale of one to ten, it rates a ten, stresses George Beller, M.D., professor of medicine and head of the Division of Cardiology at the University of Virginia School of Medicine.

Smoke increases blood levels of carbon monoxide, which displaces oxygen. And since angina is an artery-clogged heart crying out for oxygen, smoking is clearly the worst thing you can do. On the other hand, Dr. Beller notes, those who quit usually show an immediate decrease in episodes of angina.

What's more, cigarette smoke makes your blood platelets stick together, further blocking your partially blocked arteries. Last, but far from least, smoking diminishes the effects of any medication you may be taking.

Here's another fact that may help encourage you to quit. Studies have found that angina patients who quit smoking have half the death rate of those who continue.

Think "less is best" when eating. This means less salt, less fat, less calories. "Just one overly fatty, overly salty meal can cause an angina attack because it raises your blood pressure suddenly," Dr. Beller says.

To control the level of fat in your diet, most doctors and the American Heart Association suggest a diet containing less than 30 percent of calories from fat. This means cutting back as much as possible on foods containing saturated fat—the kind (such as butter) that hardens at room temperature—and cholesterol. Here are a few good ways to get started.

- Eat no more than 6 ounces of meat, seafood, or poultry daily.
- Eat only meat that is lean and trimmed of all fat, and trim it *before* cooking. Ground beef should be labeled as having no more than 15 percent fat.
- If possible, remove the skin from poultry before cooking. If not, remove it before eating.
- Learn to use meat, fish, and chicken sparingly in meals. For example, serve it stir-fried in heart-healthy monounsaturated oil (like olive oil) or polyunsaturated oil (like vegetable oil), with lots of vegetables.
- Limit your daily intake of *all* oils to 5 to 8 teaspoons. And use only monounsaturated or polyunsaturated oils.
- Eliminate cholesterol-rich organ meats, such as liver, kidney, or heart.
- Eat only nonfat or 1 percent fat milk products. And be careful when checking out the cheese counter. Some low-fat cheeses are high in salt.
- Increase your daily intake of fresh fruits and vegetables and eat more grains, particularly oat bran, which has been shown to help bring down cholesterol levels. (For more on reducing cholesterol, see page 135.)

Exercise angina away. Lots of angina patients like to sell themselves on the notion that exercise is out of the question because it exerts the heart, and since exertion brings on angina, exercise should be avoided. This just isn't so, says Dr. Beller.

Julian Whitaker, M.D., founder of the Whitaker Wellness Institute in Newport Beach, California, has firsthand knowledge of how important exercise can be for angina patients. He likes to tell the story of a group of patients awaiting heart transplants who were put on an exercise program to strengthen them for surgery. "Over a period of several months, half improved their heart function so much they no longer needed the surgery," he says.

"It's almost routine that when patients start an exercise program, they will experience angina at the beginning of a session," Dr. Whitaker says. "Angina is not a reason not to exercise."

But people with angina need to stay attuned to their bodies, Dr. Beller notes. "If they feel an attack of angina building up, they should know that if they slow down it will dissipate without their having to stop completely."

Why, you may wonder, is exercise so crucial? For one thing, exercise is a proven stress releaser, says Dr. Beller. And it will also help you lose weight. Both stress and overweight are counterproductive to heart health. "It will also lower your heart rate and reduce your blood pressure, which, in turn, will help reduce your need for medication."

Exercise produces these changes, Dr. Whitaker notes, because exercise-trained muscles can pull more oxygen out of arterial blood. "That decreases the amount of work the heart has to do to pump the same amount of oxygen to the muscles," he says.

Both Dr. Beller and Dr. Whitaker agree that exercise alone is no panacea. It takes exercise *and* diet combined to be effective.

Before you start exercising, consult your doctor and get a stress test. "That way you know what your limit is, and you can gain confidence," Dr. Beller says. "You have to have a dialogue with your doctor on what you both consider to be tolerable pain and what isn't." Always be sure to warm up gradually, Dr. Whitaker adds, especially if you're going out into cold temperatures.

Learn to relax. "Whether it's relaxation exercises or meditation, learn how to control your emotions instead of having them control you," advises Dr. Beller. "I have patients who never get angina except when they have a fight with their spouse, yet they can exercise with no problem.

"Work on resolving your conflicts and you can do as much to improve your angina as if you just took more drugs," he says.

Fat: How Low Can You Go?

Can you live a life totally devoid of butter, cream, cheesecake, and eggs? Can you steer clear of fatty foods, like ribs, and salty foods, like fries, and devote your diet to vegetables, fruits, and whole grains?

Sure you can, says Monroe Rosenthal, M.D., medical director of the Pritikin Longevity Center, Santa Monica, California, because thousands of people have done it and continue to do it, and they have shown a remarkable improvement in their heart health as a result.

"We recommend a diet in which 10 percent of calories come from fat," states Dr. Rosenthal. That means no more than 3½ ounces per day of fish, poultry, or lean meat. And since the average American diet comprises 50 percent of calories from fat, that's a pretty drastic cutback!

"Sure, it's tough," Dr. Rosenthal says. "Some people do go on the diet and fall off. But it's a great alternative to heart bypass surgery or to being apprehensive all the time that you're going to get chest pain whatever you do. The diet requires commitment, a positive attitude, and some effort."

But the payoff, he says, can be big. "Blood pressure drops, cholesterol drops, episodes of chest pain decline, and clinical symptoms improve," he says. "Frequently we can completely eliminate certain medications."

One study of 893 Pritikin patients, for example, showed that their cholesterol levels dropped an average of 25 percent after just four weeks on the diet. And 62 percent of the angina patients left, drug-free, while many others were able to reduce their need for medication after finishing the complete program of diet, exercise, and education.

How realistic is a goal of 10 percent of calories from fat? Sidney C. Smith, Jr., M.D., says it is attainable by only 10 percent of the population. The recommendations from mainstream medicine and the American Heart Association (AHA) to cut back to 30 percent of calories from fat are more realistic. "These guidelines are effective and attainable by a fairly large percentage of the population," he says. But, he adds, he'd like to eventually see the guidelines get even lower. "In my own diet I'm a lot stricter than the AHA guidelines. I've made those changes in my own life."

And that, in Dr. Rosenthal's opinion, is the bottom line. "It's not really a diet—it's a way of life."

Take an aspirin a day. For those with unstable angina (the kind that can hit you without exertion, such as when you're resting or even sleeping), aspirin can be a lifesaver, some doctors believe.

"It appears that aspirin prevents the initial activation of the blood clotting mechanism," says Dr. Beller. If your blood clots too easily, of course, it can't get through the narrowed artery and can trigger a heart attack.

In a study conducted at a Canadian hospital, researchers found angina patients reduced their chances of heart attack by 51 percent by taking four buffered or coated aspirin tablets daily. As a result of this and similar studies, many physicians recommend one aspirin daily for minimum effectiveness.

All heart patients, however, should get their doctors' approval before starting on aspirin. Even though it is an over-the-counter drug, aspirin can have side effects. In addition, it could interact with other medication you may be on.

Put your body on tilt at night. If you experience angina attacks at night, tilting the head of your bed up 3 or 4 inches can reduce the number of attacks, says cardiologist R. Gregory Sachs, M.D., assistant professor of medicine at Columbia University College of Physicians and Surgeons. Sleeping in this position makes more blood pool in your legs, so not so much returns to the heart's narrowed arteries. And it may help reduce a need for nitroglycerine.

Put your foot down. If you do get angina attacks at night, Dr. Sachs suggests an alternative to reaching for a nitroglycerine tablet. Simply sit on the edge of the bed with your feet on the floor. "It is equivalent to the effect of nitroglycerine," he says. If you don't feel your symptoms begin to subside quickly, then reach for your medication.

PANEL OF ADVISERS

George Beller, M.D., is a professor of medicine and head of the Division of Cardiology at the University of Virginia School of Medicine in Charlottesville, and chairman of the Council on Clinical Cardiology of the American Heart Association.

Monroe Rosenthal, M.D., is medical director of the Pritikin Longevity Center in Santa Monica, California.

R. Gregory Sachs, M.D., is a cardiologist in private practice in Summit, New Jersey, and an assistant professor of medicine at Columbia University College of Physicians and Surgeons in New York City.

Sidney C. Smith, Jr., M.D., is director of cardiology at Sharp Memorial Hospital in San Diego, California, and associate clinical professor of medicine at the University of California, San Diego, School of Medicine.

Julian Whitaker, M.D., is founder and director of Whitaker Wellness Institute in Newport Beach, California, where he specializes in nutritional therapies for heart disease and high blood pressure.

Arthritis

22 Remedies to Ease the Ache

Arthritis may be the oldest known ailment on earth. Mummies uncovered in Egypt had it, prehistoric man had it, dinosaurs had it. Close to 40 million Americans have it, and a million more will have it a year from now.

If you're reading this, perhaps you have it, or you know someone who does. Though new books touting new treatments with potent drugs and surgery seem to pop up every day, we're not going to tell you about any new "miracle" cures here. What we are going to tell you is how to bring about pain relief without getting a prescription filled or making a trip to the doctor. There's a lot you can do on your own, at home, without a lot of expensive equipment or pain or risk. So let's get started. (Unless otherwise noted, the following tips are helpful for all types of arthritis.)

Lose weight, gain relief. "There's no one magic food or diet that's going to do away with arthritic pain," says Art Mollen, D.O., director of the Southwest Health Institute in Phoenix, Arizona. "But if you're overweight and you lose weight, it will reduce a significant amount of the stress and pain you feel in your spinal column, knees, hips, ankles, and feet."

Reason: The more overweight you are, the more stress and pressure you place on your joints. This increases the stress on the cartilage, which interferes with the bone, thus increasing the incidence of inflammation, swelling, and pain.

Solution: Work with your doctor or nutritionist to find a diet that works for you, and stick with it.

Stretch gently for strength and mobility. When it comes to arthritis, says Mary P. Schatz, M.D., a private practitioner in Nashville, Tennessee., "moving hurts, but *not moving* destroys. Incorrect moving harms, but intelligent moving heals."

Dr. Schatz keeps that philosophy in mind when prescribing yoga for her arthritic patients. "Yoga teaches movement with proper joint alignment," she says, "which helps bring deformed joints back to normal position as appropriate muscles are lengthened and strengthened."

Consider a private session with an experienced teacher or buying a book to learn the correct poses. But remember, "Smart yoga exercise is the key to restoring health to arthritic joints," says Dr. Schatz. Work within the limits imposed by the disease, but don't let yourself be immobilized by it.

Find relief through less stress. "If you are hurting and you tense up, you hurt more," says Beth Ziebell, Ph.D., a psychologist specializing in stress and pain management in Tucson, Arizona. "People who have things in their lives under control will be better pain managers than people who don't."

Recent research confirms the importance of psychological attitude on arthritis pain relief, something Dr. Ziebell has been preaching for years. Some of her specific attitude tips include:

Don't race—pace. "People with arthritis need to learn how to pace themselves and not try to do everything they can possibly do on the days when they're feeling good," she says. "All that does is make you tired and sore the next day. Try to do a little each day, whether you are having a flare-up or not."

Learn to relax. "Take a lesson from natural childbirth classes," Dr. Ziebell advises. "Childbirth is very painful, but women learn how to deal with that pain by learning how to relax." Books and audiotapes teaching relaxation techniques are available at many bookstores, she notes. Dr. Ziebell also believes idle joints can become painful joints. "If you focus on pain, it hurts more, but if you get busy doing other things that are important to you, you're not going to feel it," she says.

Try P.M. prevention for A.M. stiffness. "Almost 90 percent of the patients I see suffer from some type of morning stiffness," says Ilya Rubinov, M.D., a physician at the Arthritis Medical Center in Fort Lauderdale, Florida.

He advises them to apply a muscle ointment at night before going to bed. "It relaxes you and gives you a psychological boost as well," Dr. Rubinov says. The reason? "People with arthritis tend to feel much better all day if they aren't stiff when they wake up in the morning."

Float pain away. Studies have shown that floating in specially designed flotation tanks, also known as isolation or sensory deprivation tanks, can relieve arthritic pain.

"You usually spend about an hour in the tank," says Roderick Borrie, Ph.D., a Brooklyn, New York, psychologist. "The pain relief is produced by stress reduction. The body is relaxing, the muscles are relaxing, and this seems to stimulate a release of endorphins, the body's natural painkillers."

Water in the tanks is heated to precisely 93.5°F, the same temperature as the skin, and the surrounding air is warm and tranquil, leading to deep relaxation.

Dr. Borrie says there are about 200 tank centers located throughout the nation. For more information, contact the Flotation Tank Association, Box 30648, Los Angeles, CA 90030.

Mix oil and water. "I have rheumatoid arthritis in my hands," says Donna King, a massage instructor at the Atlanta School of Massage. "I've taken courses in hands-on arthritis treatment, and I've also figured out what works on me—so I know this treatment works."

Her recommendation: Heat and eucalyptus ointment, in the form of a thick, oil-based product called Eucalypta-Mint, work for both osteoarthritis and rheumatoid arthritis. It's available from Therapeutic Supply and Services Company, 3931 Peachtree Road NE, Atlanta, GA 30319.

"I use that in conjunction with moist heat when I'm feeling stiff or having pain," she says. Simply rub it on and wrap the joint in plastic wrap. "The moist heat can be applied with warm towels, or you can soak your hands or feet in warm water."

Work wonders with watercise. Ask a dozen doctors about the merits of any arthritis treatment and you'll get a dozen different opinions. But ask them about exercising in water and a strange thing happens—they all agree.

"Water exercises are excellent," says Dr. Mollen, echoing the sentiments of many. "Your pain will be significantly reduced in the water, and you become much more flexible in water than you are in air. I can't say enough about water exercises!"

The Case for Copper

Sometimes longevity confers respect along with age. Artifacts that were rarely noticed in their day take on new meaning and value as they persist throughout time. Such is the case with the copper bracelet, which for decades has been worn for arthritis relief and remains popular today.

Studies have shown that some people with arthritis seem to have difficulty metabolizing copper from the food they eat, leading to increased pain. That observation led Helmar Dollwet, Ph.D., of the University of Akron to theorize that arthritis sufferers may need to get their copper from another source. "The dissolved copper from [a copper] bracelet bypasses the oral route by entering the body through the skin," he wrote in his book, *The Copper Bracelet and Arthritis.* Dr. Dollwet thought this might be the only way arthritics ever receive the copper their bodies need—copper that studies have shown can indeed relieve pain.

Physicians remain somewhat skeptical about bracelets but don't entirely dismiss them, either. "I see people wearing copper bracelets, and they're wearing them because it helps them," says Elson Haas, M.D. "I think copper may have a role. It's possible that a copper deficiency does increase joint inflammation, and it doesn't seem that supplementing copper in the diet has the same effect as wearing it."

Does that make Dr. Haas a believer? "I don't necessarily supply copper bracelets to people, but I don't discourage them from wearing one either."

The beginning exercise techniques are easy for anyone to follow. They consist of waving, walking, and bending motions performed in chest-deep water. The more advanced movements look like aquatic dance steps designed to take advantage of water's natural resistance and gentle buoyancy.

Get your spouse involved. Though it's only natural for a husband or wife to do whatever's possible to help a mate who's hurting, such help can often do more harm than good. "When a wife tries to do everything herself and is constantly asking her husband how he feels, she is reinforcing his pain," says Judith Turner, Ph.D., a psychologist with the Pain Center at the University of Washington.

Her advice: Don't be attentive and supportive only when your spouse is in pain, but also when he or she is feeling good and being active.

"That's the time to say, 'Gee, I'm really happy to see you doing things,'" Dr. Turner says. "Praise is really important and something people tend to forget to do."

Use ice to prevent pain. "I recommend cold treatments for those times when a joint's been stressed from overuse or overwork," says King. She uses a gel pack on her clients but notes that ice in a plastic bag or a bag of frozen peas will do just as well. Apply for 15 to 20 minutes, then remove for 10 to 15 minutes. "That can be repeated for hours at a time," she says, "if needed."

Use heat to reduce pain. When joints become hot, swollen, and tender, heat is the best solution, says King. "Cold would make them very painful."

Don't baby your joints. "I like people to follow an aerobic exercise program for arthritis," says Dr. Mollen. "I recommend walking, bicycling, or swimming because they don't traumatize the joints. But do whatever type of exercise you can tolerate that will elevate the pulse rate to at least 120 beats per minute and give you a beneficial effect on the heart and lungs."

Research by Susan Perlman, M.D., of Northwestern University Medical School, has shown that vigorous exercise can even be safe for patients with rheumatoid arthritis and often results in both physiological and psychological improvements. To see if symptoms such as fatigue and depression were the result of poor physical conditioning, she decided to put 54 patients through a low-impact aerobics program.

The result? The vigorous exercise did not result in joint inflammation, but it did improve the walk time, physical activity, and health status of the participants, while reducing their joint pain and swelling, as well as their general pain.

Get off addictive drugs. Sleeping pills, tranquilizers, and narcotic painkillers can become part of life for a person with arthritis—unfortunately. "It's not that these drugs don't work," says Nelson Hendler, M.D., assistant professor at the Department of Neurosurgery at Johns Hopkins University School of Medicine. "They do—but for most people they are needed in ever-increasing amounts and end up creating many more problems than they solve."

Though it may require professional help, Dr. Hendler believes such drugs should be slowly replaced with biofeedback or other forms of

Those Sometimes Helpful Herbs

The word is out about relieving arthritis pain with herbs, and the word is a strong "maybe." Some may help, but the majority probably don't.

"In the long run, the most beneficial herb probably is willow bark," says Varro E. Tyler, Ph.D., professor of pharmacognosy at Purdue University and author of *The Honest Herbal*. "That's simply because it contains salicin, which is similar to aspirin. But to treat arthritis properly, you would need a lot of bark."

Another possible arthritis herb is pokeweed berries, an Indiana favorite that's been used since pioneer times. However, Dr. Tyler cautions, there's been no research showing how pokeweed berries work or if there's any lingering toxicity.

therapy, or occasionally, with nonnarcotic pain relievers such as aspirin or ibuprofen.

Fish for relief. "Some people do indeed respond to fish oil," observes Elson Haas, M.D., the director of the Marin Clinic of Preventive Medicine and Health Education in San Rafael, California. "Not everyone, but some."

A report published by researchers at the Albany Medical Center in New York confirms that observation. It showed that patients with rheumatoid arthritis who took fish-oil capsules showed improvement in joint tenderness and fatigue.

Though fish oil has received plenty of press in the last few years, the active ingredient in fish oil—omega-3 fatty acids—has been around in the form of cod-liver oil for years. Studies have shown that 1 teaspoon per day of cod-liver oil may help alleviate symptoms of rheumatoid arthritis by providing the body with substantial amounts of vitamins D and A. Vitamin D is important for bone growth, while vitamin A may have anti-inflammatory effects. Fish oils also compete with other types of fatty acids that are believed to trigger arthritis inflammation.

Please note, both vitamins D and A can be toxic in large amounts, so limit your intake of cod-liver oil to only a teaspoon a day. Also, too much of these vitamins can cause liver damage over time. Consult with your physician if you think you need fish-oil supplements or supplemental vitamin D. Or, instead of using supplements, try a low-fat diet that includes fish such as mackerel or salmon, which contain omega-3's.

Master massage. When it comes to massage for arthritis pain, hands-on expert King offers the following advice. Work the muscles that are attached to the tendons leading to your painful joints.

"For example, if you have arthritis in your hands," she explains, "then work the forearms from the wrists to elbows, using a compression technique."

To do this, use either the heel of your hand, your thumb, or your elbow to press down on the muscle and hold it for several seconds, then release. For arthritis in the ankle or foot, work the calf and front of the leg.

Boost your vitamin C intake. "Studies have shown that people with rheumatoid arthritis are deficient in vitamin C," says Robert H. Davis, Ph.D., professor of physiology at the Pennsylvania College of Podiatric Medicine.

Dr. Davis's medical models have shown that a lack of vitamin C can aggravate rheumatoid arthritis and that strong doses of vitamin C can bring about regression of the disease.

"Vitamin C is definitely a good home remedy for someone with rheumatoid arthritis," he says. "The toxicity of vitamin C is virtually zero, and if a person took about 500 milligrams spread throughout the day, which is not excessive, that would get enough of the vitamin through to do some good." Before trying vitamin C therapy, get an okay from your doctor.

Practice food avoidance. "I think I've seen the most dramatic results when my rheumatoid arthritis patients avoid foods from the nightshade family and milk products," says Dr. Haas. The nightshade plant family consists of white potatoes, tomatoes, eggplant, tobacco, and all peppers except black pepper.

Dr. Haas suggests that arthritis sufferers develop their own personalized diet by utilizing a "food-avoidance testing plan." One testing plan worth trying calls for removing all forms of a food you crave from your diet, under the theory that you may be literally addicted to the foods you're allergic to.

If, for example, you really crave tomatoes, remove all traces of that food from your diet for a week. Make sure there is no tomato in anything you eat—which means checking labels on processed foods as well as avoiding tomatoes in their raw form. If your symptoms get worse over the next three to four days, you may have an allergy to that food, because a worsening of symptoms can be a sign of addiction. By the fifth or sixth day without the food, you should feel better. If so, this may be a good time to make an appointment with a physician for a complete allergy screening.

Cut back on vegetable oil. There's no question that vegetable oils are generally beneficial to most people, says George Blackburn, M.D., chief of the Nutrition/Metabolism Laboratory with the Cancer Research Institute at New England Deaconess Hospital in Boston. But, he cautions, studies show that people with arthritis may be a special case and may need to minimize their intake of vegetable oils while increasing their intake of oils rich in omega-3's.

That doesn't mean doing without vegetables, he says, but it does mean cutting back on oil-containing products like salad dressings, fried foods, and margarines. These foods contain high levels of omega-6 fatty acids, which have been shown to cause inflammation in those with rheumatoid arthritis. Two oils that are low in omega-6's are canola oil, made from rapeseed, and olive oil. Dr. Blackburn says these two oils can be used in moderation, noting that it's best to keep the overall level of fat in your diet at less than 30 percent of total calories.

Carry on with carrot juice. A vegetable-juice fast significantly reduces pain for many patients with rheumatoid arthritis at Dr. Mollen's clinic. "I started prescribing this type of fast several years ago and have found it very beneficial," says Dr. Mollen.

Carrot juice, celery juice, cabbage juice, or tomato juice can be used. Dr. Mollen suggests fasting on nothing but the vegetable juice for one day during the first week to get started. Follow that by alternate fasting for two days during the next week (i.e., Monday and Wednesday) and three days during the third week (Monday, Wednesday, and Friday). Don't attempt any type of fasting without a doctor's supervision, however.

PANEL OF ADVISERS

George Blackburn, M.D., is chief of the Nutrition/Metabolism Laboratory with the Cancer Research Institute at New England Deaconess Hospital in Boston, Massachusetts.

Roderick Borrie, Ph.D., is a Brooklyn, New York, psychologist who uses flotation tanks, in conjunction with more conventional psychotherapy methods, as a means of inducing deep relaxation and pain relief.

Robert H. Davis, Ph.D., is a professor of physiology at the Pennsylvania College of Podiatric Medicine in Philadelphia.

Elson Haas, M.D., is the director of the Marin Clinic of Preventive Medicine and Health Education in San Rafael, California, and author of the book *Staying Healthy with the Seasons*.

Nelson Hendler, M.D., is an assistant professor at the Department of Neurosurgery at Johns Hopkins University School of Medicine in Baltimore, Maryland.

Donna King is a massage instructor at the Atlanta School of Massage in Georgia. She also suffers from arthritis in her hands.

Art Mollen, D.O., is an osteopathic physician who is the founder and director of the Southwest Health Institute in Phoenix, Arizona, where he emphasizes proper nutrition and exercise to improve health, physical and mental fitness, and weight loss. He is the author of two books, *The Mollen Method: A 30-Day Program to Lifetime Health Addiction* and *Run for Your Life.*

Ilya Rubinov, M.D., is a physician at the Arthritis Medical Center in Fort Lauderdale, Florida.

Mary P. Schatz, M.D., is a private practitioner in Nashville, Tennessee, who views yoga as a valuable tool in the fight against arthritis pain.

Judith Turner, Ph.D., is a psychologist with the Pain Center at the University of Washington in Seattle.

Varro E. Tyler, Ph.D., is a professor of pharmacognosy at Purdue University in West Lafayette, Indiana, and the author of *The Honest Herbal.* He also serves as a *Prevention* magazine adviser.

Beth Ziebell, Ph.D., is a psychologist specializing in stress and pain management in Tucson, Arizona.

Asthma

20 Ways to Stop an Attack

"Asthma means twitchy airways," says Peter Creticos, M.D., an allergist and co-director of Johns Hopkins Center for Asthma and Allergic Disease in Baltimore, Maryland. "Your bronchial airways suddenly contract, you feel a tightness in your chest, you become short of breath, and you cough and wheeze."

"In the under-40 age group, probably 90 percent of asthma is triggered by an allergy," says William Ziering, M.D., a Fresno, California, allergist. Tree, weed, and grass pollens, animal dander, dust mites, and mold are the biggest allergic triggers for asthma. (To find out how to control these common allergens, see page 7.) "After age 40, it's about 50 percent. The other 50 percent is triggered by some form of lung disorder such as emphysema."

But no matter what the cause, asthma needn't be a life sentence. You can get your chest problems under control. "Asthma is a reversible disease," says Dr. Ziering. And you don't have to go to the Sahara desert looking for a way to reverse your asthma; there's plenty you can do right at home.

Stay out of smoke-filled rooms. People with asthma shouldn't smoke, but a recent study done in Canada found that people around asthmatics shouldn't smoke either. "This is particularly important in the winter months, when houses are closed up," says Brenda Morrison, Ph.D., a researcher and associate professor at the University of British Columbia, who conducted a study on the effects of cigarette smoking on asthma. "If someone in the house smokes, it leads to a worsening of asthma, especially in children."

Don't light a fire. Throwing another log on the fire, or in the wood stove, will also fuel asthma. "Wood stoves and fireplaces can cause significant trouble for people with asthma," says John Carlson, M.D., an allergist from Virginia Beach, Virginia. If you must make a fire, be sure the wood stove and chimney are airtight in order to reduce the amount of particulates released into your room—and lungs. Also, make sure the room is well ventilated and the fireplace draws well.

Take an antacid at bedtime. Going to sleep on a full stomach might also feed your asthma. "Asthma can be caused by stomach reflux," a condition in which acid backs up into your esophagus from your stomach. "Your stomach contents may leak out a little and drip down into your airway while you're lying down," says Dr. Creticos. "Prop your bed up and elevate the pillow to prevent the dripping, and take an antacid before bedtime to cut down on your stomach's acidity."

Stay out of the deep freeze. You open the front door, step outside, and get hit with a blast of arctic air. What can you do?

"Stay indoors when it's cold outside," says allergist Sidney Fried-laender, M.D., who is clinical professor of medicine at the University of Florida College of Medicine.

Buy a large scarf. If staying indoors isn't possible, however, make sure you keep your mouth and nose covered when going outdoors. "Cold air can trigger asthma, but when you have a scarf or mask covering your mouth and nose, you end up breathing in warm, humid air," says Dr. Friedlaender.

Don't go to Arizona for relief. "A warm, dry climate will help you, but finding the perfect climate isn't as easy as it used to be. The arid area of Arizona was once a haven for asthmatics, but that's not necessarily so anymore," says Dr. Friedlaender. The environment there has changed over the years since urbanization and irrigation. "Now you have things introduced into the air that weren't there 25 years ago, so people who have asthma frequently have as much trouble there, and sometimes even more."

How to Reduce Exercise-Induced Asthma

Does your asthma kick in at about the sixth block of your daily jog? When physically working hard, do you suddenly find yourself gasping for air? If you do, you may be experiencing exercise-induced asthma—and you're in some pretty elite company.

"At the 1984 Olympics in Los Angeles, fully 20 percent of the Olympians suffered with it," says William Ziering, M.D. "In the general population now, one in ten people is thought to have it."

And you're that one. Lucky you. Here's what Dr. Ziering recommends you do.

Open your stride, not your mouth. When you open your mouth to gasp for air when exercising hard, you're drying the back of your throat and it becomes cool, which triggers your asthma. Keep your mouth closed and breathe through your nose.

Swim to dampen your asthma. Swimming is the ideal exercise for asthmatics, says Dr. Ziering. Because of the high humidity, your mouth won't dry out. "But any sport that requires shorter bursts of exercise, such as baseball, tennis, and golf, is good."

Give yourself a breather. If you run like a deer, you're going to wear out fast. Asthmatics need to pace themselves. "Take the time to warm up, and then start out slow," he says.

Pack your asthma medicine in your gym bag. Use it before you suit up. "If you take your medicine 15 minutes before activity, you should be all right," he says.

And all you future Olympians needn't worry. Your asthma medication is sanctioned by the Olympic committee.

If you still want to move, he suggests looking for a warm, dry climate in an area that is fairly undeveloped. Then vacation there for a couple of weeks to see how your asthma—and you—can handle it.

Use auto air conditioning wisely. Air conditioning may be good for asthmatics but not if it's bringing the outside air in, warns allergist Norman Richard, M.D., a clinical assistant professor at the State University of New York at Buffalo School of Medicine and Biomedical Sciences. "Don't run the car's air conditioning on the setting that draws in outside air and cools it," he says. "Outside air brings with it pollen, and cool, pollinated air is bad for asthma. Set your air conditioner on the recirculate or maximum setting, which won't bring in pollen."

Watch what you eat. Eating the wrong foods could be the right recipe for an asthma attack. "Some of the most common types of foods that trigger asthma are milk, eggs, nuts, and seafood," says Dr. Carlson. If you're asthmatic, learn which foods can trigger an attack and avoid them.

Stay out of the kitchen. Even smelling the foods you're sensitive to can bring on an attack, says Dr. Carlson. In a study, he discovered that just a whiff of eggs frying in the pan was enough to bring on asthma attacks in a couple of his patients. "You don't have to eat the foods to be affected. Just the aroma of the food could bring on asthma in some people."

Be salt sensible. In a study conducted at the Department of Community Medicine of St. Thomas Hospital in London, researchers discovered that table salt could have a life-threatening effect on your asthma. "A strong correlation was found between table salt purchases and asthma mortality in both men and children," reported the researchers. Buying the salt wasn't killing people; eating it was.

Beware of food additives. "Food additives, especially metabisulfite and possibly MSG [monosodium glutamate], can trigger asthma," says allergist William Busse, M.D., professor of medicine at the University of Wisconsin Medical School. "Most commonly metabisulfite is found in beer, wine, shrimp, and dried fruits, particularly apricots."

Sulfites also used to be sprinkled on fruits and vegetables on salad bars to keep them looking fresh, but that practice has been banned. The best advice, according to Dr. Busse, "is to be aware of the kinds of foods sulfites are in and avoid them. When eating out, ask if MSG or metabisulfite is added to the food, and if so, request it be left out of your meal."

MEDICAL ALERT

Take New Symptoms Seriously

Asthma is nothing to wheeze at. Every year more than 4,000 people die from it. In fact, in the past few years, the death rate from asthma has gone up 23 percent.

"The mortality rate increases every year," says William Ziering, M.D., "which is sad because asthma is a reversible condition. Nobody should die from asthma."

But they do. Why is this phenomenon taking place? "One, patients don't realize the severity of the condition," he says. "Other times they let themselves run out of medicine, or they try riding out the serious attack and don't seek medical attention before it's too late."

How do you know when you need help? "Typically, if you realize your asthma is increasing and you begin to use your medicines more frequently than normal," says Peter Creticos, M.D.

"For instance, if you were normally taking one or two puffs of your inhaler a week but are now taking three or four or more puffs a day, that's a good sign that you should see your doctor. Frequency of use of medications is what to watch for," he says.

Also, the experts warn that you should seek immediate medical attention anytime you're having difficulty breathing.

Use nonaspirin pain relievers. In medical terms, it's known as the "aspirin triad," and it consists of sinusitis/nasal polyps, asthma, and a sensitivity to aspirin. For some asthmatics, taking aspirin could have life-threatening consequences. "If you have sinusitis and nasal polyps and asthma, I wouldn't recommend any nonsteroidal anti-inflammatory like aspirin or ibuprofen because it could make your asthma worse or even kill you," says allergist Richard Lockey, M.D., director of the Division of Allergy and Immunology at the University of South Florida College of Medicine, who studied the link.

This aspirin sensitivity could just suddenly develop, so it's best to stay clear of aspirin products altogether, says Dr. Friedlaender. "The problem doesn't happen when you use acetaminophen," he says.

Use inhalers correctly. An inhaler, whether prescribed by a physician or bought over the counter, can bring quick relief to an asthmatic under attack—provided it is used correctly.

"Your inhaler isn't a breath freshener. Don't spray it on the back of your throat because it won't get into your lungs that way," says Michael

Sherman, M.D., a pulmonologist at Hahnemann University Hospital in Philadelphia, Pennsylvania. "If you see the mist coming out of your mouth, you're using it wrong."

Sticking the inhaler in your mouth and taking a couple of quick hits isn't the thing to do, either. "Hold the inhaler about an inch away from your open mouth, take a slow deep breath, and just after you start breathing in—about a half second or so—depress the inhaler. Continue to breathe in after spraying and then hold your breath for 3 to 5 seconds.

"Your first puff opens up the airway, but if you take two quick puffs right away, the second puff doesn't add anything. If you wait 2 to 5 minutes, then the second puff will be of added benefit."

Count on caffeine in a pinch. You're out in the wilderness and suddenly realize that you left your inhaler at home. What do you do if you feel an attack coming on? Head for the coffee pot. "A couple of cups of strong coffee will have a beneficial effect on asthma," says allergist Allan Becker, M.D., assistant professor of medicine at the University of Manitoba, who tested the effects of caffeine on asthma.

Asthmatics given pills that contained the amount of caffeine found in two cups of coffee "could breathe better and their asthma improved," Dr. Becker found. Caffeine and the popular asthma drug Theophylline are almost identical—your body doesn't know the difference.

He cautions, however, that caffeine is not a substitute for your medication. "We don't recommend it as a treatment, but in an emergency, when you don't have your medication around, two strong cups of coffee or hot cocoa or a couple of chocolate bars would be an effective substitute medication that would buy time until you could get to your medicine or inhaler."

Enlist B$_6$ in the battle. Knowledge of the effectiveness of vitamin B$_6$ on asthma came about by accident. When researchers were studying the effects of the vitamin on those with sickle-cell anemia, they discovered that some members of the non-sickle-cell group also had a history of asthma. "When they took 50 milligrams of B$_6$ daily, it reduced the severity of their asthma attacks," says internist Clayton L. Natta, M.D., associate professor of medicine at Columbia University College of Physicians and Surgeons, who conducted the research. "Further study of asthmatics supported the effectiveness of B$_6$," adds Dr. Natta.

Megadoses of vitamin B$_6$ can be toxic and are not recommended, but Dr. Natta says for an adult, "50 milligrams is a safe dose that is given medically all the time." (For complete safety, use B$_6$ only with the approval and supervision of your doctor.)

Listen to your lungs. Of course, the best way to fight an asthma attack is to not have one in the first place. "Recognize your own pattern," says Dr. Ziering. "Be aware of what your early signs of asthma are. When you see the warning signals and you act right away, you will be able to ward it off.

"You don't suddenly have severe asthma," he notes. "That's rare. There is typically a pattern, and you can intervene in that process and stop it in its tracks." The earlier you act, the less severe the asthma will be.

PANEL OF ADVISERS

Allan Becker, M.D., is an allergist and assistant professor of medicine in the Section of Pediatric Allergy and Clinical Immunology, Department of Pediatrics, at the University of Manitoba in Winnipeg. He has done research on the effects of caffeine on asthma.

William Busse, M.D., is an allergist in private practice and a professor of medicine at the University of Wisconsin Medical School in Madison.

John Carlson, M.D., is an allergist in private practice in Virginia Beach, Virginia.

Peter Creticos, M.D., is an allergist and co-director of Johns Hopkins Center for Asthma and Allergic Disease in Baltimore, Maryland. He is also assistant professor of medicine at Johns Hopkins University School of Medicine.

Sidney Friedlaender, M.D., is an allergist and clinical professor of medicine at the University of Florida College of Medicine in Gainesville. He is also editor in chief of *Immunology and Allergy Practice,* a professional journal.

Richard Lockey, M.D., is an allergist and director of the Division of Allergy and Immunology at the University of South Florida College of Medicine in Tampa.

Brenda Morrison, Ph.D., is an epidemiologist, biostatistician, and associate professor in the Department of Health Care and Epidemiology at the University of British Columbia in Vancouver. She has done research on the effects of smoking on asthma.

Clayton L. Natta, M.D., is an internist and associate professor of medicine at Columbia University College of Physicians and Surgeons in New York City.

Norman Richard, M.D., is an allergist and clinical assistant professor of pediatrics at the State University of New York at Buffalo School of Medicine and Biomedical Sciences.

Michael Sherman, M.D., is a pulmonologist in the Division of Pulmonary Medicine at Hahnemann University Hospital in Philadelphia, Pennsylvania.

William Ziering, M.D., is an allergist in private practice in Fresno, California.

Athlete's Foot

18 Ways to Get Rid of It

Can a couch potato get athlete's foot? You bet your remote control! This fungus is an equal opportunity affliction. It doesn't care whether you're a jock or a janitor—or even a Jane. (Although men are more likely to catch this pesky infection, women are by no means immune.)

Athlete's foot is caused by an organism that lives on the skin and breeds best under warm, moist conditions. Although balmy climates probably encourage its growth, sweaty footwear is more often the culprit. Once you've got it, you'll need at least four weeks to make headway against a savage case. Worse, it will return unless you stamp out the conditions that caused it in the first place. So here are some tips on dealing with an active infection and some ways to guard against an encore.

Baby your foot. Athlete's foot can come on suddenly and be accompanied by cracked skin, oozing blisters, and an intermittent burning sensation, says Frederick Hass, M.D., a general practitioner in San Rafael, California. "When you're suffering through this acute stage, baby your

---

Is That Really Athlete's Foot?

According to Thomas Goodman, Jr., M.D., that rash probably isn't athlete's foot if:

- It's on a child's foot. (It's very rare for a child below the age of puberty to have a fungus infection of the foot.)
- It's on the top of the toes. (Eruptions on the tops of toes and the top of the foot are probably some form of contact dermatitis caused by shoe material.)
- The foot is red, swollen, sore, blistered, and oozing. (That's probably an acute form of dermatitis, and you should consult a doctor.)

foot. Keep it uncovered and at constant rest, even if you have to stay home from work or ignore your household duties to do so. Although the inflammation itself is not dangerous, it can worsen and lead to bacterial infection if you're not careful."

Soothe the sores. Use soothing compresses to cool the inflammation, ease the pain, lessen the itching, and dry the sores, says Dr. Hass. Dissolve one packet of Domeboro powder or 2 tablespoons Burow's Solution (both available without a prescription) in 1 pint of cold water. Soak an untreated, white cotton cloth in the liquid and apply three or four times daily for 15 to 20 minutes.

Look for a (salty) solution. Soak your foot in a mixture of 2 teaspoons salt per pint of warm water, says Toronto podiatrist Glenn Copeland, D.P. M. Do this for 5 to 10 minutes at a time, and repeat until the problem clears up. The saline solution helps provide an unappealing atmosphere for the fungus and lessens excess perspiration. What's more, it softens the affected skin, so antifungal medications can penetrate deeper and act more effectively.

Medicate your foot. Now's the time to apply an over-the-counter antifungal medication. According to dermatologist Thomas Goodman, Jr., M.D., an assistant professor at the University of Tennessee Center for Health Sciences in Memphis, the three main types contain either miconazole nitrate (found in Micatin products, for example), tolnaftate (Aftate or Tinactin), or fatty acids (Desenex). Two or three times a day, lightly apply one of them to the whole area involved and rub in gently. Continue for four weeks (or for two weeks after the problem seems gone).

Treat your little piggies. For athlete's foot between your toes, says Dr. Goodman, apply an aluminum-chloride solution. This clear liquid not only kills fungus but also helps to dry the area and discourage regrowth. Ask your pharmacist to make up a solution of 25 percent aluminum chloride in water. Use a cotton swab to apply the liquid between your toes two or three times a day. Continue for two weeks after the infection clears up.

One caution, says Dr. Goodman, don't use aluminum chloride on skin that is cracked or raw—it will sting like crazy. Heal the cracks first with an antifungal agent.

Rub in baking soda. For fungus on your feet, especially between the toes, apply a baking-soda paste, says Suzanne M. Levine, D.P. M., a clinical assistant podiatrist at Mount Sinai Hospital in New York City.

Take 1 tablespoon of baking soda and add a little lukewarm water. Rub that on the site of your fungus, then rinse and dry thoroughly. Finish off the treatment by dusting on cornstarch or powder.

Remove dead skin. When the acute phase of the attack has settled down, says Dr. Hass, you need to remove any dead skin. "It houses living fungi that can reinfect you. At bath time, work the entire foot lightly but vigorously with a bristle scrub brush. Pay extra attention to spaces between toes—use a small bottle brush or test-tube brush there." If you scrub your feet in the bathtub, shower afterward to wash away any bits of skin that could attach themselves to other parts of the body and start an infection there.

Pay attention to toenails. Toenails are favorite breeding spots for the fungus, says Dr. Hass. He advises that you scrape the undersides clean at least every second or third day. Be sure to use an orange stick, toothpick, or wooden match rather than a metal nail file, which could scratch the nails and provide niches for the fungus to collect in.

Keep applying cream. Once your infection has cleared up, says Dr. Goodman, you can help guard against its return by continuing to use (less often) the antifungal cream or lotion that cured your problem. This is especially prudent during warm weather. Use your own judgment in working up a schedule—anywhere from once a day to once a week.

Choose proper shoes. Avoid both plastic shoes and footwear that has been treated to keep water out, says Dr. Copeland. They trap perspiration and create a warm, moist spot for the fungus to grow.

The Alternate Route

Have a Dip of Wine

"I have a wine-loving friend who swears by this treatment for athlete's foot," says Glenn Copeland, D.P.M. "He mixes 1 ounce of sage, 1 ounce of agrimony (an herbal plant), and 2 cups of white wine. Then he simmers the mixture in a covered saucepan for 20 minutes. Let it cool, then soak the affected foot repeatedly. Here he becomes vague about timing, but I assume that when the foot hiccups, it has been soaked long enough!"

MEDICAL ALERT

Be Wise to Infection

If you assume athlete's foot will go away of its own accord, you can be in big trouble, says Suzanne M. Levine, D.P.M. An unchecked fungal infection can lead to cracks in the skin and invite a nasty bacterial infection.

Frederick Hass, M.D., recommends that you consult your physician if:

- The inflammation proves incapacitating.
- Swelling occurs in the foot or the leg at any time during the attack, and you develop a fever.
- Pus appears in the blisters or the cracked skin.

Dermatologist Diana Bihova, M.D., a clinical instructor of dermatology at New York University Medical Center in New York City, recommends that you steer clear of any tight, snug, or unventilated footwear and that you never wear boots all day. "Natural materials such as cotton and leather create the best environment for feet, while rubber and even wool may induce sweating and hold moisture. Whenever possible, such as during the summer, wear airy shoes such as sandals," she says.

Change them often. Don't wear the same shoes two days in a row, says Dean S. Stern, D.P. M., a podiatrist at Rush-Presbyterian-St. Luke's Medical Center in Chicago, Illinois. It takes at least 24 hours for shoes to dry out thoroughly. If your feet perspire heavily, change shoes twice a day.

Keep them dry—and clean. Dust the insides of your shoes frequently with antifungal powder or spray. Another good idea, says Bethlehem, Pennsylvania, podiatrist Neal Kramer, D.P.M., is to spray some disinfectant (such as Lysol) on a rag and use it to wipe out the insides of your shoes. That will kill off any fungus spores living there. Do this every time you take off your shoes, he says.

And air them out! Dr. Hass recommends giving your shoes a little time in the sun to air out. "Remove the laces and prop open the throat of each shoe. You should even leave sandals outdoors to dry between wearings. And wipe the undersides of their straps clean after every wearing to remove any fungi-carrying dead skin. The idea is to reduce even the slightest possibility of reinfection."

Sock the infection. If your feet perspire heavily, says Dr. Hass, change your socks three or four times a day. And wear only clean cotton socks, not those made with synthetic yarns. Be sure to rinse them thoroughly during laundering, because detergent residue can aggravate your skin problem. And to help kill fungus spores, says Dr. Kramer, wash your socks twice in extra-hot water.

Powder your toes. To further keep your feet dry, allow them to air-dry for 5 or 10 minutes after a shower before putting on your shoes and socks, says Dr. Bihova. To speed complete drying, hold a hair dryer about 6 inches from your foot, wiggle your toes, and dry between them. Then apply powder. To avoid the mess of loose powder, place it in a plastic or paper bag, then put your foot into the bag and shake it well.

And your footgear. Dr. Levine further recommends applying medicated powder—such as Tinactin, Halotex, or Desenex—to your shoes before you put them on.

Cover up in public places. You can decrease your exposure to the fungus, says Dr. Goodman, by wearing slippers and shower shoes in areas where lots of other people go barefoot. That includes gyms, spas, health clubs, locker rooms, and even around swimming pools. If you're prone to fungal infections, you can pick them up almost any place that is damp—so be prudent.

PANEL OF ADVISERS

Diana Bihova, M.D., is a dermatologist in private practice and clinical instructor of dermatology at New York University Medical Center in New York City. She is coauthor of *Beauty from the Inside Out.*

Glenn Copeland, D.P.M., is a podiatrist with a private practice at Toronto's Women's College Hospital. He is also consulting podiatrist for the Canadian Back Institute, podiatrist for the Toronto Blue Jays baseball team, and author of *The Foot Doctor.*

Thomas Goodman, Jr., M.D., is a dermatologist in private practice and assistant professor of dermatology at the University of Tennessee Center for Health Sciences in Memphis. He's the author of *Smart Face* and *The Skin Doctor's Skin Doctoring Book.*

Frederick Hass, M.D., is a general practitioner in San Rafael, California. He's on the staff of Marin General Hospital in Greenbrae. He's also author of *The Foot Book* and *What You Can Do about Your Headaches.*

Neal Kramer, D.P.M., is a podiatrist with a practice in Bethlehem, Pennsylvania.

Suzanne M. Levine, D.P.M., is a podiatrist in private practice and clinical assistant podiatrist at Mount Sinai Hospital in New York City. She is author of *My Feet Are Killing Me* and *Walk It Off.*

Dean S. Stern, D.P.M., is a podiatrist at Rush-Presbyterian-St. Luke's Medical Center in Chicago, Illinois.

Backache

24 Pain-Free Ideas

Here's a law of physics that you rarely hear anything about: The heavier something is, the more often you'll have to move it. Here's another law of physics: Things will look just right at the farthest spot from where you first put them.

Trying to move the suddenly immovable is the number one cause of back problems in the United States. It causes you to push, twist, bend, lift, punch, pull, and strain in ways you never thought possible. The result is often back pain—and it's not always easy to get rid of. Some back pain experts claim that four out of every five Americans experience back pain at some time in their lives. And back-related injuries cost industry more than $10 billion a year in worker's compensation claims.

So if you've heaved, and the thing you tried to lift ho ho'ed as you winced in pain, there are things you can do to get you back from a painful attack.

RELIEF FROM A BACK ATTACK

Back doctors will tell you back pain comes in two forms, acute and chronic. Acute pain comes on suddenly and intensely. It's the kind you usually experience from doing something you shouldn't be doing or from doing it in the wrong way. The pain can be from sprains, strains, or pulls on muscles in your back. It can hurt like crazy for several days, but doctors say you can be pain-free without any lasting effects by following these self-help tips.

Get off your feet. Your back will thank you for it. "For an acute problem," says orthopedic surgeon Edward Abraham, M.D., assistant clinical professor at the University of California, Irvine, California College of Medicine, "the first thing you should do is get some bed rest." In

Exercise Your Pain Away

Exercise may be the last thing you like to think about when your back is aching, but specialists say exercise is the best thing going for chronic back pain.

"For people who suffer daily from back pain, especially if the pain varies throughout the day, exercise can be very beneficial," says Roger Minkow, M.D., a back specialist and founder of Backworks in Petaluma, California.

If you're under a doctor's care for back pain, make sure you get the okay before you begin. Here are some doctor-recommended exercises.

Play press-up. Press-ups are something like half of a push-up. "Lie on the floor on your stomach. Keep your pelvis flat on the floor and push up with your hands, arching your back as you lift your shoulders off the floor," says Dr. Minkow.

This will help strengthen your lower back. Dr. Minkow recommends that you do it once in the morning and once in the afternoon.

Move into a crunch. While you're on the floor, turn over onto your back and do what's called a crunch sit-up. Lie flat with both feet on the floor and your knees bent. Cross your arms and rest your hands on your shoulders. Raise your head and shoulders off the floor as high as you can while keeping your lower back on the floor. Hold for 1 second, then repeat.

Swim on dry land. You don't need a deep-pile rug to swim on your floor. Lie on your stomach and raise your left arm and your right leg. Hold for 1 second, then alternate with your left leg and right arm as if you were swimming.

This will extend and strengthen your lower back, says Dr. Minkow.

Get into the pool. "Swimming is great exercise for the back," reports Milton Fried, M.D. "A good exercise for acute low back pain is to get into a warm pool and swim."

Put your mettle to the pedal. "Ride a stationary bike with a mirror set up so that you can see yourself," says Dr. Minkow. "Be sure to sit up straight without slouching. If you have to, raise the handlebars so that you're not bent over forward."

Remember—no pain, no gain, no brain. In doing these or any other exercises, Dr. Minkow advises that you be careful and know your limit. "If the exercise you're doing hurts or aggravates your condition, don't do the exercise anymore," he says. "You're not going to improve anything by gritting your teeth and doing one more repetition. If you feel fine the day after, or two days after you exercise, then it's safe to continue exercising."

fact, it may be the only thing you'll want to do. Any physical act, even getting up to go to the bathroom, may bring you pain. So, for the first day or two, keep activity to a minimum.

Don't lounge too long. How long you stay in bed depends on the severity of your pain, says Dr. Abraham. "If you're still in pain after two days, for example, an extra day in bed won't hurt. It's best, however, to get out of bed as quickly as possible. Let pain be your guide."

"Most people think that a week of bed rest will take away the pain," adds David Lehrman, M.D., chief of orthopedic surgery at St. Francis Hospital and founder of the Lehrman Back Center in Miami, Florida. "But that's not so. For every week of bed rest, it takes two weeks to rehabilitate."

In fact, research at the University of Texas Health Science Center bears this out. Researchers there studied 203 patients who came into a walk-in clinic complaining of acute back pain. Some were told to rest for two full days and others were told to rest for seven days. There was no difference in the length of time it took the pain to diminish in either group, reported Richard A. Deyo, M.D., who was one of the researchers and is now director of health services research at Seattle Veterans Admin-

---

MEDICAL ALERT

Some Backs Need a Doctor's Care

When does your back need medical backup? When you experience any of the following:

- Back pain that comes on suddenly for no apparent reason.
- Back pain that is accompanied by other symptoms, such as fever, stomach cramps, chest pain, or difficulty breathing.
- An acute attack that lasts for more than two or three days without any pain relief.
- Chronic pain that lasts more than two weeks without relief.
- Back pain that radiates down your leg to your knee or foot.

You shouldn't always assume that back pain is a sign that something is wrong with just your back, notes Milton Fried, M.D. It could be a sign of some other disorder.

istration Medical Center. And those who got out of bed after two days got back to work a lot sooner.

"The length of bed rest doesn't really affect recovery," says Dr. Deyo. "For some people it's just the most comfortable position for the first couple of days."

Put your pain on ice. The best way to cool down an acute flare-up is with ice, says Canadian pain researcher Ronald Melzack, Ph.D., a professor at McGill University. It will help reduce swelling and the strain on your back muscles. For best results, he says, try ice massage. "Put an ice pack on the site of the pain and massage the spot for 7 or 8 minutes." Do this for a day or two.

Try some heat relief. After the first day or two of ice, physicians recommend that you switch to heat, says Milton Fried, M.D., founder of the Milton Fried Medical Clinic in Atlanta, Georgia. Take a soft towel and put it in a basin of very warm water. Wring it well and flatten it so that there are no creases in it. Lie chest down with pillows under your hips and ankles and fold the towel across the painful part of your back. Put some plastic wrap over that, then put a heating pad turned on medium on top of the plastic. If possible, place something on top that will create pressure, like a telephone book. "This creates moist heat and will help reduce muscle spasms," says Dr. Fried.

Use heat *and* cold. For those of you who can't make up your mind which feels better, it's okay to use both methods, says Dr. Abraham. It may even have an added bonus. "An intermittent regimen of heat and ice will actually make you feel better," says Dr. Abraham. "Do 30 minutes of ice, then 30 minutes of heat, and keep repeating the cycle."

Stretch to smooth a spasm. "Stretching a sore back will actually enhance the healing process," says Dr. Lehrman. "One good stretch for lower back pain is to gently bring your knees up from the bed and to your chest. Once there, put a little pressure on your knees. Stretch, then relax. Repeat.

"Stretching will help the muscle calm down sooner than just waiting for it to calm down on its own," says Dr. Lehrman.

Roll out of bed. When you do have to get out of bed, doctors advise that you roll out—carefully and slowly.

"You can minimize the pain of getting out of bed by sliding to the edge of the bed," says Dr. Lehrman. "Once there, keep your back rigid and

Car Seat Comfort

Does your back drive you crazy every time you buckle up? It could be that what you're sitting on is the seat of your problem.

"If you have back problems, the root of your problem could be your car seat, says Roger Minkow, M.D., a back specialist and founder of Backworks in Petaluma, California, who redesigns seats for airplane and automobile manufacturers. "German cars can be the worst when it comes to backs," he says. "American cars are usually bad, too, but you can at least fix them. Japanese cars, on the other hand, have the best seats, followed by the Swedish cars Volvo and Saab."

Next time you're in the market for a car, Dr. Minkow suggests testing for cushion comfort as well as cruise-ability. The following hints will help you make a wiser choice.

Take a new car for a sit. "Look for a seat with adjustable lumbar support and adjust the support down as low as it goes," he says. "See how that feels, and if you need to adjust it, do it from the lowest level."

Get do-it-yourself comfort. If you have a car seat that does not suit your back and you drive an American-made car, you probably can fix the situation yourself with little effort. Most American cars have a zipper on the bottom of the back cushion. "Just unzip it and slip a homemade lumbar support inside the car seat," he says. Here's how to do it.

Go to an upholstery shop and buy a cushion of high-resiliency foam, which means 2.5- to 3.5-pound foam with an ILD (indent load deflection) of between 30 to 45 pounds. Cut a strip of foam 5½ inches wide by 1 inch thick with an electric carving knife. Then cut its length to fit your car seat width, being sure that you bevel the edge so that when the seat cover rolls over, it won't roll it up. Shove the foam under the seat cover, then make the necessary adjustments by either raising it or lowering it so that it fits your back over the belt line (not the small of your back). Then zip the cover back up.

"It takes about 15 minutes, costs about $3, and works as well as an $80 lumbar support," Dr. Minkow says.

then let your legs come off the bed first. That motion will act like a springboard, lifting your upper body straight up off the bed."

RELIEVING PAIN THAT LASTS AND LASTS

For some people, back pain is a part of everyday life. For whatever reason, it just lingers on and on for what can seem like an eternity. Some people suffer from recurring pain; any little movement can set it in motion. This is called chronic pain. The following tips are particularly helpful for those with chronic pain, although acute pain sufferers can benefit from them as well.

Lumber up. Lumber under the mattress will help the lumbar lying on top. "The object is to have a bed that doesn't sag in the middle when you sleep on it," says Dr. Fried. "A piece of plywood between the mattress and the box spring will end the sagging problem."

Drown pain with a waterbed. "A modern waterbed, one that is adjustable and doesn't make a lot of waves, is excellent for most types of back trouble," says Dr. Fried.

Dr. Abraham agrees. "In waterbeds you get an equalized change in the pressure on various segments of your body," he says. "You can lie in one position for the entire night because of this."

Become a "lazy S" sleeper. A bad back can't stomach lying facedown. "The best position for someone resting in bed is what we call the lazy S position," says Dr. Abraham. "Put a pillow under your head and upper neck, keep your back relatively flat on the bed, and then put a pillow under your knees."

When you straighten your legs, your hamstring muscles pull and put pressure on your lower back, he explains. Keeping your knees bent puts slack into the hamstrings and takes the pressure off your back.

Develop fetal attraction. You'll sleep like a baby if you sleep on your side in the fetal position. "It's a good idea to stick a pillow between your knees when you sleep on your side," says Dr. Fried. "The pillow stops your leg from sliding forward and rotating your hips, which puts added pressure on your back."

Take an aspirin a day. It can keep back pain away, claim the experts. Back pain is often accompanied by inflammation around the site of the pain, says Dr. Fried, and simple over-the-counter anti-inflammatory drugs, such as aspirin and ibuprofen, can help take it away. "It can even help for a fairly severe amount of inflammation," he says.

Acetaminophen is not as effective because it is not an anti-inflammatory drug.

Bark up the right tree. If you're looking for a natural anti-inflammatory, try some white willow bark, which can be found in capsule form in health food stores, says Dr. Fried. "It is a natural salicylate, the active ingredient that gives aspirin its anti-inflammatory power," says

Dr. Fried. "Taken after meals, it shouldn't hurt your stomach, and it works very well on mild to moderate back pain. Those who suffer from ulcers and heartburn, however, should not use it."

Visualize yourself pain-free. The middle of the night can be the worst time for pain. Pain wakes you up and it keeps you up. "Using visualization is a particularly good thing to do at times like this," says professor Dennis Turk, Ph.D., director of the Pain Evaluation and Treatment Institute at the University of Pittsburgh School of Medicine.

"Close your eyes and imagine a lemon on a white china plate. See a knife next to it. See yourself pick it up and slice the lemon. Hear the sound it makes cutting through. Smell the aroma. Bring the lemon up to your face and imagine its taste.

"This is just one example in how you can use your senses in visualization," says Dr. Turk. The idea is to bring as much detail to the image as possible. The more involved the image is, the more you are engaged with it and the quicker you will become distracted from the pain."

Turn your pain upside down. "Gravity inversion works wonders on back pain," says Dr. Fried. With this therapy you strap yourself to a special device that tilts back and allows you to hang upside down. "Gradually doing inversion traction with a proper, safe inversion apparatus for 5 or 10 minutes a day will really work to rid you from lower back pain," he says. You should, however, have your doctor's okay to use this kind of therapy, especially if you have disk problems. And those with a potential for glaucoma should not use it at all.

Try T'ai chi to untie muscle knots. T'ai chi is an ancient Chinese discipline of slow, fluid movements. "It's a great relaxation method that helps the muscles in your back," says Dr. Abraham, who uses the method himself. "There are a lot of breathing exercises and stretching activities that foster a harmony within the body."

T'ai chi takes time and self-discipline to learn, but Dr. Abraham feels it's worth it. "I know it's strange for an orthopedic surgeon to talk this way, but it's smart living and it will go a long way in helping people with bad backs."

PANEL OF ADVISERS

Edward Abraham, M.D., has a private practice in Santa Ana, California, and is assistant clinical professor of orthopedics at the University of California, Irvine, California College of Medicine. He originated the concept for outpatient back therapy in the United States and is the author of *Freedom from Back Pain*.

Richard A. Deyo, M.D., is director of health services research at Seattle Veterans Administration Medical Center and an associate professor of medicine and health services at the University of Washington School of Medicine in Seattle. He also holds a master's degree in public health.

Milton Fried, M.D., is the founder and director of the Milton Fried Medical Clinic in Atlanta, Georgia. He also holds degrees in chiropractic and physical therapy.

David Lehrman, M.D., is chief of orthopedic surgery at St. Francis Hospital in Miami, Florida, and the founder and director of the Lehrman Back Center, a residential facility for pain sufferers in Miami.

Ronald Melzack, Ph.D., is a professor of psychology at McGill University in Montreal. He is vice president of the International Pain Foundation and a pain researcher.

Roger Minkow, M.D., a back specialist, is founder and director of Backworks, a rehabilitation facility for people with back injuries, located in Petaluma, California.

Dennis Turk, Ph.D., is a professor of psychiatry and anesthesiology at the University of Pittsburgh School of Medicine in Pennsylvania and director of the university's Pain Evaluation and Treatment Institute.

Bad Breath

16 Ways to Overcome It

It's just after lunch and you're in the middle of an important job interview. You're sailing along, doing everything right. Answers to the interviewer's questions trip lightly from your tongue. You laugh together. You smile at each other. Your body language says you are at ease, self-assured. You've got the job—you think.

So you stand up, shake hands, and say, "I've enjoyed talking to you and I'll look forward to hearing from you."

Uh-oh.

Your interviewer grimaces just a little. His upper lip wrinkles. He smiles a tight, little smile. You can see something just went wrong. He's been bushwhacked by your bad breath.

Not exactly the lasting impression you wanted to leave. Was it your lunch? Could be. But it could also be the lunch you ate *yesterday.* To find out why—and to avoid those potentially embarrassing moments—read on.

How to Test Your Breath

How horrible is your halitosis? If you don't have a friend to tell you the truth, there are a couple of ways you can test your breath, says Eric Shapira, D.D.S.

Cup your hands. Breathe into them with a great, deep, haaaaaa. Sniff. If it smells rank to you, then it's deadly to those you come in contact with, says Dr. Shapira.

Floss. Not to clean your teeth, although that's a great idea, but to find out just how bad your breath might be, pull the floss gently between your teeth and then sniff some of the gunk you unearth. If it smells bad, you smell bad.

Don't dine with the garlic family. Highly spiced foods like to linger long after the party's over. Spices tend to stay and recirculate through essential oils they leave in your mouth. Depending on how much you eat, the odor can stay in your mouth up to 24 hours; no matter how often you brush your teeth. Some foods to avoid include onions, hot peppers, and garlic.

Meat at the deli later. Spicy deli meats such as pastrami, salami, and pepperoni also leave oils behind long after you've swallowed them. You breathe. They breathe. If an occasion calls for sweet-smelling breath, it's best to avoid these meats for 24 hours beforehand to prevent them from talking for you.

Say, "Please, no cheese." Camembert, Roquefort, and blue cheese toppings are called strong for good reason—they get a hold on your breath and don't let go. Other dairy products can have the same effect.

Don't fish for compliments. Some fish, like the anchovies on your pizza or even the tuna you tuck into your brown-bag lunch, can leave a lasting impression.

Stick with water. Coffee, beer, wine, and whiskey are at the top of the list of liquid offenders. Each leaves a residue that can attach to the plaque in your mouth and infiltrate your digestive system. Each breath you take spews traces of these back to the air.

MEDICAL ALERT

Bad Breath May Mean Major Trouble

Persistent bad breath doesn't mean you eat too many onions. Bad breath is a sign of major gum disease, says Roger P. Levin, D.D.S., president of the Baltimore Academy of General Dentistry.

"It can also be gases and odors coming up from gastrointestinal problems," Dr. Levin says. If your halitosis hangs on more than 24 hours without an obvious cause, see your dentist or doctor.

Some diseases that can also cause bad breath include cancer, tuberculosis, syphilis, dehydration, and zinc deficiency. Some drugs, including penicillamine and lithium, can cause bad breath, too.

Carry a toothbrush. Some odors can be eliminated—permanently or temporarily—if you brush immediately after a meal. The main culprit in bad breath is a soft, sticky film of living and dead bacteria that clings to your teeth and gums, says Eric Shapira, D.D.S., assistant clinical professor and lecturer at the University of the Pacific School of Dentistry. That film is called plaque. At any time, there are 50 trillion of these microscopic organisms loitering in your mouth. They sit in every dark corner, eating each morsel of food that passes your lips, collecting little smells, and producing little odors of their own. As you exhale, the bacteria exhale. So brush away the plaque after each meal and get rid of some of the breath problem.

Rinse your mouth out. When you can't brush, you can rinse. Go to the restroom after meals and get a mouthful of water, swish it around, and wash the smell of food from your mouth, says Jerry F. Taintor, D.D.S., chairman of Endodontics at the University of Tennessee College of Dentistry. Spit the water out, of course.

Eat three meals a day. Bad breath can be caused by not eating, too. One of the side effects of fasting or a poor diet is bad breath.

Swish and swallow. You're in a restaurant, and your brush and floss are at home. You can't excuse yourself from the table. So take a sip from your water glass and discreetly circulate the water across and around your teeth. Then swallow those potentially offending bits of food, says Dr. Shapira.

Gargle a minty mouthwash. If you need 20 minutes of freedom from bad breath, gargling with a mouthwash is a great idea. But like Cinderella's coach-turned-pumpkin, when your time is up, the magic will be gone and you'll be back to talking behind a hand again.

Choose your mouthwash by color and flavor. Amber and medicine-flavored mouthwashes contain essential oils such as thyme, eucalyptus, peppermint, and wintergreen, as well as sodium benzoate or benzoic acid. Red and spicy mouthwashes may contain zinc compounds. Both types will neutralize the odor-producing waste products of your mouth bacteria.

Chew a mint or some gum. Like mouthwash, a breath mint or minty gum is just a coverup, good for a short interview, a short ride in a compact car, or a very short date.

Eat your parsley. Parsley adds more than green to your lunch plate; it's also a breath-saver. Parsley can freshen your breath naturally. So pick up that sprig and chew it thoroughly.

Spice is nice. Certain herbs and spices you keep in your kitchen are natural breath enhancers. Carry a tiny plastic bag of cloves, fennel, or anise seeds to chew after odorous meals.

Brush your tongue. "Most people overlook their tongues," says Dr. Shapira. "Your tongue is covered with little hairlike projections, which under a microscope look like a forest of mushrooms. Under the caps of the mushrooms there's room to harbor plaque and some of the things we eat. That causes bad breath."

His advice? While you are brushing, gently sweep the top of your tongue, too. Don't leave food and bacteria behind to breed bad breath.

PANEL OF ADVISERS

Roger P. Levin, D.D.S., is president of the Baltimore Academy of General Dentistry and a guest lecturer at the University of Maryland in Baltimore.

Eric Shapira, D.D.S., is in private practice in El Granada, California. He is an assistant clinical professor and lecturer at the University of the Pacific School of Dentistry in San Francisco and has a master's degree in science and biochemistry.

Jerry F. Taintor, D.D.S., is chairman of Endodontics at the University of Tennessee College of Dentistry in Memphis. He is the author of *The Oral Report: The Consumer's Common Sense Guide to Better Dental Care.*

Bed-Wetting

5 Options for Sleep-Through Nights

Bed-wetting can be both uncomfortable and embarrassing for a child. Thankfully, almost all kids outgrow it in time. But chances are you will feel compelled to do something while you wait. What follows are the best bed-wetting remedies currently available—other than time.

Be realistic. "Don't praise and don't punish," says Ann Price, educational coordinator of the National Academy of Nannies, Inc. (NANI) in Denver, Colorado. "Just change the bed and don't say a word. It'll go away by itself. Kids don't do it on purpose, so don't praise them when they are dry or punish them when they are wet."

Change for the better. To help minimize psychological stress, Price recommends arranging the bedroom so the child can change the sheets himself. "And set out a felt-covered rubber pad so when he has an accident he can lay it over the wet part of the bed. Also, put out a pair of dry pajamas he can change into. That way, at least he won't feel babyish."

Don't be alarmed. "Bed-wetting alarms can work," says Bryan Shumaker, M.D., a urologist at St. Joseph Mercy Hospital in Pontiac, Michigan. "But you'd better have patience. The alarm is loud, and chances are good it'll wake up everybody in the house when it goes off."

Bed-wetting alarms emit a buzzing or ringing sound when the child is wet. The theory is that the sound will condition him to awaken when he needs to urinate. Eventually, wetting will be inhibited and bladder distension will become the signal for the child to awaken.

Most children respond to this type of conditioning strategy within 60 days, says Dr. Shumaker. Bed-wetting is considered cured when the child remains dry for 21 consecutive nights.

A new generation of alarms is much smaller and more sensitive to wetness than the bulky, complicated mats and pads of yesterday. Today's alarms run on hearing aid batteries and boast moisture sensors that attach directly to the underwear. Best of all, those who use modern alarms have relapse rates of only 10 to 15 percent, compared to the 50 percent relapse rate of older models.

Boost bladder muscles. "If the child's daytime pattern is one in which he goes to the bathroom fairly often, then bladder stretching exercises may work," says Linda Jonides, a pediatric nurse practitioner from Ann Arbor, Michigan. Her recommendation: Have the child drink lots of fluids during the daytime, then practice bladder control by holding off urination for as long as possible.

Practice patience and love. "Understand that all kids outgrow bed-wetting at a rate of 15 percent a year," says Dr. Shumaker. "Which means by the time they go through puberty, less than 1 or 2 percent will still wet the bed. So be patient and be supportive. No kid wants to wet on himself. It's unpleasant, uncomfortable, and cold, and besides 'only babies do that'—and no kid wants to be a baby. Patience and support is the bottom line."

PANEL OF ADVISERS

Linda Jonides is a pediatric nurse practitioner in Ann Arbor, Michigan.

Ann Price is educational coordinator of the National Academy of Nannies, Inc. (NANI) in Denver, Colorado, and coauthor of *Successful Breastfeeding, Dr. Mom,* and other books.

Bryan Shumaker, M.D., is a urologist at St. Joseph Mercy Hospital in Pontiac, Michigan.

Belching

10 Steps to Squelch the Problem

Belching is often caused by *aerophagia,* a medical term for swallowing air. Everyone carries a certain amount of air and other gases in the gastrointestinal tract all the time. On average, this tends to be slightly less than 1 cupful. Yet the body is constantly acquiring air and other gases throughout the day, taking some in through the mouth and producing some on its own. In all, it works out to almost 10 cupfuls of gas in 24 hours, about 9 cupfuls more than we can carry. The body constantly seeks ways to vent this excess. One of those ways is belching.

Soft drinks and beer are guaranteed to cause problems, but your saliva also contains tiny air bubbles that travel to the stomach with every swallow.

Those of us who swallow air along with our food are asking for trouble, but belching is a problem that seems infinitely curable right at home. Most of us can, with practice, control the amount of air we swallow and save the doctor for something more important.

Become aware of air. "You can swallow up to 5 ounces of air every time you swallow," says André Dubois, M.D., a gastroenterologist in Bethesda, Maryland. "And people who are nervous will do this quite frequently."

Dr. Dubois notes that some people are compulsive swallowers and create a problem simply by swallowing too much saliva. "You can improve this by learning to control your swallowing reflexes," he says. "This is best done by simply becoming *aware* of it. Ask your friends or relatives to tell you if they notice you swallowing a lot. You probably won't notice it in yourself."

Once you're aware of an excessive swallowing habit, you will automatically curb it, says Dr. Dubois. There are also some personal habits you can change to help you take in less air.

Sometimes It's Better to Belch

Many physicians see no physiological need to stifle belching. They view it simply as a natural body function.

"Some societies think belching is good for you," says Richard McCallum, M.D., professor of medicine and chief of the Gastroenterology Division at the University of Virginia Health Sciences Center. "And we have a couple of people from India and other Eastern countries who tell me that it's perfectly normal to belch in public."

Well, Doc, this ain't Calcutta—but favorable feelings about belching do make perfect sense. With this in mind, Dr. McCallum and others might suggest you remember this old saw:

'Tis better to belch
And bear the shame,
Than squelch a belch
And bear the pain.

- Avoid carbonated beverages.
- Eat slowly and chew your food completely before swallowing.
- Always eat with your mouth closed.
- Avoid chewing gum.
- Do not drink out of cans or bottles, and do not drink through a straw.
- Avoid foods with a high air content such as beer, ice cream, soufflés, omelets, and whipped cream.

Nix a nervous belching habit. It's been noted that chronic air swallowers can belch forever, since belching tends to beget more belching. Yet even chronic nervous swallowers can be helped.

Marvin Schuster, M.D., chief of the Department of Digestive Diseases at Francis Scott Key Medical Center in Baltimore, Maryland, sometimes prescribes a pencil for those who swallow air and start bloating up during tense situations.

"Clamping your teeth around a pencil, or a cork or your finger, keeps your mouth open and makes swallowing difficult," he says.

Say good-bye to gassy goodies. We will all eat a little too much a little too quickly and burp, says Samuel Klein, M.D., assistant professor of gastroenterology and human nutrition at the University of

Texas Medical School at Galveston. But that's different than people who belch hour after hour, day after day. That's chronic belching.

For those people, it may be useful to decrease their intake of foods that produce upper digestive system gas. Generally speaking, those include fats and oils such as salad oil, margarine, and sour cream.

Smash bubbles with soothing simethicone. To help alleviate a problem that already exists, digestive experts sometimes recommend over-the-counter antacids containing simethicone, such as Mylanta, Mylanta II, Maalox Plus, or Di-Gel.

"Simethicone will break large bubbles into small bubbles in the stomach, which may decrease belching," says Dr. Klein. "It does not reduce the amount of gas present."

PANEL OF ADVISERS

André Dubois, M.D., is a gastroenterologist in Bethesda, Maryland.

Samuel Klein, M.D., is assistant professor of gastroenterology and human nutrition at the University of Texas Medical School at Galveston. He is also an editorial adviser to *Prevention* magazine.

Richard McCallum, M.D., is a professor of medicine and chief of the Gastroenterology Division at the University of Virginia Health Sciences Center in Charlottesville. He does research on gastrointestinal problems.

Marvin Schuster, M.D., is chief of the Department of Digestive Diseases at Francis Scott Key Medical Center in Baltimore, Maryland, and a professor of medicine and psychiatry at Johns Hopkins University School of Medicine in Baltimore.

Bites

37 Treatment Tips

One mosquito says to another, "I heard a bum say he hadn't had a bite in a week. So I bit him."

It's a lame joke. But bites aren't all that funny if you're on the receiving end. Fortunately, most insect bites are just annoyances that itch like crazy and produce ugly little welts that go away in a day or two.

And love nips from Fifi and Fido are often more an insult than a real injury. So for those occasions when the bite is a little worse than the bark (or the buzz), doctors make the following suggestions.

FLIES AND MOSQUITOES

These pesky flying critters can make you pretty uncomfortable when they decide to munch on you. Here's what to do.

Disinfect the bite. Flies and mosquitoes can spread disease. So wash the bite area thoroughly with soap and water, says North Carolina allergist Claude Frazier, M.D. Then apply an antiseptic.

Rub in an aspirin. Herbert Luscombe, M.D., professor emeritus at Jefferson Medical College of Thomas Jefferson University, recommends an unusual aspirin treatment to help control inflammation. As soon as possible after being bitten, moisten your skin and rub an aspirin tablet right over the bite.

Relieve the itching. Fly and mosquito bites may produce swelling and intense itching that can last for three or four days. Dr. Frazier recommends the following to control these symptoms:

- An oral antihistamine. Choose an over-the-counter allergy or cold preparation.
- Calamine lotion.
- Ice packs.
- Salt. With water, moisten it into a paste and apply to the bite.
- Baking soda. Dissolve 1 teaspoon in a glass of water. Dip a cloth into the solution and place on the bite for 15 to 20 minutes.
- Epsom salts. Dissolve 1 tablespoon in 1 quart of hot water. Chill, then apply as above.

Practice prevention. You may be able to avoid a bite in the first place by using the repellents below. Keep in mind that the hotter it is, the more active flies and mosquitoes seem to be. And mosquitoes, in particular, are at their worst in damp areas, such as near ponds or in marshes. Some species are especially pesty late in the day and are attracted to outdoor lighting after dark. So don't let down your guard at sunset.

Thiamine chloride. Taken orally, this B vitamin may repel insects by being excreted through the skin, says Dr. Frazier. He does caution that it may cause itching, hives, and a rash in some people.

When the Itsy Bitsy Spider
Turns Nasty

Little Miss Muffet was no sissy—she was just savvy enough not to risk a spider bite. Basically, says paramedic Jeff Rusteen, all spiders are poisonous. It's just that most of them aren't big enough or powerful enough to penetrate the skin and do much harm. If you do get bitten, says Claude Frazier, M.D., follow these steps:

- Wash the wound and disinfect it with an antiseptic.
- Apply an ice pack to slow absorption of the venom.
- Neutralize some of the poison, adds Herbert Luscombe, M.D., by moistening the bite with water and rubbing in an aspirin tablet.

Beware, a black widow spider bite can cause intense abdominal pain that could be confused with appendicitis. Let your doctor know you've been bitten so he can administer injections of calcium gluconate, says Dr. Luscombe.

A bite from a brown recluse spider might also produce problems, he adds. If an intensely sore lump develops (sometimes weeks after the injury), consult your doctor.

DEET. He also recommends any commercial repellent containing N,N-diethyl-m-toluamide (DEET). Apply generously over all exposed skin but be careful around the eyes—it can sting badly if perspiration carries it into the eye. Do not use too often, however, especially on children.

Chlorine bleach. Dr. Luscombe recommends bathing in a very diluted solution of chlorine bleach before going out. Mix two capfuls of bleach in a tub of warm water. Soak in it for 15 minutes. Be very careful not to get the solution near or in the eyes. The repellent effect should last several hours.

Bath oil. Certain bath oils, such as Alpha-Keri and Avon's Skin-So-Soft, have a repellent effect, he says.

Sunscreen. Some sunscreens also repel insects. "PreSun, for instance, seems to work as a repellent," says Dr. Luscombe.

Vicks Vaporub. Some people have success with this strong-smelling ointment, he says.

Zinc. Illinois allergist George Shambaugh, Jr., M.D., professor emeritus at Northwestern University Medical School, recommends daily doses of zinc (at least 60 milligrams) as a natural repellent. Be aware that it takes about a month to build up enough zinc in your system to discourage insects. (Take extra supplements only with the approval and supervision of your doctor.)

TICKS
Ticks are not fussy about what type of animal provides their meals. Humans are fair game to them. Here's what to do if one latches onto you.

Remove the beast. Ticks pose a special problem because they dig their little jaws into your skin and hold on for dear life. Trying to brush away a tick as you would a fly has no effect. And forcefully plucking it out may leave its mouthparts embedded, setting the stage for infection. Here are some gentler methods for loosening a tick's grip.

Ease it out. Dr. Luscombe recommends taking a pair of tweezers and very slowly pulling the tick out. "Don't pull too fast," he cautions. "And if you're not having success, you might try applying a little heat to the tick's backside. Blow out a match and carefully touch the tick with the tip. The heat may encourage it to let go."

Irritate it. Dr. Frazier says that a drop of gasoline, kerosene, benzine, or alcohol placed on the general region of the tick's head will make it loosen its grip. But be patient—it may take 10 minutes or more to work. Note that these substances are flammable and should not be used in conjunction with a hot match.

Suffocate it. A variation on that technique, says Dr. Frazier, is to cover the tick with a drop of paraffin or fingernail polish. Either substance will close off the tiny breathing openings on its side and suffocate the tick.

Try the Benforado Method. When Joseph Benforado, M.D., professor emeritus at the University of Wisconsin–Madison, was a Boy Scout camp physician some years ago, he devised this foolproof way to remove ticks:
Take a large nail (8- or 10-penny size) and warm the tip in a match flame. Slide the flat side of a pocketknife blade under the tick's abdomen. Place the heated nail tip on the tick's back so it's sandwiched between the knife and the nail. When the tick's legs begin to wiggle in response to the heat, turn the knife blade 90 degrees so the tick is standing on its

head. Keeping it sandwiched, gently pull the tick up and away from its grip. If the legs do not wiggle, the nail is not warm enough. Try again. "The object is to annoy the tick rather than roast it," says Dr. Benforado.

Clean up. Once you've removed the tick, wash the bite area with soap and water, says Dr. Frazier. Then apply iodine or another antiseptic to guard against infection.

Be vigilant. Although June and July seem to mark the height of tick season, ticks are a danger from early spring until fall. If you're spending any time outdoors, especially in wooded or high-grass areas—even grassy dunes—take the following precautions.

- One way to discover if there are ticks in an area, says Dr. Frazier, is to tie a piece of white flannel to a string and drag it through the grass or underbrush. Examine it frequently. If ticks are present, they will cling to the cloth.
- If you're in a tick area, leave as little skin exposed as possible, says Dr. Benforado. That means wearing long pants, high socks, and long sleeves.
- Before going to bed at night, he adds, inspect your body for any freeloading ticks. Certain species can be quite small, and you might otherwise overlook them.

DOGS AND CATS
Here's what to do when a four-legged friend gets unfriendly.

Assess the damage. Seek medical help for all but the most minor wounds, say doctors.

Thoroughly wash the bite. Animal bites—especially from cats—may transmit infections, says Stephen Rosenberg, M.D., associate professor of clinical public health at Columbia University School of Public Health. He advises that you cleanse the wound thoroughly with soap and water to remove saliva and any other contamination. Continue washing for 5 full minutes.

Soak a puncture wound. If you have a puncture wound that is not bleeding, soak it in a povidone-iodine (Betadine) solution, says California paramedic Jeff Rusteen. "Add enough Betadine to a basin of warm water to turn it dark red. Soak the bite for 30 minutes."

Control bleeding. If there is any minor bleeding, cover the entire wound with thick sterile gauze or a clean cloth pad, says Dr. Rosenberg. If you have no appropriate bandage, thoroughly cleanse your hand and press it firmly against the wound. You may also put some ice against the pad (not directly on the skin) and elevate the wound above heart level to help stop bleeding.

Bandage the area. When the bleeding has stopped, says Dr. Rosenberg, cover the bite with a sterile bandage or clean cloth. Tie or tape it loosely in place.

MEDICAL ALERT

Keep Up Your Guard

Any bite could develop complications. Stay alert for these potential problems:

Infection. Examine any animal wound periodically, says paramedic Jeff Rusteen. If it gets red, painful, or hot, infection has probably developed. Get professional help.

Crush injury. Sometimes a large dog, such as a German shepherd, will bite without breaking the skin. If you can see bite marks on both sides of an extremity, there may be internal damage, says Rusteen. If tingling develops or if the extremity changes color (turns blue, for instance), there may be structural damage. Get to a hospital or call paramedics.

Rabies. All warm-blooded animals may carry rabies, says Stephen Rosenberg, M.D. Contact the animal's owner to see whether its rabies shots are up-to-date. Rabies treatment may be safely delayed as long as the animal shows no symptoms, he says, providing the bite was not too severe or too close to the head. You may be required to report all bites to the authorities, he adds; check with the police.

Rocky Mountain spotted fever. If you were bitten by a tick, a rash may develop around your wrists or ankles and spread to the rest of your body, says Herbert Luscombe, M.D. A high fever and terrible headaches can follow. The disease can be deadly, so if symptoms appear, see a doctor immediately.

Lyme disease. Also caused by ticks, Lyme disease starts as a ringwormlike spot at the site of the bite, says Dr. Luscombe. Although very serious if not treated, the organism is easily killed with antibiotics. Symptoms may not develop for a few weeks, so you should keep an eye on the bite area.

Reduce pain. Use aspirin or acetaminophen to reduce pain, says Rusteen. This is appropriate even if the bite did not break the skin. Elevate the area and apply ice if there is any swelling.

Get a tetanus shot. Any animal bite can lead to tetanus, says Dr. Rosenberg. If you haven't had a booster shot within the last five to eight years, get one now.

PANEL OF ADVISERS

Joseph Benforado, M.D., is professor emeritus of medicine at the University of Wisconsin–Madison and vice president of the U.S. Pharmacopoeia, which sets American drug standards. He spent many summers as a physician at a Boy Scout camp in northern Wisconsin.

Claude Frazier, M.D., is an allergist in private practice in Asheville, North Carolina. He is the author of *Coping with Food Allergies* and *Insects and Allergy and What to Do about Them.*

Herbert Luscombe, M.D., is professor emeritus of dermatology at Jefferson Medical College of Thomas Jefferson University in Philadelphia, Pennsylvania. He is also senior attending dermatologist at Thomas Jefferson University Hospital in Philadelphia.

Stephen Rosenberg, M.D., is associate professor of clinical public health at Columbia University School of Public Health in New York City. He is author of *The Johnson & Johnson First Aid Book.*

Jeff Rusteen is a firefighter-paramedic with the Piedmont Fire Department in Piedmont, California. He teaches emergency medical technology at Chabot College in Hayward, California. He is the author of a videotape and companion booklet called *Until Help Arrives.*

George Shambaugh, Jr., M.D., is a medical otologist and allergist in private practice in Hinsdale, Illinois, a member of the staff at Hinsdale Hospital, and professor emeritus of otolaryngology, head and neck surgery, of Northwestern University Medical School. He writes a health and nutrition newsletter that he sends to his patients.

Black Eye

5 Ways to Clear Up the Bruise

You think your black eye bugs you now? It's a good thing you didn't get your shiner back in the early 1900s! "Years ago people used to put a leech on a black eye to suck out the blood," says Jack Jeffers, M.D., an ophthalmologist at Wills Eye Hospital in Philadelphia, Pennsylvania.

Leeches got squashed as the treatment of choice once people found livestock more to their liking. "Sirloin steak is what my father used," says Jimmy, a second-generation butcher at Richard and Vinnie's Quality Meats in Brooklyn, New York. "When I was a kid, I used to get a lot of black eyes, and my father, being a butcher, used to put steaks on them. And it worked!"

Doctors no longer use leeches for treatment (thank goodness!), and it is unnecessary to waste a good steak on your eye. The best—and most effective—ways to block a black eye are much simpler than that. Here's how.

Pack it in ice. Jimmy's dad had the right idea, but it was the coldness of the steak, not the meat itself, that did the trick. In fact, a vegetarian would have gotten the same results by using iceberg lettuce!

Cold works in two ways. It helps keep the swelling down and, by constricting the blood vessels, helps decrease the internal bleeding, which is what causes the black-and-blue color.

Dr. Jeffers recommends applying an ice pack for the first 24 to 48 hours. "If your eye is swollen shut, use it for 10 minutes every 2 hours the first day," he advises. To make an ice pack for the eye, put crushed ice in a plastic bag and tape it to the forehead. This will prevent putting pressure on the eye.

Try the Tyson treatment. Champion boxer Mike Tyson has dished out lots of black eyes in his career. One of the fight doctors who has examined Tyson's battered opponents says that boxing trainers have a trick for treating black eyes that you can use outside the ring.

MEDICAL ALERT

How's Your Vision?

For a black eye, you need to see your doctor when you have a hard time seeing *any* doctor.

"If your vision is impaired, you have pain in your eye, you're light sensitive, you have double or blurred vision, or you have things floating through your field of vision," says Keith Sivertson, M.D. "that's the time you need medical care."

"It's not so much how it looks looking in but how it looks looking out," he says.

"Trainers use on the boxer's eye what looks like a small metal iron," says ophthalmologist Dave Smith, M.D., a member of the Medical Advisory Council of the State Athletic Control Board of the State of New Jersey, who has examined over 300 boxers for eye injuries. "It is extremely cold, and they use it to control the immediate hemorrhage so that the swelling is minimized. You can use the same sort of treatment by getting a cold soda can and holding it against the eye intermittently (5 to 10 minutes of every 15 minutes) until you can get some ice on it, says Dr. Smith. "Make sure the can is clean and then hold it lightly against your cheek, not your eye. Do not put any pressure on your eyeball."

Enjoy the show. Once the eye bruises, there's not a whole lot you can do except control the swelling. Even makeup can't disguise it totally. Most black eyes will last about a week, and it's a colorful week at that.

"The injury starts out black," says Keith Sivertson, M.D., director of the Department of Emergency Medicine at Johns Hopkins Hospital in Baltimore, Maryland. "Then as it starts to heal, it will turn green, then yellow, and finally it just disappears."

Avoid aspirin. Aspirin may be bad news for those with black eyes. Acetaminophen is what doctors recommend most. "Aspirin is an anticoagulant, meaning the blood won't clot as well. You'll have a harder time stopping the bleeding that causes the discoloration," says Dr. Jeffers. "You may wind up with a bigger bruise." If for some reason you need to take a pain reliever, take acetaminophen.

Don't blow your nose. If it was a severe blow that caused your black eye (something more than just bumping into a door), blowing your nose could cause your face to blow up like a balloon. "Sometimes the injury fractures the bone of the eye socket, and blowing your nose can force air out of your sinus adjacent to the socket," says Dr. Jeffers. "The air gets injected under your skin and makes the eyelids swell even more. It also can increase the chance of infection."

PANEL OF ADVISERS

Jack Jeffers, M.D., is an ophthalmologist and director of emergency services at the Sports Center for Vision at Wills Eye Hospital in Philadelphia, Pennsylvania.

Keith Sivertson, M.D., is director of the Department of Emergency Medicine at Johns Hopkins Hospital in Baltimore, Maryland.

Dave Smith, M.D., is an ophthalmologist in private practice in Ventnor City, New Jersey, and a member of the Medical Advisory Council of the State Athletic Control Board of the State of New Jersey. He is also on the medical team at the Sports Center for Vision at Wills Eye Hospital in Philadelphia, Pennsylvania.

Bladder Infections

11 Remedies for a Vexing Problem

You've been spending a lot of time groping your way to the bathroom. You need to go a *lot*. But when you get there—well, not much happens. And when it does, it *burrrrnnnns.*

What are we talking about? A health problem that's made a special sorority out of an awful lot of American women—five out of every ten will come down with a bladder infection at some point in their lives. (Men can get them, too, but it's so rare that bladder infections, also known as urinary tract infections, are considered a female malady.)

"It's absolutely one of the most common infections physicians have to treat," says David Staskin, M.D., assistant professor of urology at Boston University School of Medicine.

"Probably 50 percent of all women have at least one bladder infection at some time during their lives, and 20 percent or more will have multiple infections—it's not uncommon for many women to have one or two a year."

What's the cause?

Bladder infections are caused by bacteria known as *E. coli* that take up residence in the vagina and consequently make their way to the urethra, the tube through which urine flows, says Elliot L. Cohen, M.D., assistant professor of clinical urology at Mount Sinai School of Medicine of the City University of New York. In the vagina, the bacteria are no problem. Trouble only starts when they enter the urinary tract.

"These are bacteria normally present in all women. And the women who get UTIs (medical shorthand for urinary tract infections) aren't anatomically different from the women who don't. But for reasons we don't understand, they are more susceptible to the infection," says Dr. Cohen.

Bladder infections are really infections of the urine itself, according to Dr. Staskin, and the effect on the patient is usually relatively minor. "The bacteria irritate the wall of the bladder," he says. "In most cases, it's the bladder's equivalent of a bad sunburn."

But the infections still burn and sting and generally make life uncomfortable for those who have them. There is, however, good news.

The Alternate Route

Cranberry Juice Cure Diluted?

Every woman who's had a urinary tract infection—and every man who's gone through it with her—has heard about the cranberry juice cure. The big question: Does it work? The answer depends on whom you talk to. Some within the medical community say yes, but most say no. Over the years, several studies have documented an effect. But controversy remains on *why* it may work.

"I think it probably has as much to do with increasing fluid intake as anything else," says David Staskin, M.D. "I just don't think there's enough of anything special in cranberry juice to have an effect."

Joseph Corriere, M.D., agrees—to a point. "It's got quinolic acid (which converts to hippuric acid in the liver) in it, and it is fortified with vitamin C. Both hippuric acid and vitamin C have been shown to impact on the infection," Dr. Corriere says. "The problem is, you'd have to drink *gallons* every day to get enough to have an effect."

Although there's strong doubt that cranberry juice will *cure* your infection, there certainly is no harm in giving it a try. But remember, if it doesn't cure you, it certainly won't hurt you, either.

There's a lot you can do to make UTIs less unpleasant and to get them over with more quickly. The following doctor-tested tips tell you how.

Drink lots of fluids. This is probably the single most important tip, for two reasons: comfort and health.

"Some women get a UTI and think, 'Aha! It only burns when I go to the bathroom,' " says Dr. Cohen. "They then reason that they won't have to go if they don't drink, so they don't—which is absolutely the *worst* thing they can do."

The reason: The longer *any* amount of urine stays in the bladder, the more bacteria there are in it—*E. coli* doubles its population about every 20 minutes, according to Dr. Staskin. More bacteria mean more pain.

"Absolutely the best thing a woman can do to fight the burning is drink fluids to flush out the bacteria that are causing the inflammation," Dr. Cohen says.

"There's a very strong argument for drinking more fluid both to prevent UTIs and to treat them," Dr. Staskin says. "Studies have been performed where bacteria were mechanically introduced into the bladders of volunteers. But voiding just twice effectively *sterilized* the bladder."

Message: The more you drink, the sooner the pain will stop. And a hint: If your urine's clear, you're drinking enough. If it's colored, you're not.

Take a hot bath. "This helps relieve pain for many women," says Richard J. Macchia, M.D., professor and chairman of the Department of Urology at the State University of New York Health Science Center at Brooklyn College of Medicine. "I don't think anyone's researched the exact mechanisms involved, but a hot bath often seems to help where there's inflammation."

Take aspirin or ibuprofen. "These are anti-inflammatories, and they do help some people," Dr. Macchia says. "They reduce the inflammation in the bladder, and the less inflammation, the less burning."

Take vitamin C. "About 1,000 milligrams taken throughout the day will acidify the urine enough to interfere with bacterial growth," Dr. Macchia says. "This is a good idea if you're having problems with reinfection or have recurrence in the middle of nowhere without quick access to medical help." Caution: Some antibiotics prescribed for bladder infections don't work well in acidic urine, so tell your doctor if you're taking vitamin C. Also tell him how much you're taking. Vitamin C is not toxic, but 1,000 milligrams is considered a large dose and should have your doctor's approval.

The Signs of Something Serious

There are four major symptoms that should send anyone with a bladder infection (whether it's the first or the fifth, it doesn't matter) to the doctor. They are:

- Blood in the urine
- Pain in the lower back or flank
- Fever
- Nausea or vomiting

"About 90 percent of all women who get a bladder infection will have the bacteria gone with the first or second antibiotic pill, but the symptoms often last for two to three days," says David Staskin, M.D. "But a very small number may develop more serious problems with the kidneys. If they experience any of the above, they should see a physician *immediately.*"

The symptoms associated with a bladder infection can also be similar to something else—like cancer (especially if there is blood in the urine)—so it's important to *always* seek professional medical advice.

Back away. Wiping from front to back helps prevent infection from recurring, the doctors say. Wiping the wrong way is one of the most common causes of infection and a good way to get repeat infections. Wiping away is pure common sense, you want to move bacteria *away* from, not toward, the vagina and the opening of the urethra.

Go to the bathroom before intercourse. This helps flush out bacteria that may be present in the vagina, the experts say—bacteria that otherwise might be pushed into the bladder by intercourse.

Go to the bathroom after intercourse. This is where the myth of your partner's involvement gets its start—and like most myths, there's a grain of truth to this one, according to Dr. Staskin. A man's penis can massage bacteria present in the opening of the uretha into the bladder. Voiding effectively "rinses" the bladder out.

"There's no doubt that UTIs are more common in sexually active women," Dr. Cohen says. "But that's more the result of not knowing how to protect themselves than of sexual activity itself. If bacteria *have* been pushed into the bladder, urinating will flush most of them out."

Reconsider the diaphragm. "Diaphragms have been documented as major contributors to those who have stubborn, repeated bladder infections," Dr. Staskin says. "Two mechanisms are probably involved: Bacteria colonize the diaphragm itself, which is then inserted deep into the vagina, and the diaphragm interferes with bladder emptying, which means that bacteria already there aren't flushed out."

If this description fits you, you might want to talk to your doctor about another method of birth control.

Use pads instead of tampons. "No one's absolutely certain why certain women seem more susceptible to reinfection, but vaginal manipulation of some sort—sex, inserting the diaphragm, putting a tampon in—always seems to precede it," says Joseph Corriere, M.D., director of the Division of Urology at the University of Texas Health Science Center at Houston.

"I advise those of my patients experiencing chronic infection at the time of menstruation to quit using tampons and replace them with pads," he says.

Practice good hygiene. Good hygiene means wearing cotton underwear that keeps you dry, avoiding tight pants that decrease ventilation, and most of all, keeping clean—but *sensibly* clean.

"If you don't bathe to remove bacteria in the perineal region [between vagina and rectum], obviously you run the risk of repeated infection," Dr. Staskin says. "But too much can be as bad as too little. Douching constantly can both introduce bacteria into the vagina and rinse out the normal "friendly," noninfectious vaginal bacteria, which are then replaced with infectious *E. coli.* Irritation of the urethra may occur, which may feel like another UTI. Strong antibacterial soaps can do the same thing—and change the vaginal flora enough to make the individual more susceptible to infection."

The point: Be clean, but don't be obsessed.

PANEL OF ADVISERS

Elliot L. Cohen, M.D., is assistant professor of clinical urology at Mount Sinai School of Medicine of the City University of New York in New York City.

Joseph Corriere, M.D., is director of the Division of Urology at the University of Texas Health Science Center at Houston.

Richard J. Macchia, M.D., is professor and chairman of the Department of Urology at the State University of New York Health Science Center at Brooklyn College of Medicine.

David Staskin, M.D., is assistant professor of urology at Boston University School of Medicine in Massachusetts.

Blisters

20 Hints to Stop the Hurt

Blisters are your body's way of saying it's had enough. Be it too much friction or too much ambition, a blister—much like a muscle cramp or side stitch—is designed to slow you down and make you better prepared for physical activity.

In some cases, blisters result from the painful rigor of breaking in a new pair of badly fit shoes or spending too much time with the garden rake.

But blisters can also be viewed as a badge of initiation, a sign of someone trying something new that's hopefully worth the added effort and pain. Blisters initiate the new walker, the new racquetball player, the new cyclist. Different sports create blisters on different parts of the body, though the foot remains the site of greatest abuse.

Though the following remedies concentrate on blisters of the feet, many of these recommendations can be applied to treating friction blisters on the hands or on any other part of the anatomy where your body has said slow down.

TREATING THEM

Here's how experts recommend you deal with the discomfort of blisters you already have.

Decide whether to prick or not to prick. Once you have a blister, you have to decide what's best to do with it. That is, should you protect it and leave it alone, or should you prick it and drain the fluid?

"I think it depends on the size of the blister," says Suzanne Tanner, M.D., a private practitioner in Denver, Colorado, who specializes in sports medicine. "A purist will probably tell you not to prick it, because then you don't run any risk of infection. But I think for most people that's just not very practical."

While purists do indeed exist, our experts say you should prick large blisters that are painful, while leaving intact smaller blisters that cause no discomfort. "When you have a big blister that's in a weight-bearing area, you almost have to drain it," says Clare Starrett, D.P.M., a professor at the Foot and Ankle Institute of the Pennsylvania College of Podiatric Medicine. "They can get so full they get like a balloon."

Also, blisters that are likely to break on their own should be drained by you, our experts say. That way, you can control when and how the blister is opened, instead of leaving it to chance.

Make a moleskin doughnut. One way to protect a tender blister without draining it is to cut a moleskin pad into a doughnut shape and place it over the blister. "Leave the central area open where the blister is," says Dr. Tanner. The surrounding moleskin will absorb most of the shock and friction of everyday activity. As long as the skin is clean and dry, the moleskin will adhere by itself.

Be wise and sterilize. For those who wish to drain a blister, the first thing to do is clean the blister and surrounding skin, and sterilize your "instrument," whether it's a pin (needle) or razor blade (we'll get to that subject in a minute). "I recommend alcohol to clean both," says Nancy Lu Conrad, D.P.M., a private practitioner in Circleville, Ohio.

Other doctors advise sterilizing your instrument by flame instead of alcohol; that is, simply heat the pin or razor blade with a match until it glows red (let it cool before touching the skin, however). Either method seems equally able to kill germs, and both come equally recommended.

Stick it. "If a blister gives me pain," says Joseph Ellis, D.P.M., a private practitioner in La Jolla, California, and a consultant for the University of California, San Diego, "then I just go ahead and pop it." Use a sterilized needle and stick it in the side of the blister, Dr. Ellis says. "Just make sure the hole's big enough that you can squeeze out all the fluid."

Or slice it. "We use a sterile scalpel to drain blisters at our office," says Dr. Starrett. Not surprisingly, she recommends using a sterilized razor blade for doing the same at home. "Just make a straight incision," she says, "a little slice that's big enough to let the fluid come out."

Keep the roof on. "I think the biggest mistake most people make when treating their own blisters is that after they drain it they pull off the roof—the skin that goes over the top of the blister—and this is a

---

MEDICAL ALERT

Watch Out for Infection

"A good rule of thumb is that most wounds, no matter what they are, should get better each day," says Clare Starrett, D.P.M. That rule holds for blisters as well, she says, noting that the classical signs of infection are redness, swelling, heat, and increased pain.

"A blister is definitely infected when the fluid coming from it is not clear like water, or when it has some odor to it," she says. "That's the time to seek professional help."

Nancy Lu Conrad, D.P.M., agrees. "You can end up going too far with bathroom surgery," she warns. "Head to the doctor at the first sign of infection."

---

terrible mistake," says Richard Cowin, D.P.M., director of Cowin's Foot Clinic in Libertyville, Illinois. Always leave that roof on, our experts advise. Think of it as nature's Band-Aid.

"If you remove it, you're going to end up with a very red, raw, sore area," says Dr. Cowin. "But if you leave it on, it'll eventually harden up and fall off by itself, significantly reducing your recovery time."

Try a triple whammy for germs. Recent research has shown that triple antibiotics (such as Neosporin, to name one) can eliminate bacterial contamination from blisters after only two treatments, whereas old standbys such as iodine and camphor-phenol actually delay healing. Triple antibiotics are the choice of our experts, while iodine and camphor-phenol "are so good at killing germs that when used in high concentrations they can even kill the cells you are trying to heal," says Dr. Starrett.

Keep the dressing simple. After you've treated the blister, you'll need to keep it covered and protected while it heals. Though gauze pads and special bandages may be the first thing you'd expect a podiatrist to reach for, our experts suggest a much simpler approach.

"My first choice is a flexible fabric adhesive strip," says Dr. Cowin. Ditto for Dr. Ellis. "People will tell you to put a sterile dressing on it," he says, "but they forget that Band-Aids are sterile inside the wrapper, so you're actually putting on a piece of sterile gauze that has the adhesive already in place. It's a great dressing and very convenient."

Gauze pads, however, are recommended for blisters that are just too big for a Band-Aid to cover. Keep it in place with waterproof adhesive tape.

Use Second Skin for a second wind. If you've treated and covered your blister and find you just can't wait for it to completely heal before returning to an active lifestyle, then you'll need to know about Spenco's Second Skin dressing, a spongy material that absorbs pressure and reduces friction against blisters and surrounding skin.

"That's a good product," says Dr. Conrad, noting that a number of athletes (weekend and otherwise) apply petroleum jelly to the blister before covering it with Second Skin and taping it in place.

Give it some air. Most doctors suggest that you remove your blister dressing nightly and let it get some air. "Air and water are very good for healing," says Dr. Cowin, "so soaking it in water and keeping it open to the air at night are helpful."

Change wet dressings. Though some physicians say you can leave a dressing on for two days without worry, all agree that if a dressing becomes wet for any reason "you can consider it contaminated and it should be changed." That means you may need to change it quite often if your feet perspire heavily or you engage in activities that will lead to sweating and damp dressings.

PREVENTING THEM

Prevention is always the best option, so here's what experts recommend to keep blisters from developing in the first place.

Try a heel lift. Blisters that appear on the back of the foot usually result from the shoe's heel counter hitting the back of the heel in the wrong area, says Dr. Cowin. The fix? "All you usually have to do is put in a heel lift at the back of the shoe," he says.

Keep your socks on. "One of the fashions we're seeing again is people going without socks," Dr. Cowin says. "The people who do this suffer blisters on the back of their heels all the time." He recommends that those who want to flash some ankle without suffering the consequences invest in "footie type socks that only go around the foot area." These are available for both men and women nowadays, and they are much better than going sockless.

Powder daily. "Powder should be everybody's friend," says Dr. Conrad. "Make powdering your feet part of a daily routine."

"When people come in with shoes that fit but that still give them blisters," says Dr. Cowin. "I simply tell them to start off by applying baby powder to their feet before putting on their socks. This helps the sock to glide over the foot a little more and prevent blisters."

Coat to protect. If you're planning a long walk, run, tennis match, or whatever, one way to guard against blistered feet in new shoes is to coat blister-prone areas with petroleum jelly. "That will cut down on friction," says Dr. Conrad.

Dr. Ellis says A&D Ointment (typically used for diaper rash) is actually thicker than petroleum jelly, "and the thicker the better," he says. For walkers or runners who insist on going without socks, greasing up blister-prone areas is highly recommended.

Try new socks for new shoes. "If you've got a new pair of shoes that are rubbing up blisters, the first thing I'd do is change to different socks," says Dr. Ellis. "I recommend acrylic socks (available in sporting goods stores) because they're made in layers that are designed to absorb friction so your foot doesn't."

Cotton Up to Acrylic Socks

There's a major debate raging in the sock world that could have far-reaching consequences for millions of blister-footed Americans— weekend walkers and Olympic marathoners alike. The cause of the current "friction" among foot care specialists is a study showing that acrylic socks may actually be better at preventing blisters than socks made of cotton or other natural fibers.

For years, natural fibers and natural materials (think cotton socks and leather shoes) have been the main recommendation of most podiatrists. The recent findings about man-made acrylic offering superior protection fly in the face of conventional wisdom and go firmly against the advice of most coaches, sports physicians, and athletes alike.

But research now shows that cotton socks produce twice as many blisters in runners as acrylic socks, and that the blisters formed by cotton socks are usually three times as big as those produced by their acrylic counterparts.

"As a veteran long-distance runner and someone who treats runners for blisters every day," says Seal Beach, California, sports podiatrist and study author Douglas Richie, Jr., D.P.M., "the results don't surprise me in the least. I'm well aware that cotton fiber becomes abrasive with repeated use, and that it also loses its shape when wet. The shape of a sock is critical when it's inside a shoe.

"Many people equate acrylic with a silky, nylonlike fiber," says Dr. Richie, "yet spun acrylic feels exactly like cotton and maintains its soft, bouncy feeling even when wet."

Dr. Richie says the nonblistering property of acrylic socks holds true for any type of sporting activity, be it walking, running, tennis, etc. It could be worth a try.

Treat your feet to treated insoles. Our experts agree that many of the products made by Spenco are excellent for preventing blisters. One of the best is a chemically treated insole "that's bubbled-in nitrogen," explains Dr. Cowin. "What that does is add some cushioning to the bottom of the foot and help it glide over the bottom of the shoe better, instead of sticking in places and causing a blister."

Toughen with tannic acid. Studies have shown that applying 10 percent tannic acid to vulnerable areas of the skin twice daily for two to three weeks makes the skin tough and less prone to blisters. "If you're a hard-core athlete or distance runner, you can use something like that," says Dr. Conrad. "But weekend athletes and beginners really don't have any business using tannic acid unless it's been suggested by a physician."

Beware the terrible tube. While tube socks, those unformed heelless wonders you can slip into without thinking, are very popular, our experts advise against using them. "I personally don't believe in tube socks," says Dr. Cowin. "I don't think they ever fit properly. You need a regular, fitted sock to help prevent blisters."

PANEL OF ADVISERS

Nancy Lu Conrad, D.P.M., is a private practitioner in Circleville, Ohio. She specializes in footwear for children, as well as in sports medicine and orthopedics.

Richard Cowin, D.P.M., is director of Cowin's Foot Clinic in Libertyville, Illinois, where he specializes in the practice of minimal incision and laser foot surgery. He is a diplomate of the American Board of Podiatric Surgery and the American Board of Ambulatory Foot Surgery.

Joseph Ellis, D.P.M., is a private practitioner in La Jolla, California. He is a consultant for the University of California, San Diego and is the sports medicine consultant for the Asics-Tiger running shoe company. He also writes for *Runner's World* magazine.

Douglas Richie, Jr., D.P.M., is a sports podiatrist in Seal Beach, California, where he studies the function of socks and their effect on sporting activities. He is also a clinical instructor of podiatry at the Los Angeles County/University of Southern California Medical Center in Los Angeles.

Clare Starrett, D.P.M., is a professor at the Foot and Ankle Institute of the Pennsylvania College of Podiatric Medicine in Philadelphia.

Suzanne Tanner, M.D., is a private practitioner in Denver, Colorado, who specializes in sports medicine.

Blood Pressure

17 Ways to Keep It under Control

About 30 million people in the United States have high blood pressure (hypertension), according to the latest figures from the National Center for Health Statistics. That makes it the third most prevalent chronic condition in the nation, right behind sinusitis and arthritis.

But more important than rank is what hypertension portends for older Americans. Of all the risk factors for heart attack, high blood pressure maintains an uncanny degree of accuracy for predicting exactly who will get cardiovascular disease after age 65.

On the up side, about 70 percent of patients have what's known as mild hypertension, that is, diastolic pressure that falls somewhere between 90 and 105 mm Hg. And for this population there have been some welcome changes in treatment. The emphasis is now being placed on nondrug therapy.

"For most people with mild hypertension, just about everyone now agrees that the nondrug approach should be the first line of defense — or should at least be tried," says Norman Kaplan, M.D., a noted blood pressure authority at the University of Texas Health Science Center at Dallas Southwestern Medical School.

The remedies below are designed to help those with mild hypertension attain good control over their condition. If you're already taking medication for your blood pressure, dosage levels may need to be adjusted. So consult your physician before implementing changes.

Watch your weight. "While there are a lot of hypertensives who are not fat, obese people tend to have three times as much hypertension as people of normal weight," says Dr. Kaplan.

Twenty percent above the ideal weight for your height and bone structure is where obesity starts. But obese people need not lose anywhere near that much to reduce high blood pressure. An Israeli study

74

showed that stout people with high blood pressure can achieve normal pressures by losing only half of their excess weight, even though they remain "considerably obese."

"Even with relatively minor amounts of weight loss, one can see a measurable fall in blood pressure," Dr. Kaplan says. "We encourage obese people to lose all the weight they can. But if they can't lose a whole lot, at least whatever they *do* lose should give them some help with their blood pressure."

Shake the salt habit. The link between sodium and high blood pressure has never been proven beyond a doubt. But what is known is that a salt-sensitive subset of hypertensives probably exists, and you may be one of them.

"There's no way to know if you're salt sensitive other than putting yourself on a low-sodium diet and seeing what effect that has on your blood pressure," Dr. Kaplan says. "So we just ask *all* our hypertensives to cut down on salt to about 5 grams a day and hope it has a good effect." While that's about half the salt in the typical American diet, Dr. Kaplan notes that "most people, once they cut down, really don't find they need as much salt as they thought they did." So keep the salt low, but don't count on it to do everything.

Cut down on alcohol. Because the connection between alcohol consumption and high blood pressure has been well documented, people with hypertension should limit their alcohol consumption.

Why not advise those with hypertension to simply cut out all drinking? Doctors probably would if studies hadn't shown that those who drink a small amount of alcohol a day have lower blood pressure than those who drink more than that, or those who don't drink at all.

"Two drinks or fewer a day will probably have no detrimental effect on blood pressure," says Dr. Kaplan, "but when you go beyond that, you're looking for trouble."

Pass the potassium, please. Increased levels of this mineral may be valuable in helping control high blood pressure. "The number of hypertensives who respond to potassium seems to depend on how long the studies are performed," says George Webb, Ph.D., a professor in the Department of Physics and Biophysics at the University of Vermont College of Medicine. "In a two-week study, we find that maybe 30 percent get a reduction, but with an eight-week study, we might find that 70 percent get a reduction," he says.

Dr. Webb believes that the total amount of potassium you consume isn't as important as maintaining the correct sodium/potassium ratio

MEDICAL ALERT

Malignant Hypertension: A Deadly Pressure

If left untreated, blood pressure tends to rise slowly and steadily over a number of years.

Sometimes, however, a very high blood pressure develops quite suddenly, with diastolic pressures shooting over 130 mm Hg. for hours or days at a time. Systolic pressures can reach 250 mm Hg. or more.

Such a sharp increase could signal the onset of malignant hypertension. Though rare, this is very serious and must be treated by a physician as soon as possible. Malignant hypertension can damage blood vessels in the kidneys, eyes, or brain. Left untreated, it can be fatal within six months.

Thankfully, malignant hypertension can be brought under control very quickly with intravenous injections of the proper drugs—but rapid diagnosis and treatment are essential.

in your diet. "We believe there's a clear benefit when you get three times as much potassium as sodium," he says. "If you're on a low-salt diet and getting 2 grams of sodium (2 grams of sodium equals 5 grams of table salt) per day, then you should get 6 grams of potassium."

How do you know if you're getting enough? Well, it's virtually impossible to devise a low-salt diet that's not high in potassium. "And it's hard to avoid potassium if you eat plenty of natural foods," says Dr. Webb. Potatoes, fresh fruit, and fish are loaded with it. To calculate ratios, however, you may need to consult the tables of a nutrition reference book.

Make the calcium connection. "Calcium seems to have a favorable effect on some people," says Roseann Lyle, Ph.D., an assistant professor of health promotion and education at Purdue University. But the search to discover exactly who will respond favorably to calcium continues.

"It seems that salt-sensitive hypertensives, who may be about half the people with high blood pressure, are the same ones who respond well to calcium," says Lawrence M. Resnick, M.D., assistant professor at the New York Hospital-Cornell University Medical Center in New York City. "So if salt is bad for you, calcium's good for you."

Avoid isometrics. "Exercise, as part of a program to reduce hypertension, appears to add to the treatment," says David Spodick, M.D., director of clinical cardiology at St. Vincent's Hospital at the University of Massachusetts Medical School. But, he adds, isometric exercises such as weight lifting must be avoided. The reason is that weight-lifting exercises may cause blood pressure to temporarily skyrocket.

Try aerobic exercise instead. While numerous studies have shown the beneficial effects of aerobic exercise on high blood pressure, the primary advice for hypertensives is to proceed with caution.

"We usually start people with walking a quarter of a mile briskly," says Robert Cade, M.D., professor of medicine at the University of Florida College of Medicine. "Then we go up from there until a person can walk a mile briskly. After that we initiate running—but only after a physical exam and possibly a stress electrocardiogram."

The reason exercise works is that it forces the blood vessels to open up (vasodilate), and that makes the blood pressure come down, Dr. Cade says. "Even though it tends to go back up during exercise, it drops when exercise ends. Then when it goes back up, it doesn't go up as much."

Swimming, walking, and bike riding are all good exercises for hypertension. "You don't have to run," notes Cade. "You do about the same amount of work when you walk, it just takes longer to do it. The key thing is that it should be a brisk walk—a quarter mile in 4 minutes when you start, then later a full mile in about 15 minutes or less."

Think vegetarian. Studies have shown that vegetarians have lower blood pressure than the general population—10 to 15 mm Hg. lower for both systolic and diastolic pressures. The strange thing, however, is that nobody knows exactly why.

"But vegetarians *do* in fact have lower blood pressure," says Dr. Kaplan. "Maybe it's because people who follow vegetarian diets tend not to smoke, drink, or overeat.

Measure it yourself. "Blood pressure readings at home are to be encouraged," says Dr. Kaplan. "For anybody who has high blood pressure, it is by far the most sensible way to go about monitoring your condition."

But home monitoring can do more than just track your condition—it can help make you more aware of how diet, exercise, and medications are affecting your blood pressure. It may also help you overcome the "white coat" reaction many people experience. The minute they walk in a doctor's office, they tense up and their pressures rise dramatically.

The Lowdown
on Low Blood Pressure

For some people, the problem isn't high blood pressure but rather *low* blood pressure (hypotension). They may experience a dizzy spell—or even faint—if they stand up too fast.

Typically defined as a consistent fall of more than 20 mm Hg. systolic pressure when measured after 1 minute of standing, hypotension was once believed to afflict nearly as many elderly people as its opposite condition, hypertension. Recent studies, however, have shown that among healthy, nonmedicated elderly people, the rate of hypotension is only about 6 percent and does not increase with age after 55.

In many cases, apparently, hypotension is caused by the medications people take for hypertension, such as diuretics. Alcohol, as well as certain heart medications, tranquilizers, and antidepressants, has also been implicated.

If appropriate, and if you believe medication is causing the light-headedness, weakness, fatigue, headaches, or fainting associated with hypotension, you may need to ask your doctor to change a prescription. If that can't be done, though, there are still some things you can do on your own to help alleviate this condition.

Try a tight squeeze. Studies have shown that relatively simple physical actions that momentarily elevate blood pressure can offset hypotension. Squeezing an isometric handgrip before getting up, for example, can increase blood pressure enough to counter the momentary dip it takes upon standing.

Do some mental math. More amazingly, the researchers who documented the handgrip effect found that doing complex mental arithmetic (try counting backward from 100 by sevens as fast as you can) elevated blood pressure and offset hypotension even better than physical activity.

Eat smaller, more frequent meals. If you typically experience hypotension after meals, try eating smaller, more frequent meals throughout the day. Also, find out how much salt and fluid intake your doctor recommends. Restricting them may contribute to hypotension.

Sleep on a slant. The way you sleep may also be important in helping control hypotension. Try sleeping with the head end of your bed elevated 8 to 12 inches above the foot end (use concrete building blocks). On rising, sit up slowly and dangle your feet over the edge of the bed for a few moments before standing.

Blood-pressure kits come in three basic categories, mechanical, electronic with manual cuff inflation, and electronic with automatic cuff inflation. The manual types require the use of a stethoscope, while the electronic types eliminate the stethoscope and are somewhat easier to use.

"I think the most practical are the electronic types with manual inflation," says Dr. Kaplan. "They cost about $60 or $70, but you can get a good reading without any training at all."

Be a happy person. A study at New York Hospital-Cornell University Medical Center showed that different emotions play a very specific role in determining how high or low your blood pressure may go.

When testing unmedicated hypertensive patients around the clock with high-tech monitors, researchers found that happiness caused systolic blood pressure to drop, while anxiety caused diastolic pressure to rise. They also found that blood pressure changes were directly related to emotional intensity, so that the happier a person felt, the more the systolic pressure fell. Conversely, the more anxiety a person experienced, the higher the diastolic pressure rose.

Researchers also discovered that anxiety experienced outside the home makes blood pressure increase significantly more than anxiety experienced inside the home. The lesson in all this could be summed up as follows: Don't worry, be happy—but if you must worry, do it at home.

Try talking less. While it's hardly surprising that arguing with your spouse or fighting with the boss can make blood pressure soar, research has shown that virtually *any* communication can put blood pressure on the rise.

Researchers at the University of Maryland discovered that speaking can cause blood pressure to increase by 10 to 50 percent, with hypertensive individuals showing the greatest increase. And this effect is not restricted to the spoken word—even the use of sign language by deaf people causes dramatic increases in their blood pressure.

This has caused some scientists to speculate that a general "communicating state" may exist in humans and that this state may somehow be linked to the heart, causing its activity to increase. If true, this increased activity could result in an unintended blood pressure rise during such innocent activities as talking to your doctor.

Check your spouse's pressure, too. You've probably heard that husbands and wives start looking alike after several years of marriage, but researchers have discovered an even stranger phenomenon. The longer two people are married, the more similar their blood pressures become.

The researchers who conducted the study suggest that this mimicking effect could have something to do with shared stress or other emotional factors. "Communication, particularly handling conflict and expressing emotions, may affect blood pressure levels between spouses," says one. So the next time the doctor says your pressure is up, have him check your spouse, too. If you're in your sixties, this study predicts your blood pressures will be only a point or so apart.

"Take one dog and call me in the morning." Pliny, the Roman writer and philosopher, first wrote that prescription (or something close to it) centuries ago, but modern science is showing that it's a valid treatment for high blood pressure.

Cindy Wilson, Ph.D., associate professor and research director at the Uniformed Services University of the Health Sciences, recorded the blood pressures of 92 college students, then asked them to read aloud, read silently, or interact with a friendly dog. Reading aloud caused pressures to rise, though reading quietly or interacting with a dog resulted in blood pressure declines.

Her work only confirms the favorable feelings about pet therapy that some health professionals developed long ago. Other research has shown that coronary heart disease patients who are pet owners are more likely than nonowners to still be alive one year after discharge from a coronary care unit. And studies of children show that the presence of a pet reduces their blood pressure during reading or rest.

So what if Pliny wrote his prescription as a cure for women suffering from abdominal pains? Thanks to modern science, we now know that pets may be of benefit in hypertension, too.

PANEL OF ADVISERS

Robert Cade, M.D., is professor of medicine at the University of Florida College of Medicine in Gainesville.

Norman Kaplan, M.D., is a noted blood pressure authority at the University of Texas Health Science Center at Dallas Southwestern Medical School and coauthor of the book *Travel Well, The Gourmet Guide to Healthy Travel.*

Roseann Lyle, Ph.D., is assistant professor of health promotion and education at Purdue University in West Lafayette, Indiana, and has written a number of scientific papers about calcium and hypertension.

Lawrence M. Resnick, M.D., is an assistant professor of medicine at the New York Hospital-Cornell University Medical Center in New York City, and a prominent high blood pressure researcher.

David Spodick, M.D., is director of clinical cardiology at St. Vincent's Hospital at the University of Massachusetts Medical School in Worcester.

George Webb, Ph.D., is a professor in the Department of Physics and Biophysics at the University of Vermont College of Medicine in Burlington. He is coauthor of *The K-Factor,* a book about reducing high blood pressure through diet and exercise.

Body Odor

12 Ways to Feel Fresh and Clean

Some scientists believe that body odor, like the appendix, is a vestige of our evolution. That is, the smells we give off from certain areas of our bodies—primarily our armpits and groin—may have once served to advertise our sexuality, says Nathan Howe, M.D., Ph.D., a physician with the Department of Dermatology at the Medical University of South Carolina College of Medicine. "Of course," he adds, "whatever purpose was served by body odor then, to many Americans, it's plain objectionable now."

About this last point, there is little disagreement among doctors, or anyone else for that matter. If you want to win friends and influence people—don't stink.

Easier said than done? Actually, there are quite a few ways to take on body odor and come up smelling like a rose.

Scrub-a-dub-dub. The most basic way to hold body odor at bay is to scrub yourself with soap and water, particularly in those areas of the body that are most likely to smell, such as the armpits and groin, says Kenzo Sato, M.D., professor of dermatology at the University of Iowa.

Body odor is most often caused by a combination of perspiration and bacteria, he says. Scrubbing with soap and water will wash both culprits away.

The best type of soap for a body odor problem is a deodorant soap because it will hinder the return of bacteria. How often you need to scrub will depend on your individual body chemistry, your activities, your mood, and the time of year. If you're not sure if you're washing enough —ask a friend. Remember that perspiration glands and bacteria both work night as well as day shifts, which could mean you need to shower both morning and night.

Wash more than your body. You can wash till your skin puckers like a prune, but you'll still smell bad if your clothes aren't clean. Seven days in the same undershirt is a sure way to give offense to others, says Lenise Banse, M.D., a dermatologist with the Henry Ford Hospital in Detroit, Michigan. How often do you need to change your shirt? It depends on you as an individual. A daily change should suffice for most. On hot summer days, more than once a day might be in order.

Choose natural fabrics. Natural fabrics such as cotton absorb perspiration better than synthetic materials. The absorbed sweat is then free to evaporate from the fabric.

Play doctor. Sometimes, if you perspire a lot and have a tendency to smell bad, regular old deodorant soap may not be good enough. In this case, try an antibacterial surgical scrub, sold over the counter in most pharmacies, says Dr. Howe. Ask your pharmacist where to find them.

Antiperspirants attack best. Commercial deodorants are effective at masking underarm odor in most people, says Hridaya Bhargava, Ph.D., professor of industrial pharmacy at the Massachusetts College of Pharmacy. They leave chemicals on the skin that kill off odor-causing bacteria. But if you have a body odor problem known to friends and enemies alike, you may need an antiperspirant. "They're basically drugs," says Dr. Bhargava, that reduce the amount of perspiration the body produces. Many commercial antiperspirants combine antiperspirant with deodorant. But deodorants themselves cannot control perspiration.

Don't get irritated. If you can't use commercial deodorants or antiperspirants without developing a rash, you might try a topical antibiotic cream, sold in any drugstore. "It does the same thing as deodorants do, without any irritating perfumes," says Randall Hrabko, M.D., a dermatologist in private practice in Los Angeles, California.

Make the French connection. Another option if you can't tolerate common deodorants and antiperspirants is a product from France called Le Crystal Natural, says Dr. Hrabko. It's a chunk of mineral salts, formed into a crystal, that helps keep bacteria under control with-

---

The Alternate Route

Close Up the Sweat Shop

People with exceptionally strong body odor may find relief in an electronic device called Drionic, that can actually plug up overactive sweat ducts and keep them plugged for up to six weeks. Zapping your armpits isn't nearly as uncomfortable as it sounds, and clinical tests done at three universities prove its effectiveness at turning off faucetlike sweat glands.

The Drionic costs $125 but will save on the cost of antiperspirants and the wear and tear excessive sweating inflicts on your clothes, notes Robert Tapper, president of General Medical Company, which manufactures the device.

For more information you can ask your doctor or contact the company at 1935 Armacost Avenue, Los Angeles, CA 90025.

---

out irritating the skin. Le Crystal Natural, a product of the Burlingame, California-based French Transit company, is available in many cosmetic departments and health food stores.

Take a walk on the wild side. Forget the latest perfumes from Paris. Hunters have a way of coming up with their own fragrances. The name of the game in hunting, according to some, is to mask all trace of body odor lest the deer or bear being stalked catch wind of trouble and flee for cover.

How do hunters do it? One popular odor mask is pine soap, available in most hunting supply stores, says Dave Petzal, a veteran hunter and the executive editor of *Field and Stream* magazine. Pine soap not only masks human odor but "leaves you smelling like a pine forest," he says. If pine forest isn't your style, some hunters are using plain old glycerin soap.

Watch what you eat. Extracts of proteins and oils from certain foods and spices remain in your body's excretions and secretions for hours after eating them and can impart an odor. Fish, cumin, curry, and garlic lead the list, says Dr. Banse.

Keep calm. "Getting sexually excited or feeling anxious and nervous will make you perspire more," says Dr. Bhargava. If you anticipate a situation that is likely to upset you, no matter how much you're meditating or practicing deep breathing, consider using an extra dose of deodorant that morning.

Try the old dog trick. You've tried everything, and nothing seems to work? Maybe you haven't tried *everything*. An old folk remedy for a dog that's been skunked is to deodorize the poor pup with tomato juice. And guess what? It works for humans, too, says Alice Kilpatrick, R.N., a staff nurse at the Veterans Administration Hospital in Fort Lyon, Colorado.

Kilpatrick tried it first on her dog and then on a particularly odoriferous patient. And then on another. "It works 100 percent of the time!" she says. You don't need to fill your tub with pure tomato juice, "just pour a couple of cups in with your bath water and sit for 15 minutes," she says.

PANEL OF ADVISERS

Lenise Banse, M.D., is a dermatologist in Detroit, Michigan, where she is director of the Mole and Melanoma Clinic at the Henry Ford Hospital.

Hridaya Bhargava, Ph.D., is a professor of industrial pharmacy at the Massachusetts College of Pharmacy in Boston. He is a consultant to groups such as the World Health Organization and UNICEF.

Nathan Howe, M.D., Ph.D., is a physician in the Department of Dermatology at the Medical University of South Carolina College of Medicine in Charleston. He was formerly a zoologist with a special interest in how animals communicate using chemical smells.

Randall Hrabko, M.D., is a dermatologist in private practice in Los Angeles, California.

Alice Kilpatrick, R.N., is a staff nurse at the Veterans Administration Hospital in Fort Lyon, Colorado.

Kenzo Sato, M.D., is a professor of dermatology at the University of Iowa in Iowa City.

Boils

13 Tips to Stop an Infection

Boils are the volcanoes of the human body. They pop up like Popocatepetl and erupt like Etna, cascade like Kilauea and leave a crater akin to Krakatau (east of Java). At no time are they as fine-looking as Fuji.

The hard biological facts of a boil are these: Staphylococcus bacteria invade through a break in the skin and infect a blocked oil gland or

---

MEDICAL ALERT

The Boiling Points of Trouble

If bacteria from a boil get into the bloodstream, they can cause blood poisoning. It can be dangerous to squeeze a boil around your lips or nose because the infection can be carried to the brain. Other danger zones are the armpits, groin, and the breast of a nursing woman.

If the boil is extremely tender or under thick skin like that on the back, or if the boil victim is very young or old or sick, have a doctor treat it, says Rodney Basler, M.D. If there are any red lines radiating from it, or if you feel any general body symptoms like fever and chills or swelling of lymph nodes, he adds, see a doctor because the infection may have spread. Diabetics are especially prone to such dangerous boils, Adrian Connolly, M.D., says, and may need a course of antibiotics. Sometimes recurrent boils can be symptoms of more serious diseases.

---

hair follicle. The body's immune system sends in white blood cells to kill the invaders; the battle (inflammation) produces debris (pus). A pus-filled abscess begins to grow beneath the skin surface, rising up red with pain. Sometimes the body reabsorbs the boil; other times the boil swells to an eruption, drains, and subsides.

Boils are painful and unsightly. Sometimes they leave scars. Occasionally they can even be dangerous. But for the most part, you can treat most of them safely at home. Here's how.

Bring things to a head. "A warm compress is the very best thing you can do for a boil," says Rodney Basler, M.D., a dermatologist and assistant professor at the University of Nebraska College of Medicine. "It will come to a head, drain, and heal a lot faster."

At the first sign of a boil, place a compress — it can be just a warm, wet washcloth — over the boil for 20 to 30 minutes three or four times a day. Change it a few times during each session to keep it warm. "It's not uncommon for this to take five to seven days" until the boil breaks on its own, Dr. Basler says.

Spend extra time in Compress City. "It's important to continue the warm compresses for three days after the boil opens," Dr. Basler says. "You have to drain all that pus out of the tissues." You may also want to bandage it to keep it clean, "but it's not critical. A bandage is mainly to keep the drainage off your clothes."

The Alternate Route

Folk Remedies from the Kitchen

Food is for more than eating. Folklore has it that home remedies for boils are as close as your vegetable bin. All the following, recommended by Michael Blate, founder of the G-Jo Institute in Hollywood, Florida, are variations of the warm washcloth compress described in the beginning of the chapter. They should be changed every few hours.

- A heated slice of tomato
- A raw onion slice
- Mashed garlic
- The outer leaves of cabbage
- A bag of black tea

Go on the attack. When the boil has come to a pus-filled head, and if it's a small boil with no sign of spreading infection, Dr. Basler says, "it's certainly acceptable to sterilize a needle with a flame and make a small nick in the head. It's okay to squeeze it."

Doctors often worry that squeezing can drive the infection deeper into the skin, thus spreading it through the lymph system, Dr. Basler says, "but in reality that rarely happens. In the office we just squeeze the dickens out of them." Letting the boil break on its own can create "more of a mess," he says, because it often breaks while you're sleeping. If only the citizens of Pompeii had been able to poke a hole in Vesuvius.

Use antiseptic if you want. It's not really necessary to treat an opened boil with an antiseptic. "It's of almost no value, because the infection is localized," Dr. Basler says. "The important thing is to keep it draining." But Adrian Connolly, M.D., clinical assistant professor at the University of Medicine and Dentistry of New Jersey, recommends an OTC antibiotic ointment like Bacitracin Sterile or Neosporin as insurance against infection.

Lead staph to slaughter. If you're prone to boils, you may be able to lessen their frequency, Dr. Connolly says. "I don't think you can totally prevent them, but you can clean your skin with an antiseptic soap like Betadine," which will help keep the staph population down. Another prevention tip: Boils are usually cysts that have become infected. "Monkeying with a cyst is the surest way to get a boil," Dr. Basler says. Leave cysts alone, or have them excised by a doctor.

Don't spread it around. When a boil is draining, keep the skin around it clean, Dr. Connolly says. Take showers instead of baths to reduce the rare chance of spreading the infection to other parts of the body. After treating a boil, wash your hands well before preparing food because staph bacteria can cause food poisoning.

Try the old-timers' special. Varro E. Tyler, Ph.D., professor of pharmacognosy at Purdue University, mentions such folk remedies as poultices of warm milk and bread, burdock leaves, or the mud of a wasp's nest (which he agrees could be a little risky if the wasps aren't at work or on vacation). Any of these are applied as compresses to bring the boil to a head and are probably as effective as a warm, wet washcloth, Dr. Tyler says.

Pack on Denver mud. "It's an old folk remedy, available over-the-counter in many pharmacies," Dr. Basler says. "It's supposed to be a drying agent. You put it on at the first sign of a boil, and supposedly it draws the boil to a head quicker."

PANEL OF ADVISERS

Rodney Basler, M.D., is a dermatologist and assistant professor of internal medicine at the University of Nebraska College of Medicine in Lincoln.

Michael Blate is founder and executive director of the G-Jo Institute of Hollywood, Florida, a national health organization that promotes acupressure and oriental traditional medicine.

Adrian Connolly, M.D., is clinical assistant professor of medicine at the University of Medicine and Dentistry of New Jersey in Newark.

Varro E. Tyler, Ph.D., is professor of pharmacognosy at Purdue University in West Lafayette, Indiana, and author of *The Honest Herbal*. He also serves as a *Prevention* magazine adviser.

Breast Discomfort

16 Hints to Reduce Soreness

Maybe you're pregnant and you have trouble believing that these cartoonishly inflated and painful breasts could possibly be yours. At night, you can't find a comfortable sleeping position.

Maybe your period is around the corner and the butter-soft silk camisole you put on this morning feels like sandpaper when it shifts.

Or maybe you're still bewildered by the hard lump you found during your monthly self-exam, even though a pathologist assures you it's benign.

Welcome to the bewildering world of benign breast changes. You're not alone. An estimated 70 percent of North American women suffer from benign but discomforting breast changes during some point in their lives.

The tenderness you're apt to feel in pregnancy or just prior to your menstrual period occurs because of natural cycles of your reproductive hormones, estrogen and progesterone. These hormones signal the cells of the milk-producing glands to grow, and the areas around these glands expand with blood and other fluids to nourish the cells. These fluid-logged tissues can stretch nerve fibers, and you experience pain.

Fibrocystic changes, which include lumps and cysts, usually affect the nonworking areas: the fat cells, fibrous tissues, and other parts not involved in the making or transporting of milk.

But in either case, the same strategies can help you find relief and promote healing. Here's what our experts advise.

Switch your diet. Change to one low in fat and high in fiber—the kind of fiber in whole grains, vegetables, and beans. A study at Tufts University School of Medicine found that women who maintained this kind of diet metabolized estrogen differently. More estrogen was excreted in the stool, leaving less to circulate, says Christiane Northrup, M.D.,

---

MEDICAL ALERT

Benign?
Only Your Doctor Knows for Sure

You've already had one breast lump diagnosed as benign. Your last monthly self-exam turned up yet another lump. Is it safe to assume this one's benign, too?

No. Let this be your breast self-care rule: Whenever you find a new lump, consult your physician. The doctor may order a biopsy of the lump or use a needle to draw fluid out of a fluid-filled cyst.

About 90 percent of breast lumps are found not by doctors or nurses or mammograms, but by women during their own breast self-exam, says Kerry McGinn, R.N.

The best time to do this is one week after your menstrual period begins. That's because lumps that sometimes surface just prior to menstruation can disappear just as quickly when your period is over.

---

assistant clinical professor of obstetrics/ gynecology at the University of Vermont College of Medicine. And that means less hormonal stimulation of the breasts.

Stay slim. That means you should keep your weight within the proper range for your height. For seriously overweight women, losing weight can help relieve breast pain and lumpiness, says Kerry McGinn, R.N., author of *Keeping Abreast: Breast Changes That Are Not Cancer.*

In women, fat acts like an extra gland, producing and storing estrogen. If you've got too much body fat, you may have more estrogen circulating in your system than is good for you. And breast tissue, says Gregory Radio, M.D., chairman of reproductive endocrinology at Allentown Hospital in Pennsylvania is "very responsive to hormones."

Get your vitamins. Be sure to get plenty of foods rich in vitamin C, calcium, magnesium, and B vitamins, says Dr. Northrup. These vitamins help regulate the production of prostaglandin E, which in turn has a prohibitory effect on prolactin, a hormone that activates breast tissue.

Pass on the margarine and other hydrogenated fats.
Hydrogenated fats interfere with your body's ability to convert essential fatty acids from the diet into gamma linoleic acid (GLA), says Dr. Northrup.

Comfort from Castor Oil

To get relief from breast inflammation, try this castor oil compress recommended by Christiane Northrup, M.D. She says it helps heal minor breast infections, too.

You'll need cold-pressed castor oil, a wool flannel cloth, a piece of plastic, and a heating pad.

Fold the cloth into four layers and saturate it with the oil, but make sure it's not so wet that it will drip on the breast. Put the cloth on the breast, cover with plastic, and then apply the heating pad. Turn the setting on the pad up to moderate, and then hot, if you can stand it, says Dr. Northrup. Leave it on for an hour.

Cold-pressed castor oil contains a substance that increases T11 lymphocyte function, says Dr. Northrup. This will help speed healing of any infection.

You may need to use the compress for three to seven days to really see results. "This can often be extremely beneficial for taking away pain," she says.

GLA is important because it contributes to the production of prostaglandin E. And prostaglandin E may help keep prolactin, a breast tissue activator, in line.

Keep calm. Epinephrine, a substance produced by the adrenal glands during stress, also interferes with GLA conversion, says Dr. Northrup.

Cut out all caffeine. Caffeine's role in contributing to breast discomfort has not been proven. Some studies say it does, other studies have been inconclusive. Still, Thomas J. Smith, director of the Breast Health Center at New England Medical Center in Boston, recommends this strongly.

"I've seen women with pain and other symptoms of benign breast changes get markedly better after abstaining. You really have to cut out all caffeine," he says. And that means forgoing soft drinks, chocolate, ice cream products, tea, and over-the-counter pain relievers that contain caffeine.

Skip the pepperoni pizza. Highly salted foods make you bloated, says Yvonne Thornton, M.D., assistant professor of obstetrics and gynecology at Cornell University Medical College. This is particularly important to do about seven to ten days before your menstrual period.

Stay away from diuretics. It's true that diuretics can help flush fluid from your system. And that can help reduce the swelling in your breasts. But the immediate relief will cost you, says Dr. Thornton. Overuse of diuretics can lead to depletion of potassium, imbalance your electrolyte system, and throw off glucose production.

Reach for an OTC. Sandra Swain, M.D., director of the Comprehensive Breast Service at the Vincent Lombardi Cancer Center at Georgetown University School of Medicine, recommends ibuprofen (Advil, Nuprin) to alleviate painful breasts. "Avoid topical, steroidal anti-inflammatories," she cautions. Pregnant women, of course, shouldn't use any drug without a doctor's okay.

Apply cold. McGinn says some women find relief by dipping their hands in cold water and cupping the breasts.

Or try heat. Other women, says McGinn, find relief after using a heating pad or hot water bottle or by taking a hot bath or shower. For others, alternating heat and cold works best.

Find a good support bra. A sturdy bra, like those made for joggers, can help prevent nerve fibers in the breast, already stretched by waterlogged tissue, from stretching farther. Some women find that wearing the bra to bed at night helps, says Dr. Radio.

Consider reconsidering the pill. The estrogen level in your oral contraceptive could help or hurt your attempt to manage benign breast changes, depending upon what your particular condition is, says Dr. Radio. In general, a low-estrogen pill may help a true fibrocystic condition but aggravate fibroadenoma, a condition in which a solid but often movable lump is present.

Try massage to ease fluid accumulation. McGinn says that some women find relief with a gentle breast self-massage that helps ease extra breast fluids back into the lymph passageways. A technique developed by masseuse Carolyn Gale Anderson involves soaping the breasts, rotating the fingers along the surface in coin-size circles, and then using your hands to press the breasts in and then up.

Discover the emotional message behind your physical symptoms. "This is absolutely the first thing I look at," says Dr. Northrup. "When I ask my patients 'what's going on in your life around the issue of nurturing or being nurtured?' I often see tears.

"Breasts as the symbol of nurturance are highly charged for women," she adds. "You know that tingling feeling that accompanies the letdown of milk? Some women who have gone through menopause still feel that when they hear a baby cry. That's how closely linked breasts are to the emotions."

PANEL OF ADVISERS

Kerry McGinn, R.N., is a staff nurse at Planetree Model Hospital Unit at Pacific Presbyterian Medical Center in San Francisco and the author of *Keeping Abreast: Breast Changes That Are Not Cancer.*

Christiane Northrup, M.D., is an assistant clinical professor of obstetrics/gynecology at the University of Vermont College of Medicine in Burlington, and president of the American Holistic Medical Association. She practices medicine at Women to Women in Yarmouth, Maine.

Gregory Radio, M.D., is a practicing obstetrician/gynecologist in Allentown, Pennsylvania, and chairman of reproductive endocrinology at Allentown Hospital.

Thomas J. Smith, M.D., is chief of surgical oncology and director of the Breast Health Center at New England Medical Center in Boston, Massachusetts. He is also associate professor of surgery at Tufts University School of Medicine in Boston.

Sandra Swain, M.D., is assistant professor of medicine at Georgetown University and director of the Comprehensive Breast Service of the Vincent Lombardi Cancer Center at Georgetown University School of Medicine in Washington, D.C.

Yvonne Thornton, M.D., is a maternal fetal medicine specialist and assistant professor of obstetrics and gynecology at Cornell University Medical College in New York City. She is also director of prenatal diagnosis and an attending physician at the New York Hospital–Cornell University Medical Center.

Breastfeeding

15 Problem-Free Nursing Ideas

Wanda raised three infants on formula before she became pregnant with Julian. But when she learned about all the great things breastfeeding does for babies, she decided to give it a try.

She's glad she did.

"If I had known it was this easy, I would have done it with all of them," she says.

Choose a Good Nursing Bra

The best way to pick out a nursing bra is to go a cup size larger and a bra size bigger than your pregnancy bra, says Julie Stock of La Leche League International.

"I wouldn't overbuy bras in the beginning," she says. "It's best to wait and see. By the third or fourth day, you may be able to wear your pregnancy bras."

Here are other tips for selecting a good bra.

- Choose all cotton over nylon.
- Make sure that the opening for nursing is wide enough so it doesn't compress the breast. That could lead to clogged ducts.
- Make sure you can easily open and close the bra with one hand. That will aid discretion.
- Avoid Velcro closings on the flaps because they make too much noise.
- Make sure the straps are comfortable and the bra isn't tight across the chest.

Breastfeeding *is* easy once you know how, says Julie Stock, medical information liaison for La Leche League International, a support group for women who breastfeed. You'll be feeding more often, but when you account for the time you spend buying and preparing formula, the two probably even out, she says.

How can you make your breastfeeding trouble-free? Here's what our experts advise.

Position baby right. Our experts were unanimous that this is the key to problem-free feeding. How do you do it?

Kittie Frantz, R.N., director of the Breast-Feeding Infant Clinic at the University of Southern California Medical Center in Los Angeles, explains it this way: "The baby should face you entirely: head, chest, genitals, knees. Grip the baby so the buttocks are in one hand and the head is in the bend of your elbow. Let your other hand slip under your breast, with all four fingers supporting your breast. But don't put your fingers on the areola [the darker area around the nipple].

"Now tickle the baby's lower lip with your nipple to get the mouth open wide. When the mouth opens wide, pull the baby's body in quickly so that the mouth fixes on the areola."

The nipple should be deep in the baby's throat, adds Carolyn Rawlins, M.D., an Indiana obstetrician and a member of the La Leche League International board of directors. "This way there is no movement of the nipple when the baby sucks."

Respect your body. "It's usually unnecessary for a nursing mother to have pain," says Stock. "Form a mindset that you will not accept pain. If there's discomfort, you'll take care of it right away."

If the baby is sucking incorrectly, use your finger to break the suction and reposition him.

Interrupt baby until he gets it right. If the baby is confused by switching from the breast to a pacifier or a bottle, he may not latch onto the nipple far enough. Be sure the baby's mouth is open wide before putting him to the breast; he should latch onto the nipple so that at least an inch of the areola is in his mouth.

Leave the baby on a breast as long as he is sucking effectively, which means he is swallowing every suck or two. If you see him drifting, burp him, wake him up, and switch sides. Let him nurse on the second side as long as he wants. In general, feeding time varies from 20 to 30 minutes, Stock says.

Nurse from both breasts during each feeding. Nurse on one side until it appears that the baby is losing interest, says Stock. Then offer your baby the other side. Next time you feed, start with the side you ended with the time before.

Nurse often. "For women, there's often shock at how often a baby wants to nurse. Most doctors give instructions more appropriate to bottle feeding," says Stock. You'll probably find yourself nursing 8 to 12 times a day in the early weeks.

Human milk was designed so that a baby needs to nurse frequently, says Dr. Rawlins. That creates better bonding between mother and child.

Don't toughen the nipples. Exercises or manipulation to toughen the nipples won't help and could even do some damage, says Dr. Rawlins. "If you get the baby placed correctly, you won't have any soreness at all."

Use a breast shell for inverted nipples. It's best to start using these during the sixth or seventh month of pregnancy. Gentle suction from the device will help pull the nipple out. But don't use it for more than 15 to 20 minutes a day, says Dr. Rawlins.

Don't soap your nipples. "Use absolutely no soap on the nipples, because it dries them out," cautions Dr. Rawlins. "Do you see the little bumps around the areola? Those are glands which produce oil with an antiseptic in it. So you don't need to use soap."

MEDICAL ALERT

Dealing with Mastitis

If your breast feels inflamed, you're running a fever, or you have flulike symptoms, call your doctor. You could have mastitis, a type of breast infection.

Mastitis is usually treated with antibiotics. If that's what your doctor prescribes, be sure to finish all the medication even if symptoms disappear. This helps prevent recurrent infections.

Meanwhile, you can help speed healing on your own by "going to bed, drinking lots of clear fluids, and nursing more frequently," says Carolyn Rawlins, M.D.

"The milk isn't infected," she adds. "Besides, you're giving the baby valuable antibodies with the milk."

If you stop nursing while you have mastitis, it could lead to a breast abscess.

Let your nipples air-dry. Be sure to air-dry the nipples before you cover them, says Stock. And don't use any breast pads that retain moisture, such as those with plastic in them.

Use your milk to help heal sore nipples. "Truly 95 percent of the problem with nipple soreness comes from the way the baby sucks," says Stock. Pain stops after you correct the problem, though the damage may take a little more time to heal. To speed healing, air-dry the nipples when you finish a feeding, express a little bit of milk, and rub it in. Milk left at the end of the feeding is very high in lubricants and contains an antibiotic substance, says Stock.

Stay alert to plugged ducts. Milk ducts can clog as a result of binding clothes, the mother's anatomy, fatigue, or prolonged periods without nursing. A plugged duct can also signal the start of an infection if not dealt with promptly.

"If you feel a hard, painful-to-touch spot anywhere on the breast, get rid of it by using warmth," says Stock. Massage the breast, starting at the chest wall and working your way down with a circular motion.

Most important, however, allow your baby to nurse on that side frequently, she says. "Baby's sucking will help clear out that duct faster than anything else. Usually within 24 hours, it will be cleared up. The plug may be clear before you have physical evidence it's gone."

Use vitamin E for cracked nipples. If you notice a crack in the nipple, topical application of a small amount of vitamin E can help. When you finish nursing, says Stock, take a capsule of vitamin E, pierce it, squeeze out a drop, and rub it into the nipple. The secret, she says, is to use minimal amounts.

Try hot compresses to help with overproduction. If the baby is not keeping up with what mother is producing and you are getting overly full, put some hot, wet compresses on the breast, says Frantz. It will open the ducts so the milk flows more freely. Nurse the baby more often and longer, and take in enough fluids so that you urinate every hour.

Control leakage with a hand correctly applied. The milk production system is so sensitive to stimuli that a woman can begin to leak milk when she's out shopping and she hears a baby cry, says Stock. If that happens, take the heel of your hand and press the nipple into the chest. If you leak a lot, she says, find some good reusable breast pads you can launder yourself, preferably 100 percent cotton. "Men's cotton hankerchiefs work well," she says.

PANEL OF ADVISERS

Kittie Frantz, R.N., is director of the Breast-Feeding Infant Clinic at the University of Southern California Medical Center in Los Angeles and a pediatric nurse-practitioner. She has been working with nursing mothers since 1963. She also spent 15 years as a leader for La Leche League International.

Carolyn Rawlins, M.D., is an obstetrician in private practice in Munster, Indiana, and a member of the La Leche League International board of directors.

Julie Stock is medical information liaison for La Leche League International, a support group for breastfeeding mothers. Group headquarters is at P.O. Box 1209, Franklin Park, IL 60131–8209.

Bronchitis

9 Tips to Stop the Cough

It starts with a tickle. An invisible hand brushes a feather against the back of your throat. Then the rumblings start from deep within your chest cavity. Suddenly the volcano in your lungs erupts and you spend the next few minutes hacking up a mouthful of phlegm, the lava of your lungs.

You have bronchitis. Or more appropriately, bronchitis has you. Bronchitis usually has the upper hand because there isn't a whole lot you can do to get rid of it.

In many ways, bronchitis is a lot like a cold. It's usually caused by a virus, says pulmonologist Barbara Phillips, M.D., associate professor at the University of Kentucky College of Medicine. "So antibiotics won't do much good. Sometimes, though, bronchitis is caused by bacteria, and in that case antibiotics will work." Acute bronchitis "most times will go away by itself in a week or two," she says. But chronic sufferers can cough and wheeze for months. Although you have to let it take its course, there are things you can do to breathe easier while you have it.

Stop smoking. It's the most important thing you can do, especially if you're a chronic sufferer. Quit smoking and your chances of ridding yourself of bronchitis go up dramatically. "Ninety to 95 percent of chronic bronchitis is due directly to smoking," says pulmonologist Daniel Simmons, M.D., a professor at the University of California, Los Angeles, UCLA School of Medicine.

"Your bronchitis will improve when you stop smoking," says Gordon L. Snider, M.D., a pulmonologist and professor at Boston University School of Medicine and Tufts University School of Medicine. If you've smoked for a long time, some of the damage to your lungs may be irreversible, but "the fewer years you've been smoking, the more likely it is that you will have a complete recovery," he says.

MEDICAL ALERT

When to Call the Doctor

Bronchitis requires a doctor's attention when:

- Your cough is getting worse, not better, after a week.
- You have a fever or are coughing up blood.
- You are older and get a hacking cough on top of another illness.
- You are short of breath and have a very profuse cough.

Get active about passive smoking. Avoid those who smoke, and if your spouse smokes, get him or her to stop. Other people's smoking could be causing *your* bronchitis.

"You need to avoid all tobacco smoke," says Dr. Phillips. "Even if you don't smoke, but you're exposed to exhaled smoke, you are doing what's called passive smoking, and that can give you bronchitis."

Keep the fluids flowing. "Drinking fluids helps the mucus become more watery and easier to cough up," says Dr. Phillips. "Four to six glasses of fluid a day will do a good job of breaking it up."

Warm liquids or just plain water is best. "Avoid caffeine or alcoholic beverages," says Dr. Phillips. "They are diuretics; they make you urinate more, and you actually lose more fluids than you gain."

Breathe in warm, moist air. Warm, moist air will also help vaporize the mucus. "If you have mucus that is thick or difficult to cough up, a vaporizer will help to loosen the secretions. You could also stand in your bathroom, close the door, and then run your shower, breathing in the warm mist that steams up your bathroom."

Don't throw in the towel. Drape it over the sink. "Steam inhalation from the bathroom sink is very helpful," says Dr. Snider. "Fill the sink with hot water, put a towel over your head and the sink, creating a tent, and then inhale the steam for 5 to 10 minutes every couple of hours."

Don't expect too much from expectorants. "There is no scientific evidence that there is any medicine that works to dry up

---

Smokers: Clear the Air

Smokers plagued with chronic bronchitis may be cowed into drinking milk by the results of a scientific study done by Melvyn Tockman, M.D., a pulmonologist and associate professor at Johns Hopkins University School of Medicine.

"We found that individuals who smoked cigarettes and drank milk had a substantially lower frequency of chronic bronchitis than did people who smoked but did not drink milk." Dr. Tockman said he discovered the link when comparing health histories and lifestyles of 2,539 smokers.

The smokers who drank milk consumed on the average about one glass of it a day. So Dr. Tockman says "If you must smoke, drink your milk."

Why milk may help suppress bronchitis in smokers is still questionable, he says, but he noted that the same effect was not found in milk-drinking nonsmokers. He doesn't, however, recommend milk as the antidote for smokers who are bronchitis sufferers. "Stopping smoking is still the best way to rid yourself of chronic bronchitis," he says.

---

mucus," says Dr. Phillips. "Drinking fluids of any type is the best way to cough up secretions."

Listen to your cough. Is it a productive or nonproductive cough? "If you have a productive cough, one where you cough up sputum, you don't really want to suppress it completely because you won't be coughing up the stuff your lungs want to rid themselves of," says Dr. Simmons. His advice: Endure as best you can.

Turn down your volume. On the other hand, "If your cough is nonproductive—that is, you're not coughing anything up—then it's good to take a cough medicine designed to suppress a cough. Look for those containing the active ingredient dextromethorphan," suggests Dr. Simmons.

PANEL OF ADVISERS

Barbara Phillips, M.D., is a pulmonologist and associate professor of pulmonary medicine at the University of Kentucky College of Medicine in Lexington.

Daniel Simmons, M.D., is a pulmonologist and professor of medicine in the Division of Pulmonary Disease, at the University of California, Los Angeles, UCLA School of Medicine.

Gordon L. Snider, M.D., is a pulmonologist and chief of medicinal service at the Boston Veterans Administration Medical Center in Massachusetts. He is also a professor of medicine at Boston University School of Medicine and Tufts University School of Medicine in Boston.

Melvyn Tockman, M.D., is a pulmonologist who is associate director of occupational therapy in the Department of Environmental Health Sciences and associate professor of medicine at Johns Hopkins University School of Medicine in Baltimore, Maryland.

Bruises

6 Coverup Ideas

Unless you wrap yourself in cotton wool, you'll never be bruiseproof. But you can lessen the likelihood of large bruises and shrink and heal the bruises you occasionally incur. Here's how.

Put the chill on bruises. Use an ice pack to treat any injury that might lead to a bruise, advises emergency room physician Hugh Macaulay, M.D., of Aspen Valley Hospital in Aspen, Colorado. The ice pack must be applied as quickly as possible following the injury and treatment continued for 24 hours if you suspect that the bump will blossom into a severe bruise.

Apply the ice pack at 15-minute intervals. Don't apply heat between ice packs, but allow your skin to warm naturally.

Cooling constricts the blood vessels, and that means less blood spills into the tissues to cause that big black splotch. A cold pack also minimizes the swelling and numbs the area, so it won't hurt as much as a bruise left unchilled.

Follow ice with heat. After 24 hours, use heat to dilate the blood vessels and improve circulation in the area, says dermatologist Sheldon V. Pollack, M.D., associate professor of medicine at Duke University School of Medicine.

MEDICAL ALERT

A Bruise by Another Name

If you find you're bruising easily and can't figure out the cause, you should talk to your doctor about it. Sometimes bruises are a sign of an illness. Some disorders of the blood can cause unexplained bruises. Acquired immune deficiency syndrome (AIDS) can cause purplish bumps that seem to be bruises that won't go away.

Prop your foot up. Bruises are little reservoirs of blood. Blood, like any liquid, runs downhill. If you do a lot of standing, blood that has collected in a bruise will seep down through your soft tissues and find other places to puddle.

Add some vitamin C to your daily diet. Studies at Duke University Medical Center in Durham, North Carolina, show that people who lack vitamin C in their diets tend to bruise more easily. And their wounds heal more slowly.

Vitamin C helps build protective collagen tissue around blood vessels in the skin, says Dr. Pollack. Your face, hands, or feet contain less collagen than, say, your thighs, so bruises in those areas are often darker, says Dr. Macaulay.

If you bruise easily, Dr. Pollack suggests 500 milligrams of vitamin C three times a day to help build your collagen. Although vitamin C is not considered toxic, taking high doses should still get sanction from your doctor.

Watch those medications. People who take aspirin to protect against heart disease will find that a bump turns into a bruise very easily. Some people taking blood thinners will find they bruise easily, too. Other drugs such as anti-inflammatory drugs, antidepressants, or asthma medicines can inhibit clotting under the skin and cause larger bruises. Alcoholics or drug abusers tend to bruise easily, too. If you are taking medicine that might cause easy bruising, talk to your doctor about the problem.

You Don't Have to Bump to Bruise

Weekend warriors may notice bruises the Monday or Tuesday after a flag football game or a low-impact aerobics class. Exercise sometimes causes microtears in the blood vessels below the skin. When the tears occur, blood seeps out into the tissues and—surprise—a bruise.

If you notice bruises a day or two after exercising, use heat to begin the healing process.

PANEL OF ADVISERS

Hugh Macaulay, M.D., is an emergency room physician at Aspen Valley Hospital in Aspen, Colorado.

Sheldon V. Pollack, M.D., is an associate professor of medicine in the Division of Dermatology at Duke University School of Medicine in Durham, North Carolina.

Bruxism

10 Ways to Stop Grinding Your Teeth

Like vampires, they chomp. But sufferers of bruxism don't go for necks. Instead, they sink their upper teeth into their lower teeth, gritting and grinding—again and again and again.

They don't do it by choice. Rather, those who grit and grind usually do so because they're stressed. (Some say that clenching in reaction to stress or anger is a primal instinct.)

Though bruxism may result from stress, a mess of things can result from bruxism. Untreated, it can lead to worn-down teeth, headaches, sore necks and backs, and the whole pack of symptoms that comprise a

Dr. Goljan's 7 × 7 Solution

In Tulsa, Oklahoma, tooth-grinding patients of Kenneth R. Goljan, D.D.S., are told to go home and practice his 7 × 7.

Chomping teeth together is often a programmed response to stress, says Dr. Goljan. That is, we grit and grind when we're uptight because it's an ingrained habit. How do we break the habit?

First, identify the problem. ("Clenching and grinding my teeth is bad for me.")

Second, state why the problem is bad. ("This causes me pain and makes me sad.")

Third, state what your course of action will be. ("I will not clench and grind my teeth anymore.")

Finally, describe how this new action will be beneficial. ("This will make the pain go away and I will be happier.")

It is important, says Dr. Goljan, that you use your own words to describe your habit and your feelings about it. Copy your phrases on paper. Carry that paper with you until you memorize the phrases and repeat them seven times, seven times a day. It's that simple.

Will it stop you from grinding? "I virtually guarantee some degree of success, and in many cases, major success," says Dr. Goljan.

condition known as temporomandibular joint syndrome (TMJ). In some cases, nocturnal gnashing can even ruin a marriage.

But before you call a divorce lawyer or start sleeping with a sock in your mouth, try the home remedies provided here.

During the day, keep your mouth in the "healthy resting position." Your teeth should touch only when you're chewing food or swallowing, says Andrew S. Kaplan, D.M.D., an assistant clinical professor of dentistry at Mount Sinai School of Medicine of the City University of New York. If you practice keeping your teeth apart, it will reduce the urge to clench or grind. Set little reminders in key places around your home and office so that you won't forget. He suggests repeating the phrase "lips together, teeth apart" as a reminder.

Crunch an apple. If you grind at night, tucker out the jaw by munching on an apple, some raw cauliflower, or raw carrots before retiring. It may help calm your overactive mouth, says Harold T. Perry, D.D.S., Ph.D., professor of orthodontics at Northwestern University Dental School. This course is particularly helpful for children, for whom nocturnal clenching is common.

Apply heat to your jaws. Fold up a washcloth, run hot water over it, wring it out, and apply it against the sides of your face, suggests Kenneth R. Goljan, D.D.S., a dentist in Tulsa, Oklahoma, who has a particular interest in bruxism. Apply the heat as often and as long as you can. It will relax the clenching muscles frequently associated with head pain, he says.

For nighttime grinding, try a mouth guard. Sporting goods stores sell mouth guards that you put in hot water and then pop into your mouth and bite down on for a better fit. Sheldon Gross, D.D.S., a lecturer at Tufts University and the University of Medicine and Dentistry of New Jersey/New Jersey Medical School, says these inexpensive aids may be used temporarily to guard against nighttime chomping. If it works, tell your dentist. He can then make you a better one.

Above all else, calm down. All four of our experts agree that bruxism is most often related to stress, so the best thing you can do to stop clenching is *relax*. To do so, you should:

- Cut down on caffeine and refined carbohydrates such as candy and pastries. This will help improve your general nutrition.
- Take some warm baths.
- Ease up on yourself.
- Learn some good general relaxation techniques, such as progressive relaxation and meditation.

PANEL OF ADVISERS

Kenneth R. Goljan, D.D.S., practices general dentistry in Tulsa, Oklahoma. His practice is largely devoted to treating TMJ disorders and bruxism. He has held appointments at the University of Louisville School of Dentistry in Kentucky and the University of Medicine and Dentistry of New Jersey/New Jersey Medical School in Newark.

Sheldon Gross, D.D.S., is in private practice in Bloomfield, Connecticut. He is a lecturer at Tufts University in Boston, Massachusetts, and the University of Medicine and Dentistry of New Jersey/New Jersey Medical School in Newark. He is also president of the American Academy of Craniomandibular Disorders and a member of both the American Pain Association and the American Headache Association.

Andrew S. Kaplan, D.M.D., is an assistant clinical professor of dentistry at the Mount Sinai School of Medicine of the City University of New York and author of *The TMJ Book.* He is director of the TMJ Clinic at Mount Sinai Hospital in New York City.

Harold T. Perry, D.D.S., Ph.D., practices dentistry in Elgin, Illinois. He is a professor of orthodontics at Northwestern University Dental School in Chicago, Illinois. He is also the editor of the *Journal of Craniomandibular Disorders—Oralfacial Pain* and a past president of the American Academy of Craniomandibular Disorders.

Burns

10 Treatments for Minor Accidents

Fire! Fire!

What do you do? Put the fire out!

That's good advice for burns, too. When you catch your hand on the broiling element inside the oven, splash battery acid on your chest, take a face full of steam when you open a microwave dish, or splash a bathroom cleanser into your eyes, *put the fire out—fast!* Here's how.

Douse that flame. "The first and most important thing is to stop the burning process," says William P. Burdick, M.D., associate professor of emergency medicine at the Medical College of Pennsylvania. Flush your burns with lots and lots of cold water—15 to 30 minutes worth or until the burning stops. But *don't* use ice or ice water—they can make your burn worse.

"If it's a contact burn, run the injured part under cold water," says Dr. Burdick. "If it's hot grease or splattered hot material like battery acid or soup, remove the clothing that's saturated first, wash the grease off your skin, then soak the burn in cold water." If the clothing sticks to the burn, rinse over the clothing, then go to the doctor. Do not attempt to pull the clothing off yourself.

Once you've put the fire out, you're halfway to healing. The coolness stops the burning from spreading through your tissue and works as a temporary painkiller.

MEDICAL ALERT

Know When Your Burn
Is Too Hot to Handle

You can treat most first- and second-degree burns yourself, say doctors. But third-degree burns need medical attention. Here's how to gauge how badly you are burned.

- First-degree burns, like most sunburns and scalds, are red and painful.
- Second-degree burns, including severe sunburns or burns caused by brief contact with oven coils, blister, ooze, and are painful.
- Third-degree burns are charred and white or creamy colored. They can be caused by chemicals, electricity, or prolonged contact with hot surfaces. Usually they are not painful because nerve endings have been destroyed, but they always require a doctor's care.

Other burns that demand a doctor's immediate attention include:

- Burns on the face, hands, feet, pelvic and pubic areas, or in the eyes.
- Any burn that you aren't sure is first- or second-degree.
- Burns that show signs of infection, including a blister filled with greenish or brownish fluid, or a burn that becomes hot again or turns red.
- Any burn that doesn't heal in ten days to two weeks.

If you plan to see a doctor about a burn, says emergency medical technician John Gillies, wash it, but don't use any ointments, antiseptics, or sprays. You may, however, wrap it in a dry, sterile dressing.

Leave the butter for your bread. You wouldn't try to smother a fire with a giant slab of butter, would you? The same goes for a burn. Food on burns can hold the heat in your tissue and make the burn worse. It also might cause an infection. Don't use any of those other old-time folk remedies either; no vinegar, potato scrapings, or honey.

Inspect and measure your burn. You can usually self-treat first- and second-degree burns smaller than a quarter on a child or smaller than a silver dollar on an adult. See a doctor for larger burns or for burns on infants under 1 year old or people over 60.

Cover the burn. Gently wrap the burn in a clean, dry cloth such as a thick gauze pad.

Then do nothing. At least for the first 24 hours, leave the burn alone. Burns should be allowed to begin the healing process on their own.

Help it heal. Starting 24 hours after you burn yourself, wash your injury gently with soap and water or a mild Betadine solution once a day, suggests emergency medical technician John Gillies, program director for health services at the Colorado Outward Bound School in Denver. Keep it covered, dry, and clean between washings.

Soothe with aloe. Two or three days after you burn, break off a fresh piece of aloe and use the plant's natural healing moisture, or squeeze on an over-the-counter aloe cream. Both have an analgesic action that will make your wound feel better. Do not use aloe if you are using blood thinners or have a medical history of heart problems.

Make soothing solutions. When your burn is starting to heal, break open a capsule of vitamin E and rub the liquid onto your irritated skin. It will feel good and may prevent scarring. Or reach for an over-the-counter remedy such as sunburn-cooler Solarcaine.

Dab on an antimicrobial cream. An over-the-counter antibiotic ointment containing the active ingredients polymyxin B sulfate or bacitracin will discourage infection and speed your healing. (For a list comparing the effectiveness of various over-the-counter ointments, see page 173.)

Leave blisters intact. Those bubbles of skin are nature's own best bandage, says Gillies. So leave them alone. If a blister pops, clean the area with soap and water, then smooth on a little antibiotic ointment and cover.

PANEL OF ADVISERS

William P. Burdick, M.D., is an associate professor of emergency medicine at the Medical College of Pennsylvania in Philadelphia.

John Gillies, E.M.T., is an emergency medical technician and program director for health services at the Colorado Outward Bound School in Denver.

Bursitis

8 Ways to Wipe Out the Pain

There are 8 of them around each shoulder, 11 around each knee, and as many as 78 on each side of the body. Most of them aren't even named, and as long as they do their job, there's no reason to ever notice a single one.

But let one stop working and you'll know just how important those little sacs of fluid called bursae really are. And you'll know just how painful the condition called bursitis really is.

Bursae ensure the smooth, frictionless working of the body's many joints. They are so hard working, inconspicuous, and uncomplaining, one doctor wrote, "that even when one of them misbehaves, this is usually misattributed to some more important structure."

And there's no telling when it will happen. Bursitis strikes, it retreats, it strikes again. The on-again, off-again nature of acute bursitis is aggravating for sufferers and frustrating for those trying to determine what type of treatments actually work.

Compared with joint diseases like arthritis, bursitis is an ugly stepsister waiting for a date. Perhaps medical science will take greater notice of this wallflower affliction someday. Until then, here are some tried-and-true remedies that may bring temporary relief from this painful condition.

Rest is best. "The first thing you do with any joint pain is rest that thing," says Alan Bensman, M.D., a physiatrist at the Minnesota Center for Health and Rehabilitation in Minneapolis. "Stop the activity that's causing the pain and rest the joint. Forget that old sports adage about working through the pain."

Immobilize and ice. "I will generally use ice if the joint is hot to the touch," says Allan Tomson, D.C., of the Total Health Center for Natural Healing in Falls Church, Virginia. "Alternate 10 minutes of ice, 10 of rest, 10 of ice, and so on. As long as it is hot, do not apply heat to it."

Attract relief with opposites. If the pain or swelling is not terribly acute and the heat is gone, Dr. Tomson sometimes recommends cold-and-hot combination treatments — 10 minutes of ice, followed by 10 minutes of heat, followed by 10 minutes of ice, and so on.

Count on some OTCs. "I would recommend using an appropriate anti-inflammatory medication, as long as you're not allergic to it," Dr. Bensman suggests. "The one I like best is aspirin. Timed-release aspirin lets you build up a level in the blood without needing to take it so often. Enteric-coated aspirin (Ecotrin and Ascriptin are two examples) is absorbed through the intestines and is good for those with ulcers. But aspirin is still one of the best things going."

Calm the pain with castor oil. The acutely painful stage of bursitis will usually recede in four or five days, but it can last longer. When the pain is no longer acute, therapy must be changed. At this point, heat replaces cold and exercise replaces immobilization.

Dr. Tomson recommends a castor oil pack, which is as simple to make as it is effective. Spread castor oil over the afflicted joint. Put cotton or wool flannel over that, then apply a heating pad. That's all.

Become a swinger. If elbow or shoulder pain is the problem, doctors recommend swinging the arm freely to relieve the ache. Exercise for only a couple of minutes at first, but do it often during the day.

"You want to maintain range of motion," says Edward Resnick, M.D., director of the Pain Control Center at Temple University Hospital in Philadelphia, Pennsylvania. "You don't want to get a stiff shoulder, but you don't want to overstretch it, either."

He recommends bending forward and supporting yourself with your good arm and hand on a chair. Allow the painful arm to drop downward, then swing this arm back and forth, side to side, and finally in circles both clockwise and counterclockwise.

Try a little cat tip. The importance of exercise following a bursitis attack cannot be overemphasized. Our experts all recommend stretching techniques to return full, normal movement to the joint.

An effective primary stretching motion for stiff shoulder joints is called the cat stretch. Get down on your hands and knees. Put your hands slightly forward of your head, then keep your elbows stiff as you stretch backward and come down on your heels.

"I tell people to walk their fingers up a wall in the corner," Dr. Resnick says. "The object is to try and get your armpit in the corner. That way you know you're getting effective exercise."

Take time for ten. Some say the best cure for bursitis is one capsule of time taken daily for ten days. Sometimes less time is needed, sometimes more, but time is always the active ingredient.

If all else fails, say doctors, time will heal the wound.

PANEL OF ADVISERS

Alan Bensman, M.D., is a physiatrist at the Minnesota Center for Health and Rehabilitation in Minneapolis.

Edward Resnick, M.D., is an orthopedic surgeon at Temple University Hospital in Philadelphia, Pennsylvania, and is director of the hospital's Pain Control Center.

Allan Tomson, D.C., is a chiropractor with the Total Health Center for Natural Healing in Falls Church, Virginia.

Canker Sores

13 Cures to a Pesky Problem

Floyd Bob has a bad mouth. He eats his pizza so hot the mozzarella melts his soft palate. He loves to suck on lemon drops that etch the lining of his cheeks. When he has to think real hard (that's often, because to Floyd Bob, every day is a brand-new day), he chomps down on the inside of his lip like it was a good chaw. These habits give Floyd Bob canker sores that hurt like the time he made porcupine stew but forgot to pull out the quills. When Floyd Bob has canker sores, he's cranky, hungry, sleepy, and, as Suzy Jane will tell ya, most dee-cidedly unromantic.

Yep, this little mouth ulcer, this canker sore, can keep you from doing many of the things that make life worth living. This little ulcer is also a big mystery. No one knows why some people get canker sores and others don't. A hot pizza burn that heals in 2 or 3 days with little pain in most people, says Harold R. Stanley, D.D.S., professor emeritus at the University of Florida College of Dentistry, can set off in others "a sequence of events that leads to a lesion that won't heal for 10 to 15 days." Along

---

MEDICAL ALERT

Stubborn Sores Should Be Checked Out

A canker sore should heal within two weeks. "If the sores last a long time, or you are unable to eat, speak, or sleep properly, you should see a doctor or dentist," advises Robert Goepp, D.D.S., Ph.D. All can severely affect your health and daily life.

You will probably be given prescription topical steroids and/or oral antibiotics to treat the disease itself, not just the infection.

---

with bad habits, heredity, food, overenthusiastic toothbrushing, and emotional stress are also highly associated with canker sores. You have to be a detective to find the cause.

Whatever the cause, trying to medicate a canker sore is a difficult task, says Robert Goepp, D.D.S., Ph.D., professor at the University of Chicago Medical Center and hospital. Nothing sticks well to the skin in your mouth, and it's the most bacteria-laden place in the body. Remedies have a double-barreled aim: to kill the organisms that infect the sore (causing most of the pain and the red inflammation that surrounds the yellowish core) and to protect the sore.

There is at least one benefit to old age besides social security and senior citizen discounts. The older you get, the fewer canker sores you get. But meanwhile a cannonade of cankers can make your mouth miserable. So here are a few escape routes. Experiment until you find one that works for you.

Commit carbamide peroxide cankercide. Carbamide peroxide is the generic form of an over-the-counter medication that combines glycerin and peroxide. "The peroxide releases oxygen and cleans up the bacteria," Dr. Goepp says. "The bubbles get into the tiniest crevices. The glycerine puts on a coating and helps protect the sore." Brand names include Gly-oxide, Amosan, and Cankaid.

Punish 'em with potassium chlorate. Varro E. Tyler, Ph.D., a professor of pharmacognosy at Purdue University, suggests putting a teaspoon of potassium chlorate in a cup of water and rinsing the mouth with it several times a day. Do not swallow. "It's an old Midwest remedy," he says, "and it's feebly antiseptic."

Bring out the artillery. Look for OTC canker sore medications that contain benzocaine, menthol, camphor, eucalyptol, and/or alcohol in a liquid or gel. They often sting at first, and most need repeated application because they don't stick.

Stick to your gums. There are also pastes that form a protective "bandage" over the sore. To get pastes like Orabase to work, dry the sore with one end of a cotton swab, then immediately apply the paste with the other end. It will work only on beginning sores, however.

Trick 'em with a wet tea bag. Several experts, among them Ohio dermatologist Jerome Z. Litt, M.D., recommend applying a wet, black tea bag to the ulcer. Black tea contains tannin, an astringent that "may pleasantly surprise you" with its pain-relieving ability, he says. Tanac is an OTC medication that contains tannin.

Wash your mouth out. Dilute 1 tablespoon of hydrogen peroxide in a glass of water and swish it around in your mouth to disinfect the sore and speed healing, says Dr. Goepp. New Jersey registered dietitian Beverly D'Asaro has found her clients with cancer who get canker sores are helped by the mouthwash Folamint. It contains no stinging alcohol, but does contain healing aloe vera, folate, zinc, and vitamin C.

Attack with alum. Alum is the active ingredient in a styptic pencil, which your mother may have told you to dab on a sore that is just getting going. Alum is an antiseptic and pain reliever that can prevent the infection from getting worse, say doctors, but not truly abort a canker sore.

Get creative with Mylanta. Don't swallow your Mylanta or milk of magnesia. Instead, swish it around your mouth and allow it to protectively coat the sore. It may also have some antibacterial effect, Dr. Goepp says.

Give goldenseal a seal of approval. Make a strong tea of goldenseal root (available at health food stores) and use it as a mouthwash. Or you can make a paste of it and apply it directly. "It's antiseptic and astringent and is probably modestly effective," Dr. Tyler says.

Avoid irritation. Coffee, spices, citrus fruit, nuts high in the amino acid arginine (especially walnuts), chocolate, and strawberries irritate canker sores and cause them in some people. "If you get canker sores, you probably know darn well what you should stay away from," Dr. Goepp says. You probably already know, too, to brush your teeth carefully.

Try yogurt each day. Dr. Litt says that eating 4 tablespoons of unflavored yogurt a day might help prevent canker sores by sending in helpful bacteria to fight off those dirty mouth bacteria. Look for yogurt that contains active cultures of *Lactobacillus acidophilus.*

Be all ears. "You're going to laugh when I tell you the typical Hoosier home remedy," says Dr. Tyler. Just take a little earwax from your ear and apply it to the canker sore. It's said to be a sure cure. It may have some antiseptic value, and it may protect the sore."

Be victorious with vitamins. Virginia dentist Craig Zunka, D.D.S., president of the Holistic Dental Association, recommends you squeeze vitamin E oil from a capsule onto your canker sore. Repeat several times a day to keep the tissue well-oiled. "And at the first tingle of a canker sore," he says, take 500 milligrams of vitamin C with bioflavonoids three times a day for the next three days.

PANEL OF ADVISERS

Beverly D'Asaro, R.D., is a registered dietitian in private practice in Madison, New Jersey.

Robert Goepp, D.D.S., Ph.D., is a professor of oral pathology at the University of Chicago Medical Center and hospital in Illinois.

Jerome Z. Litt, M.D., is a dermatologist in private practice in Beachwood, Ohio, and is author of *Your Skin: From Acne to Zits.*

Harold R. Stanley, D.D.S., is a professor emeritus of dentistry at the University of Florida College of Dentistry in Gainesville.

Varro E. Tyler, Ph.D., is a professor of pharmacognosy at Purdue University in West Lafayette, Indiana, and author of *The Honest Herbal.* He also serves as a *Prevention* magazine adviser.

Craig Zunka, D.D.S., is in private practice in Front Royal, Virginia, and is president of the Holistic Dental Association.

Carpal Tunnel Syndrome

15 Coping Techniques

Three paragraphs into the letter to your grandson and the aching tingle in your writing hand makes you put down the pen.

You spent weeks finding the right paint for the kitchen, but after a few short strokes the bothersome pain in your wrist and hand makes you leave the brush in the bucket. At night you wake up with numbness in your hand and wrist for no apparent reason.

If incidents like these are happening to you, chances are you have carpal tunnel syndrome.

Carpal tunnel syndrome isn't something that happens overnight. It's a cumulative trauma disorder that develops over time due to repeated stressful movements of the hands and wrist.

Think of New York City's Holland Tunnel for a moment. Imagine what a pain it is to try to get through it during rush hour; multiple lanes of traffic aiming to get into single file. Well, your wrist, known as the carpal tunnel, is a lot like the tunnel under the Hudson River during rush hour. You don't have trucks and cabs going through your wrist, of course, but you do have a nerve and tendons, and when you use your hand in repeated stressful motions — like writing, typing, or hammering — the tendons swell and compress the median nerve that runs to your hand. The result is a big pain.

In the Holland Tunnel, when traffic swells, horns blare. In your wrist, when the tendons swell, pain flares.

Women are twice as likely as men to suffer from carpal tunnel syndrome, with the average age of onset being between 40 and 60. According to Colin Hall, M.D., professor of neurology and medicine at the University of North Carolina at Chapel Hill School of Medicine, "Symptoms normally affect one hand but can be present in both. Sometimes the affected hand will feel numb or tingle, or feel like it's 'fallen asleep.' The sensation normally is felt in the thumb and forefinger area, but it's possible to feel it throughout the whole hand."

When that feeling comes, it's time to look for relief. Here's how.

Go round in circles. "When the tingling begins," says physical therapist Susan Isernhagen of Duluth, Minnesota, "it's time to begin doing some gentle hand exercises."

One of these is a simple circle exercise that rotates the wrist. Move your hands around in gentle circles for about 2 minutes. "This exercises all the muscles of the wrist, restores circulation, and gets your wrist out of the bent position that normally brings on the symptoms of carpal tunnel syndrome," says Isernhagen.

The B₆ Benefit

Recent scientific studies are showing that physician-supervised therapy with vitamin B6 can help relieve the symptoms of carpal tunnel syndrome. In a 12-year study conducted in Louisville, Kentucky, Morton Kasdan, M.D., found that 68 percent of his 494 carpal tunnel syndrome patients improved while taking vitamin B6 daily.

John Ellis, M.D., a surgeon and family practitioner in Mount Pleasant, Texas, has been using vitamin B6 for many years to treat carpal tunnel syndrome at the Institute for Biomedical Research and in collaboration with the University of Texas at Austin. Dr. Ellis believes that "carpal tunnel syndrome is caused by a deficiency, pure and simple. In a high percentage of cases, the patients are deficient in vitamin B6."

Dr. Ellis says that over the past 26 years, he's successfully treated hundreds of patients with large doses of B6 daily and "they've had no side effects," he says.

Vitamin B6 treatment doesn't bring about immediate relief, he warns. "You have to be patient." He says it often takes about 6 weeks until the enzyme changes are sufficient enough that the symptoms gradually begin to subside. "From 6 weeks to 12 weeks you will really notice a decided difference in your hands and fingers," he says. "The numbness, tingling, stiffness, and pain in your hand subsides."

Dr. Ellis also says that "a number of people have a recurrence of carpal tunnel syndrome when they stop taking the vitamin."

Vitamin therapy for carpal tunnel syndrome, however, should be used only under the supervision of a physician. Vitamin B6 can be toxic at high levels. The U.S. Recommended Daily Allowance is 2 milligrams.

Raise your hand. Get those hands off the keyboard and up into the air. "Raise your arm above your head and rotate your arm, while rotating your wrist at the same time," says Isernhagen. This gets your shoulder, neck, and upper back in a better position and relieves the stress and tension."

Go on R & R. Take a break from what you're doing. "Rest your hands on a desk or a table and then rotate your head for about 2 minutes. Bend your neck backward and forward," recommends Isernhagen, "then tip your head to either side. Also do some neck turns, looking over your right shoulder, then your left."

Make exercise as routine as eating. It's important to exercise and relax all the muscles that are giving you problems every day, even when you're not in pain, says Isernhagen. Motion exercises, such as the ones described above, should be practiced at least four times a day.

The Straight Facts on Staying Pain-Free

The National Institute for Occupational Safety and Health estimates that carpal tunnel syndrome affects 23,000 workers a year. Some workers are affected more than others, especially meat cutters, cashiers, data processors, assembly line workers, truck drivers, and pneumatic-hammer operators—the kind of people who absolutely must use their hands on the job.

Those who work at home are at risk, too. Carpal tunnel syndrome has been known to attack homemakers who spend lots of time wringing wet laundry by hand, sweeping with a broom, dicing with a knife, or even shelling peas. Even weekend do-it-yourselfers can do themselves in. Excessive use of a staple gun over a weekend is enough to trigger the disease. But it doesn't have to.

If you're faced with a hands-on type of job, it's possible to avoid the problem —and still manage to pat yourself on the back after a job well done.

Carpal tunnel results when pressure is constantly applied to the median nerve when the wrist is flexed up or down, explains John Sebright, M.D., head of the Hand Surgery Section and director of the Microsurgery Laboratory at St. Mary's Hospital in Grand Rapids, Michigan. "If the wrist is repeatedly flexed and extended, the pressure is increased. To avoid this," he says, "keep your hands and wrists as straight as possible." It may seem unnatural at first not to bend your wrists when you're typing or driving, for example. But time and practice will get rid of that awkward feeling.

MEDICAL ALERT

It Could Be Arthritis

Wrist and hand pain is not always the result of carpal tunnel syndrome and could actually be the sign of a more serious illness, cautions physical therapist Susan Isernhagen. In fact, Isernhagen says, "if you get a crackly or crunchy feeling in your wrist when you exercise it, that's not a sign of carpal tunnel syndrome; it may be a symptom of osteoarthritis." You should have it checked out by your doctor.

Reach for the aspirin. "To reduce pain and inflammation, take a nonsteroidal anti-inflammatory medication like aspirin or ibuprofen," says Stephen Cash, M.D., an orthopedic surgeon and assistant clinical professor at Jefferson Medical College of Thomas Jefferson University. Don't take acetaminophen, though. Acetaminophen is for headaches, not carpal tunnel syndrome. According to Dr. Cash, "Acetaminophen reduces pain, but it doesn't do anything for inflammation."

Put the pain on ice. "Cold packs will work to bring the swelling down," says Isernhagen. Don't wrap your wrist in a heating pad. That will increase the swelling in the area.

Rise to the occasion. "Avoid having your hand lower than your shoulder when you take a break from work," says Isernhagen. "Sit with your elbows supported on your desk or propped on the arms of your chair. Keep your hands pointed upward. That's a good relief position."

Put the squeeze on your pain. "Gentle squeezing motions of the fingers will help relieve the tingling feeling," Isernhagen says. Press your fingers into your palm, then stretch them way back and hold. Repeat.

Stay topside at night. Keep your arms close to your body and your wrists straight while sleeping. "If you let your hand drop over the side of the bed, it can increase the pressure," says Isernhagen.

If you find yourself waking up because of the pain in your hands, Isernhagen recommends doing the same exercises at night that you do during the day. Tingling or pain might also be an indication that a night splint might help.

Go for splint second relief. To relieve symptoms of carpal tunnel syndrome, use a wrist splint to keep your wrist straight. "The splints help take pressure off the nerve," says Dr. Cash. Buying a wrist splint, though, is not as easy as buying a glove. He recommends a splint that has a metal insert and Velcro fasteners. They give support without being totally rigid. "The kind made out of plastic usually are hard and are also hot and sticky," notes Isernhagen. "Whatever kind of splint you get, it should fit into the palm of your hand, leaving the thumb and fingers free," she says.

You might want to consider having the splint tailor-made. "You should really have a professional like a physical therapist or occupational therapist fit you to make sure it fits your hand exactly," notes Isernhagen.

Don't get too tight. You don't want to completely tie up traffic in your wrist. "Don't wrap your wrist with an Ace bandage, because you could wrap it too tight and cut off the circulation," says Isernhagen.

Use the right grip. If you have to carry anything with a handle, be sure the grip fits your hand. If the grip is too small, build it up with tape or rubberized tubing. If it's too large, get another handle, says Isernhagen.

Handle with care. If you find yourself hurting after using the old drill around the house, change the way you hold it. "Don't concentrate pressure at the base of the wrist when using hand tools. Use your elbow and shoulder as much as possible," recommends Isernhagen.

PANEL OF ADVISERS

Stephen Cash, M.D., is assistant clinical professor of orthopedic surgery in the Division of Hand Surgery at Jefferson Medical College of Thomas Jefferson University in Philadelphia, Pennsylvania, and a staff member of the Hand Rehabilitation Center there.

John Ellis, M.D., is a surgeon and family practitioner in Mount Pleasant, Texas, and is on the staff of Titus County Memorial Hospital in Mount Pleasant.

Colin Hall, M.D., is professor of neurology and medicine and director of the Neuromuscular Unit in the Department of Neurology at the University of North Carolina at Chapel Hill School of Medicine.

Susan Isernhagen is a physical therapist and president of Isernhagen and Associates in Duluth, Minnesota. She acts as a consultant to industries to help reduce work injuries and rehabilitate injured workers.

John Sebright, M.D., is head of the Hand Surgery Section and director of the Microsurgery Laboratory at St. Mary's Hospital in Grand Rapids, Michigan, and an associate clinical professor in the Department of Surgery, Department of Human Medicine, at Michigan State University in East Lansing.

Cellulite

18 Ways to Fight It

To paraphrase a raven-haired monarch of fairy tale fame, "Mirror, mirror, in my hand, whose skin is fairest in the land?"

"Yours and yours alone, my queen," the loyal mirror responded.

And all was well. Until one fateful evening around bedtime when the mirror felt compelled to comment on a telltale patch of—ugh!—cellulite on the royal thighs. As you may recall, things went pretty much downhill from there. No wonder the queen was in such an evil mood when Snow White and those seven silly dwarfs came whistling down the lane!

The queen's mirror wouldn't lie, and neither will yours if you're carrying around those less-than-pleasing puckers along your thighs, on your derriere, or on the insides of your upper arms. Cellulite is actually no more than pockets of fat, says Paul Lazar, M.D., professor of clinical dermatology at Northwestern University Medical School. Its appearance is due to strands of fibrous tissue anchored to the skin, pulling the skin inward and, in the process, plumping the fat cells outward. Some people may be more susceptible to cellulite than others, Dr. Lazar says—especially women, who generally are more fatty and less muscular in the buttocks, hips, and thighs than men.

Some nonmedical skin specialists see cellulite as more than just fat. "Cellulite is a combination of fat globules, waste matter, and water imprisoned in connective tissue," says Carole Walderman, aesthetician and president of Von Lee International School of Aesthetics, in Baltimore.

Medical doctors and researchers may not agree with this theory. Neither are they likely to agree that much can be done to get rid of cellulite once it sets in. Cellulite is something you can try to avoid, says Dr. Lazar, through exercise and by keeping your weight normal. But those face-to-face with cellulite are willing to give *something* a try. We weeded through the claims, tossed out the bizarre, and came up with the following middle-of-the-road remedies. They're yours for the trying.

Peel off the pounds. Since cellulite is fat, excess weight can contribute to it, says Dr. Lazar. Lose weight gradually, he says, and "hopefully, some of what you lose will be cellulite."

Eat plenty of fresh fruit and vegetables—low in calories yet packed with nutrients—and drink fruit and vegetable juices, suggests Dolores Schneider, a nutritionist and director of Sharon Springs, a spa in upstate New York, where people go to lose pounds and detoxify their bodies.

Get back in balance by eating well. Eat a healthy, balanced diet overall, urges Kim Ulen, supervisor of the skin care department of the Cal-a-Vie Spa in Vista, California. "This returns your body chemistry to a balanced state in which cellulite is less likely to develop," she says.

Get back in balance by resting well. Relax in your bathtub, Schneider suggests, with a home mineral bath containing sea salt. Add about 2 cups of sea salt to warm bathwater and luxuriate in the soothing waters for at least 20 minutes. It will leave your skin feeling smooth.

Combat constipation. "People who are constipated on a regular basis usually have cellulite," says Ulen. Your meals move more quickly through your digestive tract when you eat plenty of high-fiber foods like green vegetables and grains every day, she says. For an extra boost, she suggests sprinkling raw bran on your foods or in your beverages at each meal. Plus:

- Practice the eating habits your mother (hopefully) taught you, like chewing your food thoroughly and forgoing late-night snacks, Ulen says.
- Drink beverages at room temperature rather than ice-cold. "Ice constricts your esophagus and stomach, hindering the flow of digestive enzymes into your stomach," she says.

Make your skin an exit ramp. Keeping your body's natural highways and byways clear gives cellulite an easier escape route, skin specialists say. They say the following techniques will open up the blood vessels in and just below your skin, and also keep your waste-removal system working properly.

- Drink lots of water. "I have found that a lot of people who have cellulite don't drink enough water," says Walderman. Drink at least six to eight glasses of bottled water—distilled or mineral— per day, she says.
- Steer clear of salt, which contributes to water retention and adds to cellulite problems, says Ulen.

The Alternate Route

Lotions and Potions

Beauty consultants believe that certain herbal formulas have restorative powers that can help smooth skin affected by cellulite. You'll have to decide for yourself how effective they really are—if at all.

Add sage, cypress, or juniper oils to your bathwater, suggests Cal-a-Vie Spa's Kim Ulen. These fragrant plant oils, frequently used for a type of massage called aromatherapy, are absorbed directly through your skin and combat cellulite from the inside out, she says. Aromatherapy oils are available in many health food stores.

- Kick the coffee and cigarette habits, says Walderman. These substances constrict your blood vessels and may actually make your cellulite more prominent.
- Dry-brush your skin. It helps improve your circulation, says Walderman. Press a soft-bristled brush gently onto your skin and rotate it in circular movements from head to toe or on cellulite areas alone, she says.

Take up muscle-toning exercises. Building stronger muscles with methods such as Nautilus or working out with weights may help fill out the tissue in cellulite problem areas, says Dr. Lazar.

Massage those trouble spots. Reinforce the benefits of exercise, says Ulen, with gentle, kneading massage you can do yourself in areas like your thighs and the insides of your knees.

Take a deep breath. Learn to breathe from deep down in your diaphragm, says Schneider. The oxygen helps burn fat. A deep breath also helps clean out toxic carbon dioxide from all your cells, says Ulen.

Stay calm. Cellulite builds up when muscles get tense, and muscles get tense when you're feeling stressed, says Walderman. You need to relax. If you're among those who find it hard to relax, the following might be of help.

- Try yoga for an ideal antistress, anticellulite remedy, she says. This discipline teaches you to breathe deeply, gives your muscles a good stretch, and relaxes you all over.

- Wipe worrisome thoughts from your mind by spending a few minutes on a slant board, Walderman suggests. Lie with your head at the low end of the board for up to 20 minutes each day. For the same benefits without a slant board, lie on the floor with your feet propped up on the wall, suggests Ulen.

PANEL OF ADVISERS

Paul Lazar, M.D., is a professor of clinical dermatology at Northwestern University Medical School in Chicago, Illinois. He is a former board member of the American Academy of Dermatology.

Dolores Schneider is a nutritionist and director of Sharon Springs, a holistic health spa in upstate New York that emphasizes weight loss and detoxification.

Kim Ulen is supervisor of the skin care department of the Cal-a-Vie Spa in Vista, California.

Carole Walderman is an aesthetician and president of Von Lee International School of Aesthetics, Inc., in Baltimore, Maryland, a clinic and professional school that specializes in skin care.

Chafing

10 Ways to Rub It Out

For ten years, the varsity wrestling team at Ohio State University practiced while wearing gray shirts made of 100 percent cotton.

Then, in 1987, the team's training uniform was changed. Wrestlers were given a 50 percent polyester, 50 percent cotton practice shirt. The shirt was thick and durable. A good buy, it seemed. They'd last through season after season.

But the wrestlers complained. The shirts rubbed against their faces and necks, leaving their skin sore and chafed. And even though the shirts were washed daily, the fabric stayed harsh and abrasive. Abrasions increase the chances of infection and in time, 8 of the 42 team members reported a herpes simplex infection on their faces or necks.

In 1988, team members again wore all-cotton shirts. Wrestlers noted few rashes. Herpes infections dropped.

The moral? When something rubs you the wrong way—and leaves a rash—there are several things you can do, including:

Get on the natural fibers team. Doctors at Ohio State University College of Medicine pointed to the heavy-duty, synthetic-blend shirt as the culprit in the wrestlers' rash problem. When the team switched back to 100 percent cotton, the problem cleared up.

Wash before you wear. Be sure to wash any new exercise clothes before you wear them, says Richard H. Strauss, M.D., a sports medicine doctor at Ohio State University College of Medicine. Washing sometimes softens fabric enough to lessen abrasion.

Wrap it up. People who are overweight or who have big thighs, which makes chafing more likely, may find relief using elastic bandages around the portions of their legs that rub, says Tom Barringer, M.D., a family physician in Charlotte, North Carolina. The bandages will shield the skin when your thighs rub together and instead of skin against skin, the rubbing will be fabric against fabric. Be sure the elastic bandage is secure so it does not move across the skin.

Keep it tight. A pair of the electric-colored, stretchy-fabric athletic tights or Lycra cycling shorts may be ideal because they are snug, yet stretch, and cause no friction against the skin, says Dr. Barringer.

Put cotton first. When your exercise outfit is made of nylon or another possibly abrasive fabric, be sure to wear cotton undies to separate the fabric from your delicate skin, says Dr. Strauss. "Lots of male athletes will put on cotton underwear and put their supporters on top of that," he adds.

Throw them away. The coarser the cloth in your outfit, the more likely it will chafe, says Dr. Barringer. "I've run from none up to 50 miles a week at times, depending on my schedule. And I've found when something chafes, sometimes the best thing to do is just toss it out and try again."

Grease your body. Petroleum jelly between your thighs, around your toes, under your arms—anywhere you chafe—will act as a lubricant and glide the rubbing skin against itself, says Robert Boyce, Ph.D., an assistant professor of exercise physiology at the University of North Carolina at Charlotte.

Find powder power. An old standby for chafing—maybe your mother used this remedy when you were a child. Talcum powder will work as a lubricant, just the way petroleum jelly does. It helps the skin slip past other skin without catching and rubbing.

Here's how to make your application easy. If you don't like powdery bathroom floors, fold your talcum into the middle of a large, soft, white handkerchief. Bind the edges together. Then, use the sack of powder like a powder puff. It will leave powder on you—not on the floor.

Block it with a bandage. Simply block the rub with an adhesive bandage. Runners, for instance, will use a bandage over irritated nipples to prevent further rubbing.

Try another sport. Overweight exercisers may find chafing a regular problem until they lose a little excess girth, says Dr. Boyce. His advice: Switch sports while your skin heals. If you have sore spots from walking, try the stationary bicycle. If the bicycle causes problems, try swimming, a virtually chafe-free sport.

PANEL OF ADVISERS

Tom Barringer, M.D., is a family physician in Charlotte, North Carolina.

Robert Boyce, Ph.D., is an assistant professor of exercise physiology at the University of North Carolina at Charlotte.

Richard H. Strauss, M.D., is a sports medicine doctor at Ohio State University College of Medicine in Columbus.

Chapped Hands

24 Soothing Tips

Where'd those scrub brushes come from? Not the ones in your hands—the ones that *are* your hands. The ones that are so red, dry, cracked, and painful you wouldn't wish them on your worst enemy. The ones that show up in time for Halloween and don't leave till after Easter. Face it, the Creature from the Black Lagoon had more attractive paws.

How did you get into this mess? Sorry to say, you probably brought it on yourself. First, the low humidity of fall and winter dries and irritates skin. (No, that's not your fault.) Second, as you age, your body just naturally produces less of the oil that keeps skin smooth and supple. (That's not your fault, either.) But bad habits, simple neglect, and lack of good skin sense conspire to make your hands rough and ready to drive you crazy. (And that is your fault!)

So what can you do to soothe those hurting hands? Here's what the experts recommend.

Don't go near the water. "The basic plan for dealing with chapped hands is to avoid water at all costs," says dermatologist Joseph Bark, M.D., of Lexington, Kentucky. "Consider water to be just like acid on your hands, because it is the worst influence for chapped hands that we know of. Repeated washing removes the skin's natural oil layer, which allows moisture within the skin to evaporate. And that's extremely drying.

"You could do what the French do to keep from getting dry skin," laughs Dr. Bark. "They don't wash their hands very often; they just hang them out the window and shake the dirt off! But seriously, always think twice about washing your hands."

Go palm up. "When you must wash your hands often, try to do just the palms," recommends dermatologist Diana Bihova, M.D., a clinical instructor at New York University School of Medicine. "You can wash the palms much more often than the backs of the hands, which have thinner skin and dry out easily."

125

Use the lotion potion. "Instead of using soap, clean your hands with an oil-free skin cleanser such as Cetaphil or SFC Lotion," says Dr. Bark. "Rub it on the skin, work it into a lather, then wipe it off with a tissue. It's a wonderful way to wash skin without any irritation whatsoever."

Try the bath oil treatment. Taking the no-soap concept one step further, Rodney Basler, M.D., assistant professor at the University of Nebraska College of Medicine, recommends washing your hands with bath oil. "They may not *feel* really clean like they might with soap, but they won't get dried out, either."

Get topical. Use some type of topical emollient every time you wash your hands and at bedtime. "Its strength would depend on the severity of your chapping," says Dr. Basler. "Lotions are the least moisturizing, followed by creams and then ointments. Try a lotion first. If that's not enough to carry you through the winter, step up to a cream, then an ointment."

Prevention Is Your Best Solution

Chapped hands are always easier to prevent than to treat, says Diana Bihova, M.D. Here are some ways to do that:

Stay out of hot water. "A good rule of thumb is to avoid hot water, detergents, and strong household solvents," says Dr. Bihova.

Avoid soaping. "Because chapped hands occur when oil is taken from the skin, you should not use a terribly harsh or alkaline soap. You're better off with a mild soap, preferably with a little cold cream in it. I often recommend Dove because it's virtually the mildest soap there is," says Joseph Bark, M.D.

Put moisture in the air. "Skin moisturizes itself from the inside out," notes Rodney Basler, M.D. "If there's moisture in the air, not as much would be drawn out through the skin. Therefore, it's a good idea to use a home humidifier."

Pamper your hands. "When you apply moisturizer to your face in the morning, immediately apply some to the hands. At night do the same," advises Dr. Bihova. "That keeps them supple and helps resist chapping. I'd say twice a day is a must. In addition, do it after each washing."

Don't throw in the towel. "If your workplace bathroom has a hot-air blower instead of hand towels, bring in a towel from home," advises Dr. Bihova. "Hot-air blowers have been associated with chapped hands. If you must use one, keep your hands at least 6 inches from the nozzle and dry them thoroughly."

Go soak your hand. Although in general you should keep your hands out of water, sometimes a therapeutic soak is in order. "For an inexpensive way to achieve the same moisturizing effects produced by skin creams, simply soak your hands in warm water for a few minutes. Then pat off excess water and apply vegetable or mineral oil to the damp surface to seal in moisture," says Howard Donsky, M.D., associate professor of medicine at the University of Toronto.

In the same vein, Dr. Basler recommends soaking in a water and oil solution. "Use 4 capfuls of a bath oil that has a good dispersant (Alpha-Keri is the best) in 1 pint of water. At the end of the day, soak for 20 minutes to get oil back into the skin. That alone will help chapped hands."

Try "Cream C." "If you want the cheapest home remedy going, use Crisco," says Dr. Bark. "It's a wonderful moisturizer that covers the skin and keeps water locked in. The key is to use very little and rub it in well so your hands don't feel greasy. Your skin needs only two molecules' worth of barrier thickness to protect it from water loss. They used to call Crisco Cream C at Duke University, where doctors dispensed it freely. It really works."

"You don't have to purchase expensive creams to get good results," agrees Dr. Donsky. "Inexpensive substitutes for people with dry and normal skin include cocoa butter, lanolin, petroleum jelly, and light mineral oil."

Double up. "When applying any type of lotion or cream, use what I call Bark's double-layer application technique," continues Dr. Bark. "Put on a very thin layer and let it soak in for a few minutes. Then apply another thin layer. Two thin ones work much better than one heavy one."

Try lemon oil. "To smooth and soothe irritated hands, mix a few drops of glycerin with a few drops of lemon oil [both are available at pharmacies]. Massage this into your hands at bedtime," says New York City skin care specialist Lia Schorr.

Dress to kill. A lot of unsuspected things around the home can act as irritants for chapped hands. "I recommend wearing plain white cotton gloves for doing any kind of dry work," says Dr. Bihova. "That

Model Your Hands after Hers

When your fingers are your fortune, you take darned good care of them. Ask Trisha Webster. She's a top hand model with the Wilhelmina agency in New York City. Those are her hands you see in many high-fashion jewelry and cosmetic ads. If they're not picture perfect, Webster is out of a job. So how does she keep her hands looking young? The same way you can.

Stop problems before they start. "I try to keep my hands out of water at all costs," says Webster, "which is why I always let someone else do the dishes (well, it's *one* of the reasons!). When I can't avoid getting my hands wet, such as during bathing, I always moisturize them immediately afterward. It takes just a few minutes for the moisture that's accumulated in the skin to evaporate. When that happens, your hands are drier than they were before."

Get protection. "I never go outdoors in the winter without protecting my hands. That means putting on a good layer of moisturizer and then gloves."

Use sun sense. "A long time ago I stopped going out in the sun because it dries and ages hands just as surely as it does your face."

If you're not ready to give up the sun, Diana Bihova, M.D., suggests using a moisturizing sunscreen on your hands. "Sunscreens moisturize hands and keep them looking younger, so make their use an everyday habit," she says. "Just stay away from gels and alcohol-based sunscreens, because alcohol is drying. Also, products containing the active ingredient PABA can be irritating if you have sensitive skin."

includes reading the newspaper and even unloading groceries. Any time you have friction against skin that's already dry, cracked, or red, you aggravate it. The advantage of cotton gloves is that they allow the skin to breathe and at the same time absorb any moisture that accumulates so it won't irritate your skin."

"In addition," according to Nelson Lee Novick, M.D., clinical associate professor of dermatology at Mount Sinai School of Medicine of the City University of New York, "cotton gloves keep the skin clean so you don't have to wash your hands so often and risk perpetuating the problem."

"If you need to get an extra-good grip on something, use leather gloves," says New York hand model Trisha Webster.

Mix rubber and cotton. "For wet work, it's extremely important to use cotton gloves under vinyl ones," says Dr. Novick. "If the cotton gloves get wet, change them immediately. Otherwise replace them with a fresh pair every 20 minutes. Perspiration, lotions, and medications on your hands accumulate inside the gloves and may become irritating rather quickly. I don't recommend rubber gloves with built-in cotton linings because it's very difficult to launder them. But you can launder separate cotton gloves in a mild detergent like Ivory Snow or Ivory Flakes."

Dr. Bihova agrees. "The biggest mistake women make when they have hand problems is wearing just rubber gloves. That only makes the hands worse. The rubber traps moisture, keeps the skin from breathing, and creates too much friction."

"Sometimes you can avoid gloves altogether," says dermatologist Thomas Goodman, Jr., M.D., assistant professor at the University of Tennessee Center for Health Sciences. "When you're doing dishes, for instance, a long-handled dish brush keeps your hands entirely out of water."

Go elegantly into the night. Dr. Goodman recommends occasionally wearing cotton gloves to bed for an extra-soothing treatment. "Moisten the fabric with about a teaspoon of petroleum jelly so the gloves won't absorb the cream from your hands. Then apply hand cream at bedtime and slip on the gloves. Leave them on overnight. Your hands remain bandaged, in a sense, and can heal."

"The important thing," adds Dr. Bark, "is not to automatically run to the sink in the morning and wash off the cream. Also I don't recommend sleeping in plastic gloves. They make your hands sweat too much overnight, so that by morning you have the most incredible case of dishpan hands you've ever seen."

Call on hydrocortisone. Over-the-counter hydrocortisone creams and ointments are of value in treating chapped hands. Use Cortaid or any other 0.5 percent cream several times a day, says Dr. Goodman. Then put a heavier, greasier product on top of that. These hydrocortisone creams don't substitute for good hand care, but they are a boost. Every time you wash your hands, reapply them.

Get a salon treatment. "Believe it or not, even shampoo can make your tender hands feel worse," says Stephen Schleicher, M.D., co-director of The Dermatology Center in eastern Pennsylvania and clinical instructor at the Philadelphia College of Osteopathic Medicine. "Either let someone else shampoo your hair or wear plastic gloves."

MEDICAL ALERT

Hands That Need a Doctor's Touch

"If you have splits and cracks on your hands, you've got hand eczema, and it's a sign you should see a dermatologist," advises Joseph Bark, M.D. "Also, if what you consider to be chapped hands starts as little blisters along the sides of the fingers, it's probably hand eczema and needs potent medication."

There are other signs that may indicate that what you have is more than a case of chapped hands. If, after two weeks of self-treatment, your hands don't clear up, you should see a dermatologist, says Dr. Bark. You may have a fungal infection or even psoriasis of the hands.

Diana Bihova, M.D., cautions that people (such as doctors, nurses, chefs, and housewives) whose occupations require them to immerse their hands for prolonged periods of time can easily contract monilial paronychia, an annoying fungal infection involving the skin around the cuticle. "Bartenders and waitresses who handle beer, which is yeasty, are particularly susceptible. When the infection strikes the finger's protective nail fold, it becomes red, swollen, and painful."

Put your hands in oatmeal. To remove the top layer of dead skin cells from chapped hands, Schorr recommends a weekly sloughing treatment. "Process 1 cup of uncooked, old-fashioned (not instant) rolled oats in a blender until you have a very fine powder. Place it in a large bowl, then rub your hands in the powder, gently removing dry skin. Rinse with cool water, pat dry, and lavish on hand cream. Wait 2 minutes and apply more cream."

Hire a cook. "The juices of raw meat and vegetables—like potatoes, onions, tomatoes, even carrots—are sometimes very toxic to skin, especially if it's already irritated. So you can either hire a cook to do all your kitchen work," quips Dr. Goodman, "or wear tissue-thin plastic gloves when handling food."

"You particularly don't want to squeeze acidic fruits like oranges, lemons, or grapefruit with your bare hands," adds Dr. Schleicher. "They're terribly irritating and will dry your hands further."

Chapped Lips

12 Tips to Stop the Dryness

Chapped lips give new meaning to the expression "crack a smile." When your lips are sore, red, and peeling, even a little grin can crack them wide open. No wonder you feel—and look—like Oscar the Grouch. So put those lips back in the pink with these tips. They'll help bring a smile to your face.

Try the palm or balm solution. "The best way to deal with chapped lips is to avoid the dry, cold weather that can cause them in the first place," says dermatologist Joseph Bark, M.D., of Lexington, Kentucky. "But since heading for the tropics is not too practical for most people, you can head for the drugstore instead."

Before you go out—and several times while you're out—coat your lips with a lip balm. Since lips don't hold anything on them very well, reapply it every time you eat or drink anything or wipe your lips.

Use a sunscreen. "Remember, too, that the sun fries lips— any time of the year," says Dr. Bark. "So you're well advised to choose a product with built-in sunscreen."

Nelson Lee Novick, M.D., clinical associate professor of dermatology at Mount Sinai School of Medicine of the City University of New York, concurs. "Sun damage to the lips can cause dryness and scaliness, the same way sun can damage the rest of your skin. In its simplest form it can harm the lower lip, which takes the brunt of ultraviolet rays."

So people should use not just any lip balm but one that contains sunscreen, such as PreSun 15, Chap Stick's Sunblock 15, or Eclipse Lip Protectant.

Wear lipstick. In addition to a sunscreen, "a creamy lipstick would help soothe lips that are already chapped," says Glenn Roberts, Elizabeth Arden's director of creative beauty in New York City. "In fact, just wearing lipstick gives some protection and may help prevent chapping in the first place."

"Because lipstick is opaque, it filters out all light, including harmful visible light," says Dr. Bark. "In addition, I believe use of lipstick is one of the reasons women seldom get lip cancer. In my 14 years of practice, I've treated maybe one or two women for lip cancer, but literally hundreds of men."

Soothe and heal. "The danger with chapped lips is that they can become infected," says dermatologist Diana Bihova, M.D., a clinical instructor at New York University School of Medicine. "To prevent infection, apply an over-the-counter antibiotic ointment such as Bacitracin or Polysporin Ointment. Over-the-counter hydrocortisone ointments can also help with chapped lips, but they would not prevent infection. If your lips are severely chapped, you may want to use both. Apply one in the morning and one at night."

B wise. "Nutritional deficiencies—such as those of B-complex vitamins and iron—can play a part in scaling of the lips. So make sure you're okay on that front with a multivitamin supplement," says Dr. Novick.

Drink up. Moisturize your lips from the inside out by drinking additional fluids in the winter. "I recommend several ounces of water every few hours," says Dr. Bihova. "As you age, the ability of your cells to retain moisture decreases, so your dryness problem may actually increase each winter. Another way to help counter wintertime dry lips is to humidify the air in your home and office."

Mind your own beeswax. "To my mind, the single best product for chapped lips is Carmex. It's an old-fashioned product that comes in a little tin and contains, among other things, beeswax and phenol," offers Rodney Basler, M.D., assistant professor at the University of Nebraska College of Medicine. "I'd say no prescription medication is better than that."

You won't get by on a lick and a promise. "Chapped lips are a dehydration problem," according to Dr. Basler. "When you lick them, you momentarily apply moisture, which then evaporates and leaves your lips feeling drier than before. Besides, saliva contains digestive enzymes. Granted they're not very strong, but they don't do your sore lips any good."

"Licking chapped lips can lead to something called lip-licker's dermatitis," cautions Dr. Bark. "It's usually seen in kids but can occur in adults, too." What happens when you lick your lips is that you scrape off any oil that might be on them from surrounding areas. (The lips themselves don't have any oil glands.) Pretty soon, you're licking not just the lips but the area around them. Eventually, you end up with a red ring of dermatitis around the mouth. The moral: Don't start licking in the first place.

If you *are* tempted to lick your lips, remember what Dr. Basler laughingly calls "the old Nebraska treatment, chicken manure applied to the lips. It doesn't make your lips better, but it sure keeps you from licking them."

Give toothpaste the brush-off. "Allergy and sensitivity to flavoring agents in toothpaste, candy, chewing gum, and mouthwash can cause chapped lips in some people," says dermatologist Thomas Goodman, Jr., M.D., assistant professor at the University of Tennessee

Center for Health Sciences. "My dentist says the new tartar-control toothpastes are even worse at drying lips than the regular ones. So I tell people to stop using toothpaste. Just use a toothbrush alone or a brush with baking soda on it."

Think zinc. "Some people have a tendency to drool in their sleep, which can dry out lips or aggravate ones that are already chapped," says Dr. Novick. "If that's a problem, they can apply zinc oxide ointment every night before bed. It acts as a barrier to protect lips."

Lay a finger alongside your nose. "Here's what I tell farmers, who may be working outside and may not have anything else handy," says Dr. Bark. "Put your finger on the side of your nose. Then rub your finger around your lips. It picks up a little of the oil that's naturally there. It's the kind of oil the lips are looking for anyway, and they usually get it from contact with adjacent skin. You couldn't get any more of a home remedy than that."

The udder alternative. Here's another idea from down on the farm. "There's a product called Bag Balm that farmers use on cows' udders when they're sore. You can use that on your lips, too," says Dr. Bihova. "It's a petroleum-based product and is available in farm supply stores, vet supply stores, and some pharmacies and health food stores." It can also be ordered directly from the Dairy Association Company, Inc., Lyndonville, VT 05851.

PANEL OF ADVISERS

Joseph Bark, M.D., is a dermatologist in private practice in Lexington, Kentucky, and author of *Retin-A and other Youth Miracles* and *Skin Secrets: A Complete Guide to Skin Care for the Entire Family.*

Rodney Basler, M.D., is a dermatologist and assistant professor of internal medicine at the University of Nebraska College of Medicine in Lincoln.

Diana Bihova, M.D., is a dermatologist in private practice and clinical instructor of dermatology at New York University Medical Center in New York City. She is coauthor of *Beauty from the Inside Out.*

Thomas Goodman, Jr., M.D., is a dermatologist in private practice and assistant professor of dermatology at the University of Tennessee Center for Health Sciences in Memphis. He's author of *Smart Face* and *The Skin Doctor's Skin Doctoring Book.*

Nelson Lee Novick, M.D., is clinical associate professor of dermatology at Mount Sinai School of Medicine of the City University of New York in New York City and author of *Super Skin* and *Saving Face.*

Glenn Roberts is director of creative beauty at Elizabeth Arden in New York City.

Cholesterol

27 Ways to Stay on the Low Side

It's not bad enough that your cheeks are chubby and your waist's a tad wide. Now your doctor says that even your blood is too fat! Well, that's not exactly what he said, but he might as well have. When your cholesterol levels are high, you've got too much of a mushy, yellow, fat-related substance circulating in your bloodstream. If the excess builds up on artery walls, it can clog your arteries and restrict blood flow, possibly leading to a heart attack, stroke, or angina pain. And you don't need a medical degree to know that's not good.

Funny thing is, cholesterol isn't all bad. Your body naturally produces it, and it performs some pretty vital jobs—helping to build new cells, produce hormones, and insulate nerves. Only when you've got too much do you have a problem.

Unfortunately, there's a lot of confusion surrounding this substance. And it's no wonder, with similar terms like dietary cholesterol, serum cholesterol, HDL cholesterol, and LDL cholesterol being bandied around, you may have trouble telling the good from the bad and the ugly. Here's how to keep them all straight.

Dietary cholesterol is what's contained in food (mostly of animal origin). One egg, for example, has 275 milligrams; an apple has none. The American Heart Association (AHA) recommends that you limit your daily intake to 300 milligrams.

Serum cholesterol is what's in your bloodstream and what your doctor measures with a cholesterol test. A reading under 200 is desirable.

HDL (high-density lipoprotein) cholesterol is a subdivision of serum cholesterol that is considered good for its artery-scouring ability. The higher your levels of HDL, the better.

LDL (low-density lipoprotein) cholesterol is HDL's artery-clogging evil twin. The lower your levels, the better.

Here's how the experts say you can lower your serum cholesterol levels.

135

Supplements That Counter Cholesterol

Can nutritional supplements lower cholesterol? Some researchers seem to think so. Here's a rundown on the supplements that have shown the most promise. But before you increase your supplemental intake of any nutrient, talk it over with your doctor.

Niacin. "Large doses of niacin (also known as nicotinic acid) may lower both total cholesterol and LDL cholesterol," says famed researcher Kenneth Cooper, M.D., of Dallas, Texas. "It's best to start off with low doses, say up to 100 milligrams a day. Then increase gradually over a period of several weeks to 1 or 2 grams three times a day, for a total of 3 to 6 grams daily."

But be aware that sudden drastic increases in niacin can produce severe overall flushing, intestinal disorders, and sometimes abnormal liver function, warns Dr. Cooper. Be sure to discuss this treatment with your doctor. Niacinamide, a form of niacin that doesn't cause flushing, has no significant effect on blood fats.

Vitamin C. Tufts University researcher Paul Jacques, found that vitamin C raised levels of protective HDL in the elderly people he studied. He estimates that 1 gram a day could increase HDL by 8 percent.

Other studies show that when extra vitamin C is added to a pectin-rich diet, cholesterol drops even lower than with pectin alone. Conveniently, many pectin-packed fruit and vegetables—such as citrus fruit, tomatoes, potatoes, strawberries, and spinach—are also rich in vitamin C.

Vitamin E. One study done by French and Israeli researchers showed that 500 international units of vitamin E a day for 90 days significantly increased HDL levels. "Our results support the use of vitamin E for people with high blood-fat levels," said the researchers.

Calcium. If you're taking calcium supplements for the sake of your bones, you may be doing your heart a favor, too. In one study, 1 gram of calcium daily for eight weeks lowered cholesterol 4.8 percent in people with mildly high levels. In another study, 2 grams a day of calcium carbonate reduced cholesterol by 25 percent in 12 months.

Watch your weight. The more overweight you are, the more cholesterol your body produces. A 20-year study in the Netherlands concluded that body weight is the single most important determinant of serum cholesterol. Every 2.2-pound rise in body weight elevated cholesterol levels 2 points. And the famous Framingham Heart Study also found a definite link between blood cholesterol and body weight.

So if your weight is up, this is one more reason to bring it down. But do so in a healthy way, says Paul Lachance, Ph.D., a professor of food and nutrition at Rutgers State University of New Jersey. "Strive for a diet that's composed of two-thirds fruit, vegetables, cereals, and whole grains. Only one-third of your calories should come from meat and dairy products, which are often high in fat and calories."

Cut the fat. "Three principal dietary factors have an impact on blood cholesterol levels," says John LaRosa, M.D., chairman of the nutrition committee of the AHA and director of the Lipid Research Center at Georgetown University School of Medicine. They are, in order of importance:

- Saturated fat, which elevates blood cholesterol
- Polyunsaturated fat, which lowers blood cholesterol
- Dietary cholesterol, which can contribute to elevated blood cholesterol to a lesser degree than saturated fat

"Of these, saturated fat has by far the greatest impact on cholesterol levels," he says.

Donald McNamara, Ph.D., a professor of nutrition and food science at the University of Arizona, agrees. "The effect of saturated fat is about three times worse than that of dietary cholesterol." So you'd be wise to cut back on such sources of saturated fat as meat, butter, cheese, and hydrogenated oil. Wherever possible, replace these items with fish, poultry, low-fat dairy products, and polyunsaturated oils, such as corn, safflower, and soybean.

Switch to olive oil. Olive oil—and certain other foods like nuts, avocados, canola oil, and peanut oil—are high in still another type of fat: monounsaturated. Previously thought to have no real effect on cholesterol levels, monounsaturates may actually lower cholesterol.

Studies by cholesterol researcher Scott M. Grundy, Ph.D., found that a diet high in monounsaturated fat lowered total cholesterol levels even more than a strict low-fat diet. What's more, his studies showed that monos selectively lowered the (bad) LDLs while leaving the (good) HDLs intact.

So strive for a low-fat diet, then "supplement" it with 2 or 3 table-spoons of olive oil (or an equivalent amount of other mono-rich food) each day. Just make sure you're *replacing* other fats with monos and not simply *adding* to them.

Go easy on eggs. But don't feel you have to cut them out of your diet entirely. Although eggs have a whopping 275 milligrams of cholesterol apiece, Dr. McNamara says that about two-thirds of the population can handle extra dietary cholesterol without experiencing a rise in their serum cholesterol levels. That's because their bodies adjust to a high intake by producing less of their own cholesterol or by excreting the excess. In one study he conducted, 50 patients ate three large eggs a day for six weeks. Less than a third of them had higher cholesterol levels during this time.

If you'd like to eat eggs but still play it safe, limit yourself to three whole eggs a week. Since only the yolks contain cholesterol, you can use egg whites freely, substituting two whites for every whole egg when baking, for example. And you can make omelets and scrambled eggs using one whole egg with two, three, or even four whites. Also, some stores now sell lower-cholesterol eggs, which may contain from 15 to 50 percent less cholesterol than usual.

Be full of beans. Nutritious and inexpensive, beans and other legumes contain a water-soluble fiber called pectin that surrounds cho-lesterol and chaperones it out of the body before it can cause trouble. Numerous studies by cholesterol researcher and professor of medicine and clinical nutrition James W. Anderson, M.D., of the University of Kentucky College of Medicine, have shown just how effective beans are in lowering cholesterol. In one experiment, men who ate 1½ cups of cooked beans a day lowered their cholesterol a whopping 20 percent in just three weeks.

Dr. Anderson says that most people would do well to add about 6 grams of soluble fiber to their diet each day. A cup of cooked beans fits the bill nicely. And you needn't worry that you'll get bored eating beans because navy beans, kidney beans, pinto beans, lima beans, soybeans, black-eyed peas, and lentils all have this cholesterol-lowering ability.

Eat more fruit. Fruit also gets the cholesterol-lowering punch from pectin. Gastroenterologist James Cerda, M.D., of the University of Florida Health Science Center, found that grapefruit pectin (found in the rind and flesh) lowered cholesterol an average 7.6 percent in eight weeks. Since a 1 percent reduction in cholesterol causes a 2 percent drop in the risk of heart disease, Dr. Cerda regards this effect as "quite significant."

To get the amount of pectin Dr. Cerda used, you'd have to eat about 2½ cups of grapefruit sections a day. But if that's a little hard to swallow, he says, "Eat lots of different fruits. If you had half a grapefruit for breakfast, an apple at lunch, and some orange sections for dinner, for example, you could probably lower your cholesterol nicely."

The Alternate Route

Potential Weapons against Cholesterol

The following substances may also help combat high cholesterol. Although they've not undergone extensive studies, initial research has been promising.

Tea. Or more precisely, the tannins found in it, may help control cholesterol. One study found that people who habitually drank tea on a high-cholesterol diet had blood cholesterol levels within the normal range.

Lemongrass oil. A common flavoring in oriental cooking, lemongrass oil lowered cholesterol by more than 10 percent in one study. It may work by interfering with an enzyme reaction and inhibiting the formation of cholesterol from simpler fats.

Spirulina. A protein-rich form of algae often sold in powdered or tablet form, Spirulina reduced both total cholesterol and LDL levels in Japanese volunteers with high cholesterol who took seven 200-milligram tablets after every meal.

Barley. Long considered a healthful high-fiber grain, barley may have the same cholesterol-lowering potential as oats. In animal studies, two chemical components of barley lowered cholesterol levels by 40 percent.

Rice bran. This fiber may prove as effective as its cousin, oat bran. Preliminary studies with hamsters showed that rice bran reduced cholesterol by more than 25 percent.

Activated charcoal. Finely ground, this substance, which is often taken to alleviate gas, may latch onto cholesterol molecules in the body and escort them safely out. In one study, patients had a 41 percent drop in LDL levels after taking ¼ ounce of activated charcoal three times a day for four weeks.

Feel your oats. Oat bran appears to lower serum cholesterol in a fashion similar to pectin-rich fruit. Numerous studies by Dr. Anderson and others show, in fact, that oat bran does as good a job as beans. To get Dr. Anderson's recommended 6 grams of soluble fiber a day, you could eat ½ cup of oat bran cooked as cereal or made into muffins. In one California study, medical students who ate two oat-bran muffins a day for four weeks had a 5.3 percent reduction in total serum cholesterol.

Although oat bran has more soluble fiber, oatmeal can also lower cholesterol. According to research at Northwestern University Medical School, when people in one study added ⅔ cup of rolled oats a day to a low-fat, low-cholesterol diet, their cholesterol fell more than on the healthy diet alone.

In response to all these studies, U.S. Department of Agriculture (USDA) scientists are breeding oat varieties that will have even higher levels of beta-glucan, the suspected cholesterol fighter.

Be a little corny. In studies conducted by nutritionist and dietitian Leslie Earll of Georgetown University Hospital, corn bran was as effective as oat bran and beans in lowering cholesterol. People with high cholesterol who had previously tried to control it with a low-cholesterol diet and weight reduction ate about 1 tablespoon of corn bran at each meal (mixed into soup or tomato juice). After 12 weeks, their cholesterol levels dropped a significant 20 percent. "This abundant low-calorie fiber is worthy of much more investigation," says the study.

Call on carrots for help. Carrots can lower cholesterol, also by way of their pectin content, says Peter D. Hoagland, Ph.D., of the USDA's Eastern Regional Research Center in Philadelphia, Pennsylvania. In fact, he says, "it may be possible for people with high cholesterol to lower it 10 to 20 percent just by eating two carrots a day." That could be enough to bring many people's levels into the safe range.

Incidentally, cabbage, broccoli, and onions also contain the ingredient thought responsible for carrots' success (calcium pectate) and may produce similar results, according to Dr. Hoagland.

Exercise! It's possible that exercise can decrease the buildup of cholesterol blockage inside arteries, says Rhode Island cardiologist Paul D. Thompson, M.D., an associate professor of medicine at Brown University. "One of the best ways to raise your levels of protective HDL," he maintains, "is through vigorous exercise, which also modestly lowers your levels of undesirable LDL.

"Exercise might also increase the body's ability to clear fat from the blood after meals," he says. "If the fat doesn't stay in the blood very long, it has less opportunity to build up on artery walls. We've found that runners are able to clear fat from their systems 70 percent faster than other people who don't exercise." So get *moving!*

Beef up your diet—sensibly. Here's a surprise. Red meat, a notorious source of saturated fat, *can* be part of a heart-healthy diet—if it's lean to begin with and then trimmed of all visible fat. British researchers put men with extremely high cholesterol on a low-fat, high-fiber diet containing 6½ ounces a day of very lean red meat. The fat content of this diet was 27 percent of total calories, which is well below the 40 percent currently consumed by most people in the United States. The men's cholesterol levels fell by a respectable 18.5 percent.

The researchers concluded, "Provided care is taken to reduce the fat content substantially, a moderate quantity of meat products may be included in a cholesterol-lowering diet."

Get a health kick from skim milk. From Aura Kilara, Ph.D., associate professor of food science at Pennsylvania State University, comes this suggestion: Drink lots of skim milk. In one experiment he conducted, volunteers added a quart of skim milk to their daily diets. At the end of 12 weeks, those with elevated cholesterol levels lowered them an average of 8 percent. Dr. Kilara believes a compound in the nonfat portion of the skim milk did the trick by inhibiting cholesterol production in the liver.

Take garlic. Researchers have long known that large quantities of raw garlic can reduce harmful blood fats. Unfortunately, raw garlic can also reduce your circle of friends. Worse yet, garlic that's been "deodorized" by heat treatment loses its cholesterol-lowering effects. But now there's an odor-modified liquid garlic extract from Japan called Kyolic that seems to lower blood fats.

When Benjamin Lau, M.D., of Loma Linda University in California, gave people with moderately high blood cholesterol 1 gram a day of the liquid garlic extract, their cholesterol levels fell an average of 44 points in six months.

Try this special seed. Fiber-rich psyllium seeds, the main ingredient of the bowel regulator Metamucil, may also lower cholesterol. In a study by Dr. Anderson, men with elevated cholesterol who took a teaspoon of Metamucil in water three times a day lowered their levels about 15 percent in eight weeks.

Dr. Anderson says Metamucil and other psyllium-seed products may be a good auxiliary treatment when diet alone doesn't bring blood cholesterol levels down.

Cut back on coffee. A study conducted by Texas researcher Barry R. Davis, M.D., has linked coffee consumption with increased cholesterol. When he studied over 9,000 people as part of a nationwide blood pressure program, he found that cholesterol levels were dramatically higher in people who drank two or more cups of coffee per day.

Although his study didn't pinpoint the ingredient in coffee that's responsible, a Finnish study showed that boiling (or perking) coffee may be part of the problem. Coffee prepared by the filter method did not increase cholesterol levels in the same way perked coffee did. In any case, caffeine—a logical suspect—does not seem to be culprit.

Don't smoke. Here's one more reason to quit smoking. In a study conducted by New Orleans researcher David S. Freedman, M.D., teenage boys who smoked as few as 20 cigarettes a week had substantial increases in blood cholesterol. In addition, a Swedish study showed that smokers tend to suffer from low levels of beneficial HDL cholesterol. When a group of habitual smokers kicked the habit, however, they all experienced rapid and pronounced increases in HDL concentrations.

So relax already. Simple relaxation can lower cholesterol, according to a study done by Margaret A. Carson, a clinical nurse specialist in New Hampshire. She found that heart disease patients on low-cholesterol diets who listened to relaxation tapes twice daily experienced significantly greater drops in cholesterol than another group that simply read for pleasure.

PANEL OF ADVISERS

James W. Anderson, M.D., is director of the endocrine section of the Veterans Administration Medical Center in Lexington, Kentucky. He is also professor of medicine and clinical nutrition at the University of Kentucky College of Medicine in Lexington. He is one of the foremost experts in cholesterol research.

James Cerda, M.D., is a gastroenterologist at the University of Florida Health Science Center in Gainesville.

Kenneth Cooper, M.D., a medical researcher, is president and founder of The Aerobics Center in Dallas, Texas, and author of *Controlling Cholesterol, Preventing Osteoporosis,* and other books.

Peter D. Hoagland, Ph.D., is a researcher with the U.S. Department of Agriculture's Eastern Regional Research Center in Philadelphia, Pennsylvania.

Aura Kilara, Ph.D., is an associate professor of food science at Pennsylvania State University in University Park.

Paul Lachance, Ph.D., is a professor of food and nutrition at Rutgers State University of New Jersey in New Brunswick.

John LaRosa, M.D., is director of the Lipid Research Center at George Washington University School of Medicine in Washington, D.C., and chairman of the American Heart Association's Nutrition Committee.

Donald J. McNamara, Ph.D., is a professor of nutrition and food science at the University of Arizona in Tucson.

Paul D. Thompson, M.D., is an associate professor of medicine at Brown University in Providence, Rhode Island, and a cardiologist at The Miriam Hospital there.

Colds

29 Remedies to Win the Battle

At one time or another, every one of us succumbs to the common cold. The bravest, the strongest, the sweetest, the smartest — our virtues matter not to these viruses as they set about reducing us to coughing, sneezing shadows of our former selves.

Worse yet, there's no cure. Antibiotics, champs at knocking out bacterial infections, are down for the count against cold viruses. So we sniffle on bravely, maybe take a cold pill or two, and hope the symptoms will disappear in the customary week or so.

But there's actually a lot more we can do to get through a cold more comfortably, say doctors who specialize in self-care medicine. Some remedies, they say, may even help us overcome a cold more quickly. Here are the best remedies the experts have to offer.

Take C and see. "Vitamin C works in the body as a scavenger, picking up all sorts of trash — including virus trash," says Keith W. Sehnert, M.D., a physician with Trinity Health Care in Minneapolis,

---

MEDICAL ALERT

It Could Be More Than a Cold

If your cold is accompanied by one or more of the following symptoms, see your doctor. Your problem may be a more serious disorder than the common cold.

- Fevers that remain above 101°F for more than three days, or any fever above 103°F. Children with high fevers should see a doctor within 24 hours.
- Any hot, extreme pain, such as earache, swollen tonsils, sinus pain, or aching lungs or chest
- Excessively large amounts of sputum, or sputum that is greenish or bloody
- Extreme difficulty swallowing
- Excessive loss of appetite
- Wheezing
- Shortness of breath

Minnesota. "It can shorten the length of a cold from seven days to maybe two or three days."

Vitamin C may also cut back on coughing, sneezing, and other symptoms. In a study conducted at the University of Wisconsin, cold sufferers taking 500 milligrams of vitamin C four times per day suffered about half as many symptoms as those not taking the vitamin.

Short-term use of such high doses shouldn't cause any side effects, says Dr. Sehnert. But you should get your doctor's okay before starting any supplement program. Better yet, simply get your additional vitamin C by drinking it. Orange, grapefruit, and cranberry juices are rich sources of vitamin C.

Zap it with zinc. Sucking on zinc lozenges can cut colds short by an average of seven days, researchers in Great Britain and the United States have discovered. Zinc can also dramatically reduce symptoms such as a dry, irritated throat, says Elson Haas, M.D., director of the Marin Clinic of Preventive Medicine and Health Education in San Rafael, California. "It doesn't work for everyone, but when it works, it works," he says.

The down side is that zinc has an unpleasant taste. There are, however, lozenges on the market that contain honey and/or citrus that are a lot easier to swallow. But do not take more than the amount recommended by your doctor. Zinc can be toxic in large doses.

The Cold Truth

So you've got a cold that won't let go, and you'd love to know just who or what to blame? Elliot Dick, Ph.D., a virologist and professor at the University of Wisconsin–Madison who has conducted research for more than 30 years on how colds are transmitted, says a lot of suspects have been taking a bum rap. They include:

- Sharing food or beverages with someone with a cold
- Kissing someone with a cold
- Not bundling up against the cold
- Sitting in a draft
- Stepping outside with a wet head

The *real* carrier, of course, is a virus transmitted through the air, says Dr. Dick. You can catch it, he says, when a cold sufferer coughs, sneezes, or does a sloppy job of blowing his nose, sending the virus floating into your path.

Be positive. A positive attitude about your body's ability to heal itself can actually mobilize immune system forces, says Martin Rossman, M.D., a general practitioner in Mill Valley, California. He teaches this theory by getting his patients to practice imagery techniques to combat colds. After bringing yourself into a deeply relaxed state, "imagine a white tornado decongesting your stuffed-up sinuses," he suggests, "or an army of microscopic maids cleaning up germs with buckets of disinfectant."

Rest and relax. Extra rest enables you to put all your energy into getting well. It can also help you avoid complications like bronchitis and pneumonia, says Samuel Caughron, M.D., a family practitioner specializing in preventive medicine in Charlottesville, Virginia.

Take a day or two off from work if you're feeling really bad, he advises. At the very least, slow down in your everyday activities and reschedule your time. "Trying to keep up with your regular routine can be draining because when you're not feeling well, your concentration is down and you'll probably need to double the amount of time it's going to take you to do things." he says.

Turn out the party lights. When you're sick, parties and other good times can wear you out physically, compromising your immune system and causing your cold to linger, says Timothy Van Ert, M.D., a physician in San Francisco and Saratoga, California, specializing in self-care and preventive medicine. Let the good times roll right on by until you feel better.

Warm up. Keep bundled up against the cold, advises Dr. Sehnert. This keeps your immune system cozily focused on fighting your cold infection instead of displacing energy to protect you from the cold.

Take a walk. Mild exercise improves your circulation, helping your immune system circulate infection-fighting antibodies, says Dr. Sehnert. "Jump on a gentle rebounder indoors for 15 minutes or take a brisk half-hour walk," he suggests. But refrain from strenuous exercise, he warns, which could wear you out.

Feed a cold—lightly. The very fact that you have a cold in the first place may point to your eating "too congesting a diet" that puts a strain on your body's metabolism, says Dr. Haas. Counteract it, he advises, by eating fewer fatty foods, meat and milk products, and more fresh fruit and vegetables.

Sip chicken soup. A long-time folk remedy is now a proven fact. A cup of hot chicken soup can help unclog your nasal passages. Researchers at Mount Sinai Medical Center in Miami Beach found that hot chicken soup, either because of its aroma or its taste, "appears to possess an additional substance for increasing the flow of nasal mucus." These secretions—what comes out when you blow your nose or sneeze—serve a first line of defense in removing germs from your system, the researchers say.

Load up on liquids. Drink six to eight glasses of water, juice, tea, and other mostly clear liquids daily, advises Dr. Sehnert. This will replace important fluids lost during a cold and help flush out impurities that may be preying on your system.

Butt out. Smoking aggravates a throat that may already feel irritated from a cold, says Dr. Caughron. It also interferes with the infection-fighting activity of cilia, the microscopic "fingers" that sweep bacteria out of your lungs and throat. So if you can't kick the habit for good, at least do it while you've got a cold.

Soothe with saltwater. Relieve an irritated throat by gargling morning, noon, and night—or whenever it hurts most, Dr. Van Ert advises. Fill a glass with warm water and mix in 1 teaspoon of salt.

Sip a hot toddy. Clear your stuffed-up nose and help yourself to a good night's sleep by drinking a "hot toddy" or half a glass of wine before bedtime, suggests Dr. Caughron. But more alcohol than that can stress your system, he says, making recovery from illness more difficult.

Get yourself in hot water. Taking a steamy shower can help clear congestion, says Kenneth Peters, M.D., an internist specializing in self-care and chronic pain in Mountain View, California. Or heat a teakettle or pot of water to boiling on your stove, turn off the flame, drape a towel in a tent over your head and the kettle, and inhale the steam until it subsides. This also relieves your cough by moistening your dry throat, he says.

Go for the grease. Relieve a nose raw from blowing by applying a lubricating layer of petroleum jelly around and slightly inside your nostrils with a cotton swab, suggests Dr. Peters.

Medicate at night. Numerous medications for colds are available without a prescription. Some treat specific symptoms. Others, like Nyquil and Contac, contain a combination of drugs—plus alcohol, in some cases—aimed at treating a wide range of symptoms. These combination drugs, however, can have many uncomfortable side effects like nausea and drowsiness, says Dr. Van Ert. "I recommend that these be taken only at night, since you won't feel the side effects while you're sleeping."

He says that if you need to take medications during the day, take only those that treat the symptoms you're suffering from. Be sure to follow the instructions carefully, he advises, and give children only a child-size dose. Here's what to reach for.

- For relief of the body aches or fever that can accompany a cold take *aspirin* or *acetaminophen* (Tylenol). But do not give aspirin to children under the age of 21. What you think is a cold may actually be flu or chickenpox, and research has shown that aspirin taken by children with certain viral infections such as these can increase their risk of developing Reye's syndrome, a relatively rare but potentially fatal disease of the brain and liver. The same goes for cold medications containing aspirin. They include Alka-Seltzer Plus cold medication tablets, Bayer children's cold tablets, Bristol Myers 4-Way cold tablets, Pepto-Bismol tablets and liquid, and St. Joseph's aspirin for children.
- To stop sneezing and dry up your runny nose and watery eyes, take an *antihistamine,* which blocks your body's release of histamine, a chemical that causes these symptoms. Look for products like Chlor-

---

The Alternate Route

Herbs and Teas

Certain herbs and teas contain special properties that are natural antagonists against colds, according to two doctors who recommend them to their patients.

Goldenseal and echinacea. "I recommend herb capsules such as goldenseal and echinacea at the early onset of a cold," says Elson Haas, M.D. Goldenseal, he says, stimulates your liver, whose partial job is to clear up infections. It also strengthens the ailing mucous membranes in your nose, mouth, and throat. Echinacea cleans your blood and lymph glands, he says, which help circulate infection-fighting antibodies and remove toxic substances. Try one or two capsules of each twice a day for up to two weeks.

Garlic. This familiar herb has an antibiotic effect, says Dr. Haas. "It can actually kill germs and clear up your cold symptoms more rapidly." He recommends two to three oil-free garlic capsules three times a day.

Herb teas can be just as effective, says Timothy Van Ert, M.D. Here's his prescription.

Licorice root tea. Dr. Van Ert says that this tea has an anesthetizing effect that soothes irritated throats and relieves coughs. Drink it daily.

Other teas. For a good night's sleep, brew a cup of hops or valarian herb teas or Celestial Seasonings Sleepytime tea, all of which have a natural tranquilizing effect. For even better results, he suggests that you add a teaspoon of honey, a simple carbohydrate that will have a sedative effect.

Monolaurian. This fatty acid, available in capsule form, has been shown in research to have an antiviral effect, says Dr. Van Ert, helping the immune system gear up in the battle against the cold virus. He recommends two capsules three times a day, taken with some food.

Trimaton, Polaraimine, Dimetane and Actidil, advises Diane Casdorph, R.Ph., a clinical instructor at the Drug Information Center of West Virginia University School of Pharmacy. Warning: Antihistamines frequently cause drowsiness, so save these for bedtime or at least for when you won't be driving or doing anything that requires coordination.

- To unstuff your nose, take a *decongestant*. Look for products that contain the active ingredients phenylproponalamine, phenylephrine, or pseudoephedrine, says Casdorph. Try Sudafed, Actifed, Dristan, Aspirin-free Congespirin or Contac.
- *Nasal sprays and drops* such as Afrin, Neosynephrine, and Coricidin are also effective decongestants. But they shouldn't be used for longer than three days, says Dr. Peters. Overuse can result in a "rebound effect," meaning your rebellious nose gets seriously stuffed up all over again.
- To relieve a cough, try *cough drops and syrups*. Look for a product that contains cough-suppressing antitussives such as dextromethorphan, diphenhydramine, or noscapine, says Casdorph. These include Benylin and Conair cough drops and Robitussin cough syrup.
- *Lozenges* can also combat coughs. Many of them contain topical anesthetics that slightly numb your sore throat, says Dr. Van Ert, which relieves your need to cough. Sucrets, Cepacol, Cepastat or Spec-T sore throat decongestant lozenges are among them.
- *Menthol or camphor rubs* have a soothing, cooling effect and may relieve congestion and help you breathe more easily, especially at bedtime. Apply Vicks VapoRub or a similar product to your bare chest, cover up, and get a good night's sleep.

Don't spread your germs. When you need to cough, go ahead and cough. When you need to blow your nose, go ahead and blow. But cough and sneeze into disposable tissues instead of setting germs free in the environment, Dr. Van Ert advises, then promptly throw the tissue away and wash your hands. Your healthy friends and family who want to stay that way will appreciate it.

PANEL OF ADVISERS

Diane Casdorph, R.Ph., is a clinical instructor of pharmacy at the Drug Information Center of the West Virginia University School of Pharmacy in Morgantown.

Samuel Caughron, M.D., is a family practitioner specializing in preventive medicine in Charlottesville, Virginia.

Elliot Dick, Ph.D., is a virologist and professor of preventive medicine at the University of Wisconsin–Madison, and has conducted research on the common cold for more than 30 years.

Elson Haas, M.D., is the director of the Marin Clinic of Preventive Medicine and Health Education in San Rafael, California, and author of the book *Staying Healthy with the Seasons*.

Kenneth Peters, M.D., is an internist specializing in self-care and chronic pain in Mountain View, California.

Martin Rossman, M.D., is a general practitioner in Mill Valley, California, and author of *Healing Yourself: A Step-by-Step Guide to Better Health through Imagery.*

Keith W. Sehnert, M.D., is a physician with Trinity Health Care in Minneapolis, Minnesota, and author of several books, including *Selfcare/Wellcare* and *How to be Your Own Doctor . . . Sometimes.*

Timothy Van Ert, M.D., is in private practice in San Francisco and Saratoga, California, where he specializes in self-care and preventive medicine.

Cold Sores

17 Hints to Heal Herpes Simplex

That tingling you feel just above your upper lip is unmistakable. Oh, cripes. You know what that is — the start of another cold sore or fever blister.

You've gone through this routine before. First it gets red. Then that itchy, tingly area puffs out. The more water the blister draws to itself, the bigger it gets, and the more embarrassed you feel.

For some reason you can't stop checking yourself out in the mirror. (Maybe you're hoping against hope each time you look that the cold sore has disappeared, that it only existed in your imagination. But no such luck.) Why, you wonder, does it have to happen to me?

Cold sores are caused by the herpes simplex virus. In all likelihood, some relative of yours infected you when you were a child by kissing you at a time when his herpes simplex was infectious.

The virus scooted right into your mouth and sought a hospitable host cell, probably a nerve cell that would let the virus move right in. The virus then "ordered" the DNA in its host cell to make lots more viruses exactly like it.

For the most part, those viruses are homebodies. They stay put. But from time to time, the virus family likes to take a little vacation. So it cruises down the nerve highways until it reaches the skin surface. And when that happens, you start to feel that awful tingling sensation that signals the start of another you-know-what.

What can you do about it?

Keep the cold sore clean and dry. "If the cold sore isn't really bothersome, just leave it alone," says James F. Rooney, M.D., a clinical virologist at the Laboratory of Oral Medicine at the National Institutes of Health. "Make sure to keep the sore clean and dry. If it becomes pussy—and this rarely happens—seek medical attention to make sure the bacterial infection is properly treated."

Replace your toothbrush. Your trusty toothbrush can harbor the herpes virus for days, reinfecting you after the present cold sore heals.

Researchers at the University of Oklahoma exposed a sterile toothbrush to the virus for 10 minutes. Seven days later, half of the disease-producing viruses remained, says Richard T. Glass, D.D.S., Ph.D., chairman of the Department of Oral Pathology at the University of Oklahoma College of Medicine and College of Dentistry.

How do you counter the infectious toothbrush? Get rid of it. Dr. Glass recommends that you throw your toothbrush away when you notice you're just beginning to get the virus. If you still develop the cold sore, throw your toothbrush away after the blister develops. That can prevent you from developing multiple sores. And once the sore has healed completely, replace your toothbrush again. Dr. Glass said that patients of his who tried this found that it cut way down on the number of cold sores they typically experienced in a year.

Don't keep your toothbrush in the bathroom. A nice wet toothbrush in a moist environment like your bathroom is as cozy an environment as the herpes simplex virus could hope for. That moisture helps prolong the life of the herpes virus on your toothbrush. That's why Dr. Glass recommends that you store your toothbrush someplace dry.

Use small tubes of toothpaste. Toothpaste can transmit disease, too, says Glass. Think how often you put the brush that's been in your mouth right up to the opening of the tube. If you use small tubes of toothpaste, you'll be sure to replace it regularly.

Protect with petroleum jelly. You can protect your cold sore by covering it with petroleum jelly, says Dr. Glass. Be sure not to dip back into the jelly with the same finger you used to touch your sore. Better yet, use a fresh cotton swab.

Zap it with zinc. Several studies show that a water-based zinc solution, applied the minute you feel that tingling, helps speed healing time.

In a Boston study of 200 patients who were followed over a six-year period, a 0.025 percent solution of zinc sulfate in camphorated water was found very effective. Sores healed in an average of 5.3 days. The solution was applied every 30 to 60 minutes during the onset of the cold sore.

Researchers in Israel also found a 2 percent water-based zinc solution, applied several times a day, to be very helpful, says Milos Chvapil, M.D., Ph.D., professor of surgery and head of the Surgical Biology Section at the University of Arizona College of Medicine.

How does zinc help? Dr. Chvapil says that zinc ions crosslink with the DNA molecule of the herpes virus and prevent the double helix from splitting. That means the virus can't get the DNA to help it replicate.

Dr. Chvapil says that zinc gluconate is kinder to the skin than zinc sulfate. The mineral is available at health food stores.

Lick it with lysine. Dermatologist Mark A. McCune, M.D., chief of dermatology at Humana Hospital in Overland Park, Kansas, advises patients who have more than three cold sores a year to supplement their daily diets with 2,000 to 3,000 milligrams of the amino acid lysine. He also recommends that they double up on the dosage when they feel the itching and tingling that signals the development of another cold sore. (Of course, don't use this or any supplement without the advice and consent of your doctor. This is especially true for pregnant women and nursing mothers. Some animal studies have shown that excess lysine can interfere with normal growth.)

Not all studies have found lysine helpful for cold sore sufferers. But in one study of 41 patients, Dr. McCune and his colleagues found a daily dose of 1,248 milligrams of lysine helped subjects reduce the number of cold sores they have in a year.

Good food sources of lysine include dairy products, potatoes, and brewer's yeast.

Identify the pattern. What was going on in your life just before you got your last cold sore? What about the cold sore prior to that? If you do some sleuthing, you just might figure out what triggers a cold sore for you. If you can find a trigger, take additional lysine when you're most prone to cold sores, says Dr. McCune.

Freeze-dry it. Some of Dr. Rooney's patients reach for ice when they first feel the tingling. "I'm not sure that it works, but if I were to speculate, I'd say that ice does decrease inflammation. And if inflammatory substances aid the reactivation process, this could help."

Dab on witch hazel. "Some patients claim that breaking a sore and using witch hazel or alcohol to dry it really helps," says Dr. Rooney.

Soften it with an OTC. There are numerous products that claim to heal cold sores. In general, they contain some emollient to reduce cracking and soften scabs, and a numbing agent like phenol or camphor.

Phenol may have some antiviral properties, says Dr. Rooney. "It does denature proteins. Theoretically, it is possible that phenol is capable of killing the virus."

Block that sun (or wind). Protecting your lips from trauma like sunburn or wind exposure was cited by all our experts as a key to preventing cold sores.

Avoid arginine-rich foods. The herpes virus needs arginine as an essential amino acid for its metabolism. So cut out arginine-rich foods such as chocolate, cola, peas, grain cereals, peanuts, gelatin, cashews, and beer.

Perfect your coping skills. Studies have shown that stress can trigger recurrences of the herpes simplex virus. High levels of stress are not necessarily the culprit, says Cal Vanderplate, Ph.D., an Atlanta psychologist specializing in stress-related disorders. "How you cope with the stress—how you perceive it—is what's important. Stress is not a tangible thing; it's a concept."

His number one stress deflator is "maintaining a loving social support system. This is the number one thing you can do to protect yourself from high stress," he says. "A sense of control is also very important. If you take a positive attitude toward your health, you'll be more able to influence your symptoms."

Relax. "By the time symptoms appear, it's too late to intervene in stress reduction," says Dr. Vanderplate. "But you may be able to reduce the severity by doing some relaxation exercise." He favors deep muscle relaxation techniques, biofeedback, visualization, and meditation.

Exercise. "There is some evidence that exercise actually helps bolster the immune system," says Dr. Vanderplate. The stronger your immune system, the better able it is to defend you against viruses. Exercise is also a super way to relax, he says.

Correct your perception. No one likes getting a cold sore. But if you've got one, focusing on it and worrying about how you look can make it worse. "Minimize any negative perceptions you have about it," says Dr. Vanderplate. "Tell yourself that 'this is just like a pimple and it won't interfere in my life in any way'."

PANEL OF ADVISERS

Milos Chvapil, M.D., Ph.D., is a professor of surgery and head of the Surgical Biology Section of the University of Arizona College of Medicine in Tucson.

Richard T. Glass, D.D.S., Ph.D., is chairman of the Department of Oral Pathology at the University of Oklahoma College of Medicine and College of Dentistry in Oklahoma City.

Mark A. McCune, M.D., is a dermatologist in Overland Park, Kansas. He is chief of dermatology at Humana Hospital in Overland Park.

James F. Rooney, M.D., is a clinical virologist and a special expert in the Laboratory of Oral Medicine at the National Institutes of Health in Bethesda, Maryland.

Cal Vanderplate, Ph.D., is a clinical psychologist specializing in stress-related disorders. He is on the clinical faculties of Georgia State University and the Emory University School of Medicine, both in Atlanta.

Colic

10 Ideas to Quell the Cries

Ancient scholars first described infantile colic in the sixth century. Modern parents have no trouble describing it today. The baby cries, pulls his knees up to his abdomen, and appears to be in great pain. He may become gassy, then become quiet, then begin crying again.

Nothing much seems to have changed over the centuries, and nothing much seems to help. Colicky babies cannot generally be quieted with feeding or a change of diapers, and episodes may last for many hours. Colic tends to be most severe at 4 to 6 weeks of age and gradually subsides by 3 to 4 months.

Though none of the remedies offered below will cure colic, most have brought some relief to suffering parents somewhere, so you might want to give them a try. And remember, this too shall pass. Colic disappears as mysteriously as it begins.

Try the colic carry. "I'm a big believer in the colic carry," says Ann Price, educational coordinator for the National Academy of Nannies, Inc. (NANI), in Denver, Colorado.

Extend your forearm with your palm up, "then place the baby [on your arm] chest down, with his head in your hand and his legs on either side of your elbow." Support the baby with your other hand and walk around the house with him in this position, Price says. "It definitely helps."

Burp that babe. "My experience is that at least some colicky babies do have more abdominal gas than the norm and may be more difficult to burp," says Linda Jonides, a pediatric nurse practitioner in Ann Arbor, Michigan.

Her recommendation: Watch the position of the baby when feeding (upright is all right), and burp frequently. When bottle-feeding, burp after every ounce, and try a variety of nipple types (some parents swear by the Playtex disposable nurser).

Cut the cow juice. Many child-care specialists believe colic is caused when cow's milk is transmitted from mother to infant through breast milk. Though some recent research casts doubt on this connection, experts agree that a maternal diet free of cow's milk may be worth a trial, especially in families with a strong history of allergies.

"I firmly believe that milk in the mother's diet is a frequent cause of colic in breastfed babies," Price says. "I recommend mothers start by eliminating milk from their diets and see what happens. If that does it, you don't have to go any further, but if not, you may need to cut back other dairy products."

Check out the diet connection. "Occasionally there may be some foods that set a baby off," says Morris Green, M.D., chairman of the Department of Pediatrics at Indiana University School of Medicine. "The breastfeeding mother may try to notice if there's any correlation between what she eats and the onset of the colic." Some potential troublemakers are caffeine-containing drinks, chocolate, bananas, oranges, strawberries, and strongly spiced foods.

Try a wrap session. "I recommend holding and swaddling a colicky baby," Jonides says, "or using a backpack to hold the baby so you can have your arms free to do other things."

For some reason, wrapping a baby snugly in a blanket has a calming effect. It's very popular in some cultures, and it does sometimes stop colic attacks. And it does not spoil an infant who wants physical contact.

Use a vacuum instead of a lullaby. Though it's true that nature detests a vacuum, colicky babies seem to love the sounds a vacuum creates. Science has failed to explain this mystery.

"The noise of a vacuum cleaner running does seem to calm a colicky baby," says Dr. Green. Parents have been known to tape-record the sound of a vacuum cleaner and play it back when baby gets fussy. Others simply start vacuuming the carpet and hope the child outgrows colic while there's still some rug left. Price suggests a more aggressive approach. "If you put the baby in a front pack and vacuum at the same time, it's a double whammy," says she. "That colicky baby goes out like a light."

Do the dryer dribble. "Put the baby in an infant seat and rest it against the side of a running clothes dryer so the baby gets that buzzing sound and vibration through the seat," suggests Helen Neville, a pediatric advice nurse at Kaiser Permanente Hospital in Oakland, California.

Sound too far-fetched? Wait until baby fusses for another 3 hours or so. "There's something about the vibration that really soothes a colicky baby," Neville says.

Warm that tummy. "A hot-water bottle or heating pad *set on low* and placed on the baby's tummy sometimes helps," Jonides says. (Place a towel between the baby and the hot-water bottle to make sure he doesn't get burned.)

Log it in. "Keeping a log would be a very good idea," Neville says. "Often, when it seems like the baby was fussing for 2 hours straight, it was really only 45 minutes. A log will help you determine just how long the baby's crying, and — more important — what might be bringing it on."

Swing into action. "Motion-type things are good for colic," says Jonides. "Many babies will at least be quiet long enough to let you get through dinner when they're swinging." Automatic swings can provide motion, and relief, for up to 20 minutes.

PANEL OF ADVISERS

Morris Green, M.D., is chairman of the Department of Pediatrics at Indiana University School of Medicine in Indianapolis.

Linda Jonides is a pediatric nurse practitioner in Ann Arbor, Michigan.

Helen Neville is a pediatric advice nurse at Kaiser Permanente Hospital in Oakland, California, where she is part of a 24-hour hotline for parents. She is author of *No-Fault Parenting*.

Ann Price is educational coordinator for the National Academy of Nannies, Inc. (NANI), in Denver, Colorado, and coauthor of *Successful Breastfeeding, Dr. Mom,* and other books.

Conjunctivitis

7 Remedies for Pinkeye

Your mother called it pinkeye, a magic word that meant no school for a couple of days. Now that you're grown up, you call it conjunctivitis. And, although it might not keep you home from work, your eyes can still use a little soothing relief. Here's how.

Wash the red away. Remember Mom sitting on the side of your bed, dipping a washcloth in a bowl and gently placing it on your eyes? Wet pillow aside, she had the right idea. "A warm compress applied to the eyes for 5 to 10 minutes three or four times a day will make you feel better," says pediatric ophthalmologist Robert Petersen, M.D., director of the Eye Clinic at Children's Hospital in Boston, Massachusetts.

Keep them clean. "A lot of times conjunctivitis gets better by itself," says Dr. Petersen. "To help the healing process along, keep your eyes and eyelids clean by using a cotton ball dipped in clean or sterile water to wipe the crusts away."

Baby yourself. A warm compress works well for children, but sometimes adults need a little something more. "Adults who have a lot of discharge should make a solution of 1 part baby shampoo to 10 parts

---

MEDICAL ALERT

Seeing a Doctor Says Eye Care

Conjunctivitis is an easily treatable problem that will usually go away on its own in about a week. You should, however, see your doctor if:

- After five days the infection is getting worse, not better.
- You have a red eye that is associated with significant eye pain, change in vision, or a copious amount of yellow or greenish discharge.
- Redness is caused by an injury to your eye. "Sometimes infections can get in the eye and scratch the cornea, leading to an ulcer or even loss of vision or loss of your eye," says Robert Petersen, M.D.

So when it comes to your eyes, don't take a wait and see attitude. Instead, see your doctor.

---

warm water," says Peter Hersh, M.D., an ophthalmologist and assistant surgeon at the Massachusetts Eye and Ear Infirmary in Boston.

"Dip a sterile cotton ball into the solution and use it to clean off your eyelashes. It works very well. The warm water loosens the crust and the baby shampoo cleans off the junction of your eyelid and eyelash."

An over-the-counter solution called I-Scrub, used the same way, is just as effective.

Throw in the towel. Toss it, the washcloth, and anything else that comes in contact with your eyes into the laundry. "This infection is highly contagious. Don't share a towel or washcloth with anyone, because it will easily spread the disease," says Dr. Petersen.

Don't chlorinate your eyes. Does swimming in a pool leave you seeing pink? "The chlorine in swimming pools can cause conjunctivitis, but without the chlorine, bacteria would grow—and that could cause it, too," says Dr. Petersen. "If you're going to go swimming and you're susceptible to conjunctivitis, wear tight-fitting goggles while in the water."

Put allergic conjunctivitis on ice. If you survive the summer swim but not the summer pollen, your conjunctivitis may be caused by allergies. "If your eye itches like a mosquito bite and you have stringy pus in your eye, most of the time that's the sign of allergic conjunctivitis," says J. Daniel Nelson, M.D., a Minnesota ophthalmologist and chief of the Department of Ophthalmology at St. Paul–Ramsey Medical Center in Minnesota. "Taking an over-the-counter antihistamine will help that, and use cold, not warm, compresses. A cold compress will really relieve the itch."

Get drugged at night. "Germ-caused conjunctivitis intensifies when your eyes are closed. That's why it tends to get worse at night when you're asleep," says Dr. Petersen. "To combat that, put any prescribed antibiotic ointment in your eyes before you go to bed. That way it will prevent crusting."

PANEL OF ADVISERS

Peter Hersh, M.D., is an ophthalmologist and assistant surgeon in the Department of Ophthalmology at Massachusetts Eye and Ear Infirmary in Boston. He is also an instructor of ophthalmology at Harvard Medical School in Boston.

J. Daniel Nelson, M.D., is an ophthalmologist and chief of the Department of Ophthalmology at St. Paul-Ramsey Medical Center in Minnesota. He is also associate professor of ophthalmology at the University of Minnesota Medical School in Minneapolis.

Robert Petersen, M.D., is a pediatric ophthalmologist and director of the Eye Clinic at Children's Hospital in Boston, Massachusetts. He is also assistant professor of ophthalmology at Harvard Medical School in Boston.

Constipation

18 Solutions to a Common Problem

What goes up must come down. Sir Isaac Newton proved that, sitting under an apple tree.

What goes in must come out. You proved that, sitting on the toilet this morning.

Well, *didn't* you?

Or was it yesterday morning that you had your last bowel movement? Or the day before? Or one cold but memorable day early last December?

Constipation is no fun. Sometimes it can be painful. But the cause of your sluggish bowels is often easy to find. It may include a lack of fiber in the diet, insufficient liquid intake, stress, medications, lack of exercise, and bad bowel habits, says Paul Rousseau, M.D., chief of the Department of Geriatrics at the Carl T. Hayden Veterans Administration Medical Center in Phoenix, Arizona.

We take a look at all of these factors, and ways to remedy the situation below.

Are you *really* constipated? You think you have a problem, but do you really? Like all of us, you have been bombarded most of your life by laxative advertisements that try to give you the impression that a daily bowel movement is essential to good health, and this just isn't so, says Marvin Schuster, M.D., chief of the Department of Digestive Diseases at Francis Scott Key Medical Center in Baltimore, Maryland.

Many Americans, he says, are subject to *perceived constipation*—they think they are constipated when they are not. In reality, the need to defecate varies greatly from individual to individual. For some, a bowel movement three times a day may be considered normal, for others three times a week may suffice.

Are you getting enough fluids? Our experts agree that the first thing a constipated individual should do is check his diet. The foremost menu items for battling constipation are dietary fiber and liquids. Lots of both are essential to keep the stool soft and to help it pass through the colon.

How much liquid and how much fiber do you need? Let's start with the liquid. A minimum of six glasses of liquid, and preferably eight, should be part of every adult's diet, says Patricia H. Harper, a registered dietitian in the Pittsburgh, Pennsylvania, area, and spokeswoman for the American Dietetic Association. While any fluid will do the trick, "the best fluid is water," she says.

Eat lots more fiber. Most Americans don't get enough fiber in their diets, says Harper. The American Dietetic Association recommends a daily consumption of 20 to 35 grams of dietary fiber for all adults and at least 30 grams for those who suffer from constipation.

Where does fiber come from? "From your complex carbohydrates—such as those in whole grains, fruit, and vegetables," says Harper. It's not

The Alternate Route

Bypass the Oil Slick

Eliminate from your diet all oils that have been removed from their sources, such as liquid vegetable, olive, or soy oil, and it may help relieve chronic constipation. says Grady Deal, D.C., Ph.D., a nutritional chiropractor in Koloa, Kauai, Hawaii.

"It's not oil per se, but eating it in its free state that causes constipation and many other digestive problems," says Dr. Deal, who bases his theory on the work of turn-of-the-century health reformer John Harvey Kellogg, M.D. (brother of the breakfast cereal magnate).

The problem with these oils, explains Dr. Deal, is that they form a film in the stomach, which makes it difficult to digest carbohydrates and proteins there and in the small intestine. "Adequate digestion is delayed up to 20 hours causing putrefaction, gas, and toxins," which back up in the colon and large intestine, he says.

But oils eaten in their natural form, locked up in such things as whole nuts, avocados, and corn, are released slowly into the body, so that no oil slicks occur to block digestion and create constipation problems. These oils, as opposed to the separated kind, are "a wholesome and nutritious element of food," says Dr. Deal.

difficult to get 30 grams in your daily diet if you choose foods carefully. One-half cup of green peas, for instance, will give you 5 grams; one small apple supplies 3 grams, and a bowl of bran cereal can give you as much as 13 grams. Tops among the fiber heavyweights, however, are cooked dried beans, prunes, figs, raisins, popcorn, oatmeal, pears, and nuts. One word of caution, though, increase your fiber intake slowly to avoid gas attacks.

Take time to go to the gym. You know that exercise is good for your heart, but did you know that it's good for your bowels? "In general, we feel that regular exercise tends to combat constipation by moving food through the bowel faster," says Edward R. Eichner, M.D., professor of medicine and chief of hematology in the Department of Medicine at the University of Oklahoma.

Take a walk, and bring your baby. Any form of regular exercise will tend to alleviate constipation, but the one mentioned most often by our experts is walking. Walking is particularly helpful for preg-

---

MEDICAL ALERT

Play It Safe; See a Doctor

Constipation itself is usually not serious, says Marvin Schuster, M.D. You should call your doctor, however, when symptoms are severe, last longer than three weeks, are disabling, or if you find blood in your stool, he says. Although it's rare, constipation can signal a serious underlying disorder.

In addition, contact your doctor if your constipation is accompanied by a distended abdomen, which may signal an intestinal obstruction, says Paul Rousseau, M.D.

---

nant women, many of whom experience constipation as their inner workings are altered to accommodate the growing fetus.

Anyone, including mothers-to-be, should walk a "good, hearty 20 to 30 minutes" a day, suggests Lewis R. Townsend, M.D., clinical instructor of obstetrics and gynecology at Georgetown University Hospital in Washington, D.C. Pregnant women should take care not to get too winded as they walk.

Toilet train yourself. Throughout our lives, many of us condition ourselves to go to the bathroom not when nature calls but when it's convenient. Ignoring the urge to defecate, however, can lead progressively to constipation. But it's never too late to improve your bowel habits, says Dr. Schuster. "The most natural time to go to the toilet is after a meal," he says. So pick a meal, any meal, and every day following that meal sit on the toilet for 10 minutes. In time, says Dr. Schuster, you will condition your colon to act as nature intended.

Slow down and take it easy. When you're frightened or tense, your mouth dries and your heart beats faster. Your bowels stop up as well. "It's part of the fight-or-flight mechanism," says John O. Lawder, M.D., a family practitioner specializing in nutrition and preventive medicine in Torrance, California. If you suspect tension is at the bottom of your constipation, take time to relax, perhaps by listening to relaxation tapes.

Have a hearty laugh. A good belly laugh can help with constipation in two ways. It has a massaging effect on the intestines, which helps to foster digestion, and it's a great reliever of stress, says Alison

Crane, R.N., president of the American Association for Therapeutic Humor. Heard any good constipation jokes lately?

Reconsider laxative tablets. Commercial laxatives often do what they are intended to do, but they are terribly addicting, warns Dr. Rousseau. Take too many of these chemical laxatives, "and your bowel gets used to them, and your constipation can get worse," he says. When should you take laxatives from a bottle? "Almost never," says Dr. Rousseau.

Know that not all laxatives are the same. In most pharmacies, right next to the chemical laxatives, you'll find another category of laxatives, often marked "natural," or "vegetable" laxatives, whose main ingredient is generally crushed psyllium seed. This is a superconcentrated form of fiber, which, unlike the chemical laxatives, is nonaddictive and generally safe, even taken over long periods, says Dr. Rousseau. He cautions, however, that these must be taken with lots of water (read the instructions on the box), or they can gum up inside you.

Try one doctor's special recipe. A problem with many of the psyllium-based laxatives is that they can be expensive. But you can make your own by buying the psyllium seeds in a health food store and crushing them yourself. Dr. Lawder suggests you grind two parts psyllium with one part flax and one part oat bran (also available in health food stores) for a super-high-fiber concoction. "Mix the ingredients up with water, and have it as a little mash every night around 9 o'clock," says Dr. Lawder.

Get fast relief—once in a while. If you're really miserable, nothing will work faster to move your bowels than an enema or a suppository. For occasional use, they are perfectly all right, says Dr. Rousseau. Use them too often, however, and you risk creating a lazy colon. That is, you could wind up worse off.

Use only clear water or saline-solution enemas, *never* soapsuds, which can be irritating, says Dr. Rousseau. And when shopping for a suppository, pick up only glycerin ones, avoiding the harsher chemical selections on the market.

Review your medications and supplements. There are a number of medications that can bring on or exacerbate constipation, says Dr. Rousseau. Among the common culprits are antacids containing aluminum or calcium, antihistamines, anti-Parkinsonism drugs, calcium supplements, diuretics, narcotics, phenothiazines, sedatives, and tricyclic antidepressants.

Beware of certain foods. Some things may constipate one person but not another. Milk, for instance, can be extremely constipating to some, while it gives others diarrhea. Foods that tend to produce gas, such as beans, cauliflower, and cabbage, should be avoided by those whose constipation is the result of a spastic colon, says Dr. Schuster. You should suspect a spastic colon if your constipation is sharply painful.

Eat small meals. Those with spastic colons should also avoid large meals that distend the digestive tract, thus worsening constipation, says Dr. Schuster.

Be cautious about herbs. Herbal remedies for dealing with constipation abound. Among those touted are aloe (juice, not gel), senna, rhubarb (medicinal), cascara sagrada, dandelion root, and plantain seeds. Some, such as cascara sagrada, can be very effective, says Dr. Lawder, but you need to be careful. Certain herbal laxatives, just as chemical ones, should not be overused.

Don't strain. As tempting as it may be to huff and puff your way out of constipation, it is not wise to do so. You risk giving yourself hemorrhoids and anal fissures, which not only are painful, but can also aggravate your constipation by narrowing the anal opening. Straining can also raise your blood pressure and lower your heartbeat. Dr. Rousseau says he has known several elderly patients to black out and fall off the toilet, sometimes suffering fractures as a result—which brings us back once again to Sir Isaac Newton and those immutable laws of gravity.

PANEL OF ADVISERS

Alison Crane, R.N., is president of the American Association for Therapeutic Humor. She is also vice president of Strombach, Crane & Associates, a consulting firm in Skokie, Illinois, that specializes in stress reduction programs for hospitals.

Grady Deal, D.C., Ph.D., is a nutritional chiropractor and psychotherapist in Koloa, Kauai, Hawaii. He is also the founder and owner of Dr. Deal's Hawaiian Fitness Holiday health spa in Koloa.

Edward R. Eichner, M.D., an expert in the effects of exercise on the human body, is a professor of medicine and chief of hematology in the Department of Medicine at the University of Oklahoma in Oklahoma City.

Patricia H. Harper, R.D., is a spokeswoman for the American Dietetic Association and a nutrition consultant in the Pittsburgh, Pennsylvania, area.

John O. Lawder, M.D., is a family practitioner specializing in nutrition and preventive medicine in Torrance, California.

Paul Rousseau, M.D., is chief of the Department of Geriatrics at the Carl T. Hayden Veterans Administration Medical Center in Phoenix, Arizona. He is also an adjunct professor in the Adult Development and Aging Section of Arizona State University in Tempe.

Marvin Schuster, M.D., is chief of the Department of Digestive Diseases at Francis Scott Key Medical Center in Baltimore, Maryland, and professor of medicine and psychiatry at Johns Hopkins University School of Medicine in Baltimore.

Lewis R. Townsend, M.D., is in private practice in Bethesda, Maryland, and is a clinical instructor of obstetrics and gynecology at Georgetown University Hospital and director of the physician's group at the Columbia Hospital for Women Medical Center, both in Washington, D.C.

Corns and Calluses

20 Ways to Smooth and Soothe

You can have the strength of Hercules and the wits of Zeus, but if your feet hurt, you've got an Achilles' heel. Indeed, painful corns and calluses can sweep you right off your feet—the hard way.

These ugly little bumps and lumps are a veritable trash heap of discarded—but hardly forgotten—dead skin cells, the result of friction and irritation between your feet and your shoes or even between adjacent bones on the same foot.

"Calluses are your body's way of protecting you from pressure," says Neal Kramer, D.P.M., a podiatrist from Bethlehem, Pennsylvania. "When the pressure gets extreme, the callus gets thicker and thicker. If it develops a hard core, it becomes a corn. Soft corns, which form between toes and remain soft from foot perspiration, happen when two bones from adjacent toes become overly friendly. The skin between them thickens in an attempt to protect you from the constant pressure."

"People can live with calluses more easily than with corns," says Richard Cowin, D.P.M., director of Cowin's Foot Clinic in Libertyville, Illinois. "If you get painful corns on your toes, it's like having a bad toothache. It can ruin your day." To start *your* day—every day—on the right foot, heed these tips.

Stay away from sharp instruments. First and foremost, say the experts, don't play surgeon. Resist the temptation to pare down corns and calluses with razor blades, scissors, or other sharp instruments.

"Bathroom surgery is extremely dangerous," says Circleville, Ohio, podiatrist Nancy Lu Conrad, D.P.M. "It can lead to infections and worse. I've seen so many horrible things happen to people who thought they could be their own surgeons." And diabetics should *never* treat their own foot problems (see "When to Keep Your Hands Off Your Feet," on page 168).

Approach medicated pads with caution. If you use corn plasters or other over-the-counter salicylic-acid products, which come in liquid, salve, and disk form, religiously follow the advice of New York City podiatrist Suzanne M. Levine, D.P.M., clinical assistant podiatrist at Mount Sinai Hospital there. Apply them *only* to the problem area, not surrounding skin. If treating a corn, first put a doughnut-shaped non-medicated pad around the corn to shield adjacent skin. Never use such a product more than twice a week, and see a doctor if there's no sign of improvement after two weeks.

Better yet, avoid them completely. Dr. Kramer says unequivocally, "I don't recommend corn plasters or any other over-the-counter medications. Those things are nothing more than acid, which doesn't know the difference between corns and calluses and normal skin. So although they may work on your corn or callus, they will also eat away normal skin, causing burning or even ulcers."

Enjoy a good soak. "Your corn pain may be coming from a bursa, a fluid-filled sac that becomes inflamed and enlarged at the site between the bone and the corn," says Dr. Levine. "For temporary relief of the pain, soak your feet in a solution of Epsom salts and warm water. This will diminish the size of the bursa sac and take some pressure off the nearby sensory nerves. But be aware that if you put your feet back into tight shoes, the bursa will soon swell up again to its painful size."

Have a tea party. If you have a lot of callused tissue, Dr. Levine recommends that you soak your feet in very diluted chamomile tea. The tea will both soothe and soften hard skin. Although the brew will stain your feet, it comes off easily with soap and water.

Be a little abrasive. Before treating a callus, soak your foot in comfortably hot water for several minutes. Then, says Dr. Cowin, use a callus file or pumice stone to lightly abrade the area and rub off the top layers of skin. Finish by applying some hand cream, such as Carmol 20, which contains 20 percent urea and helps dissolve hard skin. If you have bad calluses, make this part of your daily routine after showering or bathing.

But the doctor cautions you not to use abrasive action on hard corns, because that will make the area very tender and more painful than it was before.

Bag your callus. For a large or cracked callus, especially on the heel, try this suggestion from Marvin Sandler, D.P.M., chief of podiatry surgery at Sacred Heart Hospital in Allentown, Pennsylvania. On a piece of foil or waxed paper, mix equal amounts of Whitfield's Ointment and hydrocortisone cream, both of which can be purchased without a prescription. Apply to the foot at night. Place a plastic bag over the foot and then a sock. Leave in place until morning. Then rub off as much callus as you can with a coarse towel or firm brush. Do this regularly to control a difficult heel callus.

Take five aspirin tablets—but don't swallow them. Another way to soften tough calluses, says Dr. Levine, involves crushing five or six aspirin tablets into a powder. Mix into a paste with a tablespoon each of water and lemon juice. Apply this to all the hard-skin spots on your foot, then put your entire foot into a plastic bag and wrap a warm towel around everything. The combination of the plastic and the warm towel will make the paste penetrate the hard skin. Sit still for at least 10 minutes. Then unwrap your foot and scrub the area with a pumice stone. All that dead, hard, callused skin should come loose and flake away easily.

Work fast. It's best to take action when a corn first takes shape, says Frederick Hass, M.D., a general practitioner in San Rafael, California. At that point, your corn is a hardening small circle of skin that produces little or no pain. You should immediately gently massage the area with lanolin to soften the corn and make it less responsive to pressure. And then pad the area to relieve pressure.

Give 'em space. Because soft corns are caused by bones from two adjacent toes rubbing together, says Dr. Cowin, "you need to put something soft there to separate the toes. You can buy toe separators or toe spacers, which are simply little pieces of foam that you place between the toes."

Be a lamb. Or use good-quality lamb's wool between toes, suggests Elizabeth H. Roberts, D.P.M., professor emeritus of the New York College of Podiatric Medicine in New York City. But don't get the coarse

---

MEDICAL ALERT

When to Keep Your Hands Off Your Feet

People with diabetes or any kind of reduced feeling in their feet should never treat themselves, says Neal Kramer, D.P.M. Diabetes affects tiny blood vessels throughout the body, including those in the feet. That leads to decreased circulation and a tendency for wounds not to heal or resist infection.

"Anyone with a circulation disorder is okay if his skin remains intact," says Dr. Kramer. "But if he gets any kind of cut or opening in the skin, it becomes very dangerous. And anyone who can't feel pressure or pain very well may not know he cut himself or may not realize the full severity of an injury and could wind up with a nasty infection."

---

type found in beauty parlors. Draw the strands into a thin, even layer, and wrap it loosely around one of the toes. Remove the wool before bathing.

Mark D. Sussman, D.P.M., a podiatrist in Wheaton, Maryland, advises against using cotton between the toes because it will harden and cause increased irritation—just the opposite of what lamb's wool does.

Make horseshoes. To cushion corns, says Dr. Roberts, don't use corn pads with an oval opening. The oval will cause pressure on the surrounding area, making the corn or callus bulge into the opening. If you've got that type of pad, cut a wedge out of it to make a horseshoe shape. Position the pad far enough behind the corn so that as you walk—if your foot slides forward in your shoe—the pad won't rub against the corn it is supposed to protect.

Get spot relief. Even better than a corn pad, says Dr. Roberts, is a spot-type Band-Aid, which also has the advantage of a sterile gauze center. But avoid bandages that must be wrapped completely around the toe. The bulk may lead to irritation and discomfort.

Pad the area. An easy way to take pressure off a callus, says Dr. Roberts, is to place a little gauze or absorbent cotton over the area, then cover it with a thin piece of moleskin. She recommends removing the covering each night, as well as when bathing, so the skin can breathe and so excessive moisture doesn't accumulate under the pad.

When you remove the moleskin, be sure to hold the skin of the sole of your foot taut while you *slowly* pull the moleskin back toward the heel. If you pull quickly or in the opposite direction, you risk tearing the skin.

Customize your insoles. Dr. Sussman recommends this easy way to modify insoles to relieve pressure on calluses: Buy a pair of foam-rubber insoles and wear them for a week. Your calluses will leave impressions, indicating the areas of greatest stress and showing you the areas *around which* each insole needs to be built up to even out the pressure.

If the callus is in the middle of the ball of the foot, cut ⅛-inch-thick foam or felt into two strips (each ½ inch wide by 2 inches long). Glue them on either side of the depression. Take another strip (2 inches wide by 2 inches long), and position it behind the depression. If the callus is off to one side, use appropriate combinations of strips. When you wear the insoles, the pads will redistribute weight away from the callus and provide relief.

Stretch your shoes. Sometimes relief of a painful, hard corn can be had by stretching your shoes to remove the pressure that caused the friction. Your shoemaker can do the stretching, or you can take this home approach from Dr. Sandler. Apply Stella's Stretch All or another leather-stretching solution to your shoes. This allows the leather fibers to stretch while you are walking. Apply the solution many times, and walk in the shoes (while the leather is still wet) until the shoe becomes comfortable.

Go to a bar. For calluses at the base of the foot, you can modify your shoes by getting your shoemaker to attach a rubber, or leather metatarsal bar to the sole of the shoe, says Dr. Sandler. It's placed so that the ball of your foot rocks over the bar without pressing on the bones in that area. Be sure to replace the bar when it becomes worn down.

Be careful though—these bars can catch on stairs, carpets, or curbs and cause you to trip. For this reason they may not be suitable for older folks. The elderly may be better off with a safer but less effective bar that is flat and continuous with the sole. Remember, however, that these bars do not prevent the metatarsal bones from pressing painfully against the *inside* of your shoe, so you may need a removable inlay there.

Be well-heeled. "I see a lot of problems in women because of high heels," says Dr. Conrad. "I've heard good shoe fitters say that any pump has to be fit short and narrow to keep it on. And that's true. Oxfords, on the other hand, have a tie that holds the shoe on and keeps the back of the foot firmly in the shoe. That keeps the foot from slipping forward and putting pressure on the forefoot as you walk. With a pump, your foot slides right to the forepart of the shoe, jamming everything together in a space that is too small."

To avoid problems, says Dr. Cowin, wear well-fitting shoes that don't have exceptionally high heels. "Men aren't too much of a problem; you can get them to wear pretty good shoes. With women, I recommend midheight heels rather than high ones for work. For special occasions, high heels won't hurt, but for everyday situations lower shoes are better."

"If you must wear high heels," adds Dr. Levine, "look for ones with extra cushioning in the forefoot area, or have your shoemaker put extra foam cushioning there. And if you have bad calluses on the backs of your heels, avoid open-backed shoes until the area heals."

And get a proper fit. "The most important thing when buying a shoe is fit," says Terry L. Spilken, D.P.M., a podiatrist in New York City and Edison, New Jersey. "Whether a shoe costs $20 or $200, if it doesn't fit correctly, it's going to give you problems. Make sure it's the proper length; you want a thumb's-width distance from the end of your longest toe to the end of your shoe. (And your longest toe isn't necessarily the big toe.) You should have enough width across the ball of the foot and enough room in the toe box so there's no pressure across the toes.

"Look for natural materials, like leather, that breathe. And remember that it's just as harmful for the foot to get a shoe that's too big as one that's too small. If the shoe's too big, the foot will slide in it and cause friction. And the friction of the skin rubbing can cause a callus or corn just as easily as a tight shoe that pinches."

Calluses: Who needs 'em? Maybe you do. Sometimes a little callus is good. "People who go barefoot a lot develop calluses across their soles," says Hass. "And that's desirable. They protect the skin from rough terrain or ground heat. If sufficiently developed and toughened, they can even ward off cutting by sharp objects. These calluses are rarely painful."

Sometimes a callus develops as a safeguard against an ingrowing toenail. As the sharp-edged nail bites into the adjoining tissue, the skin thickens and hardens to prevent further intrusion.

Should you develop this kind of callus, you must leave it in peace, says Dr. Hass. If it proves painful, get temporary relief by soaking the foot in warm, soapy water, but do not ever attempt to hone it. If it becomes too painful, consult a doctor to have the ingrowing nail fixed.

Cuts and Scrapes

13 Ways to Soothe a Sore

You're trotting up the stairs, proud of yourself for avoiding the escalator. Your feet tap a rhythm against the concrete and steel. Then suddenly, your foot misses a beat and you begin to fall.

Your hands swing to the front to block, your knees bend to catch. Just as suddenly, it's over. You survey the damage as you peel each appendage from the rock-hard floor.

Bandage Busters

Got a boo-boo? Bandage made it all better? Until you have to pull the adhesive strip off, that is.

Here are a couple of tricks to help you remove adhesive bandages painlessly. The first two tips are courtesy of a New England high school nurse, and the last comes from Ed Watson, corporate spokesman for Johnson & Johnson.

- Use a tiny pair of scissors to separate the bandage part from the adhesive sections. Pull it gently away from your scrape. Then remove the adhesive strips.
- If your scab is stuck to the bandage, soak the area in a mixture of warm water and salt—about a teaspoon of salt to a gallon of water. Have patience. The dressing will eventually let go.
- If the bandage is stuck on your forearm, leg, or chest hair, pull in the direction of hair growth, says Watson. Use a cotton swab saturated in baby oil or rubbing alcohol to moisten the adhesive fully before pulling away from the skin.

The palms of your hands look like beavers have chewed on them, they're scraped with a dozen tiny scratches now welling with blood.

Your knees did a great job of breaking the fall. But one knee is cut and beginning to ooze dark red rivulets. And for a second—before the stinging edges into your consciousness—it reminds you of the scabby knees you wore when you were 10.

Life is full of unpleasant little surprises like this fall. You slice a finger instead of a cucumber when making a salad; your dog gets too affectionate and accidentally scratches your arm; your hand slips while you're doing a home repair, and the wrench wrenches you instead of a bolt.

But you can do your own home repairs on these little cuts and scrapes of life with items you probably have stored in your kitchen or medicine cabinet. Here's the first-aid information you need to do the work.

Stop the bleeding. The fastest way to stop bleeding is to apply direct pressure. Place a clean, absorbent cloth—a bandage or a towel—over the cut, then press your hand against it firmly. If you don't have a cloth, use your fingers. This will usually stop the bleeding within a minute or two. If blood soaks through your first bandage, add a second one and press steadily. Add new bandages over old ones because removing a cloth may tear off coagulating blood cells.

Choosing
an Over-the-Counter Ointment

Look under "First Aid" on any pharmacy shelf. It can be a consumer's nightmare. What to choose? An antibacterial ointment? Perhaps something labeled "first-aid cream." Or should you choose the spray the advertisements claim doesn't sting?

In one study, James J. Leyden, M.D., compared the effectiveness of nine over-the-counter products on wound healing. He found that some products are faster than others when it comes to the time it takes to mend minor cuts, scrapes, and burns. Here's what the research showed.

- Polysporin (active ingredients: polymyxin B, bacitracin ointment): 8.2 days
- Neosporin (active ingredients: neomycin, polymyxin B, bacitracin ointment): 9.2 days
- Johnson & Johnson First Aid Cream (wound protectant with no antibiotic agent): 9.8 days
- Mercurochrome (active ingredient: merbromin): 13.1 days
- No treatment: 13.3 days
- Bactine spray (active ingredient: benzalkonium chloride): 14.2 days
- Merthiolate (active ingredient: thimerosol): 14.2 days
- Hydrogen peroxide 3%: 14.3 days
- Campho-Phenique (active ingredients: camphor, phenol): 15.4 days
- Tincture of iodine: 15.7 days

If applying pressure doesn't stop the bleeding, elevate the limb above the level of the heart to reduce the pressure of blood on the cut. Continue applying pressure all the while. This should stem the bleeding.

Clean the wound. This is important to prevent infection and to decrease the chance of permanent discoloration, or tattooing. Wash the area with soap and water or just water, says Hugh Macaulay, M.D., emergency room physician at Aspen Valley Hospital in Aspen, Colorado. The object is to dilute the bacteria in the wound and remove debris. Also, if you don't remove stones or sand from the cut, they can leave pigment under the skin, which acts like a tattoo. Gently clean your cut twice a day.

Strap it up. When the bleeding stops or slows, tie the wound firmly with a cloth or wrap with an elastic bandage so there is pressure against the cut, *but do not cut circulation off,* says John Gillies, an emergency medical technician and program director for health services

---

MEDICAL ALERT

Doctor Your Wound with Professional Advice

First aid isn't always enough. See a doctor when:

- Bleeding is bright red and spurting. You may have punctured an artery.
- You can't wash all the debris out of the wound.
- The cut or scrape is on your face or any other area where you want to minimize scarring.
- Your wound develops any red streaks, weeps pus, or redness extends more than a finger width beyond the cut.
- The wound is large and you "can see way down inside," says Hugh Macaulay, M.D. You may need stitches. But don't attempt home-stitchery, even if you are stranded far from medical help.

---

at Colorado Outward Bound School in Denver. If the cut is on an arm or leg, you can check circulation to that area by squeezing a fingernail or toenail. The nail should turn white, then when you release it, pink again. If necessary, loosen the bandage a little.

Go for extra pressure. If the cut continues to bleed, it is more serious than you thought and you probably need to see a doctor immediately. Until you get there, add a pressure point to your efforts. Press on the point nearest the cut but between the wound and the heart. The pressure points are places you might think of when taking a pulse: inside your wrists, inside your upper arm about halfway between the elbow and armpit, and in the groin where your legs attach to your torso. Press the artery against the bone. Stop pressing about a minute after the bleeding stops. If bleeding starts again, reapply pressure to the pressure point.

Don't use a tourniquet. With most everyday cuts and scrapes, first aid is plenty. Tourniquets are extreme and dangerous. "Once you apply a tourniquet, the person may end up losing that limb because you cut off all circulation," cautions Gillies.

Smear on an over-the-counter antibiotic ointment. Broad-spectrum antibacterial ointments work best, according to James J. Leyden, M.D., professor of dermatology at the University of Pennsylvania. (See "Choosing an Over-the-Counter Ointment," on page 173.)

People who use a triple antibiotic ointment and the right kind of bandage heal 30 percent faster, says Patricia Mertz, research associate professor at the University of Miami School of Medicine, who studies how wounds heal.

Still, Mertz warns, be wary of over-the-counter drugs that contain neomycin or ointments that contain a lot of preservatives. They can cause an allergic reaction. If you have an allergic reaction to the ointment, your scrape will get red and itchy and may become infected.

"In our tests," Mertz says, "we found Polysporin ointment was the best performer and Merthiolate the worst offender for irritation."

Keep it undercover. When exposed to air, cuts form scabs, which slow down new cell growth, says Mertz. She recommends a plastic bandage similar to food wrap. They come in all sizes. Most bandage

---

The Alternate Route

Healing Can Be a Sweet Success

Got a cut or wound? You can speed up the healing process with a little table sugar, says Richard A. Knutson, M.D., an orthopedic surgeon at Delta Medical Center in Greenville, Mississippi. He's treated more than 5,000 serious wounds over the past ten years with a mixture of tamed iodine and sugar, healing a variety of mishaps from cuts, scrapes, and burns to amputated fingertips. (Raw iodine will burn the skin.)

Sugar, he says, leaves bacteria without the nutrients necessary to grow or multiply. Wounds usually heal quickly, without a scab and often with little scarring. Keloids (irregular, large scars) are kept to a minimum.

Brew one of Dr. Knutson's sugary ointments by mixing household table sugar with Betadine (an iodine-based antibacterial wash available at any local pharmacy). To make a blend, mix ½ ounce of Betadine solution, 5 ounces of sugar, and 1½ ounces of Betadine ointment. Pack a cleaned wound with the homemade ointment and cover carefully with gauze. Four times a day, rinse the area gently with tap water and hydrogen peroxide and pack on fresh ointment. Taper off as healing progresses.

Caution: Make sure the wound is clean and the bleeding has stopped before applying the mixture. Sugar will make a bleeding wound bleed more. Don't use powdered sugar or brown sugar, Dr. Knutson advises. They will work, but the starch in them neutralizes the iodine. Wounds treated with those sugars will form crusts.

manufacturers make them. Or, she says, look for gauze impregnated with petroleum jelly. Both types of bandages trap healing moisture in the wound but allow only a little air to pass through. Cells regenerate more rapidly when moist.

Top it off with a tetanus shot. Cut your thumb on a sharp knife? Nick your hand on a rusty nail? Scrape your knee on the concrete? Small or large cuts should remind you to keep your immunizations current. If you haven't had a tetanus shot in the past five years, you need a booster, says Dr. Macaulay. Local health departments usually give them for a minimal fee or for free, he adds. If you don't remember when you had your last booster, it's a good idea to have one within 24 hours of the injury.

PANEL OF ADVISERS

John Gillies, E.M.T., is an emergency medical technician and program director for health services at the Colorado Outward Bound School in Denver.

Richard A. Knutson, M.D., is an orthopedic surgeon at Delta Medical Center in Greenville, Mississippi.

James J. Leyden, M.D., is a professor of dermatology in the Department of Dermatology at the University of Pennsylvania in Philadelphia.

Hugh Macaulay, M.D., is an emergency room physician at Aspen Valley Hospital in Aspen, Colorado.

Patricia Mertz is a research associate professor in the Department of Dermatology and Cutaneous Surgery at the University of Miami School of Medicine in Florida.

Dandruff

18 Tips to Stop Flaking

Sometimes it's good to be a little "flaky." You know, a little offbeat. A little creative. It gives you character. Makes you unique—memorable. But if all that people remember about you is your flaking dandruff, your flakiness is off in the wrong direction.

And you are not alone. Some hairdressers say dandruff is the single most common scalp complaint their patrons have. And dermatologists agree that virtually everyone has the problem to some degree.

So if you're just itching to get to the root of this head-scratching problem, listen to the experts.

Don't ignore it. Whatever you do, don't ignore your dandruff or fall into a scratch-and-itch cycle, says Maria Hordinsky, M.D., a dermatologist and assistant professor at the University of Minnesota Medical School–Minneapolis. Ignoring the condition lets the scaling build up on your scalp. That in turn can cause itching, which can lead to scratching. Scratching too vigorously can wound the scalp and leave it open to infection.

Shampoo often! The experts are unanimous on this point: Wash your hair often — every day if necessary. "Generally, the more frequently you shampoo, the easier it is to control the dandruff," says New Orleans dermatologist Patricia Farris, M.D., a clinical assistant professor at Tulane University School of Medicine.

Start mild. Often a mild, nonmedicated shampoo is enough to control the problem. Dandruff is frequently caused by an overly oily scalp, says New York City hair care specialist Philip Kingsley. Shampooing daily with a mild brand diluted with an equal amount of distilled water can control the oil without aggravating your scalp.

Then get tough. If regular shampoos aren't doing the job, switch to an antidandruff formula. Dandruff shampoos are classified by their active ingredients, which work in different ways. According to Diana Bihova, M.D., New York City dermatologist and clinical instructor at New York University Medical Center, those with selenium sulfide or zinc pyrithione work fastest, retarding the rate at which scalp cells multiply. Those with salicylic acid and sulfur loosen flakes so they can be washed away easily. Those with antibacterial agents cut down bacteria on the scalp and reduce the chance of infection. Those with tar retard cell growth.

Beat the tar out of it. "For very stubborn cases, I recommend tar-based formulas," says Dr. Farris. "Lather with the tar shampoo and then leave it on for 5 or 10 minutes so the tar has a chance to work." Most people rinse dandruff shampoos off too quickly, she says.

If you've avoided tar shampoos because you remember them as having unpleasant smells, be aware that many newer formulas are much more pleasant.

Don't be too harsh. If tar-based shampoos — or any other dandruff preparations — are too harsh for everyday use, alternate them with your regular shampoo, says Dr. Farris.

MEDICAL ALERT

Is It Dandruff or Dermatitis?

Severe dandruff is actually a disease known as seborrheic dermatitis, which requires prescription medications. See a doctor if you have:

- Scalp irritation
- Thick scale despite regular use of dandruff shampoos
- Yellowish crusting
- Red patches, especially along the neckline

Don't mix black with blond. If you have blond or silver hair, you might want to think twice about tar-based shampoos. They can give light hair a brownish stain, says Dr. Farris.

Lather twice. Always lather twice with a dandruff shampoo, says R. Jeffrey Herten, M.D., assistant clinical professor of dermatology at the University of California, Irvine, California College of Medicine. Work up the first lather as soon as you step into the shower so the shampoo has sufficient time to work. Leave it on until you're just about finished with your shower. Then rinse your hair very thoroughly. Follow that with a quick second lather and rinse. The second rinse will leave just a bit of the medication on your scalp so it can work until your next shampoo.

Cap it. Dr. Bihova has still another approach to improving the effectiveness of medicated shampoos. After you lather up, put a shower cap on over your wet hair. Leave it on for an hour, then rinse as usual.

Switch-hit. If you've found a brand of shampoo that works well for you, keep using it, says Toronto dermatologist Howard Donsky, M.D., an associate professor at the University of Toronto. Be aware, however, that your skin can adapt to a shampoo's ingredients, so you'd be wise to change your brand every few months to maintain its effectiveness.

Massage it in. When shampooing, says Dr. Farris, gently massage your scalp with your fingertips to help loosen scales and flakes. But don't scratch your scalp, she warns. That can lead to sores that are worse than the dandruff.

Flake off. Louisville dermatologist Joseph F. Fowler, Jr., M.D., an assistant professor at the University of Louisville, recommends an over-the-counter product called P&S Liquid for people with particularly stubborn scaling and crusting. Apply it to your scalp at bedtime and cover your hair with a shower cap. Wash it out in the morning. Although you can use this preparation every night, Dr. Fowler recommends once-a-week treatments. "It's just too messy for daily use," he says.

Invest some extra thyme. Thyme is reputed to have mild antiseptic properties that can help alleviate dandruff, says New York City hair stylist Louis Gignac. Make an effective rinse by boiling 4 heaping tablespoons of dried thyme in 2 cups of water for 10 minutes. Strain the brew and allow it to cool. Pour half the mixture over clean damp hair, making sure the liquid covers the scalp. Massage in gently. Do not rinse. Save the remainder for another day.

Steer clear of beer. If you use beer as a rinse and styling lotion, it may be causing your dandruff, says Gignac. Beer can dry out your scalp and eventually lead to dandruff, he says.

Get into condition. Although dandruff shampoos are effective on your scalp, they can be a little harsh on your hair, says Dr. Farris. So be sure to apply conditioner after every shampoo to counteract their effects.

Strike oil. Although excess scalp oil can cause problems, an occasional warm-oil treatment helps loosen and soften dandruff scales, says Dr. Herten. Heat a few ounces of olive oil on the stove until just warm. Wet your hair (otherwise the oil will soak into your hair instead of reaching your scalp), then apply the oil directly to your scalp with a brush or cotton ball. Section your hair as you go so you treat just the scalp. Put on a shower cap and leave it on for 30 minutes. Then wash out the oil with a dandruff shampoo.

Let the sun shine. "A little sun exposure is good for dandruff," says Dr. Fowler. That's because direct ultraviolet light has an anti-inflammatory effect on scaly skin conditions. And it may explain why dandruff tends to be less severe in summer.

But by all means, says Dr. Fowler, use sun sense. Don't sunbathe; just spend a little time outdoors. Limit sun exposure to 30 minutes or less per day. And wear your normal sunscreen on exposed skin. "You have to balance the sun's benefit to your scalp against its harmful effect on your skin in general," he advises.

Calm down. Don't overlook the role emotions play in triggering or worsening skin conditions such as dandruff and other forms of dermatitis. These conditions are often made worse by stress, says Dr. Fowler. So if your emotions are overtaxed, look for ways to counteract the stress. Exercise. Meditate. Get away from it all. And don't worry so much about your dandruff!

PANEL OF ADVISERS

Diana Bihova, M.D., is a dermatologist in private practice and clinical instructor of dermatology at New York University Medical Center in New York City. She is coauthor of *Beauty from the Inside Out.*

Howard Donsky, M.D., is an associate professor of medicine at the University of Toronto and staff dermatologist at Toronto General Hospital. He is author of *Beauty Is Skin Deep.*

Patricia Farris, M.D., is a dermatologist in private practice in New Orleans, Louisiana. She is also clinical assistant professor of dermatology at Tulane University School of Medicine in New Orleans.

Joseph F. Fowler, Jr., M.D., is a dermatologist in private practice in Louisville, Kentucky. He is also assistant professor of dermatology at the University of Louisville. In addition, he is a member of the North American Contact Dermatitis Group, an elite skin-allergy research group.

Louis Gignac is a New York City hair stylist who is the owner of the Louis-Guy D Salon. He is also the author of *Everything You Need to Know to Have Great-Looking Hair.*

R. Jeffrey Herten, M.D., is assistant clinical professor of dermatology at the University of California, Irvine, California College of Medicine.

Maria Hordinsky, M.D., is a dermatologist in private practice in Minneapolis. She is also assistant professor of dermatology at the University of Minnesota Medical School–Minneapolis.

Philip Kingsley is a trained trichologist (hair care specialist) who maintains salons in New York City and London. He is the author of *The Complete Hair Book.*

Denture Troubles

14 Ideas for a More Secure Smile

Everyone knows George Washington sported a set of dentures. But did you know that troublesome tusks ruined a world cruise for President Ulysses S. Grant? The bearded president, perhaps while admiring the whitecaps, leaned over the rail and, oops, down went his dentures into the briny deep.

You have to pity those poor denture wearers of yesterday. Before the age of super-sticky denture creams and pastes, artificial teeth were so loose, many people removed them while they were eating.

Thank goodness things have changed. Or have they? If you're wearing a new set of dentures, you may be wrestling with some of the age-old problems: sore mouth, difficulty in eating or talking, dentures that slip, and a feeling that perhaps they just don't look real.

Today, denture wearers have several choices of dental ware. There are partial and full dentures, those that can be removed, and those that are implanted into the bone and become like real teeth.

All of them, like any artificial body part, take some getting used to, says prosthodontist George A. Murrell, D.D.S., of Manhattan Beach, California, who teaches at the University of Southern California School of Dentistry. He and other specialists have some suggestions.

Look in the mirror. Smile. Frown. Be happy. Be sad. Be serious. Practice what you look like so you'll be more confident in front of other people, says Dr. Murrell.

Practice talking. Say your vowels. Recite your consonants, says Jerry F. Taintor, D.D.S., chairman of endodontics at the University of Tennessee College of Dentistry. Practice will help you learn to talk around the appliance in your mouth.

Make a video. Videos are valuable for several reasons, says Dr. Murrell. They give you a stranger's-eye view of how you look. Plus you can show the tape to a dentist, who can use the pictures to decipher problems in jaw muscles or lip movements.

Watch out for toothpicks. Those tiny wooden spikes are especially dangerous for denture wearers, says Dr. Taintor. "You lose a lot of your tactile sense with dentures. You bite into a toothpick, but you don't know it because you can't feel it. You can get it lodged in your throat."

Read a book. And read aloud. "Having dentures is like having a prosthetic limb," Dr. Taintor says. "You have to practice using it to use it well." Read out loud to yourself, he says. Listen to your pronunciation and your diction and correct what doesn't sound right.

Use an adhesive. If you feel your new teeth are a less-than-perfect fit, says Dr. Taintor, "There's nothing wrong with using a denture adhesive during that adjustment period. It's when you have to use the adhesive all the time that you need to have the denture refitted." You can find over-the-counter denture adhesives—a type of soft paste that will form a vacuum between your gums and your dentures to temporarily "glue" them together—in any drugstore.

Start soft and slow. No, you're not doomed to baby foods the rest of your life, but start soft, says Dr. Taintor. Gradually increase the texture and hardness of your food so your gums and your ability to use the dentures build on good experience.

Scrub with soap and water. When you're finished eating, take your dentures out and scrub them with plain soap and lukewarm water.

Get those choppers clean. If you wear implants, you'll need to set up a twice-daily cleaning ritual just like you had when you were caring for your original teeth, says Dr. Murrell. "We can do beautiful dentistry, but it won't last if it isn't taken care of." Some of the brushes may be a little different, but the idea is still the same. Get those choppers clean.

Baby your mouth. "Babies are born with plaque in their mouths," says Eric Shapira, D.D.S., a dentist in El Granada, California, and assistant clinical professor and lecturer at the University of the Pacific School of Dentistry. "Even if you have no teeth, you need to wash your gums to remove the plaque." Use a soft brush and gently whisk away at your gums, he says. You shouldn't brush hard enough to make the inside of your mouth sore. A good cleaning will lessen the possibility of bad breath and help your gums stay healthier, he says.

Try a lozenge. One common complaint, says Dr. Murrell, is excess saliva during the first few weeks of wearing dentures. Solve this problem neatly by sucking on a lozenge frequently for the first couple of days. This will help you swallow more frequently and get rid of some of the excess.

Massage your gums. Place your thumb and index finger over your gums (index on the outside) and massage them, says Richard Shepard, D.D.S., of Durango, Colorado. This will promote circulation and give your gums a healthy firmness.

Rinse with salty water. To help clean your gums, rinse your mouth daily with a glass of warm water mixed with a teaspoon of salt, says Dr. Taintor.

Give your gums a rest. When you can, take out your teeth and let your gums do nothing for a while, says Dr. Taintor.

PANEL OF ADVISERS

George A. Murrell, D.D.S., is a prosthodontist in private practice in Manhattan Beach, California, who teaches at the University of Southern California School of Dentistry in Los Angeles.

Eric Shapira, D.D.S., is in private practice in El Granada, California. He is an assistant clinical professor and lecturer at the University of the Pacific School of Dentistry in San Francisco and has a master's degree in science and biochemistry.

Richard Shepard, D.D.S., is a retired dentist in Durango, Colorado. He edits the newsletter for the Holistic Dental Association.

Jerry F. Taintor, D.D.S., is chairman of endodontics at the University of Tennessee College of Dentistry in Memphis. He is author of *The Oral Report: The Consumer's Common Sense Guide to Better Dental Care.*

Depression

22 Ways to Beat the Blues

Life (oweeeee!) might be compared to a roller coaster. Rich man, poor man, beggar man, thief. Doctor, lawyer, Indian chief. *Everyone* has ups and downs. Why, even top experts on depression occasionally get bottomed out.

But what these depression experts know from experience is that nearly all cases of depression can be reversed—even the most serious ones. And for the not-so-serious ones (call them the blues, the blahs, or the I-just-don't-want-to-get-out-of-bed days), some very simple techniques can work wonders.

So if you're feeling down in the dumps, melancholy, like life is dragging you down and dragging you out, try one of these proven methods for making your spirits soar.

Sit back and enjoy (or at least tolerate) the tumble. Benjamin Franklin said that nothing is certain in this world but death and taxes. He missed something: sadness.

"Realize that feeling a little bad is no big deal," says William Knaus, Ed.D., a private practice psychologist in Long Meadow, Massachusetts. Psychologist Fred Strassburger, Ph.D., associate clinical professor of psychiatry at the George Washington University School of Medicine, adds: "Understand that the down feelings are temporary—don't get sadder because you're sad."

Do something active. Hanging around the house and moping is sure to make you more depressed. So this home remedy involves getting *away* from home. It doesn't matter much what you choose to do, as long as it's something *active*, says Jonathan W. Stewart, M.D., a research psychiatrist at the New York State Psychiatric Institute in New

York City. Go for a walk, take a bike ride, visit a friend, play a game of chess, read a book, or become a Big Brother. Turning the knob on the television set, however, is *not* being active.

Search your memory for fun things to do. The best way to pick an activity is to start by jotting down a list of things you enjoy. The problem, of course, is that nothing looks too enjoyable when you're down and out. What to do? List activities that you *used* to enjoy, suggests C. Eugene Walker, Ph.D., a professor of psychology and director of training in pediatric psychology at the University of Oklahoma Health Sciences Center. Then, pick one—and do it!

Talk it out. "It's always helpful to share your feelings with someone," says Bonnie R. Strickland, Ph.D., a professor of psychology at the University of Massachusetts at Amherst. "Find friends who care about you and tell them what's on your mind."

Helping Others through Depression

What's the best thing to do if someone close to you gets depressed?

"Listen," says family therapist Robert Jaffe, Ph.D., "more than anything, your friend needs an ear."

If someone you care about seems depressed and hasn't said anything about it, go ahead and ask, "Do you feel depressed?" suggests Dr. Jaffe. Follow up with open-ended questions, like "When did you first start feeling this way?" This is a good question, says Dr. Jaffe, because determining when a depression began often helps uncover the incident or incidents that might have sparked it.

Here are other helpful hints Dr. Jaffe recommends.

- As your friend opens up and starts talking about his depression, do your best to create a safe environment. *Don't* trivialize the situation by saying things like "Oh, cut it out, you have no reason to be depressed."
- *Don't* offer easy solutions like "You know, all you need is . . ." Instead, let the person find *his own* solutions, using you as a sounding board for ideas.
- *Do* try to get the depressed person involved in physical activities like exercise.
- *Do* try to keep the person interested in finding solutions. "Remember," says Dr. Jaffe, "depression could be defined as a loss of interest in all things."

Have a good cry. If talking about your problems leads to tears — let them flow. "Crying is a wonderful release — especially if you know what you're crying about," says Robert Jaffe, Ph.D., a marriage and family therapist in Sherman Oaks, California.

Sit down and analyze the situation. "A lot of times, if you can pinpoint the source of your depression, you'll feel a lot better," says Dr. Strassburger. "Once you understand the problem, you can begin to figure out what you need to do about it."

Try and try again—then quit. "As kids and adolescents, we have ideas of what life will bring, and sometimes we hang on to them even when life dictates that these ideas are unrealistic," says Arnold H. Gessel, M.D., a private practice psychiatrist in Broomall, Pennsylvania. Chasing elusive goals can lead to depression, he says. This is when you simply have to say "I've given it my best shot" — and give up.

The Alternate Route

The Nutrition Prescription

Nutrition—more than anything else—controls your state of mind, claims Priscilla Slagle, M.D., an associate clinical professor at the University of California, Los Angeles, UCLA School of Medicine. The most beneficial nutrients for battling depression? Above all, she says, it's B vitamins and certain amino acids. Here's her formula.

If you're feeling down, try 1,000 to 3,000 milligrams of the amino acid L-tyrosine first thing in the morning (on an empty stomach), followed by a B-complex vitamin supplement 30 minutes later, with breakfast, suggests Dr. Slagle.

L-tyrosine converts in the brain to norepinephrine, a chemical that promotes positive moods and gives us motivation and drive, she says. The B-complex vitamins, particularly vitamin B6, allow the body to metabolize amino acids.

"I don't know anyone with a mild problem who hasn't responded to this treatment," says Dr. Slagle. However, you should get your doctor's approval before starting supplement therapy.

Representatives from both the American Medical Association and the American Psychiatric Association say they haven't seen enough research to give either a thumbs-up or a thumbs-down to Dr. Slagle's claims.

Exercise. Numerous studies show that exercise can help overcome the blues. If you *already* exercise regularly and are in good physical shape but poor mental shape, consider "going for total exhaustion," suggests Dr. Gessel. "It's a good way to discharge your tensions."

Pick up a box of crayons. A great way to express your feelings is by writing them down, or better yet, by *drawing* them, says Ellen McGrath, Ph.D., chairwoman of the American Psychological Association's National Task Force on Women and Depression and clinical associate professor at New York University. If you sit down immediately after something upsets you and start to draw, you might be surprised at the insight you'll gain into your emotions, she says. Use lots of color. A choice of red could suggest anger; black, sadness; and gray, anxiety.

Adjust the facts, ma'am. "Sometimes when you start to gauge your assumptions against reality, you may find things aren't as you think they are," says Dr. Knaus. For instance, if you suspect your lover

---

MEDICAL ALERT

When It's Time to Seek Help

If you're feeling down and out and the feeling persists—even though you've tried all you know to beat it—it may be time to see a mental health professional.

Experts at the National Institute for Mental Health suggest that anyone who experiences *four or more* of the following symptoms *for more than two weeks* should seek help.

- Persistent sad, anxious, or "empty" feelings
- Feelings of hopelessness and/or pessimism
- Feelings of guilt, worthlessness, and/or helplessness
- Loss of interest or pleasure in ordinary activities, including sex
- Sleep disturbances (including insomnia, early-morning waking, and/or oversleeping)
- Eating disturbances (changes in appetite and/or weight loss or gain)
- Decreased energy, fatigue, and/or a feeling of being "slowed down"
- Thoughts of death or suicide, or suicide attempts
- Restlessness and/or irritability
- Difficulty in concentrating, remembering, and/or making decisions

may be cheating on you (a good reason to be depressed)—go ahead and ask. You may be wrong.

Find something really boring to do. What you may need to snap you out of the blues is simply something to distract you, to shift your attention away from your woes. To do this, "pick something dreadfully boring to do and do it," suggests Dr. Knaus. For instance? Clean your bathroom tiles with a toothbrush. Or study the same leaf, again and again and again.

Slow down. Life in the twentieth century can be mighty hectic at times. If you suspect that overscheduling is at the root of your depression, then you may simply need to relax, says Dr. Strickland. "Give yourself more time for things like warm baths or massages."

Avoid making major decisions. "You can't really trust your judgment when you're depressed," says Robert S. Brown, Sr., M.D., Ph.D., professor of psychiatry at the University of Virginia School of Medicine. He advises that major life decisions should be put off till you're feeling better, lest you make the *wrong* decisions, which, of course, can only drag you down further.

Treat others with respect. Being depressed, you may be inclined to be snippy with other people, says Dr. Knaus. Don't do it, he warns, for others may be snippy right back—the last thing you need when you're down.

Stay out of department stores. Just as snapping at other people can have a boomerang effect on your depression, so can shopping binges, says Dr. Knaus. That is, while they can be loads of fun, they can come back to haunt you when the bills come in.

Close the refrigerator. Eating binges also have a boomerang effect, warns Dr. Knaus. While a binge might make you feel good at the moment, it can add depressing inches to your waistline. Get out of the house, if you have to, to fight the urge to eat.

PANEL OF ADVISERS

Robert S. Brown, Sr., M.D., Ph.D., is a professor of psychiatry at the University of Virginia School of Medicine in Charlottesville and a psychiatrist in private practice there.

Arnold H. Gessel, M.D., is a psychiatrist in private practice in Broomall, Pennsylvania. He specializes in disorders of stress and tension, and works with many Vietnam veterans.

Robert Jaffe, Ph.D., is a marriage and family therapist in Sherman Oaks, California. He holds a master's degree in counseling therapy.

William Knaus, Ed.D., is a private practice psychologist in Long Meadow, Massachusetts. He is the author of seven books, including *How to Get Out of a Rut* and *The Illusion Trap.*

Ellen McGrath, Ph.D., is a psychologist in private practice in New York City, a clinical associate professor of social sciences at New York University, and chairwoman of the American Psychological Association's National Task Force on Women and Depression.

Priscilla Slagle, M.D., is an associate clinical professor at the University of California, Los Angeles, UCLA School of Medicine and a psychiatrist in private practice in Los Angeles. She is author of *The Way Up from Down.*

Jonathan W. Stewart, M.D., is a research psychiatrist with the Depression Evaluation Service at the New York State Psychiatric Institute in New York City. He is also associate professor of clinical psychiatry at Columbia University College of Physicians and Surgeons there.

Fred Strassburger, Ph.D., is a psychologist in private practice and an associate clinical professor of psychiatry and behavioral sciences at the George Washington University School of Medicine in Washington, D.C.

Bonnie R. Strickland, Ph.D., is a professor of psychology at the University of Massachusetts at Amherst. She is a past president of the American Psychological Association.

C. Eugene Walker, Ph.D., is a professor and director of training in pediatric psychology at the University of Oklahoma Health Sciences Center in Oklahoma City.

Dermatitis and Eczema

23 Clear-Skin Remedies

Maybe the first question you asked yourself after the doctor diagnosed your condition was, "Why me? Why am I stuck with the itching and dryness of eczema? Why do I have to suffer the redness and irritation of dermatitis?"

Your doctor is perhaps best qualified to answer that question, difficult as it can be, but it may help to know that you're not alone. The latest government statistics show that close to nine million Americans suffer from some form of dermatitis every year. That's a lot of scratching.

The following tips are designed to help those with physician-diagnosed conditions of eczema or dermatitis control the itching and dryness that typically accompany those afflictions.

The experts tell us that, in general, the best way to treat the itching of eczema and dermatitis at home is to keep dry, patchy skin moist and well lubricated. For that reason, many of the remedies offered in Dry Skin and Winter Itch, beginning on page 224, may help with this problem as well.

Got a Nickel Rash?

"Nickel dermatitis is probably the most common contact dermatitis going," says Howard Donsky, M.D. "But people often don't suspect that that's the problem —they think they've got a problem with gold."

Nickel dermatitis occurs ten times more often in women than men, and is often triggered by ear piercing. Strangely enough, having the ears pierced can cause rashes to occur in other areas of the body whenever the person comes in contact with nickel-containing metal. Suddenly, bracelets, necklaces, and other jewelry the person has worn for years can bring on a contact rash.

If this sounds like what's happening to you, the following tips might help.

Buy posts of stainless steel. Newly pierced ears should be studded only with steel posts until the earlobes heal (about three weeks).

Stay cool. Since perspiration plays a big role in nickel dermatitis—it leaches out the nickel in nickel-plated jewelry—stay out of the heat if you're wearing this type of jewelry. Or don't wear it if you're going out in the heat.

Go for the gold. Buy only quality gold jewelry, says Dr. Donsky. "If it's less than 24-karat gold, there's some nickel in there," he says, "and the lower the karat the higher the nickel."

Don't go nickel nuts. Some European dermatologists are advising nickel-sensitive patients to watch what they eat. Having observed that nickel dermatitis can occur without any apparent contact with the metal, these doctors are telling folks to avoid apricots, chocolate, coffee, beer, tea, nuts, and other foods high in nickel.

While intriguing, the "nickel-nut" theory hasn't garnered a great following on this side of the Atlantic. "The jury's still out on foods high in nickel causing a reaction," Dr. Donsky confirms. "But if you're highly sensitive to nickel, there might be some validity to it."

Beware of dry air. Dermatitis is aggravated by dehumidified air, especially during winter months when forced-air heat circulates in the home.

"Forced-air heat is a bit more drying than other types of heat," says Howard Donsky, M.D., staff dermatologist at Toronto General Hospital in Toronto. Since dry air tends to aggravate the itching of eczema or dermatitis, keeping indoor air moist should be a primary concern of sufferers and their families. "If you can counter dry air with a good humidifier, then forced-air heat's not as much of a problem," Dr. Donsky notes.

But, the experts caution, don't expect a single room humidifier to do it all. "People think that if they put a humidifier in their place, that'll take care of it," says Hillard H. Pearlstein, M.D., a private practitioner and assistant clinical professor of dermatology at Mount Sinai School of Medicine of the City University of New York. "But humidifiers are like air conditioners—you really need a big unit to do anything. If you sleep next to it, however, that's okay. Put it next to your bed."

Like it lukewarm. The long-held belief that people with dermatitis should avoid bathing is coming under increased scrutiny. While some physicians feel excessive bathing can aggravate the condition, others feel that regular bathing reduces the chances of infection and helps soften the skin.

Our experts generally fall into the second category. "Bathe, but bathe in lukewarm water," says Dr. Donsky. "Avoid water that's either too hot or too cold."

Go for the grease. Regular soap need not be avoided in your bath as long as a moisturizer is applied after its use to keep the skin from drying out. "You can't bathe too frequently unless you grease up afterward," says Dr. Pearlstein. "The grease is what holds the water in, and dry skin is a function of water loss, not of oil loss."

Some favorite after-bath emollients (or greases, as dermatologists typically call them) include Complex-15, Eucerin, Keri, Lubriderm Lotion, or Moisturel Lotion. If your skin still seems dry after using one of those products, move up to creams such as Lubriderm Cream, Purpose, or Moisturel Cream, or ointments such as Aquaphor, Eucerin, Nivea, or Petrolatum White.

Take an oatmeal bath. For an additional soothing treat, Dr. Donsky recommends adding colloidal oatmeal like Aveeno to the bath, and even using oatmeal as a soap substitute. For the bath, pour 2 cups of colloidal oatmeal (available at pharmacies) into a tub of lukewarm water.

The term *colloidal* simply means the oatmeal has been ground to fine powder that will remain suspended in water. For use as a soap substitute, wrap colloidal oatmeal in a handkerchief, place a rubber band around the top, dunk it in water, wring it out, and use as you would a normal washcloth.

Avoid antiperspirants. Metallic salts such as aluminum chloride, aluminum sulfate, and zirconium chlorohydrate are the active ingredients in many antiperspirants, and these have been known to cause irritation in people with sensitive skin. "Usually it's the antiperspirant, as opposed to the deodorant, that's irritating," Dr. Donsky says. "I recommend that people use a product called Aqueous Zephiran, an over-the-counter product available in drugstores." Or, if you plan to continue using commercially produced antiperspirants, look for those that contain such anti-irritants as allantoinate, zinc oxide, magnesium oxide, aluminum hydroxide, or triethanolamine.

Try this OTC. Topical creams, ointments, and lotions containing cortisone are often used to alleviate the itching and inflammation of dermatitis or eczema. Hydrocortisone is the mildest member of the cortisone family of steroid hormones, and it is available as a nonirritating emollient at drugstores.

"Half-percent hydrocortisone cream is available without a prescription," says Dr. Pearlstein, "and that can help. You've got to start somewhere, and going to the drugstore and getting 0.05 percent hydrocortisone cream won't hurt you." Stronger cortisone creams can have serious side effects, however, and should not be used without a doctor's direct supervision.

Take comfort in cotton. "Cotton clothing worn next to the skin is much better than either wool or polyester, especially wool," says dermatologist John F. Romano, M.D., a clinical instructor at New York Hospital–Cornell University Medical Center. The bottom line: Avoid synthetics or itchy fabrics, as well as tight- or ill-fitting clothes. In addition to looking tacky, such clothing can trigger itching.

Stay away from fake nails. Recent research at the Cleveland Clinic Foundation has shown that acrylic manicure products can cause "frequent and obvious cases of dermatitis." Such acrylics may be present in artificial fingernails, fingernail extenders, or sculptured nails, and can cause eye, nose, and respiratory irritation in addition to allergic contact dermatitis.

MEDICAL ALERT

A Wolf in Sheep's Clothing

There once was a time when wolves roamed freely across the face of Europe and the vast continent of Asia. Occasionally, humans were attacked. Those who survived sometimes bore upon their faces the red marks of the wolf—the mark of the lupus. Other people bore similar marks but had been ravaged by no animal. These people were known to have the disease of *lupus,* the attack of the wolf.

Today, we know that lupus is actually an attack of the body upon itself. It can take two forms, sometimes affecting only the skin, other times attacking both the skin and many vital organs throughout the body. It can be brought on by exposure to sunlight, certain drugs, or emotional crisis.

Lupus always leaves its mark; a patchy, red skin rash, roughly resembling a butterfly, that appears typically on the cheeks or the bridge of the nose. As one patch heals, a new one forms. These lesions itch and form scales. The person may suffer from severe arthritic joint pain, fever, and lung inflammation. If you recognize these symptoms, contact your physician immediately. This wolf cannot be tamed at home.

Such products were once limited to salons, but they have become available for application at home. Even so, "Probably most people don't have a problem with artificial nails," says Dr. Donsky. "The problem was that the first fixatives had formaldehyde in them, and some of them still do. You can have a contact problem with that, as well as with the other polymers in artificial nails."

If you suspect an allergic reaction from such products, avoiding contact with them may be the only cure.

Compress to soothe. Cold, wet dressings can help soothe and relieve the itching associated with contact dermatitis. "I tell people to try cold milk instead of water," says Dr. Romano. "It seems to be a lot more soothing."

His recommendation: Put milk into a glass with ice cubes and let it sit for a few minutes. Then pour the milk onto a gauze pad or thin piece of cotton and apply it to the irritated skin for 2 or 3 minutes. Resoak the cloth and reapply, continuing the process for about 10 minutes.

Though Dr. Romano doesn't recommend this treatment for cases of generalized eczema or dermatitis, eczema can sometimes get so bad that it begins to ooze. This condition is known as weeping eczema, and some doctors believe it responds well to cold compresses applied several times a day. If the condition does not respond, however, consult your physician as soon as possible.

Cool with calamine. "Calamine lotion is good for many types of rashes that ooze and may need to be dried out," Dr. Romano says. "Also, calamine lotion with menthol or phenol added to it can be purchased over-the-counter at drugstores, and that seems to help itching better than calamine lotion alone."

Put your diet to the test. "Food allergies can play a big role in atopic dermatitis during childhood," says Dr. Pearlstein. "They are intimately related before age 6, and you can manipulate an infant's diet and do well in helping his skin."

Traditionally, eggs, orange juice, and milk have been implicated as eczema aggravators in children. But, says Dr. Pearlstein, "I certainly wouldn't incriminate those foods wholesale." That means parents will need to consult their physicians about trying elimination diets, just to be sure. Such diets seem to work best in infants less than 2 years old, Dr. Pearlstein says. "After age 6, we've found that food plays a minimal role in most people."

For adults, Dr. Pearlstein says he leaves diet manipulation largely in the hands of his patients. If you think there's any food you eat that has an adverse effect on your skin, avoid it and see what happens, he says. If your problem clears up, you may have a food allergy.

Avoid quick changes in air temperature. "If you have eczema," says Dr. Donsky, "then rapid temperature changes can be a problem." Going from a warm room out into cold winter air, or even from an air-conditioned room to a hot shower, can trigger itching. Wearing layers of clothing—cotton clothing—is the best way to protect yourself in the first instance, says Dr. Donsky. And, of course, persons with eczema should always avoid hot baths or showers. A little forethought can help cut down on this type of itch trigger.

Use white to wipe. For controlling the itch of contact dermatitis, "white toilet paper's best," Dr. Donsky says. "It's the dyes that irritate."

Beware of baby lotions. "Sometimes baby lotions aren't the best thing for childhood eczema," Dr. Romano says. "They have a high water content, and that can further dry and irritate the skin as evapora-

The Primrose Path

The early research looked promising. A study published in the British medical Journal *Lancet* showed a significant improvement in eczema when patients took high doses of evening primrose oil (EPO) in capsule form. Other studies, however, were unable to confirm those results and the battle over EPO is still raging.

"Evening primrose oil has gotten a lot of press," says Hillard H. Pearlstein, M.D., "but we don't think there's anything to it. There's no scientific evidence that it does anything." John F. Romano, M.D., is likewise skeptical. "There have been some reports that EPO can help in cases of atopic dermatitis, but I don't know that I'm convinced."

Those who are still tempted to try EPO should be advised that it takes a rather large number of these expensive capsules to produce results and it can take at least six months to see any results. Also, cases of "imposter EPO" have been discovered, so beware of discount prices and "no-name" brands. You can find EPO in health food stores.

tion takes place." Some of the fragrances and active ingredients in baby lotions (lanolin and mineral oil) are common causes of skin allergy.

"What you want instead are creams or ointments," he says. "Something like Eucerin Cream, Aquaphor, or Vaseline Dermatology Formula."

Rub some urea on me. "Emollients that contain urea are pretty good for relieving the itch of eczema or dermatitis," says Dr. Pearlstein. "Urea is a sloughing agent, and it's a good product. We usually use it when the skin is a little thick from rubbing and scratching."

A couple of urea-containing products to try include Carmol 10 or 20, or Ultra Mide 25. Emollients that contain lactic acid (LactiCare 1 percent or 2 percent, Aqua Lacten, or Lac-Hydrin) are also recommended.

Use antihistamines for atopics. Antihistamines block the release of histamine from mast cells, thereby reducing such classic allergy symptoms as headaches, runny nose, and itching. For that reason, "over-the-counter antihistamines such as Benadryl are good for eczema," says Dr. Romano.

Antihistamines reduce itching by preventing histamine from reaching and swelling sensitive skin cells. A note of caution, however, antihistamines must sometimes be taken in large doses to bring relief. Drowsiness can result, leading to possible problems with driving or handling dangerous machinery.

Wash once, rinse twice. When it comes to doing laundry for people with eczema or dermatitis, "it's not the detergent so much as the rinse," says Dr. Romano.

"You've got to make sure the detergent is washed out thoroughly," he says. "Don't overdetergent your clothes when washing, and always use a second rinse cycle to get all the soap out."

Get to know your eye doctor. In a 20-year study of 492 people at the Mayo Clinic in Rochester, Minnesota, 13 percent of those with atopic dermatitis developed cataracts. "There is a higher incidence of cataracts in people with atopic dermatitis," Dr. Pearlstein confirms. "Atopics should be seen by an ophthalmologist more frequently than other people."

PANEL OF ADVISERS

Howard Donsky, M.D., is an associate professor of medicine at the University of Toronto and staff dermatologist at Toronto General Hospital. He is author of *Beauty Is Skin Deep.*

Hillard H. Pearlstein, M.D., is a private practitioner and assistant clinical professor of dermatology at the Mount Sinai School of Medicine of the City University of New York in New York City.

John F. Romano, M.D., is a dermatologist and an attending physician at St. Vincent's Hospital and Medical Center of New York. He is also clinical instructor in medicine at New York Hospital–Cornell University Medical Center in New York City.

Diabetes

51 Ways to Keep It under Control

Yenta, the matchmaking insulin hormone, attaches herself to lonely, befuddled Mr. Glucose, a bachelor sugar molecule, and goes knocking at Miss Cell's door. Familiar with Yenta's knock, the spinster Miss Cell opens the door. "Have I got a match for you," Yenta tells Miss Cell, and pushes Mr. Glucose inside. Together, Mr. Glucose and Miss Cell make beautiful energy.

That is how the body's energy production is supposed to work. But for 11 million Americans with adult onset (Type II) diabetes, it doesn't. Yenta the matchmaker can't find the door (the cell's receptor) because there isn't one, or there aren't enough matchmakers to handle all the bachelor sugar molecules, or the would-be matchmakers aren't very good at their jobs. Adult onset diabetes mellitus is the result.

As a person with diabetes, you know that you are at risk for heart disease, kidney disease, atherosclerosis, nerve damage, infection, blindness, and slow healing. Each person reacts to diabetes in his own way. This means each person has to be under a doctor's care and constantly monitored. This need cannot be overstated. What's good for your diabetic friend may be bad for you.

But every diabetic's goal is to maintain his or her blood sugar and blood fat as close to normal levels as possible. A diabetic regimen has three cornerstones: nutrition, weight control, and exercise. The good news is that you can virtually eliminate all symptoms of diabetes—in other words, "control" it—by carefully following the regimen you and your doctor work out.

Here's how to begin. If you're planning any changes in your current regimen, talk it over first with your doctor.

Start with the ADA diet. The American Diabetes Association (ADA) revised its nutritional guidelines in 1986. Although knowledge of dietary needs is continually expanding, these guidelines are based on current consensus thinking. "Each person's diet should be tailored to fit individual needs and lifestyles," says registered dietitian Marion Franz, M.S., R.D., vice president of nutrition at the International Diabetes Center in Minneapolis, Minnesota. The ADA diet includes the following principles:

Load up on carbohydrates. The ADA recommends that a Type II diabetes diet include *up to* 50 to 60 percent of calories from carbohydrates. "Generally, the recommendation will be somewhere around 50 percent,"

MEDICAL ALERT

Three Dangers for Diabetics

There are three potentially dangerous acute effects of diabetes needing medical attention: hypoglycemia, hyperglycemia, and wounds. And diabetics need a doctor's care in certain circumstances when they have the flu. Here's what the experts say.

Hypoglycemia occurs when blood sugar drops too low. You can treat mild symptoms yourself (See "Self-Treatment for Mild Hypoglycemia" on page 203). Severe symptoms include headache, confusion, combative behavior, or unconsciousness. Get to a hospital emergency room immediately, where a doctor will give you intravenous glucose. "If you're having frequent hypoglycemic reactions," says Karl Sussman, M.D., American Diabetes Association past president, "see your doctor because you may need to change your regimen."

Hyperglycemia is when blood sugar rises too high. Its mild symptoms are excess urination, excess appetite or thirst, blurred vision, or dizziness. "You can be hyperglycemic and not have any symptoms, so you won't even know unless you're monitoring your blood glucose," Dr. Sussman says. Severe hyperglycemic symptoms include loss of appetite, stomach cramps, nausea and vomiting, dehydration, fatigue, deep rapid breathing, and coma.

Wounds and sores, especially on the feet and legs, get infected easily in a person with diabetes. Have them treated by a doctor.

When you think you have the flu, call your doctor right away; or get to a hospital emergency room if:

- You're vomiting or having abdominal pain.
- You have large amounts of sugar and acetone in your urine.
- Your blood sugar levels are above 200 milligrams.
- Your temperature is 100°F or more.

Franz says. Carbohydrates are either simple (sugars) or complex (starches). Each gram of carbohydrate produces 4 calories.

Go easy on the protein. The ADA says protein should amount to about 12 to 20 percent of your calories. Each gram of protein equals 4 calories.

Face the fats. The ADA wants you to cut the fat out of your diet budget. Calories from fat should account for *no more* than 30 percent of your calories. Each gram of fat produces 9 calories. Every chance you get, replace artery-clogging saturated fat with polyunsaturated or, better yet, monounsaturated fat, or with complex carbohydrates, Franz says.

Eat food with fiber. Natural fiber in food has been found to have a host of beneficial effects for everyone. That goes double for people with diabetes. The ADA advises you to gradually head for 40 grams a day. Whole wheat products, barley, oats, legumes, vegetables, and fruit are the best sources of fiber, as well as essential nutrients.

One possible benefit fiber provides diabetics is lower cholesterol levels. "The water-soluble fibers found in legumes, oats, barley, and fruit, when eaten in a low-fat diet, have been shown to lower blood fat levels," Franz says. "Because they form a gel in the gastrointestinal tract," they may also cause the energy (sugar) in food to be absorbed at a slower rate, giving your insulin a chance to keep your blood sugar on a more even keel.

Fiber also helps keep you from feeling hungry. "I think one of the main benefits of fiber is that it adds bulk to the diet," Franz says. "For Type II people who are trying to control their weight and so are on restricted calories, bulk lets people feel fuller."

Besides giving you that pleasantly satiated feeling, fiber foods are good for you. "They're often high in important vitamins and minerals," Franz says.

Cut your cholesterol. The ADA recommendation is that you should eat no more than 300 milligrams of cholesterol daily. This means cutting way down on organ meat and egg yolks and restraining yourself when it comes to meat and dairy fats. It also means adding fiber to your diet. (For more information, see Cholesterol on page 135.)

Substitute for sugar. Research shows that sucrose and table sugar, when used in equal amounts with starches, doesn't hike blood sugar levels any more than other starches, such as potatoes and wheat. Thus the ADA says you can have modest amounts of refined sugars if

Don't Let Your Feet Fail You

Except for insulin, a diabetic's weakest link is the foot. Nerve damage from diabetes lessens the sensation of pain, so diabetics may not know they've injured their feet. Blood vessel damage means injuries and infections don't heal like they should—a little sore can become gangrenous, leading to amputation. "And once you lose one leg as a result of a diabetic amputation," says podiatrist Marc A. Brenner, D.P.M., past president of the American Society of Podiatric Dermatology, "there's a 75 percent chance you'll lose the other leg within three to five years." As a diabetic, you have to develop foot consciousness. And here's how to keep your feet doing what they should—walking off weight, walking on fitness.

Take a load off the dogs. Need another reason to lose weight? Consider the pounding your feet take. "Obviously, if the feet are your foundation and you have more weight on that foundation, you're going to have more wear and tear on that foundation," Dr. Brenner says. "We in podiatric medicine see more heavy people than thin people by far."

Become a foot inspector. "Inspect your feet two or three times a day," Dr. Brenner says. "Have someone else do this for you if you don't have good eyesight." Make sure there's no redness, bruises, cuts, blisters, cracks, heat, swelling, or infection.

Keep them clean. Wash your feet well with mild soap and pat them dry every day.

Keep them dry. Use a good foot powder between the toes, and change your socks frequently.

your diabetes is under control and you're not too overweight. But otherwise, check out alternative sweeteners. "They're certainly safe to use," Franz says. The ADA has approved noncaloric sweeteners, like aspartame and saccharin, and sweeteners with calories, like fructose and sorbitol.

Proceed with caution. People with well-controlled diabetes can use fructose and sorbitol with little problem, the ADA says. Fructose raises blood sugar the least of the caloric sweeteners. But, warns New York City practitioner Stanley Mirsky, M.D., an associate clinical professor at Mount Sinai School of Medicine of the City University of New York, "in people with low insulin reserves, fructose will raise triglyceride levels."

Keep them well-maintained. Cut your toenails short and straight across. Treat athlete's foot and other minor problems promptly. Never go barefoot. Buff your calluses with a pumice stone. Don't soak your feet for prolonged periods.

Keep them warm on cold days. But don't use a hot-water bottle or heating pad because they can burn you without your knowing it.

Make sure your shoes fit well. Research has indicated that the running shoe may be better for protecting the feet of people with diabetes than expensive custom-made shoes costing hundreds of dollars. "The research and development put into both running and walking shoes has far exceeded that of the dress shoe industry," Dr. Brenner says. The running or walking shoe of today is part of the whole "foot-support system," he says. "As a result of the research put into them, you're buying a very biomechanically sound piece of equipment for your feet."

Don't forget the socks. Before you slip on one of those biomechanically sound shoes, however, make sure your socks are up to the task. "Socks are also part of the foot-support system," Dr. Brenner says. For athletic or casual wear with either walking or running shoes, Dr. Brenner recommends Thor-Lo socks, which come in 11 sports-specific varieties. Most boast thick, cushioned heel and toe pads that help protect the feet of those with diabetes.

While there are no dress socks currently being made for people with diabetes, Dr. Brenner says it's quite possible a specialized dress sock will be developed in the near future.

And in large amounts, Dr. Mirsky says, both fructose and sorbitol can cause diarrhea.

Beware: calories ahead. Calorie-rich fructose and sorbitol, both found in fruit (sorbitol breaks down in the body to form fructose), are *not* exchanges for the noncaloric sweeteners. So if you've added fructose and taken out saccharin, you've still added calories to your diet.

Eat smaller meals more often. The diabetic body can handle smaller meals more easily because the smaller the meal, the less insulin is needed to handle the glucose influx from each meal, Franz says. Less glucose equals less insulin equals more constant blood sugar levels. Some diabetes meal plans call for three meals a day or three small meals plus one or two small snacks between meals. Franz says she favors more actual meals because "often if people go too long between meals they get so hungry they can't control what they eat at the next meal." She also recommends snacks like a piece of fruit or a couple of crackers between meals.

Use care with alcohol. The ADA recommends you drink no more than 2 ounces of liquor twice weekly. That's 3 ounces of distilled beverage, 8 ounces of wine, or 24 ounces of beer. Take your drink with food. Light beer and dry wine may be the way to go because they have fewer carbohydrates.

Treat booze like fat. Exchange alcohol calories for fat calories, the ADA says, because alcohol is high in calories per gram and because it's metabolized like fat.

Don't take fish oil. Omega-3 capsules may help prevent atherosclerosis, another diabetes complication. "But it's been shown to increase blood glucose levels if you take too much of it, simply because it's high calorie," says New York City physician Ronald Hoffman, M.D., medical director of the Hoffman Center for Holistic Medicine. One study showed what the researchers called a "rapid metabolic deterioration" when 5.5 grams of omega-3 were taken daily for a month. But eating fatty fish is encouraged.

Lose weight. "Weight loss is the number one priority," Dr. Mirsky says. Eighty percent of Type II diabetics are overweight. They tend to live a sedentary life and eat a lot. Obesity may obliterate insulin receptors so sugar can't enter the cells and remains in your blood. If you're overweight, diet and exercise will almost certainly help you lose some weight and get your blood sugar back to normal, and that may be all you need, Dr. Mirsky says. "Sometimes, all you have to lose is 5 or 10 pounds and you're fine."

Don't go to extremes. Maybe you've tried every fad diet, even tried fasting, and still haven't lost weight. There's some evidence that it might be harder for a person with diabetes to shed pounds than for a person without diabetes, Franz says. She prefers to advise weight *control*, "which may or may not include weight loss, but always includes improved eating habits and exercise. And that helps control blood sugar and blood fat levels."

Self-Treatment for Mild Hypoglycemia

Hypoglycemia occurs when blood sugar drops too low. Because keeping their blood sugar at normal levels requires quite a balancing act, diabetics are particularly prone to hypoglycemia. People with adult-onset diabetes usually get hypoglycemia from skipping or delaying meals, or from unplanned-for strenuous exercise.

Symptoms of mild hypoglycemia include numbness in the mouth, cool wet skin, a fluttering feeling in the chest, and hunger.

To treat it yourself, says American Diabetes Association past president Karl Sussman, M.D., associate chief of staff for research and development at the Veterans Administration Hospital in Denver, Colorado, "you need to take some form of sugar that's readily available." Drink something sweet like orange juice or soda, or eat a candy bar, he says, and be ready for it by carrying candy or mints with you.

Don't let frustration drive you to a fad diet, Franz warns. "If all the fad diets worked, we wouldn't need new ones all the time. They may not be nutritionally sound, and they may be so restrictive people can't stick with them. Plus, they don't help you change your eating behavior in the long run."

For a Type II diabetic who isn't on insulin or oral antidiabetic drugs, "fasting for a day is probably no more dangerous than it is for anyone," Franz says. If you're controlling your diabetes with diet and exercise, fasting "won't hurt, but it probably won't help either. You won't lose even 1 pound of fat by fasting for a day, and the danger is that you'll often overcompensate the next day by eating too much."

Nor should you skip meals in hopes of losing weight, Franz says. This "mini-fasting" is ultimately self-defeating. "So many people skip breakfast and lunch. Then they go on an eating binge later." Fads, fasting, and skipping meals won't work, and sooner or later you could end up losing control of your diabetes altogether.

Make it a family affair. "If the whole family doesn't make these nutritional changes to improve eating habits and control weight," Franz says, "it will be hard, if not impossible, for the person with diabetes to do it alone."

The Alternate Route

One Doctor's Supplement Regimen

While the American Diabetes Association diet is adequate in Recommended Dietary Allowances of vitamins and minerals if followed carefully, says Ronald Hoffman, M.D., diabetes increases the need for certain nutrients to help maintain normal blood sugar levels and prevent complications.

Depending on your individual needs, *as determined in consultation with your doctor,* you may want to take one or more of these supplements. Always take them immediately after meals, unless otherwise noted. Aware that these supplements can have potent, even toxic, effects, Dr. Hoffman monitors his diabetic patients closely. Don't even consider taking these supplements without your doctor's approval and close supervision. Also, don't exceed your doctor's recommended dose.

Chromium G.T.F. G.T.F. stands for glucose tolerance factor, Dr. Hoffman says. It's sold in health food stores. "What it seems to do is enhance the effect of insulin," he says. Dr. Hoffman recommends chromium picolinate, the form that's most "bioavailable." Many forms of chromium are from brewer's yeast, "so those with candida or with yeast allergy should avoid yeast sources of chromium."

Niacin. This important B vitamin "helps potentiate the effects of chromium," Dr. Hoffman says. Take it in the middle of your meals. He warns, however, that high levels of niacin can be harmful, especially to people with diabetes, so limit your intake and have it monitored by a physician.

Inositol. Another B vitamin, found in lecithin, "inositol is helpful in protecting the nerves from damage by high sugar levels," Dr. Hoffman says.

Exercise. The benefits of regular exercise for everybody, diabetic or not, are well recognized. But diabetics have even more reason to get their arms and legs moving and their hearts pumping. Exercise strengthens the heartbeat, helps control blood sugar levels, and increases circulation to the body's extremities. Exercise can cut the level of cholesterol and triglycerides while raising the level of high-density lipoproteins (the "good" cholesterol that protects against heart disease). It helps you control your weight, increases your stamina, and lets you sleep more soundly. And it really helps shore up your emotional fortitude. "Regular exercise has been shown to have beneficial effects on mood, especially for

Anthocyanic acid. Also called blueberry extract, anthocyanic acid lowers blood sugar, he says.

Vitamin C. This vitamin helps fight infection, heal wounds, and form collagen (the body's building blocks of protein, found in all tissues).

Zinc. "It's very important in diabetes," Dr. Hoffman says. "It's helpful for immunity and tissue repair." The picolinate or gluconate form is best.

Magnesium. "Diabetics tend to lose magnesium through the kidneys," he says. "Magnesium is very important for cell energy production." Take the chelated form.

Vitamin B$_6$. "B$_6$ is an important co-factor in many cellular reactions, and many diabetics seem to have a higher requirement for it," Dr. Hoffman says. B$_6$, however, is toxic in high doses and its use must be monitored by a physician.

Thiamine (vitamin B$_1$.) "B$_1$ is especially important in sugar metabolism," he says.

Garlic. "Diabetics tend to develop yeast infections more because yeast thrives in a high-sugar environment," Dr. Hoffman says. "Garlic suppresses yeast," he says. Deodorized capsules are best.

Acidophilus. This organism "helps keep the intestinal flora away from favoring yeast multiplication," Dr. Hoffman says. It comes in capsule form.

depression," says health psychologist Paula Hartman-Stein, Ph.D., of the Akron General Medical Center in Ohio.

There's also some evidence that exercise increases the number of insulin receptors on cell surfaces, which means insulin can find a place to put glucose where it's needed—inside the cells. In fact, to a person with diabetes, exercise is like a dose of insulin.

Repetitive, rhythmic movements involving your large muscles —arms and legs—are best for diabetics. That means walking, jogging, swimming, rowing, or bicycling. You have to exercise regularly and at least three times a week for 20 to 30 minutes, the experts say. Your doctor may even prescribe exercise five to seven times a week. Studies show that even a two- or three-day layoff from exercise reverses its beneficial effects in diabetics.

Start walking. "The best exercise for people with diabetes is brisk walking," says diabetes specialist Henry Dolger, M.D., former chief of the Diabetes Department at Mount Sinai Medical Center in New York City. "It's by far the safest, least stressful, and most productive of all exercises. It improves the efficiency of every unit of insulin taken in or produced by the body," Dr. Dolger explains. "That means you get more effectiveness out of every gram of food you eat than you would without exercise. It also gives you a great sense of well-being and requires no equipment." If you walk a mile a day, burning 100 calories, in a year you'd shed more than 10 pounds.

Check with your doctor. If your diabetes isn't under control or you have complications, exercise can make it worse. If you have high blood pressure, that also needs to be controlled first. Your doctor may want you to take a stress test. He'll want to judge the effects of any medication you're taking.

Exercise not to do. Don't lift weights or anything else that involves pushing or pulling heavy objects. It raises your blood sugar levels and blood pressure, and can make diabetic eye disease worse.

Take care of your teeth. "A diabetic has to maintain an absolutely immaculate mouth," says Roger P. Levin, D.D.S., president of the Baltimore Academy of General Dentistry. "Because diabetics are much more susceptible to infection, they are also more susceptible to gum disease, which is a bacterial infection." Everything a nondiabetic person should do for dental health, a diabetic person should do even more conscientiously. This means more frequent visits to your dentist and especially conscientious brushing and flossing to control plaque and tartar. (See Tartar and Plaque on page 583.)

A perfect fit is important. "Restorations must be very well contoured in a diabetic," Dr. Levin says. Poorly fitting dentures, bridges, or crowns can cause mouth sores, which can become serious because of inefficient wound healing. And because wounds don't heal well, the diabetic is not a candidate for the newer techniques like dental implants.

Reduce stress. "Stress and anxiety can destabilize diabetic control in two ways," Dr. Hartman-Stein says. "Some people's blood sugar can skyrocket, others' goes way down. And when diabetics are depressed or anxious, frequently they don't adhere to their regimen very well," relapsing into a fat and sugar pig-out and couch potatohood.

Diabetes, with its constant emotional and physical demands, is a stressful disease. "If a person is having some very stressful life events they're having trouble coping with, they should seek the help of a mental health professional," Dr. Hartman-Stein says. Here are some ways you can help yourself relieve stress.

Relax. Dr. Hartman-Stein tested relaxation therapy and cognitive therapy for diabetes control and found these techniques "may be helpful." Relaxation techniques focus on controlled breathing and visualization, and can be learned from professionals or books.

Learn how to think. Cognitive therapy teaches you to "recognize the kinds of thinking you engage in that might be affecting your mood," she says. "You might have thoughts like, 'My legs are really ugly because of the marks from injecting insulin' or 'I feel like a freak every time I have to test my urine.' You can turn those negative thoughts about the regimen into a more rational way of looking at it. You can instead think, 'Nobody's noticing those little marks in my skin but me', or 'Testing my urine is a chemistry experiment.' Dr. Hartman-Stein recommends a self-help book by David Burns, *Feeling Good.* "It's very good for mood problems," she says.

Improve your perspective. You are more than a case of diabetes. "Some people do focus on it too much. They label themselves as having this chronic illness, and it colors everything," Dr. Hartman-Stein says. "Well, it doesn't have to color *everything.* You do have to be more disciplined about your daily life in terms of your eating schedule, but it doesn't have to hamper you. You need to add uplifts to your daily life for a better perspective. Those with diabetes can't eat a box of cookies to make themselves feel better. One lady told me she rents video tapes and indulges herself when she's feeling depressed or stressed. Do something you enjoy doing—buy yourself something new, call a friend you haven't talked to in a long time, any little treat that isn't expensive and you don't have to plan weeks for, but that you can do on a daily or weekly basis."

Test your blood. Over-the-counter blood glucose testing kits can run into money—up to $750 a year if you test your blood four times a day. "But it's very worthwhile," Franz says. "Urine testing for Type II diabetes is quite inaccurate, because you can get quite a high blood sugar level before sugar spills into the urine," especially if you're older. Blood testing can tell you when you have hyperglycemia (high blood sugar) without symptoms. If your diabetes is mild or controlled, Franz says, you may not need to test your blood as often as four times a day. But you do need to know *how* often and how to test accurately.

Use care with OTCs. Some over-the-counter drugs (OTCs) contain sugar and other ingredients that can disturb blood sugar levels. Dr. Mirsky offers a simple warning: "Watch out for over-the-counter stuff." Always check the label for any warning directed to people with diabetes, but don't stop there. Ask the pharmacist if you're not sure, and be sure to monitor your reactions after taking any OTC medication. And, of course, check with your doctor.

Here are a few ingredients to be wary of.

Aspirin. Large quantities of aspirin taken for chronic pain can lower blood sugar levels. Occasional small amounts, such as two tablets for a headache, are not enough to worry about.

Caffeine. The main ingredient in OTC appetite suppressants is caffeine, which can raise blood sugar levels when taken in large amounts. Many headache and cold medications also are loaded with caffeine.

Ephedrine or epinephrine. These are used in preparations that treat respiratory illnesses, but they can increase blood sugar in people with Type II diabetes. So can phenylephrine, a drug found in nasal sprays and cold preparations.

PANEL OF ADVISERS

Marc A. Brenner, D.P.M., has a private practice in Glendale, New York, is past president of the American Society of Podiatric Dermatology, and author of *The Management of the Diabetic Foot.*

Henry Dolger, M.D., is former chief of the Diabetes Department at Mount Sinai Medical Center in New York City.

Marion Franz, M.S., R.D., a certified diabetes educator, is vice president of nutrition at the International Diabetes Center in Minneapolis, Minnesota, and chairman of the Council on Nutritional Sciences and Metabolism of the American Diabetes Association.

Paula Hartman-Stein, Ph.D., is a clinical psychologist in the departments of Medicine and Surgery at the Akron General Medical Center in Ohio, specializing in health psychology with a focus on diabetes.

Ronald Hoffman, M.D., is a nutritional physician and medical director of the Hoffman Center for Holistic Medicine in New York City. He is host of a weekly radio show in New York City and is coauthor of the book *Diet-Type Weight-Loss Program.*

Roger P. Levin, D.D.S., is president of the Baltimore Academy of General Dentistry and a guest lecturer at the University of Maryland in Baltimore.

Stanley Mirsky, M.D., is a private practitioner in New York City and an associate clinical professor at Mount Sinai School of Medicine of the City University of New York.

Karl Sussman, M.D., is associate chief of staff for research and development at the Veterans Administration Hospital in Denver, Colorado, and professor of medicine at the University of Colorado Health Sciences Center School of Medicine in Denver. He is past president of the American Diabetes Association.

Diaper Rash

5 Easy Solutions

Diaper rash can interrupt the peaceful routine of an otherwise carefree baby, and it won't do much for your quality of life, either. Babies have this knack for making their problems your problems, and if baby has diaper rash, you have it, too.

During the first two to three years of life, just about every parent on the planet gets to share in the diaper rash experience at least once. Thankfully, nearly 50 percent of all diaper rashes go away by themselves within one day. What about the other 50 percent? They can last ten days or more (though it's likely to seem longer).

If you're reading this, you're probably sharing the diaper rash experience right now. Here's some trivia to welcome you to the club. Did you know that breastfed babies have less diaper rash than bottle-fed babies? Even better, research has shown that this resistance continues long after a baby has been weaned.

What? Your obstetrician didn't tell you about that? Well, he didn't tell us either. But we found one that did. Here's what else we found out.

Give 'em some air. The oldest advice is sometimes still the best. "Give that baby's bottom some air," says Ann Price, educational coordinator for the National Academy of Nannies, Inc. (NANI), in Denver, Colorado.

Simply take the baby's diaper off and lay him chest down, with his face turned to one side, on towels underlaid with a waterproof sheet. Leave the baby that way for as long as you're there to keep an eye on him. Remember: An unwatched, undiapered baby is trouble waiting to happen.

Superdiapers to the rescue. "These new superabsorbent diapers seem to be a good idea," says Morris Green, M.D., chairman of the Department of Pediatrics at Indiana University School of Medicine. "I think they're the best thing there is for preventing diaper rash."

Recent studies confirm Dr. Green's observation. Diapers containing absorbent gelling material (Ultra Pampers, for example) have been shown to significantly reduce skin wetness and leave skin closer to its normal pH than either conventional disposable diapers or cloth diapers.

Blow-dry that baby. Keeping the diaper area clean promotes healing, but drying with a towel can irritate sensitive skin. Option? "Try a blow dryer," says Linda Jonides, a pediatric nurse practitioner in Ann Arbor, Michigan. Dry the diaper area with a hair dryer set on "low," which avoids abrasion to wet skin. After the area is dry, zinc oxide ointments such as A&D or Desitin may be applied.

Give cloth diapers a vinegar rinse. "Adding vinegar to the final rinse when washing diapers will help bring the pH of cloth diapers into line with [that of] the baby's skin," says Price. She notes that diaper rash enzymes are most active in a high-pH environment, which often exists in cloth diapers after washing. Add 1 ounce of vinegar to 1 gallon of water during the final rinse.

The "Bead Bottom" Mystery

A medical journal article tells of parents calling pediatricians to report a strange diaper rash that looks like "small, shiny beads" covering their babies' bottoms. Pediatricians investigating the mysterious outbreak of "bead bottom" noticed that the afflicted infants all wore superabsorbent disposable diapers. Was there a connection?

Yes. The "beads" are actually the gelling material that makes superabsorbent diapers "super." Apparently, small, loose quantities of the material may occasionally pass through a break in the top sheet of the diaper and transfer to the infant's skin. Physicians say the material is nontoxic and presents no reason for concern.

"Actually, I believe there's a lot to be said for diaper services," Price notes. "They go to a lot of trouble to get the pH balance right, and they're not all that expensive either. If you're using cloth diapers and your baby has a bad rash, I recommend giving them a try."

The cranberry connection. When urine and feces mix in the diaper area, the result is a high pH that irritates the skin and promotes diaper rash.

Unorthodox as it may sound, Jonides notes that 2 to 3 ounces of cranberry juice given to older infants will leave an acid residue in the urine, helping lower pH and reduce irritation.

PANEL OF ADVISERS

Morris Green, M.D., is chairman of the Department of Pediatrics at Indiana University School of Medicine in Indianapolis.

Linda Jonides is a pediatric nurse practitioner in Ann Arbor, Michigan.

Ann Price is educational coordinator for the National Academy of Nannies, Inc. (NANI), in Denver, Colorado, and coauthor of *Successful Breastfeeding, Dr. Mom,* and other books.

Diarrhea

16 Remedies to Deal with It

"Acute diarrhea is one of your body's best defense mechanisms," says Lynn V. McFarland, Ph.D., a research associate with the Department of Medicinal Chemistry at the University of Washington. "It's your body's way of getting something nasty out of your system."

That thought may or may not be of comfort to you right now, but it helps explain why doctors today will tell you to "tough it out" instead of automatically trying to stem the tide of this annoying, but hopefully short-lived, illness.

"It used to be that when somebody had diarrhea," Dr. McFarland explains, "doctors would quickly prescribe some type of antidiarrheal medication. Today we think the best medicine is to simply let it run its course, if you'll pardon the pun."

David A. Lieberman, M.D., associate professor of medicine at Oregon Health Sciences University School of Medicine, seconds that opinion. "I don't recommend antidiarrheal medications when a patient has acute diarrhea unless he or she has an urgent need for control—like a very important business meeting that just can't be missed. Otherwise, I think the purge is probably beneficial and helps speed recovery."

Because of that thinking, most of the tips below are designed to help you weather the discomfort of diarrhea and make a speedy recovery, rather than try to halt the course of diarrhea and risk prolonging the illness. For those who may have "an urgent need for control" while stricken, we've listed some medications to help stem the tide while you take care of other business.

Make the milk connection. "One of the leading causes of diarrhea in this country is lactose intolerance," says William Y. Chey, M.D., professor of medicine at the University of Rochester School of Medicine and Dentistry.

While few of our experts agree that lactose intolerance is the *leading* cause (most say viral infection), all agree that it is a *major* cause of diarrhea among unsuspecting adults.

"Lactose intolerance can have its onset when you're just a baby, or it can kick in suddenly during your adult years," says Dr. Chey. "You're drinking milk and the next thing you know—bam!—you have gas, pain, and diarrhea."

The cure, of course, is to avoid lactose-containing foods, which means staying away from most dairy products, with the exception of yogurt and some aged cheeses, such as cheddar. "Once you do that," says Dr. Chey, "it stops by itself."

Take the tolerance test. Given the dose-related nature of lactose intolerance, as well as its ability to kick in unexpectedly, how can you be sure whether or not milk products are responsible for your current troubles?

"What I do is have patients completely abstain from milk products for a week or two and see if that helps," says Dr. Lieberman.

If a week without milk helps, he says, "then I have them gradually add back milk products with the knowledge that at some point they may reach a level where the intolerance symptoms will return." But, Dr.

MEDICAL ALERT

When Diarrhea Demands an M.D.

Diarrhea should usually disappear in one or two days and leave you only slightly worse for wear. In infants, small children, elderly people, or those already sick or dehydrated from another illness, however, acute diarrhea can be particularly severe and demands prompt medical attention.

Medical help is also needed if diarrhea does not subside within one or two days, or if it's accompanied by fever and severe abdominal cramps, or if it occurs with rashes, jaundice (yellowing of the skin and whites of the eyes), or extreme weakness. If blood, pus, or mucus is found in the stools, call your doctor.

"The most immediate risk associated with acute diarrhea is dehydration," says Harris Clearfield, M.D. "So if an individual is having a major bout of diarrhea and isn't taking in any food or drink during that time, you're looking at a medical emergency." Seek help, he says.

Lieberman notes, once a person knows what that level is, he can avoid lactose-induced diarrhea by keeping consumption beneath it. (For more tips, see Lactose Intolerance on page 407.)

Think about your medications. Our experts say there's a good possibility that the diarrhea you have now was caused by the heartburn you had earlier today. Not because of a direct connection between stomach and bowel, but because of the antacid you may have taken to soothe your burning belly.

"Antacids are the most common cause of drug-related diarrhea," says Harris Clearfield, M.D., professor of medicine and director of the Division of Gastroenterology at Hahnemann University Hospital in Philadelphia, Pennsylvania. "Maalox and Mylanta both have magnesium hydroxide in them that acts exactly like milk of magnesia does, which makes these antacids a common cause of diarrhea."

To avoid future bouts of heartburn-related diarrhea, he suggests trying antacids that contain only aluminum hydroxide, with no magnesium added. "These are less likely to cause diarrhea," Dr. Clearfield says, "but they're less effective, too."

Besides antacids, antibiotics, quinidine, lactulose, and colchicine may also cause diarrhea. Consult your doctor if you suspect that these or any other medications may be causing problems for you.

Diarrhea at a Dangerous Age

Diarrhea in babies and small children can be dangerous. Infants are easily dehydrated, and they lack the ability to tell you exactly how they feel. To help you treat cases of acute diarrhea in infants and young children, we consulted Loraine Stern, M.D., a private practitioner in New Hall, California. These are her recommendations.

Reach for the right stuff. "Water and fruit juice really aren't the best fluids for rehydrating a baby," says Dr. Stern. What does she recommend? "Rehydration solutions are good for infants and toddlers during the acute phase of diarrhea. You can make your own rehydration solution [add 1 teaspoon of sugar and a pinch of salt to 1 quart of water], but if you make a mistake, you can overload the baby with salt. If you can afford to buy the commercially available ones (Pedialyte, ReSol, Lytren, etc.), you're much better off. These are available at drugstores without prescription."

Continue feeding. "You should continue to feed a child," says Dr. Stern, "but you should probably avoid milk for a day if the diarrhea is severe. What you feed a child depends on the age of the child, but for infants I recommend rice cereal, apple sauce, and bananas for a day or two. These foods tend to be a bit binding. For older children, stick with plain dry toast, plain crackers, chicken without the skin, and other bland foods."

Know when to quit. "The biggest mistake most people make is in not knowing when to quit treatment," Dr. Stern says. "Children may have loose stools for quite a while after the initial illness—perhaps one or two watery stools a day for the next couple of weeks. If they are otherwise okay, it's not necessary to keep them on a restricted diet. Only do that for a couple of days."

Try the carrot cure. "Some people think strained carrots are the greatest thing in the world for a child with diarrhea," she says. "You can include these in the diet if you wish." (Carrots may help enhance recovery by replacing electrolytes and minerals lost during diarrhea.)

Put bacteria back in. "After the first couple of days, yogurt tends to repopulate the bowel with good bacteria," says Dr. Stern. "It isn't a bad idea to feed it to them. Three ounces a day should do it."

Remember Mother's advice. "Chicken broth or beef broth is fine for a child over a year old," she says. "For some children the high salt content of broth is good because it makes them drink when they might not want to. But I wouldn't use it more than once or twice a day."

Consume a clear diet. Okay, so you didn't eat a second bowl of ice cream and you didn't travel to Mexico last week, but you've got diarrhea anyway. Now you're hungry as well as cranky and there's just one thing you need to know—is it safe to eat food? Yes, our experts say, but with a few cautions.

"Start with a 'clear-liquid' diet," says Dr. Chey. "By clear I mean chicken broth, Jell-O, or other foods and fluids you can look 'clear' through." The reason, he explains, is that the bowel needs rest during the time you have diarrhea, "and that's why you should stick with a diet like this until it subsides. You don't want to force your system to handle more than it already has to."

After you've tested the waters with broth and Jell-O, rice, bananas, applesauce, or yogurt can be introduced gradually as your symptoms improve.

Keep liquid levels high. "The type of food you eat doesn't really matter that much," says Dr. McFarland. "The most serious thing is to make sure your fluid intake is high." Though many folks don't feel like consuming large amounts of liquids during bouts of diarrhea, all our experts agree that increasing your fluid intake is vital to ward off dehydration.

Fluids that contain salt and small amounts of sugar are particularly beneficial, as they help the body replace glucose and minerals lost during diarrhea. A good "rehydration fluid" can be easily made by adding 1 teaspoon of sugar and a pinch of salt to 1 quart of water.

A more complex but tastier mix can be made by adding ½ teaspoon of honey or corn syrup and a pinch of table salt to 8 ounces of fruit juice. Stir well and drink often.

For those who don't feel like making anything, Gatorade comes highly recommended. It contains glucose and electrolytes in sufficient quantities to replace those being lost by your body. (Now if you can just get somebody to run to the store.)

Avoid these foods. While eating may not be as important as drinking for riding out diarrhea in the best possible shape, there are some foods that should be avoided because of their, um, well, potentially explosive nature. Obvious ones to pass up include beans, cabbage, and brussels sprouts.

Other foods containing large amounts of poorly absorbed carbohydrates can aggravate diarrhea. A short list includes bread, pasta, and other wheat products; apples, pears, peaches, and prunes; corn, oats, potatoes, and processed bran.

And, just in case you were reaching for that carton of ice cream, all our experts say you should avoid dairy products during a bout of diarrhea. Whether or not milk products caused the problem, they tend to aggravate diarrhea after you have it.

Avoid the bubble, bubble toilet trouble. "I'd suggest avoiding carbonated beverages as well," says Dr. Clearfield. "The gas they contain may add additional explosiveness to a delicate situation."

Stay out of the kitchen. While we're still on the subject of food, you or any member of your family who has diarrhea should not prepare food for other members of the household until diarrhea subsides. Also, good hand washing by you and other household members will help keep a parasitic infection from spreading. (If your job involves contact with large numbers of people or food handling, state law may require you to stay off the job until all symptoms subside.)

If you must—take something to stem the tide. Our experts insist that letting diarrhea "run its course" is the best medicine going. If, however, you absolutely must go someplace and be in control of your bodily functions while there, an over-the-counter product called Imodium, available in capsule or liquid form, is probably your best bet for slowing the flow.

"Imodium is very effective," says Dr. Clearfield. "It works by causing the bowel to tighten up, and by doing so, it prevents things from moving along."

Imodium isn't your only choice. Hydrophilic (*hydro* means water, and *phili* means love) products, such as Kaopectate and Pepto-Bismol may be useful in the treatment of mild diarrhea.

Aluminum hydroxide antacids, unlike their magnesium counterparts, have hydrophilic abilities and may be effective for reducing the symptoms of diarrhea. Amphojel and Alternagel are two to try.

Food remedies not to rely on. Such things as pectin, acidophilus tablets, carob powder, barley, bananas, Swiss cheese, and a host of exotic foods, teas, and other folk remedies have been used by some as a treatment for diarrhea. "They work to bind the bowel and slow the course of the diarrhea," says Dr. McFarland. "But that's not what you want to do. You're just increasing the time that whatever is causing the problem will stay inside you. What you want to do is get it out."

Your best bet, he says, is to let nature take its course.

Diverticulosis

21 Self-Care Techniques

Once upon a time — say before 1900 — diverticulosis was just another of the many "rare" medical conditions doctors had heard about but seldom seen. And in Third World nations, diverticulosis is rare even today.

But not in the United States, where people can easily live on a diet of processed foods.

"Diverticulosis is a problem that is acquired," says Paul Williamson, M.D., a general and colon and rectal surgeon at Orlando Regional Medical Center in Florida. "It's come about with the advance of processed foods — foods that are low in fiber." (Fiber is important because it helps reduce tension on the colon and helps it expand when eliminating waste.)

A lot has changed since 1900. Studies now indicate that more than half of those over the age of 60 have diverticulosis — which is characterized by tiny, grapelike pouches or sacs (diverticula) along the outer wall of the colon.

Putting More Fiber into Your Diet

You know that getting enough fiber in your diet (30 to 35 grams daily) is the most important thing you can do to treat and prevent diverticulosis. But what you may not know is how much fiber is in the recommended high-fiber foods, or, how to inject more fiber into your diet without sitting down to a bowl of raw bran.

Here are some tips for making the transition to a high-fiber diet.

- Make a habit of eating whole-grain bread instead of white bread.
- Answer your sweet tooth with fruit desserts—berries, bananas, peaches.
- Eat more vegetarian meals.
- Leave the skins on apples, peaches, and pears when you bake them.
- Add dried fruits, such as raisins and apricots, to your meals.
- Substitute beans for beef in chili or casseroles.
- Add barley to vegetable soups.

These pouches show up on x-rays, but many people never have this area x-rayed and don't even know that they have diverticulosis, says Samuel Klein, M.D., an assistant professor of gastroenterology and human nutrition at the University of Texas Medical School at Galveston.

Of those who do have diverticulosis, Dr. Klein says, only about 10 percent will ever get diverticulitis—a painful inflammation that can become serious. So having diverticulosis does not mean you are destined for severe pain and a hospital stay.

And fortunately, you can take an active role in treating and preventing diverticulosis. Here's what our experts suggest.

Bulk up on fiber. The average American gets about 16 grams of fiber daily, or only half of what he should be getting, says Marvin Schuster, M.D., chief of the Department of Digestive Diseases at Francis Scott Key Medical Center in Baltimore, Maryland. "Bran fiber appears to be the most effective," he says.

Fiber draws water into the stool, making movements smoother. Whole wheat bread and all-bran cereals are excellent sources of bran. Sprinkling raw bran over foods is also an option.

Vegetables and fruit are other good sources of fiber, adds Dr. Klein. "If it's fiber you're after, eat an apple instead of drinking apple juice. The juice typically doesn't have any fiber."

Increase your fiber intake slowly. "Do this gradually over six to eight weeks," Dr. Klein suggests. "You need time for your digestive system to adapt."

You can expect bloating and gas the first few weeks, Dr. Schuster says. "But most people will get over this."

If you can't get enough fiber in your diet, take a supplement. "Take psyllium seed supplements (such as Metamucil)," says Dr. Schuster. "They're natural, too."

Drink a lot of liquids. "Drink six to eight glasses of water a day," advises Dr. Klein, adding that the liquid is an important partner to fiber in combating constipation, which is associated with diverticulosis.

"If you have to strain a great deal when having a bowel movement," Dr. Schuster says, "you tend to expand those little diverticula through the muscle walls of the colon."

Go when you have to go. If you don't yield to nature's call, you defeat the purpose of adding more fiber to your diet and drinking more liquids. "Don't suppress the need to move your bowel," Dr. Williamson advises.

MEDICAL ALERT

From the Benign to the Serious

If you live long enough, chances are you will get diverticulosis. Even so, odds are you won't get diverticulitis—painful inflammation that is potentially serious. Still, you should be aware of the warning signs.

Fever and severe pain in the lower left portion of the abdominal region are good indicators that diverticulosis has advanced to diverticulitis, says Marvin Schuster, M.D.

This change shouldn't be taken lightly.

"You can have rupturing or bleeding," says Albert J. Lauro M.D. And while it doesn't happen often, people can die from diverticulitis.

So act on those warning signs and get to a doctor fast. And stay calm—the odds are still in your favor. "If it's just an infection," Dr. Lauro says, "it usually can be handled with rest, diet, and antibiotics. You'll be okay."

Exercise. It tones more than your legs and hips. Exercise also tones the muscles in your colon. "It helps bowel movements; you don't have to strain as much," says Dr. Klein.

Don't use suppositories. While they may offer a quick fix to constipation, they aren't the best choice for stimulating bowel movements.

"Your system can get addicted to it," Dr. Klein explains. "And then it becomes a vicious circle—you need more suppositories."

Go natural. "Prunes, prune juice, and herbal teas are very effective natural laxatives," Dr. Schuster says. Specially formulated teas can be found in most health food stores.

Don't smoke. Harmful in so many ways, smoking also may aggravate diverticulosis, says Albert J. Lauro, M.D., director of emergency medical services at Charity Hospital in New Orleans, Louisiana.

Eat highly processed foods only in moderation. This is good general health advice, but also applies to treating diverticulosis. If you eat a lot of low-fiber processed foods, says Dr. Klein, you won't have room to eat the high-fiber foods you need.

Chew seeds extra well. Foods such as nuts and popcorn contain seeds or other hard particles that could become lodged in the diverticula and cause inflammation, Dr. Klein says.

"And if you've ever had an acute attack of diverticulitis," Dr. Lauro adds, "you should keep away from foods that have seeds."

Drink only in moderation. "Alcohol in moderation—a drink or two a day—will actually relax spasm of the colon and could improve the situation a little bit," says Dr. Schuster.

Avoid caffeine. "Coffee, chocolate, teas, colas—all tend to irritate," Dr. Williamson says.

Look for a pattern. Certain foods may disrupt your bowel habits or cause loose stools, Dr. Williamson says. Try to identify those foods and avoid them.

PANEL OF ADVISERS

Samuel Klein, M.D., is an assistant professor of gastroenterology and human nutrition at the University of Texas Medical School at Galveston. He is also an editorial adviser to *Prevention* magazine.

Albert J. Lauro, M.D., is director of emergency medical services at Charity Hospital in New Orleans, Louisiana.

Marvin Schuster, M.D., is chief of the Department of Digestive Diseases at Francis Scott Key Medical Center in Baltimore, Maryland, and professor of medicine and psychiatry at Johns Hopkins University School of Medicine in Baltimore.

Paul Williamson, M.D., is a general surgeon and colon and rectal surgeon at Orlando Regional Medical Center in Florida.

Dry Hair

10 Solutions for a Manageable Mane

The average human head has 150,000 hairs, and, conformists that they are, when one's dry, they're *all* dry. But unlike a dry flower garden or polished rice, the solution is not simply to add water. Water, in fact, may be responsible for the hair's parched condition, particularly if we're talking about water of the salty, chlorinated, or sudsy variety.

Swimming and overshampooing are two common causes of arid, fly-away locks, says Jack Myers, director of the National Cosmetology Association. Other culprits, he says, can include colorings, permanents, electric curlers, excessive blow-drying, and too much exposure to wind and sun.

Whatever the culprit, your poor, abused hair needs help—badly. You can almost hear all 150,000 of them down on their little split ends, pleading, "Save me! Save me!" Here's a quick course on how to rescue dried-out hair.

Shampoo with care. "It's in vogue these days to shampoo every day, but shampooing doesn't only wash away dirt, it washes out the hair's protective oils," says Thomas Goodman, Jr., M.D., a dermatologist from Memphis, Tennessee, and assistant professor at the University of Tennessee Center for Health Sciences. If you've dried your hair out from too much lather, give your hair a needed break—try washing less often. And use only a mild shampoo, one labeled "for dry or damaged hair."

A Topical, Tropical Blend

If you've ever wondered what the hairdresser to big Hollywood stars uses to condition her own hair, wonder no more. "I take old bananas, rotten and black, and mash them together with mushy, rotten avocado," says Hollywood hairdresser Joanne Harris.

"I came back from the beach one day, and there was no conditioner in the house, but I did have an old banana and an old avocado. I tried it and I loved it! It has lots of nutrients, so it feeds my hair and nurses it," says Harris.

She recommends you leave the tropical puree in your hair for 15 minutes, and then wash it out in the *kitchen* sink—preferably one with a garbage disposal to avoid clogging the pipes.

Use a conditioner. When hair becomes dry, the outer layers, called cuticles, peel off from the central shaft. Conditioners glue the cuticles back to the shaft, add lubricant to the hair, and prevent static electricity (which creates frizz). Pick a conditioner that works well for you and use it after every shampoo, says Dr. Goodman.

Go heavy on the mayo. "Mayonnaise makes an excellent conditioner," says Steven Docherty, senior art director at New York City's Vidal Sassoon Salon. He advises you to leave the oily white goo in your hair for anywhere from 5 minutes to an hour before washing it out.

Snip off those frayed ends. Dry hair tends to suffer most at the ends. The answer? Snip 'em off, says Anja Vaisanen, a hair stylist at New York City's stylish Suga Salon. Once every six weeks or so should keep those frayed ends under control.

Design your hair without heat. Heat is what makes the desert a desert; it also contributes to dried-out hair. Two of the most intense sources of heat are curling irons and electric curlers, says Joanne Harris, a hairdresser in Los Angeles whose clients include many Hollywood stars. She suggests you rediscover those (unheated) plastic cylinder rollers from years gone by. For straightening, wrap slightly moist hair under and around rollers (like a page boy hairdo) for about 10 minutes. For curling or adding wave, try using sponge rollers overnight or sleeping with moist braids.

Protect your hair from the elements. "Whipping wind can fray your hair just like a piece of fabric," says Docherty. Sun, too, takes a mighty toll. Solution: Wear a hat, both on breezy, balmy summer days, and gusty, frosty winter days.

Don't swim bare headed. "Chlorine is one of the most destructive things to hair," says Docherty. So make a rubber cap part of your regular swim attire. For extra protection, he says, first rub a little olive oil into your hair.

Have a beer. "Beer is a wonderful setting lotion. It gives a crisp, healthy, shiny look, even to dry hair," says Docherty. The trick is to spray the brew onto your hair using a pump bottle after you've shampooed and towel-dried, but before you blow-dry or style. And don't worry about smelling like a lush — the odor of the beer quickly disappears, says Docherty.

Consider a trip to the beauty parlor. Our experts agree that a professional moisturizing treatment can work wonders for your dried-out head of hair. "A real good steam treatment with oils and creams lasts about an hour, and afterward you can *really* tell the difference," says Claudia Buttaro, manager of the Watergate Beauty Salon in Washington, D.C. The cost at the Watergate is around $20.

PANEL OF ADVISERS

Claudia Buttaro is the manager of her family-owned salon, the Watergate Beauty Salon in Washington, D.C. She's been in the business for 20 years.

Steven Docherty is the senior art director of New York City's Vidal Sassoon Salon. He cares for the hair of some of New York's top magazine and television models.

Thomas Goodman, Jr., M.D., is a dermatologist in private practice and assistant professor of dermatology at the University of Tennessee Center for Health Sciences in Memphis. He is author of *Smart Face* and *The Skin Doctor's Skin Doctoring Book*.

Joanne Harris is hairdresser to many of Hollywood's top actors and actresses, such as Angie Dickinson and Justine Bateman. She operates the Joanne Harris Salon in Los Angeles, California.

Jack Myers, a professional cosmetologist for the past 30 years, is director of the National Cosmetology Association. He is also the owner and operator of the Owensboro School of Hair Design and Jack Myers Hair Styles in Owensboro, Kentucky.

Anja Vaisanen is a hair stylist at New York City's well-known Suga Salon. Trained in Finland, she's been a stylist for ten years.

Dry Skin and Winter Itch

10 Cold-Weather Options

If you're reading this book at your home in Miami Beach, you can probably skip this chapter. Go out and bask in the warm, moist air. Give your skin a good drink of tropical humidity. Enjoy yourself. Have a nice day.

Okay, now that they're gone, the rest of us can get down to the business of keeping our skin from flaking off in a bunch of little piles while we scratch away the remaining months until spring. Yes, those of us who live in cold, dry climates—where the forced-air heater runs day and night—are the ones who know the agony of dry skin and winter itch.

Well, what to do about it? Easy. Turn down the heat and move to Florida. Can't move? Then at least turn down the heat; that's a big step along the path to healthier winter skin. There are plenty more steps you can take, and we've listed many of them here. They all follow one basic premise, however, and it's this: Dryness results from a lack of *water* in your skin—not oil. Keep that in mind as you read this and as you go about your daily routine this winter, and your skin will thank you for it.

Don't try to drink dryness away. Many beauty books and glamour magazines recommend drinking "at least seven or eight glasses of water per day" to keep the skin hydrated and prevent dryness. Don't believe it.

"If you're totally dehydrated, your skin will become dry," says Kenneth Neldner, M.D., a professor and chairman of the Department of Dermatology at the Texas Tech University Health Sciences Center School of Medicine. "But if you are normally hydrated, you cannot possibly counteract or correct dry skin by drinking water."

224

Put water where it counts. "The best way to get water into the skin is by soaking in it," says Hillard H. Pearlstein, M.D., assistant clinical professor of dermatology at the Mount Sinai School of Medicine in New York City. He recommends a 15-minute soak in *lukewarm* water, not hot water. And forget the notion that you should bathe every day. The rule of thumb for dry skin is: Bathe less and use cooler water.

Lubricate the skin. "Follow each bath with a moisturizer," says Dr. Pearlstein. "The tendency is for all the moisture that soaked into the skin to evaporate. If you bathe frequently, a moisturizer is doubly important. The moisturizer is what holds the water in.

Dr. Pearlstein says many people think the reason for applying moisturizers is to put oil back into the skin, but that's not totally true. "Just remember that dry skin is a function of water loss, not of oil loss," he says.

"Everybody knows how easy it is to cut the toenails or fingernails after they've been in water," he explains. "That's a good example of hydration, of what happens to the skin when you bathe." Moisturizers applied after the bath help keep water in the skin and therefore prevent drying.

Dry yourself damp—then stop. "It's much more effective to apply moisturizer to damp skin immediately after bathing than to put it on totally dry skin," says Dr. Neldner.

That's not to say you have to hop from the tub or shower soaking wet and immediately apply lotion. "But a couple of pats with a towel will make you as dry as you want to be before you apply the lotion," he says. "You're trying to trap a little water in the skin, and that's the fundamental rule in fighting off dryness."

Don't get greased by ad hype. "Nothing beats plain petroleum jelly or mineral oil as a moisturizer," says Howard Donsky, M.D., associate professor at the University of Toronto and staff dermatologist at Toronto General Hospital. In fact, for those who don't mind the feeling, virtually any vegetable oil (sunflower oil, peanut oil) or hydrogenated oil (Crisco) can be used to combat dry skin and winter itch. They are effective, safe, and pure skin lubricants. They are very inexpensive as well.

Those products do have one drawback, however. All of them tend to be greasy. "People like things that smell good, feel good, and don't make them feel like a greased pig," Dr. Pearlstein says. "It all depends on how much you want to spend, what you want to smell like, and how you want to feel. All moisturizers do the same basic thing, and there's no scientific way to prove that any one of the commercially available products is any better for you than another. It's strictly your personal decision."

Use oatmeal to heal. Some researchers believe people first discovered the skin-soothing effects of oatmeal nearly 4,000 years ago. Many folks are still discovering it today. "Oatmeal can work in the bath as a soothing agent," says Dr. Donsky. Just pour 2 cups of colloidal oatmeal (like Aveeno, available at pharmacies) into a tub of lukewarm water. The term *colloidal* simply means the oatmeal has been ground to fine powder that will remain suspended in water.

"You can also use oatmeal as a soap substitute," he says. Tie some colloidal oatmeal in a handkerchief, dunk it in water, squeeze out the excess water, and use as you would a normal washcloth.

Select superfatted soaps. "Most soaps have lye in them," says Dr. Pearlstein, "and while lye is great for cleaning, it's very irritating to dry skin." He recommends that people with dry skin avoid strong soaps such as Dial or Ivory and reach instead for "superfatted" soaps like Basis, Neutrogena, or Dove. Superfatted soaps have extra amounts of fatty substances—cold cream, cocoa butter, coconut oil, or lanolin—added during the manufacturing process.

"A product like Dove, for instance, isn't really a soap at all," Dr. Pearlstein says. "It's more like a cold cream." But such are the trade-offs in the skin game. Though they don't clean as well, "the superfatted soaps are less irritating to dry skin," he says, "and they do make a difference."

Don't soap as often. "There's nothing therapeutic about soap," says Dr. Pearlstein. "We in America are the great overwashed, overdeodorized society, and we as dermatologists see more problems from the overuse of soap than we ever do from the lack of it." His advice: If it's not dirty, don't wash it.

Let a humidifier help. "Part of the problem with dry skin and itching is dry heat in the wintertime," says Dr. Pearlstein. Furnace-heated air can reduce the humidity level inside your house to 10 percent or less, whereas 30 to 40 percent is closer to ideal for keeping moisture in your skin. For that reason, our experts all recommend the use of humidifiers during those dry winter months—but with a caution.

"People think that if they put a humidifier in their place, that'll take care of it," says Dr. Pearlstein. "But humidifiers are like air conditioners— you would really need a huge unit to do the whole house. However, if you put a smaller unit next to your bed, that can help."

"If you put a humidifier in your bedroom," Dr. Neldner adds, "then be sure you close the door to keep moisture in."

Does it help to do things like leaving the bathroom door open when you take a shower? "It might help for a little while," Dr. Neldner says, "because every little bit of humidity helps. When you're running that furnace in the winter, you're really sucking the moisture out of the air."

Keep it cool. One good way to combat winter itch is as easy as reaching for your thermostat and turning it down. "Keeping your house on the cool side in the winter might help," says Dr. Pearlstein. "That's because cool air has an anesthetic effect—it makes your skin feel good." When you heat your house too much, he explains, it makes blood vessels dilate, and when blood vessels dilate, the itch/tingle cycle begins. "But when you cool skin, either by cool water or cool air, it feels good," Dr. Pearlstein says. "And skin tends to be less itchy if you keep it on the cool side."

PANEL OF ADVISERS

Howard Donsky, M.D., is an associate professor of medicine at the University of Toronto and staff dermatologist at Toronto General Hospital. He is author of *Beauty Is Skin Deep*.

Kenneth Neldner, M.D., is a professor and chairman of the Department of Dermatology at the Texas Tech University Health Sciences Center School of Medicine in Lubbock.

Hillard H. Pearlstein, M.D., is a private practitioner and assistant clinical professor of dermatology at the Mount Sinai School of Medicine of the City University of New York in New York City.

Earache

12 Ways to Stop the Pain

It's a fact. Earaches *are* worse at night. And it's not just because finding medical help is harder after everyone has gone to bed.

Plugged eustachian tubes (which lead from the back of the throat to the middle ear) are the most common cause of earache for children and adults, explains Dudley J. Weider, M.D., an otolaryngologist at Dartmouth–Hitchcock Medical Center in Hanover, New Hampshire. And the situation is usually aggravated by a cold, sinus infection, or allergy.

During the day, you hold your head up and your eustachian tubes drain naturally into the back of your throat. Also, as you chew and swallow, the muscles of the eustachian tubes contract, opening them and allowing air into the middle ear.

But at night when you sleep, things change. You fall asleep feeling just fine. But those tubes no longer drain naturally. And you're not swallowing as often, so they aren't getting as much air. The air already in the middle ear is absorbed and a vacuum occurs, sucking the eardrum inward. Then about midnight you awaken with the feeling that someone has jammed a hot poker through your ear.

Other things cause earaches, too. Infections, such as swimmer's ear, can trigger pain. Atmospheric pressure from airplane travel and deep-sea diving can also cause your ears to ache. Odd things, like tiny clippings from a haircut, can fall into the ear canal and irritate your ears. Then there's referred pain—a problem that exists somewhere else—that makes your ears tingle. Those earaches can originate in your teeth, tonsils, throat, tongue, or jaw.

When your ears ache, you need to see a doctor. But until you get there, here are some quick pain stoppers.

Sit up. A few minutes upright will decrease swelling and start your eustachian tubes draining. Swallowing will help ease the pain. If you can, prop up your head slightly while you sleep to get better drainage, says Dr. Weider.

Turn on the hair dryer. Granddad's trick of blowing smoke from his pipe into painful ears had a basis in fact. It wasn't the smoke that relieved the pain, it was the warmth of the smoke, says Dan Drew, M.D., a family physician in Jasper, Indiana. To do the same trick without putting your lungs in jeopardy, turn your hair dryer to a low, warm setting. Then, holding the dryer 18 to 20 inches from the ear, aim that warm air into your aching ear.

Wiggle your ear. Here's a test to help determine whether you have otitis externa (an external problem like swimmer's ear) or otitis media (middle ear infection). Grab your outer ear, says Donald Kamerer, M.D., chief of the Division of Otology at the Eye and Ear Institute in Pittsburgh, Pennsylvania. If you can wiggle it without pain, the problem is probably in the middle ear. If moving your outer ear causes pain, then the infection is probably in the outer ear canal.

Warm some oil to body temperature. Place a bottle of baby oil or mineral oil in a pan of body-temperature water, says Dr. Weider. Let the oil sit in the water until it, too, is at body temperature. Placing a drop or two of oil in the offending ear will help lessen the pain. Caution: Never drop fluids into your ear if you think the eardrum may be ruptured or punctured.

Chew a wad of gum. Most people know this is one way to open their ears on an airplane flight, but have you considered it at midnight? The muscular action of chewing will do the trick by opening the eustachian tubes.

Yawn. Yawning moves the muscle that opens the eustachian tube even better than chewing gum or sucking on mints.

Hold your nose. If you are flying at 32,000 feet when your ears begin to ache, there's help, according to the American Academy of Otolaryngology/Head and Neck Surgery. Pinch your nostrils shut. Take a mouthful of air and then, using your cheek and throat muscles, force the air into the back of your nose as if you were trying to blow your fingers off the end of your nose. A pop will tell you when you have equalized the pressure inside and outside your ear.

Don't sleep during an airplane descent. If you must doze off while flying, close your eyes at the beginning, not the end of the trip, recommends the academy. You don't swallow as often when you're asleep, so your ears won't keep up with pressure changes during the descent and they may hurt.

Head off trouble. Before you get into trouble, use an over-the-counter decongestant. For instance, if you have to fly and you know your sinuses are going to back up and block your ears, take a decongestant or use nose drops an hour before you land, Dr. Weider says. At home, use a decongestant at night before you climb in bed with a stuffy head to avoid the middle-of-the-night ache.

Get the squeeze off your face. Like people who fly, scuba divers must be able to equalize the pressure inside their ears with that of the water around them or they can suffer ear trouble. Shallow diving, according to *The Physician and Sports Medicine* journal, is more likely to cause an earache because "the greatest changes in air volume occur in relatively shallow water [less than 33 feet]." Avoid super snug earplugs and wet suits with tight-fitting hoods that prevent equalization of pressure during descent, recommends Gary D. Becker, M.D., a staff physician at Kaiser Permanente Medical Center in Panorama City, California.

For recreational swimmers, swimming on the surface puts less pressure on the eardrums than swimming under the water, says Dr. Drew. He recommends that swimmers not dive deeper than 3 or 4 feet to avoid putting stress on the eardrum.

Avoid the pain. If nothing else seems to work, avoid flying or diving when your head is stuffy.

Count on painkillers. Don't forget, an over-the-counter pain-killer (aspirin, acetaminophen, or ibuprofen) will usually buy you time until you can get to a doctor, says Dr. Kamerer.

PANEL OF ADVISERS

Gary D. Becker, M.D., is a staff physician at Kaiser Permanente Medical Center in Panorama City, California.

Dan Drew, M.D., is a family physician in Jasper, Indiana. He is the inventor of the Goggl'Cap, a swim cap-goggle combination.

Donald Kamerer, M.D., is chief of the Division of Otology at the Eye and Ear Institute in Pittsburgh, Pennsylvania. He also is a professor of otolaryngology at the University of Pittsburgh School of Medicine.

Dudley J. Weider, M.D., is an otolaryngologist at Dartmouth–Hitchcock Medical Center in Hanover, New Hampshire.

Ear Infection

10 Ideas to Ease the Symptoms

The baby rolls around in her crib in a restless, relentless bad dream. You check the clock. Midnight. You sigh and pull the covers up tighter and try to sleep.

She kicks the end of the crib. She rearranges her body with a snort and a sigh and a heavier-than-usual thud. She whimpers without waking.

You hear it all. You aren't asleep and, deep down, wonder if you will sleep at all tonight. Instead of counting sheep, you're counting little sensations of guilt. What could I have done to help her sleep better?

"Mommmmmy. Daddddy." Her cries signal time for the midnight ear infection blues.

Children get middle ear infections for several reasons. Their eustachian tubes, the canals that lead from the back of the throat to the middle ear, are wider and shorter than those in adults. Or the nerves to the area may not be fully mature yet, which can also affect the eustachian tubes. Also, children in day care centers may be more exposed to colds, which can lead to ear infections.

And just because you're sleeping in a bed instead of a crib, don't think that you're immune. Take one adult with plugged sinuses and give him a ride in an airplane or let a cold and drippy nose hang on a couple of days too long and *Pow!* Instant ear infection.

The usual symptoms of a middle ear infection are pain and hearing loss, but adults and children can get ear infections without pain, says George W. Facer, M.D., an otolaryngologist at the Mayo Clinic in Rochester, Minnesota. Once infection hits, the best thing to cure it is antibiotics, although some clear up on their own. Your ears will be good as new in a week to ten days.

But what are you going to do tonight? And how can you prevent the next ear infection?

TENDER LOVING CARE

When you or your child is in pain, you want relief. Here's what the experts advise.

Try acetaminophen. This kind of pain reliever (Tylenol, Panadol, Tempra) is a doctor's first choice. A dose at bedtime may be enough to put the pain to sleep while you or your child dream. (No one under age 21 should be given aspirin because of the risk of Reye's syndrome, a life-threatening neurological disease.)

Keep your head up. When your head is upright, your eustachian tubes clear naturally, says Dudley J. Weider, M.D., an otolaryngologist at Dartmouth-Hitchcock Medical Center in Hanover, New Hampshire. This is one reason children with an ear infection don't seem to be in pain during the day. They're busy playing and running around and their eustachian tubes are draining into the backs of their throats.

Take a drink. Sipping water—swallowing—triggers the muscular action that helps your eustachian tubes open and drain, says Dr. Weider. Open tubes mean less pain.

MEDICAL ALERT

Don't Wait for Pain

If you have hearing loss or your ears stay plugged up for more than a couple of days after a cold, see your doctor. You could already have an ear infection or fluid in the middle ear, says George W. Facer, M.D.

Left untreated, an ear infection can cause a permanent hearing loss in children and adults, he says. Ten to 14 days of antibiotics is the usual treatment.

Decongest at bedtime. Children and adults who seem to get a lot of ear infections may benefit from a dose of an over-the-counter oral decongestant right before they go to sleep. If there's fluid inside their ears waiting to haunt them, the medicine will dry it up and help them sleep.

Spray your nose, dry your ears. Adults may want to try a decongestant nose spray before bed in addition to an oral decongestant or antihistamine, says Dr. Facer. But use nose drops for only a day or two. Overuse can create a rebound effect, making a clogged nose worse.

PREVENTIVE CARE

While you can't really prevent ear infections, there are some things you can do that might help lessen the chances of getting them.

Breastfeed your baby. Some experts believe this will lessen your baby's chances of ear problems.

A study of 237 infants in Helsinki, Finland, showed that 6 percent of breastfed babies and 19 percent of formula-fed babies had developed middle ear infections by the end of the first year. By age 3, only 6 percent of those breastfed developed an infection compared with 26 percent of those fed formula.

Why the big difference? Researchers believe that breast-fed infants have an enhanced immune response to respiratory infections.

Quit smoking. Smoking can push an adult with ear problems toward an infection by littering the air with irritants, which in turn leads to eustachian tube congestion, says Dr. Weider. Second-hand smoke, which is also pollutant-filled, can be just as hard on children prone to ear problems.

Douse the fire in your wood-burning stove. For the same clean-air reasons you should quit smoking, you'll want to put out the fire in your woodstove. Soot and smoke from the fire in your stove load the air with hard-to-breathe and hard-to-tolerate toxins.

Choose child care carefully. Children exposed to large groups of other children are more likely to come into contact with the bugs that cause ear infections. Parents who need day care for a child prone to ear infections may want to consider a small group setting, such as a family day-care home, until the child outgrows ear infections, says Dr. Weider.

Be patient. Some children outgrow ear infections by age 3, says Dr. Facer. Then you both can sleep.

PANEL OF ADVISERS

George W. Facer, M.D., is an otolaryngologist at the Mayo Clinic in Rochester, Minnesota.

Dudley J. Weider, M.D., is an otolaryngologist at Dartmouth–Hitchcock Medical Center in Hanover, New Hampshire.

Earwax

4 Steps to Irrigate Your Ears

You should feel lucky—you probably never had to have a doctor pull a cockroach out of your ear after it decided your ear canal was a perfect sleeping bag. That *can* (but rarely does) happen, says David Edelstein, M.D., an otolaryngologist at Manhattan Eye, Ear, and Throat Hospital in New York City. The more common problem is earwax that's formed a hard little plug next to the eardrum and has to be removed by a doctor. Here's how to prevent that from happening.

Stick nothing in your ear. That old cliché, "Never put anything smaller than your elbow into your ear," is one ear doctors swear by. Never stick anything sharp—a bobby pin, a pencil tip, a paper clip—into your ear, because you could tear your eardrum. Don't use a cotton-tipped swab or finger, either, says George W. Facer, M.D., an otolaryngologist at the Mayo Clinic in Rochester, Minnesota. Even while you think you're cleaning out your ear, you are really ramming the wax deeper so it acts like a plug over your eardrum.

Drop in a softening fluid. A few drops of some liquids you probably already have at home can soften your earwax. Try hydrogen peroxide, mineral oil, or glycerin for inexpensive cleaning, says Dr. Facer. Or buy an over-the-counter cleaner such as Debrox or Murine Ear Drops, says Dr. Edelstein.

Add a drop or two of one of the liquids to each ear. Allow the excess to flow out of your ear. The liquid left inside will bubble away at the wax and soften it. Try this for a couple of days.

Once the wax is soft, you're ready to rinse. Fill a bowl with body-temperature water, says Dr. Facer. Fill a rubber bulb syringe with the water, then, holding your head over the bowl, squirt the water *gently* into your ear canal. The stream of water should be under very little pressure. Turn your head to the side and let the water run out.

Blow-dry your ears. Don't rub your ears dry, say doctors. Instead, dry your ear with the hair dryer or drop a little alcohol in each ear to complete the drying. Do this after the procedure and also every time you shower.

Make it a habit. A once-a-month ear wash is plenty for anyone, says Dr. Edelstein. More than that and you're washing away your protection.

PANEL OF ADVISERS

David Edelstein, M.D., is an otolaryngologist at Manhattan Eye, Ear, and Throat Hospital in New York City.

George W. Facer, M.D., is an otolaryngologist at the Mayo Clinic in Rochester, Minnesota.

Emphysema

24 Remedies for Easy Breathing

When your doctor told you, it was quite a blow. Emphysema. The diagnosis fell like a dark curtain around you, separating you from the things you love to do, the people you love, the feeling that—for better or worse—you can count on your body.

What you learned next didn't help. Emphysema itself is very rare. Usually it's complicated by chronic bronchitis or asthma. And there's no medical cure for emphysema, no way to reverse the damage that's been done to your airways. In short, you're stuck with these lungs that have aged beyond your chronological years.

That was the worst of it.

But then you discovered something else about yourself. You're tougher than your emphysema. You're smarter than this disease. And so you made a decision.

This is the year you take control of your health, learn to work smarter, and live more simply. From now on, you're saving your energy for the things you want to do.

Here's how to make that happen.

Stop smoking now! Yes, your doctor already told you. But the point can't be stressed enough.

"It's never too late to stop," says Henry Gong, M.D., professor of medicine at the University of California, Los Angeles, and associate chief of the Pulmonary Division at UCLA Medical Center. "Even if you stop in your fifties or sixties, you'll help slow down the deterioration in your lungs." Another plus: You may immediately increase your capacity to exercise.

The leading theory on how smoking causes emphysema is this: Cigarette smoke incites neutrophils, the disease-battling warriors of the white blood cells, to migrate selectively to the lungs. "Apparently, they extrude their enzymes, which can digest lung tissue," says Dr. Gong. "In normal people, there is a balance between that enzyme and antitrypsin, the one that blocks."

In rare cases, nonsmokers get emphysema too. Victims of a rare inherited protein disorder, they lack sufficient levels of antitrypsin.

Stay away from passive smoke. If the smoke from your own cigarettes can harm you, so can the smoke from your spouse's cigarette or air in a smoky dance hall. A nonsmoking spouse can develop lung cancer by inhaling the cigarette smoke from a smoking spouse after many decades of living together, says Dr. Gong.

Avoid allergens. If you have known allergies and they affect your breathing, it's doubly important to stay away from them when you have emphysema, says Dr. Gong. (For more on allergy control, see Allergies, page 7.)

Control what you can. You can't repair your airways. What you can do, says pulmonary specialist Robert Sandhaus, M.D., Ph.D., consultant for the National Jewish Center for Immunology and Respiratory Medicine and other health facilities in Denver, Colorado, is increase how efficiently you breathe, use your muscles, and approach your work. If you can rearrange your kitchen, for instance, so that you can do in five steps what used to take you ten steps, so much the better, he says.

Exercise. All our experts agree that regular exercise is vitally important to the emphysema sufferer. What kinds are best?

"Walking is probably the best overall exercise," says private practitioner Robert B. Teague, M.D., a clinical assistant professor of medicine at Baylor College of Medicine. "You should also exercise to tone the muscles in your upper extremities. Try using 1- or 2-pound hand weights, and work the muscles in the neck, upper shoulders, and chest." This is important, he says, because people with chronic lung diseases use their neck and upper respiratory chest muscles more than other people.

People who have asthma and emphysema seem to really benefit from swimming, because the activity allows them to breathe very humidified air, says Dr. Teague.

Eat a little and often. As emphysema progresses and there is more obstruction to airflow, the lungs enlarge with trapped air. These enlarged lungs push down into the abdomen, leaving less room for the stomach to expand.

That's why six small meals will make you feel better than three large ones. Your best bet, says Dr. Teague, is to reach for foods that pack a lot of calories into a small volume, like high-protein selections.

Be aware, too, that prolonged digestion draws blood and oxygen to the stomach and away from other parts of the body, which may need them more.

Maintain your ideal body weight. Some emphysema sufferers gain a lot of weight and tend to retain fluid, says Dr. Teague. It takes more energy to carry extra body weight. The closer you are to your ideal weight, the better for your lungs.

"The true emphysema patient tends to be very skinny," adds Dr. Teague. "Because they have to breathe harder, they expend more energy." If you're underweight, conscientiously add calories, says Dr. Teague. High-protein foods are a good source of calories.

Become a champion breather. There are several things you can do to get the maximum oomph from each breath you take. They include:

Make your breathing uniform. When Dr. Teague and his colleagues studied 20 patients with advanced emphysema, they found that even under normal conditions their subjects had "very chaotic breathing patterns. Their breathing was all over the map—big breaths, little breaths. We taught them normal breathing patterns and it helped, at least in the short term.

Breathe from your diaphragm. This is the most efficient way to breathe. Babies do it naturally. If you watch them, you'll see their bellies rise and fall with each breath.

Not sure whether you're breathing from your diaphragm or your chest? Francisco Perez, Ph.D., a clinical assistant professor of neurology and physical medicine at Baylor College of Medicine, tells his patients to lie down, put City of Houston–size phone directories on their bellies and watch what happens to them when they breathe.

Keep those airways open. You can strengthen your breathing muscles if you blow out slowly through pursed lips for 30 minutes a day, says Dr. Gong. Try to exhale twice as long as it took you to breathe in. This will help you rid the lungs of stale air, so fresh air can get in.

You can also buy a device from your pharmacy that offers resistance when you blow against it. "It looks like a little plastic mouthpiece with a ring on the end," says Dr. Sandhaus. "When you turn the ring, the opening at the mouthpiece changes size. You start with the largest opening, take a deep breath in and blow out. Once you master one setting, you move on to another one."

Try vitamins C and E. Dr. Sandhaus advises his emphysema patients to take a minimum of 250 milligrams of vitamin C twice a day, and 800 international units of vitamin E twice a day. (Of course, don't practice this or any vitamin therapy without your doctor's okay and supervision.)

Dr. Sandhaus says that the vitamin therapy is unproven, but it can't hurt. He thinks vitamins C and E may be helpful because they're antioxidants. "We know that the oxidants in cigarette smoke are what damage the lungs," he says.

Allow yourself to grieve. Your life with emphysema won't be the same as your life before emphysema. Allow yourself to move through each stage of the grieving process, says Dr. Perez. "There are some losses. But then you recognize that you have control over it.

"The ultimate stage in adapting is compromising," he says. "That involves give and take, instead of seeing things in black and white."

Relax. "If you cognitively view the disease as a threat, you'll arouse some physiological mechanisms that can make your emphysema worse," says Dr. Perez. "When you're in a constant state of alarm, you're demanding a lot of oxygen in the process. Alarm is created by the thought process, which you can control. That means you can also control the physiological mechanisms."

Shift your focus to the present. When you find yourself feeling guilty that you brought on your disease, shift your orientation to the present and concentrate on what's happening now, says Dr. Perez. "You can't deal with events that happened in the past. You can only learn from them."

Anger and self-blame are normal, he says. Your best bet is to talk about it and then let it go.

Set small goals. One way to shift your focus from "emphysema is incapacitating" to "emphysema is something I have control over" is to set realistic small goals for yourself, says Dr. Perez.

Exercise is a great way to boost your confidence, he says. "Set some real objective goal based on the physical evidence. Use charts and graphs to measure your progress. This gives you a very objective measure of your ability to do something."

Join a rehabilitation group. Consider joining a pulmonary rehabilitation group, says Dr. Gong. If you can't find one locally, contact your nearby American Lung Association chapter. A group can educate you about your condition and provide social support. "Statistics show that these programs can decrease the number of hospitalizations," says Dr. Gong.

Have a family member play "coach." Have your significant other become your coach and help you through those times when you're short of breath, suggests Dr. Perez. "A coach can help you go through the basic relaxation technique. They can sit down with you and ask you about your thought processes just before and during the attack. Psychologically, emphysema patients are very normal," he says. "Once they verbalize what they're thinking, they can see it's pretty ridiculous. The moment they start laughing, they relax and their breathing comes back."

Don't isolate yourself socially. "You need to avoid generalizing about the shortness of breath," says Dr. Teague. "Some emphysema sufferers think, 'Well, I probably can't do this.' Because they're scared they might get out somewhere and get short of breath, they quit going places they'd normally enjoy." Don't let it isolate you.

Pace yourself. "The other thing emphysema sufferers have to learn to do is to take their own time," says Dr. Teague. "They really can do what they want to do but they have to do it at their own pace. That is not an easy thing to do, to learn to walk slower."

Work smarter. Little things can make a big difference. Can you rearrange your work spaces so you can get more done with less effort? What about setting your table with dishes directly from the drying rack instead of putting them away?

The American Lung Association also suggests that you obtain a three-shelf utility cart to help you with your housework. Small efficiencies like these pay you back with extra energy.

Coordinate your breathing to your lifting. According to the American Lung Association, housework will be easier if you remember to lift while you exhale through pursed lips. Inhale while you rest. Similarly, if you have to climb steps, climb while you exhale through pursed lips and inhale while you rest.

Don't use unnecessary sprays. You don't need to add to your respiratory problems by inhaling unknown substances, says the American Lung Association. Use liquid or gel-type hair dressings and roll-on or solid deodorants. Avoid aerosol-spray household cleaners.

Let loose. On your clothing, that is. Choose clothing that allows your chest and abdomen to expand freely. That means no tight belts, bras, or girdles, says the American Lung Association. Women may find camisoles more comfortable than bras. Men and women might substitute suspenders for tight belts.

PANEL OF ADVISERS

Henry Gong, M.D., is professor of medicine at the University of California, Los Angeles, and associate chief of the Pulmonary Division of the UCLA Medical Center.

Francisco Perez, Ph.D., is a clinical assistant professor of neurology and physical medicine at Baylor College of Medicine in Houston, Texas. He is coauthor of a paper on managing chronic pulmonary disease.

Robert Sandhaus, M.D., Ph.D., is in private practice in Denver, Colorado. A pulmonary specialist, he is a consultant for the National Jewish Center for Immunology and Respiratory Medicine, as well as Porter Memorial Hospital, Swedish Medical Center, Craig Hospital, and Littleton Hospital in Denver.

Robert B. Teague, M.D., is in private practice in Houston, Texas, and is a clinical assistant professor of medicine at Baylor College of Medicine in Houston. He is also coauthor of a paper on managing chronic pulmonary disease.

Endometriosis

14 Coping Techniques

For years, pain has crept through your days like a cat burglar, stealing time, peace of mind, and happiness. Many days, your lower back hurts for no apparent reason. Bowel movements and intercourse are painful. For the first day or two of your period, intense cramping keeps you doubled into a ball on your bed.

Your gynecologist has named this insidious intruder endometriosis. Endometrial tissue, which is supposed to line the inside of the uterus

The Effects of Pregnancy

Doctors say pregnancy and breastfeeding have been shown to induce hormonal changes in women with endometriosis and can, for a time, end some of the symptoms of the painful uterine disease. But studies show women with endometriosis are more likely to be infertile than otherwise healthy women. Those who conceive may have a higher rate of miscarriage and a higher rate of ectopic pregnancy, where the fertilized egg implants outside the uterus.

And, even though the symptoms of endometriosis may disappear during pregnancy, they often recur after the baby is born, reports the Endometriosis Association.

and be shed each month with the menstrual cycle, is growing outside your uterus on your ovaries, around your fallopian tubes, or across the ligaments that support your uterus. Where it lands, it weaves weblike scars as it anchors itself in your internal tissues. Then, like normal endometrial tissue, it swells and bleeds during menstruation, leaving a discharge that can't exit the body and that can cause inflammation and scarring.

Your doctor is probably trying one of several different medical approaches to controlling your endometriosis. In the meantime, there are some things you can do to help yourself and ease the discomfort.

Share your pain. Call your local women's center and find a support group, says Mary Lou Ballweg, co-founder of the international Endometriosis Association with headquarters in Milwaukee, Wisconsin. She founded the association when she needed help with endometriosis.

"Sometimes it helps just to hear you aren't all alone, knowing that other people are going through the same thing," says Mary Sinn, R.N., WomanCare coordinator at Gnaden Huetten Hospital in Lehighton, Pennsylvania. "It's an information source, too. Not everything works for everyone, but there will be ideas to try. Some women will say, 'I tried that pain reliever and it really worked for me.'"

"You will have to work on building knowledge of your disease," says Ballweg. "If you rely solely on your physician, you won't do as well. Women who look for solutions for themselves seem to do the best."

Women with fertility problems caused by endometriosis may find additional help from infertility support groups, adds Sinn.

Keep a calendar. Chart your cycle. Note when your symptoms are worse and when they are barely noticeable. Observe your diet and activity. Then consider how what you eat and how much you exercise affects your cycle, says Kay Evans, a Littleton, Colorado, psychotherapist who has endometriosis. You'll be able to take charge of some of your symptoms by avoiding things that cause pain and by seeing what makes you feel your best.

Block the prostaglandin. One of the reasons for cramping, especially at the time of your period, is that your body produces too much prostaglandin, a hormone in the uterine lining. It overstimulates your uterine muscles, forcing them to work overtime. And, like any muscle that works too hard, they cramp. Aspirin, an anti-inflammatory drug, may relieve cramps, but the best over-the-counter pain relievers are anti-prostaglandins such as Advil, Medipren, or Nuprin. Take two tablets at a time, says Camran Nezhat, M.D., an Atlanta, Georgia, gynecologist and fertility expert who is an adviser to the Endometriosis Association.

Eat more fish. Add a natural antiprostaglandin to your diet with fish, advises Dr. Nezhat. Fish contains omega-3 fatty acids, which suppress prostaglandin production.

Add some heat. Some of the old-time remedies for menstrual cramping and low back pain will bring relief to women with endometriosis, says Sinn. Try bed rest, moist heat, or a heating pad and warm drinks to relax the cramping muscles in your abdomen.

Try a cold pack. If warmth doesn't work, you may be one of the women who finds more relief from cold than heat, Sinn adds. Place the ice pack on your lower abdominal area.

Exercise for relief. Exercise reduces estrogen levels, which may slow the growth of endometriosis. Exercise also increases the body's production of endorphins, natural pain-blocking substances. Try gentle exercise such as walking, because jarring exercise can pull on adhesions and scar tissue.

Nancy Fletcher, who was diagnosed as having endometriosis in 1980 and is the support program and development coordinator for the Endometriosis Association, walks 2 miles a day and runs about 4 miles three times a week. She finds that exercise, along with a positive outlook on life, has an impact on alleviating her symptoms.

Cut your caffeine. Caffeine, in soda, tea, or coffee, seems to aggravate the pain in some women, according to Dr. Nezhat. He advises women to avoid caffeine.

Stay carefree. Keeping the menstrual flow free and unobstructed may help prevent endometriosis, says Dr. Nezhat. Tampons may contribute to menstrual cramping by plugging the vagina like a cork. Use napkins instead of tampons, especially if you have a narrow vagina or small vaginal opening.

Take a new position. Women with endometriosis may also have a tipped uterus and often find intercourse painful, Dr. Nezhat says. During intercourse, the man's penis pushes against the uterus, which bumps nerves. The solution is to try new positions, he says. One he suggests, which allows for penetration without pain, places the man on his knees behind the woman, who positions herself on her hands and knees.

Use a natural lubricant. Extra lubrication may be necessary to ease painful intercourse, Dr. Nezhat says. And women who are having a hard time getting pregnant, a frequent problem in endometriosis, should

---

The Alternate Route

A Tip from the Chinese

Some women report that a Chinese healing technique can relieve the painful symptoms of endometriosis, says psychotherapist Kay Evans, who also suffers from the disease.

The method is called moxibustion, and here's how it works. Moxa sticks—the herb mugwort rolled tightly into a sticklike cigar—are lit at one end until they glow. Then the burning white leaf-stick is held close enough to acupressure points that correspond to painful areas, until the skin turns pink and feels very hot but is not burned.

Relief, report women who have used this treatment, lasts for hours. Before you try this, you must be taught where to place moxa sticks and how to use them properly, says Evans. The sticks can be found in some health food and oriental stores. An acupuncturist can give you information on getting proper instruction.

use egg whites instead of petroleum jelly. "Petroleum jelly could kill the sperm," he says, "but the egg whites won't. The whites may encourage the sperm to race toward the ovum."

Call for help. For self-help information, or help in finding a knowledgeable doctor or a support group, call the Endometriosis Association. In the United States, call 1-800-992-3636. In Canada, 1-800-426-2363.

Press when it hurts. Acupressure relieves pain without drugs. That's important to Susan Anderson, president of the Los Angeles, California, chapter of the Endometriosis Association. When pain begins, there are two spots she presses for relief.

One spot is located on the inside of your leg, about 2 inches above your ankle bone. You'll have found the right spot if it feels a little tender, Anderson says. The other pressure point is at the base where the bones of your thumb and your index finger meet. Press as hard as possible.

PANEL OF ADVISERS

Susan Anderson is president of the Los Angeles, California, chapter of the Endometriosis Association.

Mary Lou Ballweg is co-founder of the Endometriosis Association, a self-help organization in Milwaukee, Wisconsin. She is the author of *Overcoming Endometriosis.*

Kay Evans is a psychotherapist in Littleton, Colorado. She has endometriosis and is a former officer in the San Diego, California, chapter of the Endometriosis Association.

Nancy Fletcher is the support program and development coordinator for the Endometriosis Association. She was diagnosed as having endometriosis in 1980.

Camran Nezhat, M.D., is a gynecologist and fertility expert in Atlanta, Georgia, and the director of the Fertility and Endocrinology Center there. He has been an adviser to the Endometriosis Association since 1985.

Mary Sinn, R.N., is coordinator of the WomanCare unit at Gnaden Huetten Hospital in Lehighton, Pennsylvania.

Eye Redness

5 Ways to Wipe It Out

Do the whites of your eyes have more red lines than a road map? If so, here's what you can do.

Water your eyes. "It seems obvious, but if your red eyes are a result of not getting enough sleep, find a way to catch up on your rest," says Mitchell Friedlaender, M.D., a California ophthalmologist and director of corneal and external diseases in the Division of Ophthalmology at Scripps Clinic and Research Foundation in La Jolla, California. "Closing your eyes for 7 to 8 hours helps to rehydrate them. Without sleep the eyes can dry out. And dry eyes are red eyes."

Treat your eyelids. If your eyes are red when you wake up, the problem may not be in your eyes but on your eyelids. "It's called blepharitis, and it's a low-grade infection of your eyelids," says Dr. Friedlaender. "You

---

Look for the Red Badge of Aging

There's a patch of blood in the white of your eye, and you can't remember anything happening. There's no swelling, no pain, no loss of vision, nothing. Just a blotch of red.

If that's the case, then relax. "It's a common occurrence, especially if you're over 40," says Michael Marmor, M.D., an ophthalmologist and chairman of the Department of Ophthalmology at Stanford University Medical Center in California. "The blood will go away by itself. You can't do anything for it. Eyedrops won't do any good. It will go away by itself in one to two weeks. The hardest part of the whole thing will be trying to think up a story to explain to your friends how it happened."

MEDICAL ALERT

Protect Your Pupils

When you see blood in the white of your eye, that's okay, but it's not okay if you see blood covering your pupil. "Anytime there is blood inside the eye, over the pupil, that's serious and you need to see a doctor right away," says Michael Marmor, M.D., an ophthalmologist and chairman of the Department of Ophthalmology at Stanford University Medical Center in California.

"Many times you won't actually see the bleeding, but your eye will hurt, your vision will be blurred, or you'll have a pinkish haze. If any of these symptoms is present, you know something is wrong, and you need medical treatment."

---

can treat it by washing your eyelids with warm water at night before you go to bed. Make sure you cleanse the lids so that the debris, oils, bacteria, makeup, and dandruff on the lashes are all removed."

Use drops sparingly. "Drops designed to get the red out have an agent in them that works to constrict your blood vessels," says Dr. Friedlaender. "They take the redness out by shrinking the blood vessels in your eye, which makes your eye look whiter for the time being.

"The problem is, most of those drops have a rebound effect so that when they wear off in a couple of hours, the redness comes back worse than it was in the first place."

The best advice: Use eyedrops sparingly.

Shed crocodile tears. Do you arrive at work bright-eyed, but leave in the red? "Redness that comes on during the day is caused by dryness," says Dr. Friedlaender. "If that's the case, over-the-counter artificial tears can be used to moisten the eyes." Unlike other eyedrops, artificial tears do not shrink blood vessels.

Get your eyes to cool it. "Use a cool, wet washcloth and lay it over your closed eyes," says Dr. Friedlaender. "The cold will constrict the blood vessels without the rebound effect, plus the water will add moisture to your eyes."

Eyestrain

10 Tips to Avoid It

"Around age 40 or 45, your focusing power starts to go and it can lead to eyestrain," says Samuel L. Guillory, M.D., a New York City ophthalmologist and assistant clinical professor at Mount Sinai Medical Center of the City University of New York. "It's a gradual process that happens to everyone."

But you can get eyestrain at *any* age if what you're staring at all day is a video display terminal (VDT).

If you find your eyes straining to read your birthday cards or a VDT screen, here are some suggestions that might help.

Pay attention to lighting. "It doesn't hurt your eyes to read in dim light, but you can strain them if the light doesn't provide enough contrast," says Dr. Guillory. "Use a soft light that gives contrast, but not glare, when you read. And don't use any lamp that reflects light directly back into your eyes."

Try reading glasses. You can get them from your doctor or even from your drugstore. "If you have good distance vision in both eyes and just have trouble seeing up close, go to your local drugstore and buy the reading glasses they have on display there," says ophthalmologist David

---

MEDICAL ALERT

Problems That Need a Doctor

Sometimes the cause of eyestrain is a lot more serious than just passing your fortieth birthday. "Strain can also be caused by eye misalignment, where one eye starts to turn in or out," says David Guyton, M.D. "If that's the case, the problem needs to be treated by an ophthalmologist who can suggest specific exercises, prescribe special prism glasses, or—if necessary—even perform eye muscle surgery to realign the eyes."

All the experts agree that if you have pain in your eye or sensitivity to light, you need to see an ophthalmologist right away.

Guyton, M.D., a professor at Johns Hopkins University School of Medicine. "They're sold in all 50 states, cost from $10 to $20, and are impact-resistant, good-quality glasses that will help you."

Pick the right power. You are the best judge of which reading glasses work best for you. "Pick the weakest, or least powerful, ones that will allow you to read at the distance you want," says Dr. Guyton. "If you buy ones that are too powerful, you will see fine up close, but things will be blurred beyond that distance."

Interrupt your work. Save and store what's on your VDT screen every once in a while. "If you use the computer for 6 to 8 hours," says Dr. Guillory, "take a break every 2 to 3 hours. Do some other work, get coffee, go to the bathroom—just take your eyes off the screen for 10 to 15 minutes." Also consider working from a printout of your screen.

Darken your screen. Those aren't just letters and numbers on your screen. They're also tiny light bulbs that send light directly into your eyes. You need to turn the wattage down, so to speak. "Don't make the letters too bright," advises Dr. Guillory. "Turn the brightness down to a dim level and then adjust the contrast to make up the difference." An added tip: Take a pencil and make a mark on the knob you adjusted. Then make a corresponding mark on the computer. That way you'll just have to realign the marks if somebody changes the setting on your computer when you're not there.

The Alternate Route

Yoga—And Beyond

For Meir Schneider, yoga wasn't only the key to gaining spiritual insight. It also was the key to simply gaining sight. "Yoga helped cure my blindness," claims Schneider, who was born blind. He credits daily yoga exercises for helping bring back his vision, which he says is now 20/60. "And it's still improving."

The techniques Schneider teaches at his Center for Self Healing in San Francisco, California, and in his book *Self Healing: My Life and Vision,* are influenced by the controversial work done by turn-of-the-century ophthalmologist and eye-exercise proponent Dr. William Bates. "I took the Bates Method and added a bit of my own work to it," says Schneider. While it might be straining science a bit to say it cures blindness, some of his techniques may be helpful in handling eyestrain.

Take a tea break. But don't drink it; put it on your eyes instead. "Take a towel and soak it in eyebright tea," says Schneider. "Lie down and place the warm towel over your closed eyes and leave it there for 10 to 15 minutes. It will make your eyestrain go away." Be very careful not to pour tea into your eyes, though. And also let the tea cool down a bit after the pot boils before you soak the towel in it.

Try a different sort of eye/hand coordination. If you want to help your eyes, Schneider says, you need to lend them a hand. "Take your hands and rub them together until they are warm. Then close your eyes and put your palms on your eye orbits. Don't press on your eyes, just cover them. Breathe deeply and slowly and visualize the color black. Do this for 20 minutes every day."

Put your eyes "on the blink." Your eyes have their own personal masseuse—the eyelids. "Make it a point to consciously blink your eyes 300 times every day and not squint," says Schneider. "Each blink cleanses your eyes, and gives them a tiny little massage." And it's free.

Work in the shade. When it comes to relieving eyestrain, it's best to keep your computer in the dark. "Shade your screen by creating a hood over it," Dr. Guillory suggests. "Go to an art supply store and buy a sheet of heavy black cardboard. Put it on top of your terminal and fold both sides down over it. That will allow you to slide it back and forth.

What you've done, essentially, is put your machine in a black box. So now you can turn the brightness down to a very low level."

Shut out the light by shutting your eyes. Our experts say the best way to relieve eyestrain is to rest your eyes. And that's easier than you may think. "You can do it while you're on the phone," says Dr. Guillory. "If you don't need to read or write, just close your eyes while you're talking. Depending on how much time you spend on the phone each day, you may be able to rest your eyes for almost an hour or two daily. People who practice this technique say their eyes really feel better, and it helps rid them of eyestrain."

PANEL OF ADVISERS

Samuel L. Guillory, M.D., is an ophthalmologist and assistant clinical professor of ophthalmology at Mount Sinai Medical Center of the City University of New York in New York City.

David Guyton, M.D., is an ophthalmologist and professor of ophthalmology at Johns Hopkins University School of Medicine in Baltimore, Maryland.

Meir Schneider is director of the Center for Self Healing in San Francisco, California. He is author of *Self Healing: My Life and Vision.*

Fatigue

35 Hints for a High-Energy Life

Be honest. When you first heard the words "energy crisis," did you think of Arab oil embargoes or yourself?

If you thought of yourself—struggling to start your inner engine in the morning, desperate to keep it humming after lunch in the afternoon, and only too willing to let it sputter to a stop in the evening—you are not alone.

Everyone, at one time or another, feels fatigued. And who wouldn't like to have more energy than they now have?

Unfortunately, having more energy is a lot like having more money—it's easier to talk about it than to get it. Yet it's also easier to increase your energy than you probably realize. Of course, the broad prescription from doctors is still the same: Get plenty of rest, eat a balanced diet, and exercise. But here physicians and other authorities on fatigue go beyond these generalities and offer more specific, high-octane suggestions.

So, ladies and gentlemen, please start your engines.

Warm up. "Give yourself an extra 15 minutes in the morning before you start your day," says Vicky Young, M.D., an assistant professor in the Department of Preventive Medicine at the Medical College of Wisconsin. "That way you don't start off feeling rushed and tired."

Eat a three-piece breakfast. The three components of a good breakfast are carbohydrates, proteins, and fats, advises Rick Ricer, M.D., assistant professor of clinical family medicine at Ohio State University College of Medicine. Of course you don't want to *add* fat to your breakfast table. You will get plenty of fats, a good form of storable energy, in the proteins you eat.

But even cereal (a complex carbohydrate) with milk (a source of protein) can get your day off to a good start. Wheat toast and muffins are also good complex carbohydrate options. For protein, you might want to consider low-fat yogurt and cottage cheese, or a small piece of chicken or fish.

Meanwhile, Dr. Ricer warns not to eat an ultra-high carbohydrate breakfast laden with simple sugars. "You can actually overactivate your insulin and your blood sugar will drop; that can leave you jittery." So avoid the doughnut shop between home and office.

Know where you're going. If you don't, you will probably be too tired to get there. "Take time each morning to set specific goals for the day," says David Sheridan, M.D., an associate professor in the Department of Preventive Medicine at the University of South Carolina School of Medicine. "Determine what you want to do; don't let the routine control you."

Arrest the energy robbers. "If it's a problem on the job, or if it's a family feud, you've got to resolve it," says M. F. Graham, M.D., a Dallas, Texas, consultant to the American Running and Fitness Association and author of *Inner Energy: How to Overcome Fatigue.*

But if you can't resolve your problem, "at least take a vacation from the situation," Dr. Ricer suggests. So if you're trying to hold down a second job, quit it or take a leave of absence. And if relatives have overstayed their welcome, politely suggest they visit again—in about three years.

Turn off to turn on. Television is famous—make that infamous—for lulling human beings into lethargy. "Try reading instead," Dr. Ricer says. "That has to be more energizing."

Work out to rev up. "Exercise actually gives you energy," Dr. Young says. Study after study supports those words, including one by the National Aeronautics and Space Administration. More than 200 federal employees were placed on a moderate, regular exercise program. The results: 90 percent said they had never felt better. Almost half said they felt less stress, and almost one-third reported they slept better.

Dr. Young recommends giving yourself a dose of energetic exercise—brisk walking is enough—three to five times a week, for 20 to 30 minutes each time and no later than 2 hours before bedtime.

Remember—honesty is the best policy. For all the good exercise can do, it can be addictive. And you can overdose if you're not honest about what your body is telling you.

"I have to work at telling myself that it will be good for me, that I will gain by taking time off," says Mary Trafton, a hiker, marathoner, and skier who works for the Appalachian Mountain Club in Boston, Massachusetts.

Tackle one thing at a time. "Make lists," Dr. Sheridan says. "Many times, people feel fatigued because they think, 'I have so much to do I don't know where to start.' " By setting priorities and charting your progress as you make your way through the list, you can remain focused and energetic.

Take one a day. If you are guilty of missing meals, dieting, or not eating properly, Dr. Young says, taking one multivitamin and mineral supplement a day is a good idea. "A lack of good nutrition can cause fatigue, and a supplement can help make up for the missing nutrients. But don't look to a vitamin to give you instant energy," says Dr. Ricer.

"It's a fallacy that when you're tired you just take more vitamins and feel better," Dr. Ricer says. Only eating properly can do that.

Teach your body to tell time. Circadian rhythms act as our bodies' internal clocks, raising and lowering blood pressure and body temperature at different times throughout the day. This chemical action

---

MEDICAL ALERT

When Tired Means Sick

Fatigue may be just a signal that you need to manage your life better, or that a cold or flu is coming on.

But it also can be a warning sign of serious illness. "Anything that's chronic —diabetes, lung disease, anemia—will cause fatigue," says Rick Ricer, M.D.

Fatigue is also a symptom of many other illnesses, including hepatitis, mononucleosis, thyroid disease, and cancer. So if your tiredness persists, don't try to diagnose yourself. See a doctor.

---

causes the "swings" we experience — from feeling alert to feeling mentally and physically fogged in.

So why are some people's natural peak times so inconvenient — like late at night? "I think sometimes people, perhaps without even knowing it, work themselves into a particular time cycle," says William Fink, an exercise physiologist and assistant to the director of the Human Performance Laboratory at Ball State University.

Fink suggests changing your schedule, as much as practically possible, to complement your circadian rhythms. This can be done simply by getting up a little sooner or a little later — say 15 minutes — until you feel comfortable with it. Keep it up until you reach your desired schedule.

Put out the fire. Doctors always advise giving up smoking, but add this to the list of reasons: Smoking adversely affects the delivery of oxygen to tissues. The result is fatigue.

When you first quit, however, don't expect an immediate energy boost. Nicotine acts as a stimulant, and withdrawal may cause some temporary tiredness.

Make exercise an all-day activity. Whether you work out early, at lunchtime, or in the evening, don't save all your exercising for one block of time. "Get up and move around at least every couple of hours," Dr. Sheridan says.

The options are limitless: the executive who rides a stationary bicycle in the privacy of his office, the medical resident who runs hospital stairs, and the researcher who does isometric exercises sitting at her desk.

Just say no. "Learn to delegate," Dr. Sheridan says. If too many obligations or commitments are wearing you out, learn to say, "I will not serve on that committee."

Shed. As in pounds. "If you're obese—if you need to drop 20 percent of your weight or more—losing weight will be a great help," Fink says. Of course, make sure you follow a sensible diet in combination with exercise. Losing a lot of weight quickly isn't healthy and will wear you down.

Get fewer zzzzzzs. You can get too much of a good thing, even sleep. "If you oversleep, you tend to be groggy all day," Fink says. "Usually 6 to 8 hours of sleep per night is enough for most people."

Blow out the candle. Burning the candle at both ends—not going to bed until 2:00 A.M. and getting up at 5:00 A.M., for example—will leave you feeling burned out. Don't shortchange yourself on sleep.

Get 20 winks. Naps aren't for everybody, but they might help recharge older people who aren't sleeping as soundly as they used to, Dr. Ricer says. Younger people with very hectic schedules and short nights also might consider taking naps. If you do decide to take naps, try to take them at the same time each day and for no more than an hour.

Breathe deeply. It's one of the best ways to relax and energize at the same time, according to doctors and athletes.

Just have one. Alcohol is a depressant, notes Dr. Ricer, and will calm you down, not rev you up. Limit your alcohol intake to one drink, Dr. Ricer suggests, or don't drink at all.

Eat a light lunch. Some doctors advise a light lunch to avoid a severe case of the post-lunch-I-want-to-sleep-on-my-desk blues. And for some people, this is probably the advice to follow. Soup and salad and a piece of fruit is light but nutritious.

Make lunch your big meal of the day. If soup and salad and a piece of fruit don't satisfy you, Dr. Young suggests eating your largest meal of the day at lunch and following it up with a 20-minute walk. Eating most of your calories early in the day will give you the fuel you need to keep perking. But you've got to be selective in the type of fuel you choose. Carbohydrate, for example, is a fast burner. Fat, on the other hand, burns slowly, meaning it'll slow you down, too.

Say adios. "In a lot of cases, taking a vacation is almost mandatory," Dr. Ricer says. "If you haven't had a vacation in a long time, a vacation can be the perfect energy booster." That's *real* good advice.

Divert your energy. Strong emotion is mentally draining, but it can be physically draining, too, says Dr. Young. Redirect strong emotions, such as anger, and apply that energy to your job or a workout.

Open Your Mind to Energy

Where your mind goes, your body goes. That the mind can influence the body is now generally accepted. But have *you* accepted it? Are you aware that your thoughts can have a lot to do with how tired you feel?

Well, they can. So here are some beneficial attitudes that can affect your energy level.

Think positive. Championship athletes do it, successful corporate executive officers do it, and you should do it.

"It's important to think positively," says Mary Trafton, an avid hiker and marathoner. "If I step in a huge puddle while hiking, I don't think, 'Ah, I'm going to be cold and tired.' I think about the wool socks I have on for protection and warmth."

Be motivated. When you think about it, it's pretty hard to do much of anything if you're not motivated. But it's next to impossible to accomplish tasks that require mega-energy if your spirit just isn't in it.

Take E. Drummond King, for example. He participates in the grueling Iron Man competitions in Hawaii—where competitors swim, bicycle, and run long distances for hours on end. He says when he has been too far behind to win his age group (50–54), he has finished the race by walking instead of running. Yet when there's a chance to win, or a bet riding on how long it takes him, he somehow finds the energy to continue running.

Be confident. Chances are good that if you feel you *can* do it, you will have the energy to do it. And once you've proven to yourself that you've got the energy, you will become even more confident.

That's the way they feel at the University of Miami, where winning on the football field is expected. "We encourage our athletes by telling them that they're in better shape than their opponents and that the fourth quarter is ours," says Bill Foran, head strength and conditioning coach at the university.

Color your world. "If you live in a dark, dark house, you're going to feel fatigued," Dr. Ricer says. He suggests a little sunshine—literally or figuratively. Several studies have shown that lots of color and lots of variety are important in keeping energy levels high. Red, for example, is good for short-term, high-energy stimulation, while green is good at eliminating distractions and maintaining focus for long periods of time.

Tune in. Music can light your fire, Dr. Ricer says. Listen to U2, Willie Nelson, Frank Sinatra—whatever and whoever peps you up.

Give yourself a target. Some people simply need deadlines to keep moving forward, Dr. Sheridan says. If you're like that, give yourself both short and long deadlines—so neither becomes too routine.

Make a splash. When fatigue starts to drop one New York stock-broker, he doesn't buy or sell. He stops—long enough to hit himself in the face with splashes of cold water.

But if he were home, perhaps a cold shower would restore his energy even better. Cascading water emits negative ions in the air, which surround the body. Negative ions are thought to make some people feel happier and more energetic.

Drink up. Not booze but water. The day before you're going to be out in the hot sun and physically active—say a day at Disney World with the grandchildren—doctors advise that you drink plenty of water and continue to do so on the day of the activity. This will guard against dehydration, which in turn can cause fatigue.

E. Drummond King, an over-50 triathlete, learned the hard way that it's best to start drinking a lot of fluids the day before his body is going to need them.

"The major problem is dehydration and the fatigue that comes with it," he says. "Now I spend the day before walking around with a water bottle in my hand."

Rethink your medications. Do you really need to take all those prescription and over-the-counter medicines? If not, you may be shocked at what eliminating or reducing dosages of certain medications may do for you.

Sleeping pills, for example, are notorious for their next-day hang-over effects. But also among the villains, according to doctors, are high blood pressure medicines and cough and cold medicines.

If you suspect a medication is guilty of grand theft energy, discuss it with your doctor. Maybe he can change your prescription, or better yet, take you off the medicine altogether. But never stop taking a prescription medication without your doctor's approval.

If it feels good, do it. There's no denying the pleasures of massages, whirlpools, and steam baths. "It's hard to study scientifically whether or not they lessen fatigue," says Fink. "But there are those who swear by them. I'm convinced, too—if people feel better, they'll perform better."

Change and explore. Sometimes fatigue can be caused by being in a rut. Even the simplest of changes, says Dr. Ricer, can make the difference. If you always start your day by reading the paper, for example, try reading something inspirational. If you always eat fish for Monday dinner, reel in chicken next Monday instead. If you're a daily runner, try interspersing some scenic bicycle rides.

Curb your caffeine. One or two cups of coffee can work to kick you into gear in the morning, says Dr. Ricer, but its benefits usually end there. Too much caffeine is just as bad as too much of anything. Drinking it throughout the day for an energy boost can actually backfire.

Caffeine is a magician, Dr. Ricer says. "It makes you feel like you have more energy, but you really don't."

Dr. Ricer advises at least cutting back on caffeine to reduce the roller-coaster effect. "If someone is looking for an energy boost," Fink says, "I would hesitate to recommend caffeine."

PANEL OF ADVISERS

William Fink is an exercise physiologist and assistant to the director of the Human Performance Laboratory at Ball State University in Muncie, Indiana.

Bill Foran is head strength and conditioning coach at the University of Miami in Coral Gables, Florida.

M. F. Graham, M.D., is a pediatrician in Dallas, Texas, and a consultant to the American Running and Fitness Association. He is also author of *Inner Energy: How to Overcome Fatigue.*

E. Drummond King is a triathlete and a lawyer in Allentown, Pennsylvania.

Rick Ricer, M.D., is assistant professor of clinical family medicine at the Ohio State University College of Medicine in Columbus.

David Sheridan, M.D., is an associate professor in the Department of Preventive Medicine at the University of South Carolina School of Medicine in Columbia.

Mary Trafton is a hiker, marathoner, and skier and information specialist for the Appalachian Mountain Club in Boston, Massachusetts.

Vicky Young, M.D., is an assistant professor in the Department of Preventive Medicine at the Medical College of Wisconsin in Milwaukee.

Fever

26 Coping Tactics

"Man, are you hot!"

In some circles that's quite a compliment. At the moment, however, it's just a cold, hard fact: Your temperature's up, and you are quite uncomfortable. Right now, compared with you, the devil is a real cool dude. But before you take steps to douse the fire, listen to what doctors say.

Make sure you actually have a fever. Although 98.6°F is considered the norm, that number is not etched in stone. "Normal" temperature varies from person to person and fluctuates widely throughout the day. Food, excess clothing, emotional excitement, and vigorous exercise can all elevate temperature, says Donald Vickery, M.D., a corporate-health consultant and assistant clinical professor at Georgetown University School of Medicine. "In fact, vigorous exercise can raise body temperature to as high as 103°F. Furthermore, children tend to have higher temperatures than adults and greater daily variations.

"So here's a general rule: If your temperature is 99° to 100°F, start thinking about the possibility of fever. If it is 100° or above, it is a fever," he says.

Leonard Banco, M.D., an associate professor of pediatrics at the University of Connecticut School of Medicine, adds that often a person's appearance is a better indicator of his condition than hard-and-fast numbers. "A child with a raised temperature who looks ill needs attention sooner than one who looks and acts well."

Don't fight it. If you do have a fever, remember this: Fever itself is not an illness—it's a symptom of one. In fact, it's one of the body's defense mechanisms against infection, says public-health authority Stephen Rosenberg, M.D., an associate professor of clinical public health at Columbia University School of Public Health. And fever may even serve a useful purpose: shortening an illness, increasing the power of antibiotics,

MEDICAL ALERT

Know the Danger Signs

Donald Vickery, M.D., recommends that you see a doctor for:

- Fever in a child less than 4 months old.
- Fever associated with a stiff neck.
- Fever above 105°F if home treatment fails to reduce it at least partly.
- Fever above 106°F under any condition.
- Fever that lasts more than five days.

Stephen Rosenberg, M.D., warns that in children under 6 an oral temperature of 102°F or higher can trigger convulsions. And adults with chronic illnesses, such as heart or respiratory disease, may not be able to tolerate prolonged high fevers.

and making an infection less contagious. These possibilities should be weighed against the discomfort involved in letting a slight fever run its course, he says.

If you feel the need for extra relief, try the following steps.

Liquefy your assets. When you're hot, your body perspires to cool you down. But if you lose too much water—as you might with a high fever—your body turns off its sweat ducts to forestall further water loss. That makes it more difficult for you to cope with your fever. The moral of this story: Drink up, mateys, or your ship will be sunk. In addition to plain water, doctors favor the following.

Fruit and vegetable juices. These are high in vitamins and minerals, says nutrition counselor Eleonore Blaurock-Busch, Ph.D., president and director of Trace Minerals International in Boulder, Colorado. She particularly favors nutrient-dense beet juice and carrot juice. If you're thirsty for tomato juice, notes pharmacology professor Thomas Gossel, Ph.D., R.Ph., chairman of the Department of Pharmacology and Biomedical Sciences at Ohio Northern University, choose one that is low in sodium.

One doctor's botanical tea. Although any tea will provide needed fluid, several are particularly suited for fever, says Dr. Blaurock-Busch. (Look for the following unusual botanicals in health food stores.) One mixture she likes combines equal parts dried thyme, linden flowers, and chamomile flowers. Thyme has antiseptic properties, chamomile reduces inflammation, and linden promotes sweating, she says. Steep 1 teaspoon of the mixture in 1 cup of boiling water for 5 minutes. Strain and drink warm several times a day.

Linden tea. This tea by itself is also good, she says, and can induce sweating to break a fever. Use 1 tablespoon of the flowers in 1 cup of boiling water. Prepare as above and drink hot often.

Willow bark. This bark is rich in salicylates, which are aspirin-related compounds, and is considered "nature's fever medication," says Dr. Blaurock-Busch. Brew into a tea and drink in small doses.

Black elder. Another old-time fever treatment, black elder is preferable to willow bark if you can't tolerate aspirin, she says. Again, brew into a tea and drink as desired.

Ice. If you're too nauseated to drink, you can suck on ice. For variety, freeze fruit juice in an ice-cube tray. To entice a feverish child, embed a grape or strawberry in each cube.

Get compressed relief. Wet compresses help reduce the body's temperature output, says Dr. Blaurock-Busch. Ironically, she says, hot, moist compresses can do the job. When the patient starts to feel uncomfortably hot, remove those compresses and apply cool ones to his forehead, wrists, and calves. Keep the rest of his body covered.

But if the fever rises above 103°F, she says, do not use hot compresses at all. Instead, apply cool ones to prevent the fever from getting any higher. Change them as they warm to body temperature and continue until the fever drops.

Sponge off. Evaporation also has a cooling effect on body temperature. Philadelphia, Pennsylvania, nurse clinician Mary Ann Pane, R.N., recommends cool tap water to help the skin dissipate excess heat. Although you can sponge the whole body, she says, pay particular attention to spots where heat is generally greatest, such as the armpits and groin area. Wring out a sponge and wipe one section at a time, keeping the rest of the body covered. Body heat will evaporate the moisture, so you don't need to towel off.

Thermometer Ins and Outs

Your mother could gauge your temperature just by feeling your forehead. If you didn't inherit the knack—or if you don't have much confidence in this hands-on approach—you'll need to rely on thermometer readings. Here's how to get the most accurate results:

- Before using a glass and mercury thermometer, hold it by the top end (not the bulb) and shake it with a quick snap of the wrist until the mercury is below 96°F. If you're concerned about dropping and breaking the thermometer, do this over a bed, says Stephen Rosenberg, M.D.

- Wait at least 30 minutes after eating, drinking, or smoking before taking an oral reading, he says. These activities alter mouth temperature and will cause inaccurate readings.

- Place the thermometer under your tongue in one of the "pockets" located on either side of your mouth rather than right up front. These pockets are closer to blood vessels that reflect the body's core temperature.

- Hold the thermometer in place with your lips, not your teeth. Breathe through your nose rather than your mouth, so the room temperature doesn't affect the reading. Leave the thermometer in place for at least 3 minutes (some experts favor 5 to 7 minutes).

- In children under 5, take rectal readings rather than oral ones. Rectal temperature is generally 1 degree warmer than oral. Recognize rectal thermometers by their shorter, rounder bulb.

- To use a rectal thermometer, place your child, stomach down, on your lap and hold one hand on his buttocks to prevent movement, says Donald Vickery, M.D. Lubricate the end of the thermometer with petroleum jelly. Carefully insert it about 1 inch, but never use force. The mercury will start rising within seconds. Remove it when the mercury is no longer rising, after 1 or 2 minutes.

- If a thermometer breaks in the mouth or rectum, don't panic. The mercury is not poisonous, and usually the only harm done is a superficial scratch of the mouth or lining of the rectum. But do call a doctor if you can't find all the pieces of glass.

- After use, wash a glass thermometer in cool, soapy water. Never use hot water. And never store it near heat.

- Use a digital thermometer according to the directions that accompany it. Afterward, wash the tip with soap and lukewarm water or with rubbing alcohol. Do not immerse the instrument completely or splash water on the readout; you risk ruining the thermometer. Be prepared to change the battery every two years.

Doctors warn that although alcohol evaporates more rapidly than water, it can be uncomfortable for someone with a fever. What's more, there's the danger of inhaling the vapors or even absorbing them through the skin.

Take a dip. "Often when I have a fever, I really start to shiver," says Dr. Gossel. "At that point I'm most comfortable getting into a tub of warm water."

Dr. Banco advises room-temperature baths for babies. An alternative treatment, he says, is to sandwich the child between wet towels and change them every 15 minutes.

Don't suffer. If you're very uncomfortable, take a pain reliever. For adults Dr. Vickery recommends either two aspirin or two acetaminophen tablets every 4 hours. The advantage of acetaminophen, he says, is that fewer people are allergic to it.

Since aspirin and acetaminophen exert their effects in slightly different manners, he notes, you might want to pair them up if one alone is not effective in controlling the fever. Take two aspirin *plus* two acetaminophen (a total of four tablets) every 6 hours. Or stagger the medications so you take two aspirin at one time and two acetaminophen 3 hours later. Make sure this therapy gets your doctor's approval.

Give children acetaminophen. Where those under 21 are concerned, avoid aspirin. That's because aspirin can trigger Reye's syndrome, a potentially fatal neurological illness, in feverish children. Instead, says New Orleans pediatrician George Sterne, M.D., a clinical professor of pediatrics at Tulane University School of Medicine, use 5 to 7 milligrams of acetaminophen per pound of body weight. Repeat every 4 hours. "There is no reason to give it more frequently," he says. "And excessive doses over a period of days are dangerous."

Dress the part. Use common sense as far as clothing and blankets go, says Pane. If you're very hot, take off extra covers and clothes so body heat can evaporate into the air. But if you have a chill, bundle up until you're just comfortable.

Be especially careful to monitor infants, who cannot undress themselves if they become overheated, cautions Dr. Sterne. In fact, he says, overdressing a child or leaving him in a hot place (such as a car) can actually *cause* a fever.

Create a healing atmosphere. Do your best to make the sickroom conducive to healing, says Dr. Blaurock-Busch. Don't overheat it—German doctors generally recommend that the temperature not exceed 65°F, she says. Allow just enough fresh air to promote recuperation but not to create a draft. And keep the lighting subdued so it's properly relaxing.

Eat—if you want to. Don't fret over whether you should *feed* a fever or *starve* one. Some doctors, like Dr. Blaurock-Busch, prefer juice fasting until the fever is reduced nearly to normal. Others feel that you should eat during a fever because the body's increased heat uses up calories. Ultimately, of course, the choice is yours and hinges on your appetite. Just remember to keep up your fluid intake.

PANEL OF ADVISERS

Leonard Banco, M.D., is an associate professor of pediatrics at the University of Connecticut School of Medicine in Farmington. He is also director of pediatric ambulatory services and assistant director of the Department of Pediatrics at Hartford Hospital in Connecticut.

Eleonore Blaurock-Busch, Ph.D., is president and director of Trace Minerals International, Inc., a clinical chemistry laboratory in Boulder, Colorado. She is also a nutrition counselor specializing in the treatment of allergy and chronic diseases at the Alpine Chiropractic Center there, and is the author of *The No-Drugs Guide to Better Health*.

Thomas Gossel, Ph.D., R.Ph., is a professor of pharmacology and toxicology at Ohio Northern University in Ada and chairman of the university's Department of Pharmacology and Biomedical Sciences. He is an expert on over-the-counter products.

Mary Ann Pane, R.N., is a nurse clinician in Philadelphia, Pennsylvania. She is affiliated with Community Home Health Services, an agency catering to people who require skilled health care in their homes.

Stephen Rosenberg, M.D., is associate professor of clinical public health at Columbia University School of Public Health in New York City. He is author of *The Johnson & Johnson First Aid Book*.

George Sterne, M.D., is a pediatrician in private practice in New Orleans, Louisiana. He is also clinical professor of pediatrics at Tulane University School of Medicine there.

Donald Vickery, M.D., is president of the Center for Corporate Health Promotion in Reston, Virginia. He is also assistant clinical professor of family medicine and community medicine at Georgetown University School of Medicine in Washington, D.C., and associate clinical professor of family medicine at the Medical College of Virginia in Richmond. He is the author of *Life Plan for Your Health* and coauthor of *Take Care of Yourself*.

Fissures

14 Soothing Solutions

The similarities between anal fissures and hemorrhoids are largely superficial. Hemorrhoids are generally swollen veins. In contrast, fissures are ulcers, or breaks in the skin, which just happen to occur in the same general area.

Fissures are very much like those painful tears that sometimes develop at the corners of your mouth, says J. Byron Gathright, Jr., M.D., chairman of the Department of Colon and Rectal Surgery at the Ochsner Clinic in New Orleans, Louisiana, and an associate professor of surgery at Tulane University. Both the oral and anal variety occur where skin meets delicate mucous membrane. In the anus, a common cause of such tears is the passing of a large, hard stool, says Dr. Gathright.

If you have fissures, you know that these little sores can make your life—or at least your sitting life—miserable. They burn, they sting, they often bleed. Below, the experts tell you how to get to the bottom of the problem as quickly as possible.

Ban hard stools with fiber and fluid. The anal opening was never meant to accommodate large, hard stools. Generally a by-product of a Western diet lacking in fiber, rock-hard stools tug and tear at the anal canal, which can result in anal fissures as well as hemorrhoids.

The solution? Adapt yourself to a diet high in fiber and fluids that will produce soft bowel movements. Eating more fruit, vegetables, and whole grains, and drinking six to eight glasses of water a day is "the best remedy and preventive measure," you can use for anal fissures, says Dr. Gathright. Once your stool is soft and pliable, your anal fissures should begin to heal on their own.

Try the petroleum solution. Eating more fiber will soften your stool, but you can also protect your anal canal by lubricating it before each bowel movement. A gob of petroleum jelly inserted about ½ inch

---

MEDICAL ALERT

Signs of Something Serious

Fissures are generally not dangerous. "The real caution with fissures is not to put them off forever—an ulcer that doesn't heal may be a cancer," says Lewis R. Townsend, M.D., a clinical instructor of obstetrics and gynecology at Georgetown University Hospital in Washington, D.C.

"If you have fissures that don't heal within four to eight weeks, go get them evaluated," says Dr. Townsend. "Remember that a sore that will not heal is one of the seven classic warning signs of cancer."

In addition, if you notice a mucous discharge from your anus, have it checked out by a doctor. "Abscesses can be very serious in that area," says John O. Lawder, M.D.

---

into the rectum may help the stool pass without causing any further damage, says Edmund Leff, M.D., a proctologist in private practice in Phoenix and Scottsdale, Arizona.

Buff yourself with talcum. Following each shower or bowel movement, brush yourself with baby powder. This will help keep the area dry, which can help to reduce friction throughout the day, says Marvin Schuster, M.D., chief of the Department of Digestive Diseases at Francis Scott Key Medical Center in Baltimore, Maryland, and a professor of medicine and psychiatry at Johns Hopkins University School of Medicine.

Watch out for diarrhea. It may seem odd, but not only can hard, constipated stools worsen anal fissures—so too can diarrhea. Watery stools can soften the tissues around them, and they also contain acid that can burn the raw anal area and give you a form of "diaper rash" to add additional misery to your condition, says Dr. Schuster.

Keep your nails away. Anal fissures may make you want to scratch. Fight the urge. Running sharp fingernails over your tender anus can tear at the already sore tissue, says Dr. Lawder.

Shed those excess pounds. The more weight you carry, the more you're likely to sweat. Perspiration between the cheeks of your rump will only slow your fissures' healing, says Dr. Lawder.

Use a little dab. Nonprescription topical creams containing hydrocortisone can be very helpful in reducing the inflammation that often comes with anal fissures, says Dr. Gathright.

Try a vitamin cream. Particularly helpful for soothing pain and helping to heal fissures are those nonprescription ointments available at the drugstore containing vitamins A and D, says Dr. Schuster.

Jump into a hot tub. Whether you fill your bathtub with hot water or slip into an outdoor hot tub, warm water will help to relax the muscles of the anal sphincter and so reduce much of the discomfort of fissures, says Dr. Leff.

Steer clear of certain foods. While no food will cause fissures, some foods may provide excess irritation and discomfort to the anal canal as they pass through the bowels. Beware of hot, spicy foods and pickled foods, says Dr. Schuster.

Buy yourself a special pillow. Sitting on anal fissures can be unpleasant, to say the least. You can help ease the pain by picking up one of a number of either doughnut-shaped or liquid-filled pillows available at many pharmacies and medical supply stores, says Dr. Lawder.

Wipe yourself oh-so-gently. Rough toilet paper and overzealous wiping will impede healing of your fissures. So wipe gently and don't skimp when picking a brand of toilet paper. Be particularly choosy when it comes to color (you want only white) and scent (you don't want one). Perfumes and colorings can provide irritation to the already irritated area, says John O. Lawder, M.D., a family practitioner in Torrance, California, specializing in nutrition and preventive medicine. Dampen each wad of paper under the faucet before wiping to remove most of the scratchiness, says Dr. Lawder.

Treat yourself to the best. The Rolls Royce of toilet paper isn't a toilet paper at all. Facial tissues coated with moisturizing lotion offer the least amount of friction to your fissure-plagued bottom, says Dr. Lawder.

Try liquid toilet tissue. Rubbing dry toilet paper over a tender bottom can be a most unpleasant experience. But there is an alternative.

From Hepp Industries of Seaford, New York, comes ClenZone, a small tool that diverts water from your bathroom faucet to underneath your toilet seat. A narrow stream of water, aimed right where you need it most, does all your "wiping" for you. There's no need for toilet paper, except for one or two sheets to pat yourself dry.

"This is a neat little appliance that offers a real nice way to get clean after a bowel movement," says John A. Flatley, M.D., a colon-rectal surgeon in Kansas City, Missouri, and clinical instructor of surgery at the University of Missouri–Kansas City School of Medicine. Dr. Flatley, who says he uses a ClenZone in his own home, maintains that this product, intended for both fissures and hemorrhoids, "is not a cure," but it does offer "a gentle, soothing way of cleaning. I'd suggest it for anybody."

The ClenZone costs about $22 and is available through Hepp Industries, Inc., 687 Kildare Crescent, Seaford, NY 11783.

PANEL OF ADVISERS

John A. Flatley, M.D., is a colon-rectal surgeon in Kansas City, Missouri, where he also serves as a clinical instructor of surgery at the University of Missouri–Kansas City School of Medicine.

J. Byron Gathright, Jr., M.D., is chairman of the Department of Colon and Rectal Surgery at the Ochsner Clinic in New Orleans, Louisiana, and an associate professor of surgery at Tulane University in New Orleans. He is also president of the American Society of Colon and Rectal Surgeons.

John O. Lawder, M.D., is a family practitioner specializing in nutrition and preventive medicine in Torrance, California.

Edmund Leff, M.D., has a private practice in colon and rectal surgery in Phoenix and Scottsdale, Arizona.

Marvin Schuster, M.D., is chief of the Department of Digestive Diseases at Francis Scott Key Medical Center in Baltimore, Maryland, and professor of medicine and psychiatry at Johns Hopkins University School of Medicine in Baltimore.

Lewis R. Townsend, M.D., has a private practice in Bethesda, Maryland. He is a clinical instructor of obstetrics and gynecology at Georgetown University Hospital, and director of the physicians' group at Columbia Hospital for Women Medical Center, both in Washington, D.C.

Flatulence

5 Ideas for Getting Rid of Gas

It's tough to be serious about flatulence, though we promise to try. It's tough because even the scientists who study the subject poke fun at their own research, writing of failed experiments that ended "without even a whiff of success."

Yes, the pun was intended and was in very bad taste, but such is the nature of this science—even at the highest levels. Consider Michael D. Levitt, M.D., one of the top researchers in the field. His peers know him as "the man who brought status to flatus and class to gas." In his own words, Dr. Levitt describes his work as "an attempt to pump some data into a field filled largely with hot air."

Hot air, perhaps, and a colorful history as well. Hippocrates investigated flatulence extensively, and ancient physicians who specialized in it became known as "pneumatists." In early American history, such great men as Benjamin Franklin taxed their minds seeking a cure for "escaped wind."

In more recent times, Stephen Goldfinger, M.D., a digestive disease expert, wrote that "glaring at the next guy, when all else fails, can make life easier." Yes, it's tough to be serious about flatulence, but we promise to try. Read on.

Lay off the lactose. "If you are lactose intolerant, you could have flatulence problems from eating dairy foods," says Dennis Savaiano, Ph.D., associate professor of food science and nutrition at the University of Minnesota–Minneapolis. (For more tips, see Lactose Intolerance on page 407.) Lactose-intolerant people have a low intestinal level of the enzyme lactase, which is needed to digest lactose, the type of sugar found in many dairy foods.

But you don't necessarily need to be diagnosed as lactose intolerant to have unwanted repercussions. Some people can only handle certain amounts and different kinds of milk products with comfort. If you or your doctor suspects that your favorite dairy product is causing your problem, try eating it in smaller servings or along with a meal for a day or two until you notice where gas begins to be a problem.

Avoid gas-promoting foods. The primary cause of flatulence is the digestive system's inability to absorb certain carbohydrates, says Samuel Klein, M.D., assistant professor of gastroenterology and human nutrition at the University of Texas Medical School at Galveston.

Though you probably know that beans are sure fire flatus producers, many people don't realize that cabbage, broccoli, brussels sprouts, onions, cauliflower, whole wheat flour, radishes, bananas, apricots, pretzels, and many more foods can also be highly flatugenic.

Fight off fiber-induced flatus. "Although we often encourage fiber in the diet for digestive health, some high-fiber vegetables and fruits may increase gas," says Richard McCallum, M.D., a professor of medicine and chief of the Gastroenterology Division at the University of Virginia Health Sciences Center.

If you're adding fiber to your diet for health reasons, start with a small dose so the bowel gets used to it. That lessens the increase of flatus, and doctors have found that most people's flatus production returns to normal within a few weeks of adding fiber.

Use charcoal to help you reach your goal. Some studies have found that activated charcoal tablets are effective in eliminating excessive gas. "Charcoal absorbs gases and may be useful for flatulence,"

Bean Cuisine: Getting the Gas Out

If you love beans and legumes but hate living with the consequences, there is a solution.

Clearly, beans and legumes cause flatulence, although the better they're cooked, the less the problem. Indeed, beans seem to lose a lot of their gas-producing properties in water. Studies have shown that soaking beans for 12 hours or germinating them on damp paper towels for 24 hours can significantly reduce the amount of gas-producing compounds. In fact, soaking followed by 30 minutes of pressure cooking at 15 pounds per square inch reduced the compounds by up to 90 percent in one study.

says Dr. Klein, "It's probably the best available treatment—after appropriate dietary changes have been made and other gastroenterological diseases have been treated or ruled out." Check with your doctor if you're taking any medication because charcoal can soak up medicine as well as gas.

Get quick relief with popular OTCs. While many physicians are recommending activated charcoal for relief of intestinal gas, pharmacists say simethicone-containing products are still the most popular with consumers. Among the over-the-counter favorites: Gas-X, Maalox Plus, Mylanta II, and Mylicon.

Unlike activated charcoal's absorbent action, simethicone's defoaming action relieves flatulence by dispersing and preventing the formation of mucous-surrounded gas pockets in the stomach and intestines.

PANEL OF ADVISERS

Samuel Klein, M.D., is an assistant professor of gastroenterology and human nutrition at the University of Texas Medical School at Galveston. He is also an editorial adviser to *Prevention* magazine.

Richard McCallum, M.D., is a professor of medicine and chief of the Gastroenterology Division at the University of Virginia Health Sciences Center in Charlottesville. He does research on gastrointestinal problems.

Dennis Savaiano, Ph.D., is associate professor of food science and nutrition at the University of Minnesota–Minneapolis.

Flu

21 Remedies to Beat the Bug

Do you feel like a truck ran over you—repeatedly? Are you so sick you're afraid you'll die? More to the point, are you so sick you're afraid you *won't* die?

If your head throbs, your muscles ache, and your brow's on fire, you've probably been bitten by the flu bug. And it will continue to bite until it's good and ready to stop.

Cold Facts about the Flu

How can you tell a cold from the flu? This isn't a riddle. Or maybe it is. Although similarities exist between the two illnesses—and their treatment—they're caused by entirely different organisms. The worst part of a cold might last longer, but the flu generally causes more discomfort. Here, according to Ohio Northern University pharmacology and toxicology professor Thomas Gossel, Ph.D., is a comparison of common symptoms and the differences between them, depending on whether they are caused by a cold or the flu.

Fever. With flu, it's characteristic and comes on suddenly; with a cold, it's rare.

Headache. It's a prominent symptom of flu but rare with a cold.

General aches. In flu, aches are usual and often severe; in a cold, they're slight.

Fatigue. Fatigue is extreme in flu and can last two to three weeks; a cold leaves you mildly fatigued.

Runny nose. Sometimes you'll have a runny nose with flu, but it's common with a cold.

Sore throat. A sore throat sometimes accompanies flu; it's a common symptom of a cold.

Cough. It's common with flu and can become severe; a cold brings a mild to moderate hacking cough.

This insidious virus might better be called the beast of a thousand faces. Although there are just three main types (influenza A, B, and C), they have unlimited ability to mutate into different forms. So while it's true that a bout with one strain gives you immunity to that particular virus, its mutant offspring can lay you low next year—or even later this season.

Is there no escape? It depends. Yes, there are some precautions you can take to lessen future susceptibility (see "Outsmart the Flu Bug" on page 272). But no, when the flu's got you in its clutches, you're down for the count.

If you're counting on antibiotics for relief, you're out of luck. That's because the flu is a viral infection, and antibiotics simply can't kill viruses. The best you can do is ease your misery. Here's how.

Stay home. The flu is a very infectious disease that spreads like wildfire, says Pascal James Imperato, M.D., professor and chairman of the Department of Preventive Medicine and Community Health at the State University of New York Health Science Center at Brooklyn College of

Outsmart the Flu Bug

Individual immunity and the particular strain of flu virus circulating in a given year play a large role in determining who will knuckle under to the flu. Still, there are steps you can take to reduce your susceptibility to this virulent bug.

Get a flu shot. Every year, scientists develop a vaccine against the most recently circulating strain of the virus. "So the best thing you can do to protect yourself against flu is to be vaccinated in the fall or very early winter," says epidemiologist Suzanne Gaventa. She particularly advises shots for residents of nursing homes, those with chronic conditions such as heart or lung disease, anyone over 65, and most medical personnel.

In cases where the shot doesn't prevent the flu, it considerably lessens the disease's severity. Don't wait until the flu's in town before acting, because the vaccine takes about two weeks to work. And don't get a flu shot at all if you're allergic to eggs—the vaccine is made from them.

Avoid crowds. Because the virus spreads easily, stay away from movies, theaters, shopping centers, and other crowded places during an epidemic, says Pascal James Imperato, M.D. And keep your distance from people who are sneezing or coughing, even if it means getting off an elevator or giving up a seat on the bus.

Come in from the cold. Prolonged exposure to wet and cold weather lowers your resistance and increases your risk of infection.

Give up bad habits. Smoking and alcohol can also impair your resistance. Smoking, in particular, injures the respiratory tract and makes you more susceptible to the flu, Dr. Imperato says.

Kiss at your own risk. Kissing is one of the most efficient ways for the flu to spread. And just sleeping in the same room with a sick spouse is asking for trouble. So, if possible, move to another room for the duration, he advises.

Keep up your strength. Don't get tired or run-down. Paint the living room, clean the attic, or build a basement playroom *some other time,* not during flu season.

Medicine. So don't be a workaholic or a martyr. Stay home from work—and anywhere else—until at least one day after your temperature has returned to normal. And keep your children home from school until they have fully recovered.

Get some rest! You shouldn't have much trouble following this advice, since you're probably too sick to do much else. Bed rest is essential, says Dr. Imperato, because it lets your body put its energy into combating the flu infection. Being active while you're still quite ill weakens your defenses and leaves you open to possible complications.

Drink up. Liquids are especially important if you have a fever because dehydration can occur. In addition, fluids can provide needed nutrients when you're too sick to eat. Thin soups are good, as are fruit and vegetable juices. Nutrition counselor Eleonore Blaurock-Busch, Ph.D., president of Trace Minerals International in Boulder, Colorado, favors beet juice and carrot juice, both of which are rich in vitamins and minerals.

Jay Swedberg, M.D., an associate professor of family practice at the University of Wyoming College of Health Sciences, recommends that you dilute fruit juice half and half with water. "A little sugar provides necessary glucose, but too much can cause diarrhea when you're ill," he says. "Also dilute ginger ale and other sugar-sweetened soft drinks. And allow them to go flat before drinking because their bubbles can create gas in the stomach and make you more nauseated."

Reach for pain relief. Aspirin, acetaminophen, or ibuprofen can reduce the fever, headache, and body aches that so often accompany the flu. Take two tablets every 4 hours, says Virginia corporate-health consultant Donald Vickery, M.D., an assistant clinical professor at Georgetown University School of Medicine. Because symptoms are often most pronounced in the afternoon and evening, he says, take the medication regularly over this period.

Do not give aspirin to children. Be sure *not* to give aspirin or medications that contain aspirin to anyone under 21 who has the flu, says epidemiologist Suzanne Gaventa of the Centers for Disease Control in Atlanta, Georgia. Studies have shown that aspirin increases a flu-stricken child's risk of developing Reye's syndrome, a life-threatening neurological illness. Give children acetaminophen as directed by your doctor.

Think twice about other drugs. Over-the-counter cold medicines might give you some temporary relief of symptoms, says Dr. Imperato. Those with antihistamines, for instance, can dry up a runny nose. But be careful—these drugs may suppress your symptoms to the point where you have a false sense of recovering. Prematurely resuming your normal activities can bring on a relapse or trigger serious complications.

Gargle with salt water. A sore or scratchy throat is apt to accompany the flu. Get some relief—and wash out any secretions that are collecting in your throat—by gargling with a salt-water solution, says Philadelphia, Pennsylvania, nurse clinician Mary Ann Pane, R.N. Dissolve 1 teaspoon of salt in 1 pint of warm water. This concentration approximates the pH level of body tissues and is very soothing, she says. Use as often as needed, but try not to swallow the liquid because it's so high in sodium.

Do something sweet. Sucking on hard candy and lozenges can also keep your throat moist so it will feel better, says Pane. In addition, these products contain calories that your body can use at a time when you're probably not eating much.

Humidify the air. Raising the humidity of your bedroom will help reduce the discomfort of a cough, sore throat, or dry nasal passages. "A humidifier or vaporizer may also be helpful if there is chest congestion or nasal stuffiness," says Calvin Thrash, M.D., founder of Uchee Pines Institute, a nonprofit health education facility in Seale, Alabama.

Pamper your nose. If you've been blowing your nose a lot, it's probably pretty sore. So lubricate your nostrils frequently to decrease irritation, says Pane. A product such as K-Y Jelly is preferable to petroleum jelly, which dries out quickly.

Take some heat. One characteristic of the flu is tired, achy muscles. Warm them and ease their pain with a heating pad, says Pane.

Warm your feet. Soaking your feet in hot water may help if you have a headache or nasal congestion, says Dr. Thrash.

Breathe fresh air. Make sure your sickroom has a good supply of fresh air at all times, says Dr. Thrash. But avoid a draft. And prevent chills by using warm, close-fitting bedclothes.

MEDICAL ALERT

Don't Underestimate the Flu

Influenza can be as deadly today as it was in 1918, when the Spanish flu killed over 20 million people worldwide. So, advises Pascal James Imperato, M.D., see a doctor if:

- Your voice becomes hoarse.
- You develop pains in your chest.
- You have difficulty breathing.
- You start bringing up yellow- or green-colored phlegm.

Also be aware that prolonged vomiting can lead to dehydration, which is especially serious in the very young and in elderly people, says Mary Ann Pane, R.N. And abdominal pain can be the sign of another problem, such as appendicitis. If the pain or vomiting don't subside after a day, see a doctor.

Get rubbed the right way. A back rub may help activate the immune system to fight the flu, says Dr. Thrash. And it's very comforting.

Eat lightly and wisely. During the worst phase of the flu, you probably won't have an appetite at all. But when you're ready to make the transition from liquids to more substantial fare, put the emphasis on bland, starchy foods, says Dr. Swedberg. "Dry toast is fine. So are bananas, applesauce, cottage cheese, boiled rice, rice pudding, cooked cereal, and baked potatoes, which could be topped with yogurt." For a refreshing dessert, peel and freeze very ripe bananas, then puree them in a food processor.

PANEL OF ADVISERS

Eleonore Blaurock-Busch, Ph.D., is president and director of Trace Minerals International, Inc., a clinical chemistry laboratory in Boulder, Colorado. She is also a nutrition counselor specializing in the treatment of allergy and chronic diseases at the Alpine Chiropractic Center there, and is the author of *The No-Drugs Guide to Better Health.*

Suzanne Gaventa, is an epidemiologist in the Division of Viral Diseases of the Centers for Disease Control in Atlanta, Georgia.

Thomas Gossel, Ph.D., R.Ph., is a professor of pharmacology and toxicology at Ohio Northern University in Ada and chairman of the university's Department of Pharmacology and Biomedical Sciences. He is an expert on over-the-counter products.

Pascal James Imperato, M.D., is professor and chairman of the Department of Preventive Medicine and Community Health at the State University of New York Health Science Center at Brooklyn College of Medicine. He is the editor of the *New York State Journal of Medicine* and author of *What to Do about the Flu*. He has served as New York City's Commissioner of Health.

Mary Ann Pane, R.N., is a nurse clinician in Philadelphia, Pennsylvania. She is affiliated with Community Home Health Services, an agency catering to people who require skilled health care in their homes.

Jay Swedberg, M.D., is an associate professor of family practice at the University of Wyoming College of Health Sciences in Laramie.

Calvin Thrash, M.D., is the founder of Uchee Pines Institute, a nonprofit health education facility in Seale, Alabama. He is also coauthor of *Natural Remedies: A Manual*.

Donald Vickery, M.D., is president of the Center for Corporate Health Promotion in Reston, Virginia. He is also assistant clinical professor of family medicine and community medicine at Georgetown University School of Medicine in Washington, D.C., and associate clinical professor of family medicine at the Medical College of Virginia in Richmond. He is the author of *Life Plan for Your Health* and coauthor of *Take Care of Yourself.*

Food Poisoning

23 Controlling Methods

What a grand-slam picnic! You could hardly wait for the softball game to end so you could dig into the feast seductively arrayed on the picnic table in the summer sun—the tangy barbecued chicken, the buttery steamed clams, the potato salad, and the topper, that luscious cream pie.

It's now a few hours later, though, and you feel as if you've been hit in the gut by a fastball. You're dizzy and queasy. You vomit. You have diarrhea. You're definitely benched for the rest of the day.

What has happened? Chances are, the food you ate was tainted with toxic bacteria of one kind or another, giving you what is commonly known as food poisoning. Perhaps the potato salad was prepared by unclean hands that transferred staphylococcus bacteria onto your food. Or maybe the chicken was not barbecued long enough to kill contami-

---

MEDICAL ALERT

Some People Need Special Care

With a normal case of food poisoning, the symptoms—cramps, nausea, vomiting, diarrhea, dizziness—will disappear in a day or two, says Lynne Mofenson, M.D. "But for the very young, the elderly, or someone suffering a chronic condition or immune disorder, food poisoning can be very serious. These people should contact a doctor at the first signs of food poisoning."

Even if you don't fall into this category, call a doctor immediately if your symptoms are also accompanied by:

- Difficulty swallowing, speaking, or breathing; changes in vision, muscle weakness, or paralysis, particularly if this occurs after eating mushrooms, canned food, or shellfish.
- Fever above 100°F.
- Severe vomiting—meaning you can't even hold down any liquids.
- Severe diarrhea for more than a day or two.
- Persistent, localized abdominal pain.
- Dehydration—you have extreme thirst, a dry mouth, or decreased urination, and when you pinch the back of your hand, the skin stays pinched.
- Bloody diarrhea.

---

nating salmonella organisms. And that great-tasting cream pie left sitting in the sun? It might have served as a perfect petri dish for multiplying bacteria.

In any case, once inside you, these bad bugs attack your intestines—and, for a day or so, you feel wretched as your body tries to battle back. Here's what the experts say you can do to help your body fight a case of food flu.

Fill up on fluids. The bacteria irritate your intestinal tract and trigger a great deal of fluid loss, possibly from both ends. You'll need to drink lots of fluids to prevent becoming dehydrated. Water is the best replacement fluid, followed by other clear liquids like apple juice, broth, or bouillon. Soft drinks are okay, too, provided you drink them flat, says Vincent F. Garagusi, M.D., professor of medicine and microbiology and director of the Infectious Disease Service at Georgetown University Hospital in Washington, D.C. Otherwise the carbonation can further irritate the stomach. And defizzed Coca-Cola, for reasons yet to be determined, has an added bonus—it works to settle the stomach.

Don't Let It Happen Again!

You can't always blame the diner across town for your tummy troubles. The truth is, says Daniel Rodrigue, M.D., "many cases of food poisoning probably come from carelessness in your own home." Follow these common-sense rules and you'll significantly decrease your chances of getting food poisoning.

- Wash your hands before preparing food to avoid passing on bacteria such as staphylococcus (commonly found on the skin and in the throat) or shigella (passed from fecal matter). Wash again after handling raw meat and eggs.
- Don't eat raw protein food like fish, fowl, meat, milk, or eggs. Avoid sushi, oysters on the half shell, Caesar salad made with raw eggs, and unpasteurized eggnog. Don't use cracked eggs. Raw food can harbor bacteria.
- Heat or chill raw food. Bacteria can't multiply above 150° or below 40°F.
- Cook meat until the pink disappears, poultry until there are no red joints, and fish until it flakes. Complete cooking is the only way to ensure that all potentially harmful bacteria have been killed.
- Use a meat thermometer, especially when microwaving large meat and fowl. This also ensures that they are cooked thoroughly.
- Don't taste test the raw pork sausage stew, the fish chowder, or even the cookie batter before it's done.
- Don't let raw meat juice drip onto other food. It can taint otherwise harmless food.

Dr. Garagusi says you can get the bubbles out of soft drinks quickly by pouring the soda back and forth between two glasses.

Sip a little, slowly. Trying to gulp down too much at once may trigger more vomiting, says Dr. Garagusi.

Try a food flu cocktail. Vomiting and diarrhea can flush out important electrolytes—potassium, sodium, and glucose. You can replace them by sipping commercially prepared electrolyte products like Gatorade, suggests Lynne Mofenson, M.D., associate branch chief for clinical research at the National Institutes of Health. Or try this rehydration recipe: Mix fruit juice (for potassium) with ½ teaspoon of honey or corn syrup (for glucose) and a pinch of table salt (sodium chloride).

- Use a separate chopping board and utensils when handling raw meat and sanitize them with soapy water or bleach after use. It'll help prevent cross contamination.
- Scrub can openers and countertops and always clean out crevices. It will prevent bacteria from hiding there.
- Replace sponges often and use paper towels to wipe off counters.
- Don't leave food at room temperature for more than 2 hours, and avoid eating anything that you suspect may have been unrefrigerated for that long. Bacteria thrive in warm protein food made with meat or eggs, cream-filled pastries, dips, potato salad, and so forth.
- Thaw meat in the refrigerator. Bacteria can multiply on food surfaces while the center is still frozen.
- Immediately refrigerate leftovers, even if they are still hot. Cool down large stews by refrigerating in smaller portions.
- Never pick and eat wild mushrooms. Some carry toxins that attack the nervous system and can be deadly. Picking wild mushrooms should be left for the experts.
- Never taste home-canned food before boiling for 20 minutes. If not properly canned, food contains bacteria that can produce a dangerous toxin.
- Don't taste any food that doesn't smell or look right. Avoid cracked jars or swollen, dented cans or lids, clear liquids that have turned milky, or cans and jars that spurt or have an "off" odor when opened. They could contain dangerous bacteria. Make sure you discard them carefully so that household pets cannot come in contact with them.

Save the antacids for heartburn. They can reduce the acids in your stomach and weaken your defense against bacteria. "Possibly," says Dr. Mofenson, "bacteria could multiply in greater numbers and more rapidly if you take an antacid."

Don't interfere with progress. Your body is trying to flush the toxic organism out of your body, explains Daniel Rodrigue, M.D., a medical epidemiologist with the Centers for Disease Control in Atlanta, Georgia. "In some cases, taking antidiarrheal products [like Imodium or Lomotil] may interfere with the body's ability to fight the infection." So stay away from them and let nature take its course. If you feel it's necessary to take something, consult your doctor first.

Don't induce vomiting. Don't let the word poisoning scare you into sticking your finger down your throat, says Bonnie Dean, assistant director of the Pittsburgh Poison Control Center of Childrens Hospital of Pittsburgh, Pennsylvania. "There's just no need to do so."

Reintroduce bland foods. Usually within a few hours to a day after the diarrhea and vomiting have subsided, you'll be ready for some "good" food. But go easy. Your stomach has been attacked; it's weak and irritated. "Start with easily digestible foods," suggests Dr. Mofenson. Try cereal, pudding, soda crackers, or broth. Avoid high-fiber, spicy, acidic, greasy, sugary, or dairy foods that could further irritate the stomach. You should do this for a day or two; then your stomach will be ready to get back to its routine.

PANEL OF ADVISERS

Bonnie Dean is assistant director of Pittsburgh Poison Control Center of Childrens Hospital of Pittsburgh, Pennsylvania.

Vincent F. Garagusi, M.D., is a professor of medicine and microbiology and director of the Infectious Disease Service at Georgetown University Hospital in Washington, D.C.

Lynne Mofenson, M.D., is an associate branch chief for clinical research at the National Institutes of Health. She was formerly assistant commissioner of the Division of Communicable Disease Control for the state of Massachusetts, Massachusetts Department of Public Health.

Daniel Rodrigue, M.D., is a medical epidemiologist for the Enteric Disease Branch of the Center for Infectious Diseases, Centers for Disease Control in Atlanta, Georgia.

Foot Aches

18 Feet Treats

Oh, pity those poor dogs of yours. No, not Fifi and Pierre. You treat *them* with respect. You cosset, coddle, and pamper them like royalty. You never squeeze them into high heels and make them shop till they drop. You never force them to cram a month's worth of sightseeing into five measly days. You never walk all over them—day after day, year after year.

MEDICAL ALERT

Set Foot in the Doctor's Office

According to Mark D. Sussman, D.P.M., you should definitely see a doctor if:

- You have pain in your feet that continually increases during the day.
- Your feet get to the point where you can't keep your shoes on.
- You have trouble walking first thing in the morning—"the first three or four steps are killers."

Also be aware that painful burning in the feet can be a sign of poor circulation, athlete's foot, a pinched nerve, diabetes, anemia, thyroid disease, alcoholism, or other problems.

But your feet! Well, friend, they're another story. Oh, you're not the only one who takes *those* dogs for granted. Few of us think about our feet at all until they hurt. The rest of the time, we simply use them like there's no tomorrow.

So what can you do at the end of a long, hard day when your feet cry uncle? You can't just throw them out and get a new set. No, siree, it's one pair to a customer, and you have yours. If you expect them to last as long as you do, you'd better sit down and heed some advice from the experts.

Elevate those babies. "The best thing you can do for your feet when you get home from work is to sit down, get your feet up, and exercise your toes to get the circulation going again," says orthopedic surgeon Gilbert Wright, M.D., of Sacramento, California, spokesman for the American Orthopedic Foot and Ankle Society. So elevate your feet at a 45-degree angle to your body and relax for 20 minutes.

Soak 'em. A tried-and-true foot revitalizer is to soak your feet in a basin of warm water containing 1 or 2 tablespoons of Epsom salts, says Maryland podiatrist Mark D. Sussman, D.P.M. Rinse with clear, cool water, then pat your feet dry and massage in a moisturizing gel or cream.

Run hot and cold. Dr. Sussman recommends a treatment popular at European spas. Sit on the edge of the bathtub and hold your feet under running water for several minutes (alternate 1 minute of comfortably hot water with 1 minute of cold, ending with the cold). The contrasting baths will invigorate your whole system. If you have a shower-massage attachment, use it for an even more stimulating workout. But as always, if you have diabetes or impaired circulation, don't expose your feet to extremes of temperature.

Find the essence of relaxation. A variation on this technique comes from aromatherapist Judith Jackson of Cos Cob, Connecticut: Soak your feet for 5 minutes in a shallow tub of hot water containing 6 drops of eucalyptus oil and 6 drops of rosemary oil. Slosh your feet in the water and let the eucalyptus essence relax you. Then drain the water and pour some cold water over your feet. Follow that with hot water from the tap and then more cold. For an entirely different experience, use 6 drops each of juniper oil and lemon oil in the initial bath. (Look for essential oils in health food stores.)

Brew up a tea party. If you don't have any essential oils, says Jackson, make a strong brew of peppermint or chamomile tea. Steep four tea bags in 2 cups of boiling water. Add the brew to 1 gallon of hot water. Soak your feet as above, then follow with the alternating cold and hot rinses.

Massage away your aches. "A really nice thing is to have somebody massage your feet with baby oil," says Dr. Sussman. If you can't find a willing partner, take matters into your own hands. Either before or during a soak, says Jackson, give yourself a nice little foot massage. Work over the whole foot, squeezing the toes gently, then pressing in a circular motion over the bottom of your foot. One really effective movement is to slide your thumb as hard as you can in the arch of the foot.

Get relief on ice. Another way to refresh tired feet is to wrap a few ice cubes in a wet washcloth, then rub it over your feet and ankles for a few minutes. Ice acts to relieve any inflammation and it also serves as a mild anesthetic, says Bethlehem, Pennsylvania, podiatrist Neal Kramer, D.P.M. Then dry your feet and swab them with witch hazel, cologne, alcohol, or vinegar for a cooling and drying effect.

Exercise! We don't mean aerobics or any other heavy-duty activity. But many doctors recommend that you exercise your feet and leg muscles throughout the day to ward off aches and keep the circulation going. Try these ideas from experts at the Kinney Shoe Corporation.

- If your feet feel tense and cramped anytime during the day, give them a good shake, as you would your hands if they felt cramped. Do one foot at a time, then relax and flex your toes up and down.

- If you must stand for long periods of time, walk in place whenever you can. Keep changing your stance, and try to rest one foot on a stool or step occasionally. If possible, stand on carpeting or a spongy rubber mat.
- To relieve stiffness, remove your shoes, sit in a chair, and stretch your feet out in front of you. Circle both feet from the ankles ten times in one direction, then ten times in the other. Point your toes down as far as possible, then flex them up as high as you can. Repeat ten times. Now grasp your toes and gently pull them back and forth.
- For a nice mini-massage, remove your shoes and roll each foot over a golf ball, tennis ball, or rolling pin for a minute or two.

New York City skin care specialist Lia Schorr recommends these foot-reviving workouts:

- Scatter a few pencils on the floor and pick them up with your toes.
- Or, she says, put a handful of dried beans in moccasin-style slippers, slip them on, and walk around the room several times—you'll get a massagelike workout on the soles of your feet.

Save your soles. Try wearing shoes with thick, shock-absorbing soles to shield your feet from rough surfaces and hard pavements. Don't let your soles become too thin or worn because they just won't do the job they're supposed to do. Women's thin-soled, pointy-toed high heels are classic villains, says Dr. Wright. If you must dress up for work, ease foot strain by wearing walking or athletic shoes to and from the job and switching to heels at the office.

Change heel heights. Wearing high heels tightens the calf muscles, which leads to foot fatigue, says John F. Waller, Jr., M.D., an attending surgeon in orthopedic surgery at Lenox Hill Hospital in New York City. So changing heel heights from high to low during the day is an excellent idea.

Wear insoles. High heels have the added disadvantage, says Dr. Waller, of causing your foot to pitch forward as you walk, putting painful pressure on the ball of your foot. To prevent this discomfort, wear a half insole to help keep your foot in place. And be sure to take the insoles with you to the shoe store to ensure that they'll fit comfortably in your new shoes.

Stretch your shoes. When you add insoles to shoes you already have, says Dr. Sussman, make sure they don't cramp your toes. If things are tight, you may be able to stretch the shoes to accommodate the insoles. Fill a sock with sand, stuff it into the shoe's toe box, and wrap the shoe with a wet towel. Let it dry out over the next 24 hours. Repeat once or twice, if needed.

PANEL OF ADVISERS

Judith Jackson is a health and beauty consultant in Cos Cob, Connecticut. She is also a certified aromatherapist with a degree in massage and aromatherapy. She is author of *Scentual Touch: A Personal Guide to Aromatherapy.*

Neal Kramer, D.P.M., is a podiatrist in private practice in Bethlehem, Pennsylvania.

Lia Schorr is a skin care specialist in New York City and author of *Lia Schorr's Seasonal Skin Care.*

Mark D. Sussman, D.P.M., is a podiatrist in Wheaton, Maryland. He is coauthor of *How to Doctor Your Feet without the Doctor* and *The Family Foot-Care Book.*

John F. Waller, Jr., M.D., is an orthopedic surgeon specializing in the foot and ankle. He is attending surgeon in orthopedic surgery at Lenox Hill Hospital in New York City.

Gilbert Wright, M.D., is an orthopedic surgeon in Sacramento, California, and spokesman for the American Orthopedic Foot and Ankle Society. He is also director of the Sacramento Orthopedic Foot Clinic.

Foot Odor

19 Deodorizing Secrets

What *is* that smell? It couldn't be your, er, your *feet*, could it? No, no, of course not. That would be so embarrassing. It must be, um, something else. Like maybe a piece of Limburger fell behind the sofa—last month. Yeah, that's it. Cheese. Behind the couch. Been there awhile.

Well, thank goodness that's settled. Now you won't even have to read these odor-eating tips from the experts. Now you can go and do something else.

But first, could you maybe put your shoes back on—and stick around for the following advice?

Wash—often. It may sound elementary, the experts agree, but you should keep your feet scrupulously clean. Use warm, soapy water and wash your feet as often as needed—several times a day if you perspire a

---

Do Your Feet Work Harder Than You Do?

Believe it or not, says Bethlehem, Pennsylvania, podiatrist Neal Kramer, D.P.M., sometimes feet perspire a lot because they simply *work* harder than they should. A structural defect (such as flat feet) or a job that keeps you hopping all day could be the underlying culprit. Either would increase the activity of your foot muscles. And the harder your feet work, the more they perspire in an attempt to cool themselves.

Although feet that perspire don't necessarily smell bad, the wetness is an open invitation for bacteria that do produce odor.

"If you correct the underlying problem with an arch support or some other orthotic shoe insert," says Dr. Kramer, "you can actually cut down on the amount of sweat produced. If the muscles don't have to work as hard, they just don't give off as much heat."

---

lot or notice an odor. Scrub gently with a soft brush, even between your toes, and be sure to dry your feet thoroughly.

Powder your toes. After washing, apply foot powder, cornstarch, or an antifungal spray. Another good method for keeping feet cool and dry, says private practice podiatrist Suzanne M. Levine, D.P.M., clinical assistant podiatrist at Mount Sinai Hospital in New York City, is to treat your shoes—sprinkle the insides with talcum powder or cornstarch.

Use an antiperspirant. The key to controlling odor is to use either an antiperspirant or a deodorant right on your feet. You can buy foot deodorants or simply use your underarm brand. Be aware, however, that although deodorants eliminate odor, they don't stop perspiration. Antiperspirants take care of both problems. Dr. Levine recommends products that contain aluminum chloride hexahydrate.

But don't use an antiperspirant if you have active athlete's foot lesions, says Stephen Weinberg, D.P.M., director of podiatry at Columbus Hospital's Running and Sports Medicine Clinic in Chicago, Illinois, because it will sting. "In addition, I recommend roll-on products rather than sprays because most of a spray's antiperspirant action is lost in the air. Use the product two or three times a day in the beginning, then gradually cut back to once a day."

Change your socks—often. The logical approach to excessively sweaty, odoriferous feet, says Glenn Copeland, D.P.M., a podiatrist practicing at Toronto's Women's College Hospital, is to change socks as frequently as possible—even three or four times a day. And always wear socks made of natural fibers, such as cotton, because they are far more absorbent than synthetic materials.

Double up on them. You may also be able to reduce perspiration by wearing two pairs of socks at a time, says Frederick Hass, M.D., a general practitioner in San Rafael, California. At first glance this might seem like a contradiction, but the air spaces that form between the two layers of material actually enhance cooling. Wear cotton socks next to the skin and a woolen pair on the outside. Avoid synthetics because they only encourage perspiration.

Show shoe sense. "Closed shoes aggravate sweaty feet and set up a perfect environment for bacteria to grow, leading to more odor and more sweat," says Dr. Levine. Choose sandals and open-toed shoes when appropriate, but stay away from rubber and plastic shoes, which don't allow feet to breathe easily. And never wear the same shoes two days in a row. It takes at least 24 hours for shoes to dry out thoroughly.

Sleep on it. Maryland podiatrist Mark D. Sussman, D.P.M., recommends this nighttime treatment to help dry up feet: Wash your feet thoroughly with rubbing alcohol to dry and cool them. Then apply a heavy-duty deodorant such as Mitchum to the bottom of each foot. Cover the foot with plastic wrap (to induce sweating so the deodorant can penetrate the foot better). Pull a sock over the wrap and sleep with it on. In the morning, wash off the excess powder. Repeat every night for one week, then once or twice a week as needed.

Take frequent soaks. Various soaking agents can help keep the feet dry, which may also control odor.

Tea. Tannin, which can be found in tea bags, is a drying agent. Boil three or four tea bags in 1 quart of water for about 10 minutes, then add enough cold water to make a comfortable soak, instructs dermatologist Diana Bihova, M.D., clinical instructor of dermatology at New York University Medical Center in New York City.

Soak your feet for 20 to 30 minutes, then dry them and apply foot powder. Dr. Bihova says to do this twice a day until you get the problem under control. Repeating it twice a week thereafter should keep odor from recurring.

Kosher salt. For extra-sweaty feet, Dr. Levine recommends soaking in a solution of ½ cup kosher salt (which is coarser than ordinary table salt) in 1 quart of water.

Aluminum acetate. Try soaking once or twice daily in a solution of cool water and aluminum acetate, which has drying properties, says Dr. Hass. To use, dissolve either 1 packet Domeboro powder or 2 tablespoons Burow's Solution (both available over-the-counter) in 1 pint of water, then soak for 10 to 20 minutes at a time.

Sodium bicarbonate. This makes the foot surface more acidic, thereby cutting down on the amount of odor produced, says Dr. Levine. Dissolve 1 tablespoon baking soda in 1 quart of water. Soak twice a week for about 15 minutes at a time.

Vinegar. Another acid footbath Dr. Levine recommends is ½ cup vinegar in 1 quart of water. Soak for 15 minutes twice a week.

Hot and cold water. Alternate hot and cold footbaths, says Dr. Levine. This procedure constricts the blood flow to your feet, reducing perspiration. Then fix yourself a third footbath of ice cubes and lemon juice. Finally, rub your feet with alcohol to cool and dry them. In hot weather, when your feet perspire a lot, you could probably do this every day. Warning: Diabetics and those with impaired circulation should not use this treatment.

Heed sage advice. Europeans sometimes sprinkle the fragrant herb sage into their shoes to control odor, says Dr. Levine. Perhaps a dash of these dry, crumbled leaves will do the trick for you.

Try inserts. Some shoe inserts, such as Johnson's Odor-Eaters, contain activated charcoal, which absorbs moisture and helps control odor. Dr. Levine says these products have helped some of her patients.

Stay cool. The sweat glands in your feet, similar to those in your armpits and palms, respond to emotions, says Richard L. Dobson, M.D., head of the Department of Dermatology at the Medical University of South Carolina College of Medicine. Stress, whether good or bad, can trigger excessive sweating. That, in turn, can increase bacterial activity in your shoes, leading to extra odor. So try not to get frazzled.

Watch what you eat. As bizarre as this may sound, says Dr. Levine, when you eat spicy or pungent foods (such as onions, peppers, garlic, or scallions), the essence of these odors can be excreted through the sweat glands on your feet. So, yes, your feet can end up smelling like your lunch!

PANEL OF ADVISERS

Diana Bihova, M.D., is a dermatologist in private practice and clinical instructor of dermatology at New York University Medical Center in New York City. She is coauthor of *Beauty from the Inside Out.*

Glenn Copeland, D.P.M., is a podiatrist with a private practice at Toronto's Women's College Hospital. He is also consulting podiatrist for the Canadian Back Institute, podiatrist for the Toronto Blue Jays baseball team, and author of *The Foot Doctor.*

Richard L. Dobson, M.D., is head of the Department of Dermatology at the Medical University of South Carolina College of Medicine in Charleston.

Frederick Hass, M.D., is a general practitioner in San Rafael, California. He is on the staff of Marin General Hospital in Greenbrae. He is the author of *The Foot Book* and *What You Can Do about Your Headaches.*

Neal Kramer, D.P.M., is a podiatrist in private practice in Bethlehem, Pennsylvania.

Suzanne M. Levine, D.P.M., is a podiatrist in private practice and clinical assistant podiatrist at Mount Sinai Hospital in New York City. She is author of *My Feet Are Killing Me* and *Walk It Off.*

Mark D. Sussman, D.P.M., is a podiatrist in Wheaton, Maryland. He is coauthor of *How to Doctor Your Feet without the Doctor* and *The Family Foot-Care Book.*

Stephen Weinberg, D.P.M., is director of podiatry at Columbus Hospital's Running and Sports Medicine Clinic in Chicago, Illinois.

Forgetfulness

24 Handy Ways to a Better Memory

Do you have a hard time remembering names, phone numbers, and important dates? Are you constantly losing your car in parking lots? When you leave for vacation, do you have to turn around 20 miles down the road to make sure you shut off all the appliances? Do you sometimes forget how to spell common words? If you can answer yes to most of these questions, here's some very good news: Forgetfulness is curable!

MEDICAL ALERT

Keep These Symptoms in Mind

Most skin lumps are not cancer, and most slips of memory are not Alzheimer's disease. "But people tend to be hard on themselves, particularly so as they get older," says Stanley Berent, Ph.D.

When is your forgetfulness so serious that you should see a professional about it? Dr. Berent suggests the following guidelines:

- Do you lose contact with reality? It's one thing to forget today's date, another to forget the year. If you lose track of where you are, can't remember if it's evening or morning, or have forgotten the name of your spouse (as opposed to someone you just met), a doctor should be consulted.
- Are you uncomfortable with yourself? If you're feeling anxious about your recent memory lapses, don't sweat it out—seek a doctor's advice.
- Are you performing your day-to-day roles efficiently? If forgetfulness is affecting your work, your role as a parent or grandparent, or any of your other life activities, you may need help.

Above all, says Dr. Berent, know that your memory doesn't have to be perfect to be okay. Some forgetfulness is just part of life.

Er, let's see, where were we? Ah, yes. We checked with a few professional memory experts, and a few whose professions require excellent memories. We even checked with a 13-year-old national spelling bee champion. They told us their secrets for building an iron-clad memory.

"With a few simple devices, it's within most people's power to have a super memory," says memory expert Michael Pressley, Ph.D., professor of human development at the University of Maryland.

What kinds of devices? Glad you asked.

Think of remembering as re-membering. Say you're appearing on a television game show and you're on the verge of winning an all-expense-paid trip around the world. All you need to do is remember the name of the battle in which Napoleon was defeated. You know the answer. It's on the tip of your tongue. How to get it off?

"Try to reinstate as much as possible of what you know surrounding the issue," says Robin West, Ph.D., a professor of psychology at the University of Florida. Thus, Napoleon may lead to Josephine, to France,

Are There Any Pills for Forgetfulness?

Scientists have long looked for relationships between nutrients and your brain's ability to learn and remember. They know that a lack of certain nutrients can lead to memory and other cognitive failures, but whether supplemental nutrients can lead to supplemental memory is still a mystery.

Research over the past several years has focused on the following nutrients, all of which seem related to memory: vitamins B_1 (thiamine), B_6, B_{12}, and C, choline, folate, niacin, calcium, copper, iodine, iron, magnesium, manganese, potassium, zinc, and—above all—lecithin.

Some research from the Institute of Physiology in Sofia, Bulgaria, raises questions and hopes about a new, exotic nutrient. Scientists there, experimenting with mice and ginseng, have determined that something in the root of the Chinese plant improves both learning and memory. At least with mice.

So it appears that the day may come when forgetfulness can be cured by popping a pill every morning. Of course, some of us will inevitably forget to take our pills.

to the Napoleonic Code, to battles, and (eventually) to Waterloo. "The more connections you make, the better your chances of finding the right pathway," says Dr. West.

Take a picture. The average American, in the course of a lifetime, spends *a full year* looking for misplaced objects. Want to save yourself a year of your life? You can. Take a good look at those keys as you place them on the table. "Raise your hands to your eyes, miming a camera, and click the button," suggests Joan Minninger, Ph.D., in her book *Total Recall: How to Boost Your Memory Power.*

Talk to yourself. Go ahead, don't be shy. Give yourself an aural as well as a visual image to remember. If you leave your car at the end of the parking lot, under the huge oak tree, go ahead and say, "I'm leaving my car at the far end of the parking lot, under the huge oak tree." Say it out loud. "It's another way to reinforce the memory," says Irene B. Colsky, Ed.D., a memory expert and adjunct professor in the Department of Teaching and Learning at the University of Miami.

Tie a yellow ribbon around the old oak tree. Afraid you'll remember your car is under an oak tree, but you'll forget *which* oak tree? Use physical reminders—they are "very efficient ways to remember," says

Forrest R. Scogin, Ph.D., an assistant professor of psychology at the University of Alabama. The "yellow ribbon" on the oak tree could just as well be a rubber band around your wrist (to remind yourself to buy tissues), a wristwatch on the "wrong" arm (to remind yourself of Aunt Bertha's birthday)—or just about anything you can think of.

Make lists. Wherever and whenever possible, jot down on paper what you need to remember. "Our short-term memory has limited capacities—there's only so much space available," says Dr. Scogin. By making lists, you not only are assured of remembering what you wrote down, but it frees your mind for more important things.

Categorize. When pencil and paper are unavailable, you'll have to list things in your head—but don't do so randomly, says Dr. Scogin. If you're on your way to the grocery store and you know you need 20 items, you'll probably never remember all 20 unless they are logically grouped. Think: five vegetables, four paper goods, three fruits, etc.

Chunk. "Chunking" is like categorizing, but you do it with numbers. If, for instance, you had to remember the numbers 2, 0, 2, 4, 5, 6, 1, 4, 1, 4, you'd probably have a rough time of it. Remembering (202) 456-1414 (the phone number of the White House) is quite a bit easier. Phone numbers come naturally chunked, as do social security numbers (001-00-1000). You are free, of course, to "chunk" not only these but any numbers you like.

Make up a silly story. If you've got several items to remember and you're afraid you never will—no problem. Just make up a tale involving your items, says Dr. Pressley. Say you're on your way to the market and you need pork chops, apricots, milk, and bread. Tell yourself a story in which a pig is drinking milk, in a wheat field, under the shade of an apricot tree.

To remember names, think of faces. Perhaps the most difficult memory task we're faced with is remembering the names of people we've just met, says Dr. Scogin. The trick is to etch in your mind a permanent association between the name and the face. Better yet, find a prominent feature on the face and focus in on that. If Budd Luzinski, that new guy in the office, happens to have a long nose—visualize a tiny man skiing down that long nose. Imagine that little man losing (*Luzinski*) those skis.

How to Avoid Stage Fright

For most of us, keeping a dozen or so phone numbers, an occasional shopping list, and the starting times of our favorite television shows under our cap is about all we demand of our short-term memory.

But what do you do when you have to remember a sales pitch, a speech, or the lines of a play? Or how to spell at a moment's notice any word in the English language? Professional Shakespearean actor Edward Gero and 13-year-old national spelling bee champion Rageshree Ramachandran of Sacramento, California, have a few tips for remembering words and their spellings.

From Edward Gero:

- "Before I memorize my lines, they have to make sense to me. I will read Shakespeare's lines to myself, putting them into my own words."
- "I look for rhythm patterns. 'To be, or not to be' . . . dum de, dum dum de dum."
- "I look for any alphabetical keys. For instance, in *MacBeth,* I had to say the following line: 'But I have none; the king-becoming graces, as justice, verity, temp'rance, stableness . . .' It helped me to remember the order by knowing that the first two, justice and verity, are in alphabetical order, and that the second two, temp'rance and stableness, are in reverse alphabetical order."
- "I try to associate lines with movements, so that in *The Merchant of Venice,* I say, 'and let my liver rather heat with wine' as I'm reaching for a glass of wine."

From Rageshree Ramachandran:

- "A lot of spellers just try to memorize a list of words for spelling bees— that doesn't work. It's not just memorizing, it's learning the words. I make a new word part of my everyday vocabulary."
- "Spelling is mostly logic. If a word is unfamiliar, I'll look for a part of it that I can understand. I can spell *elegiacal,* for instance, because I know it comes from *elegy.* (Elegiacal means expressing sorrow.) I can spell *mhometer* because I know that *mho* is the reciprocal of *ohm,* and a mhometer measures ohms (a measure of electricity)."
- "A lot of memory is visual. It helps me to remember a new word if I write it down several times."
- "There are often little tricks to help spell a word. Take *curliewurly* (a little squiggly shape). I had to remember that it was curl*ie*wurly, and not curlywurl*ie*. The solution was simple: *ie* comes before *y* in the word—just like in the alphabet."

Make name associations. It's always easier to remember names if you have something to associate the name with. If you have to remember the name of someone who has no big nose or mole on the cheek, make up a little story. Picture someone named Bruce Taylor sitting in front of you with a pair of scissors, a measuring tape, and a piece of chalk. Someone named Feinstein, you might picture sitting before you holding a huge stein full of beer. Someone named Pressley? Imagine him reading the *Pittsburgh Press* or shaking hands with Elvis, says Dr. Pressley.

Look for "markers." Things that happened to you long ago did not happen in isolation from other events, says Dr. Pressley. Say, for instance, you forgot when it was that you worked at the ABC Construction Company. Think of any markers or cues that might help your focus. You may recall that you were dating so-and-so at the time, and that so-and-so and you would often go to the movies, and that one movie you saw together was *Jaws*. You may then recall (or your local librarian can help you find out) that *Jaws* appeared in the theaters in 1975.

Outline your thoughts. Many college students become intimately involved with a pink, yellow, or green highlighting marker. But you don't need a highlighter to outline your thoughts. You can do it mentally. "Select what is important and what is not," says Dr. Pressley. You're far less likely to forget what you read, he says.

Read, read, and read. If your problem is forgetting words, it's probably because you don't use them enough, says Frederic Siegenthaler. As a senior interpreter at the United Nations, he must store an enormous vocabulary in his memory and keep it ready to pull out at any moment. In English alone (and Siegenthaler is also fluent in French, German, Russian, and Spanish), there are as many as 200,000 words available, although we typically use fewer than 5,000 on a daily basis. So if you can't seem to find the right word, your vocabulary is likely to be a bit rusty.

Solution? "Do as much reading as you can," says Siegenthaler. "I recommend good fiction, particularly classics of the English language, such as those of Charles Dickens, Jane Austen, or Somerset Maugham."

Test yourself. "People generally aren't very good at knowing how good they are at remembering," says Dr. Pressley. "It's very common that someone may think he remembers something, but he doesn't." You've probably experienced this in the middle of an exam. The way to make sure it doesn't happen again is to give yourself a quiz before the exam, says Dr. Pressley. "A practice test will let you know if you have it down or not."

Keep calm. Stress and anxiety can clearly disrupt memory performance, says Dr. Pressley. "You need your consciousness to encode things. Anxiety eats that up."

If you're a forgetful person, it may be that your mind could use a vacation. Patricia Sze of Berlitz International Language School in New York City claims that her school's success in teaching students foreign languages lies largely in the nonthreatening environment of soothing colors, no grades, and no testing.

Check your medicine cabinet and liquor cabinet. Dozens of things have the potential to contribute to forgetfulness, says Stanley Berent, Ph.D., director of the Neuropsychology Program and an associate professor in the Department of Psychology, Psychiatry, and Neurology at the University of Michigan Medical School. At the root of your forgetfulness may be the booze you're drinking or certain drugs you're taking, such as diet pills, blood pressure medication, or antihistamines.

PANEL OF ADVISERS

Stanley Berent, Ph.D., is director of the Neuropsychology Program and an associate professor in the Department of Psychology, Psychiatry, and Neurology at the University of Michigan Medical School in Ann Arbor.

Irene B. Colsky, Ed.D., is an adjunct professor in the Department of Teaching and Learning in the School of Education at the University of Miami, Florida, where she also teaches "Brainpower," a popular course on learning and memory techniques to students, business professionals, and members of the community.

Edward Gero is a professional actor who has played major roles, such as Henry V and MacBeth, in many of Shakespeare's plays. He performs at the Shakespeare Theatre at the Folger in Washington, D.C.

Michael Pressley, Ph.D., is a professor of human development at the University of Maryland in College Park.

Rageshree Ramachandran of Sacramento, California, is the winner of the 1988 Scripps-Howard National spelling bee.

Forrest R. Scogin, Ph.D., is an assistant professor of psychology at the University of Alabama in Tuscaloosa, where he teaches courses on memory.

Frederic Siegenthaler is a senior interpreter at the United Nations. He has been a professional interpreter for the past 25 years.

Patricia Sze is an executive with Berlitz International Language School in New York City.

Robin West, Ph.D., is a professor of psychology at the University of Florida in Gainesville. West is author of *Memory Fitness over Forty.*

Frostbite

17 Safeguards against the Cold

When Tod Schimelpfenig was 18, he and a friend wanted a winter adventure. So they went hiking and mountain climbing in the northern Vermont wilderness.

"We were out trying to be mountaineers and ended up going to the school of hard knocks," Schimelpfenig says now, almost 20 years later.

Schimelpfenig, in fact, took an advanced course in frostbite. The toes of his right foot turned white and hard. "It looked like a frozen steak," he recalls with a laugh.

Of course, he wasn't laughing then. Fortunately, he and his companion found a place to camp for the night and he was able to stay off the frozen foot for a while. But to prevent even more serious injury, he had to make sure the foot didn't thaw and refreeze. So while keeping the rest of his body in a warm sleeping bag, he kept the frostbitten foot outside the bag and frozen. And he had to stay awake all night to do it.

"I walked out 8 miles the next morning and I was fine," he says. "I still have all my toes."

Schimelpfenig, who, ironically, is now safety and training manager for the National Outdoor Leadership School in Lander, Wyoming, and a volunteer emergency medical technician, readily admits he needlessly put himself in a dangerous situation. But less severe forms of frostbite can occur quickly in very cold weather when you're simply shoveling snow or changing a tire.

And there are plenty of instances of outdoorsmen and motorists getting lost, and then stranded, and having to face the cold. So here's what you need to know about frostbite—from treating mild pain on the tip of your nose to preventing it in the first place.

Know the signs. Frostnip is the least severe form of frostbite and typically leaves skin somewhat numb and white.

The cheeks, tip of the nose, and ears are most frequently frostnipped, says Bruce Paton, M.D., a clinical professor of surgery at the University of Colorado at Denver. Peeling and blistering, he adds, are also possible after the affected area is warmed.

Peeling and blistering after warming are more likely with superficial frostbite, a more serious condition. Frostbite is an injury in which the tissues of the body freeze, causing damage to the tissue. The skin is also frozen harder than with frostnip, but not so deeply that all resiliency is lost.

"Frostbite is the body's way of trying to preserve heat by shutting down circulation to an extremity," says Ruth Uphold, M.D., medical director of the emergency department at Medical Center Hospital of Vermont in Burlington. "Unfortunately, as you develop frostbite," she warns, "you might not even know that you have it because of the numbness."

MEDICAL ALERT

Hypothermia: The Cold Inside

The human body was designed to operate at an internal temperature of 98.6°F. A 6½-degree drop—hardly noticeable in air temperature—could be enough to kill a human being. "Below 92°, cardiac arrest can occur," says James Sturm, M.D.

Hypothermia, simply defined as low body temperature, begins in its mildest stage at about 96°, Dr. Sturm says. Symptoms of hypothermia include shivering, slow pulse, lethargy, and a general decrease in alertness. If body temperature drops low enough, muscles turn rigid and the person may lose consciousness.

Falling into an icy pond would bring on hypothermia in less than an hour, but most cases result from prolonged exposure to cold temperatures. Elderly people are at increased risk for hypothermia, because their bodies regulate temperature less effectively.

If hypothermia occurs, Dr. Sturm recommends taking the following steps, and getting the person to a doctor as soon as possible.

- Move the person to a warmer place.
- Wrap the person with blankets.
- Give the person warm liquids. But don't give any alcohol, Dr. Sturm says. "Alcohol just gives an artificial feeling of warmth."

Hide from the wind. Obviously, getting out of the elements into a warm place is a good idea. But if that's impossible, at least get out of the wind—windchill factors contribute significantly to frostbite.

Think before warming. Don't use dry, radiant heat, such as a heat lamp or campfire, Dr. Paton says, if your skin appears to be frostbitten. Frostbitten skin is easily burned.

Use yourself. If you can't get inside, take advantage of your own body heat. To warm fingers and hands, for example, place them under your armpits. "Rolling yourself into a ball also makes you more energy efficient," Schimelpfenig says.

Don't rub with snow. "It just causes friction with the skin," Dr. Uphold says. "Plus, you lose more heat when you get extremely wet."

Frostbite: Don't Delay Action

Severe frostbite demands professional medical attention. Tissue is dying. And that opens the door to some dark possibilities—infection and loss of fingers or toes, and in extreme cases, loss of an arm or leg.

With deep frostbite, the skin is cold, hard, white, and numb. When rewarmed, the skin may turn blue or purple. It also may swell, and blisters might form. The idea, of course, is to treat frostbite quickly and effectively so none of that happens. While waiting for medical attention, here's what you should do.

Thaw quickly. "The trend now is to thaw severe frostbite as fast as is safely possible, which is very painful," says Ruth Uphold, M.D. Typically this is done in warm water—104° to 108°F. "Water," she says, "conducts heat better than air."

Do not allow a frostbitten part to refreeze. "Never," emphasizes Dr. Uphold. "The water crystals are bigger when the part refreezes, which causes even more tissue damage."

Use your head to save your foot. It's not advisable to walk on frozen feet, but it's better than allowing a frozen foot to thaw and refreeze, so if you think walking may be your only route to survival, don't take a shoe or boot off a frostbitten foot, says Bruce Paton, M.D. "The foot could blister and swell," he says, "and you wouldn't be able to get the boot back on."

Don't get wet. Heat loss is greatly accelerated by contact with water, says Dr. Paton.

Make Mom proud. "Wear mittens instead of gloves—mittens are warmer—and wear a stocking cap to protect your ears," advises James Sturm, M.D., an emergency medicine physician at St. Paul-Ramsey Medical Center in Minnesota.

Don't drink. "You only *think* alcohol is warming you from the inside out. Alcohol actually causes more heat loss," says Dr. Uphold.

Don't smoke. Smoking decreases peripheral circulation, Dr. Uphold says, thereby making the extremities more vulnerable.

Hang loose. To protect circulation, wear loose clothing and don't wear any jewelry on your fingers, says Schimelpfenig.

Don't delay. Schimelpfenig learned the hard, cold way. He says, "You can get into a trap saying, 'Well, my feet [or my hands] are kind of cold, but I'm going to get inside in a little while anyway.' Now I make sure I can honestly say my feet and hands are still *warm*."

Use the "buddy system." You watch a friend's face—specifically the ears, nose, and cheeks—for any noticeable change in color, and he or she does the same for you.

Avoid contact with metal. Just a few moments with your bare hand on a metal wrench can lead to frostbite in severe cold.

Stay in your vehicle. If you get stranded in your vehicle on a subfreezing night, it's best to stay put and not venture out into the unknown, says Schimelpfenig. You could risk developing hypothermia or an abnormal drop in body temperature (see "Hypothermia: The Cold Inside" on page 296). "Many of the people we've found who were stranded and tried to walk for help were dead," he says.

PANEL OF ADVISERS

Bruce Paton, M.D., is a clinical professor of surgery at the University of Colorado at Denver.

Tod Schimelpfenig is safety and training manager for the National Outdoor Leadership School in Lander, Wyoming. He also is a volunteer emergency medical technician.

James Sturm, M.D., is a staff physician in the Emergency Medicine Department at St. Paul–Ramsey Medical Center in Minnesota.

Ruth Uphold, M.D., is medical director of the Emergency Department at Medical Center Hospital of Vermont in Burlington.

Genital Herpes

17 Managing Strategies

You played sexual Russian Roulette and you lost. You have burning sores on your genitals. You are feverish and weak. The doctor runs a few tests and says you have genital herpes, also known as herpes simplex II. He says the disease is incurable—you will have it forever. You feel like you've just been handed a one-way ticket to hell.

But you haven't been, so stop feeling so bad. In fact, here's your ticket back home.

Keep your chin up. Why? First, if you're like most people, once your initial attack of herpes comes and goes (usually in two to three weeks), subsequent attacks will be infrequent and usually not nearly as severe as the first one. Second, if you're among those for whom herpes seems destined to bring misery, there is now a prescription medication called acyclovir that can reduce the frequency of attacks up to 90 percent. In short, "either by the natural progression of the disease or by therapeutic intervention, herpes is far from a hopeless condition," says Will Whittington, M.D., a research investigator with the Sexually Transmitted Diseases Division at the Centers for Disease Control in Atlanta, Georgia.

Beef up your immune system. Experts do not know exactly what causes the herpes virus to lie dormant for long periods and then abruptly awake to create havoc. But many think that a weakened immune system, like a drunken sheriff in an old western town, invites the little

The Mind/Body Connection

Why do some people carry the herpes virus for years without an attack, while others carrying the virus experience regular attacks?

The answer is largely in the mind, says Christopher W. Stout, Ph.D., of Denver, a clinical psychologist specializing in psychoneuroimmunology. "People who are more tense, depressed, carry more hostility, and are more easily aroused to anger, seem to suffer more frequent outbreaks," says Dr. Stout. "These kinds of attitudes are thought to suppress the body's immune system."

Judy Hurst, R.N., says "I don't care how much research is done over the next 1,000 years, I'm convinced that stress will always be the number one factor."

But if you weren't subject to stress *before* you learned you had herpes, you're certainly feeling stress now. This can create a situation in which your stress contributes to outbreaks, which contributes to stress, which—on and on. The question is—how do you get off this roller coaster?

Learn all that you can. Read about herpes, speak to your doctor, try to make as much sense out of, and gain as much control over your situation as you can, says Dr. Stout.

Join a support group. Every major city has one. They offer camaraderie, emotional support, and a place to talk confidentially and share information, says Hurst. The American Social Health Association can help you find one in your area. Call (919) 361-2742.

Consider short-term therapy. Upon learning you have herpes, you may experience sadness, depression, anger, and guilt. A good professional psychotherapist, in only a few sessions, should be able to help you gain some perspective, says Dr. Stout.

Learn relaxation techniques. There's a wide variety out there, including meditation, relaxation therapy, visualization, and biofeedback. Find an approach that works for you, says Dr. Stout.

---

bandits to return. However strong this connection may be, it would be wise for you to keep your immune system sober and armed with a well-rounded diet, lots of rest and relaxation, and regular exercise.

Use soap and water. Your inclination upon discovering sores on your genitals may be to bombard them with everything in your medicine cabinet. Don't. As with any sores, you do need to be concerned

---

MEDICAL ALERT

A Drug to Aid Healing

If you have a stubborn case of herpes or are experiencing many recurrences, you might want to consider seeing your doctor for a prescription of acyclovir, a drug that has been proven to speed healing time and limit the severity of the attack, says Stephen L. Sacks, M.D. If you are having your first attack or your recurrences are frequent, or if you *believe* them to be frequent, your doctor can most probably help you.

If you are pregnant, it is very important for you to inform whoever is handling your pregnancy, as herpes can infect newborns, says Dr. Sacks.

A strong link was once suspected between genital herpes and cervical cancer. That link is not as strong as once thought, but it would still be wise for women with herpes to get a yearly pap smear, says Will Whittington, M.D.

---

about developing a secondary (bacterial) infection, but soap and water is all you need or want to keep the area germ-free, says Dr. Whittington. You won't kill the virus with anything in your medicine cabinet anyway, and lots of things in there may make matters worse. "Acyclovir is the *only* medication that has been shown to have clear benefits for people with herpes," says Dr. Whittington.

Steer clear of ointments. Genital sores need lots of air to heal. Petroleum jelly and antibiotic ointments can block this air and slow the healing process, says Stephen L. Sacks, M.D., an associate professor of medicine at the University of British Columbia and the founder and director of the UBC Herpes Clinic. *Never* use a cortisone cream, which can inhibit your immune system and actually encourage the virus to grow, he says.

Warm the discomfort away. During your primary attack or bad secondary attacks, taking a bath or shower to get warm water over the genital area three or four times a day may prove soothing. (It does to most people, but some find they don't like it.) When you get out of the shower or bath, blow the genital area dry with a hair dryer set on low or cool, being careful not to burn yourself. The air from the dryer will also prove soothing and may possibly speed up the healing process by help- ing the sores dry out, says Dr. Sacks.

Wear loose-fitting, cotton undies. As air is essential to healing, wear only underpants that allow your skin to breathe—that is, wear cotton, not synthetics, says Judith M. Hurst, R.N., coordinator and medical adviser to Toledo HELP, a support group for people with herpes in the Toledo, Ohio, area. If you wear nylon panty hose, make sure the crotch is made of cotton. If you want to wear a bathing suit without compromising fashion, consider cutting the cotton crotch out of a pair of undies and sewing it into the swimsuit, says Hurst.

Ease painful urination. Urination for people having a first herpes outbreak can bring intense pain as acidic urine passes over open sores. This is particularly true for women. Try directing the urine stream away from your sores with a bit of rolled-up toilet tissue, suggests Dr. Sacks. Or, consider urinating in the tub when you finish bathing, says Hurst.

Don't touch. Although the disease is called *genital* herpes, it is possible to pass the virus to other parts of the body by touching an open sore and then bringing your fingers into contact with, say, your mouth or eyes. For this reason, it is important not to touch your sores, says Sandy Moy, coordinator of the Herpes Resource Center at the American Social

---

The Alternate Route

Can You Beat Herpes with Castor Oil?

Apply castor oil packs to your abdomen? Why? Because a strong immune system can keep the herpes virus from acting up, and castor oil packs fortify your immune system.

So says C. Norman Shealy, M.D., Ph.D., head of the Shealy Institute for Comprehensive Pain and Health Care in Springfield, Missouri. Dr. Shealy bases his theory on the writings of deceased psychic healer Edgar Cayce, and, he says, on as yet unpublished current research at a major university.

For maximum beefing-up of your immune system, says Dr. Shealy, start with 1 cup of castor oil, with which you thoroughly soak two thicknesses of flannel cloth. Place the saturated cloth on top of your tummy, and cover with plastic. Over the plastic, apply a heating pad, set as high as is comfortable, and leave it on for 1 hour. Initially, do this once a day, every day for a month. Continue the treatments three times a week, increasing use of the packs during a herpes attack.

Health Association (A.S.H.A.). If you think you might scratch at night, cover your sores with protective, breathable material such as gauze, she says.

Consider these supplements. Some people and even some doctors say that such things as zinc in ointment form or capsules, the amino acid lysine, or the food-additive butylated hydroxytoluene (BHT) taken as a supplement, can fight off herpes attacks. But despite spotty studies on their effectiveness, these are unproven remedies, according to the vast majority of doctors. If you decide to try any of these, know that high dosages may be dangerous and should only be taken under a doctor's supervision.

Call for help. If you have any questions regarding your condition, help is available, says Moy. A.S.H.A. runs two hotlines that offer free advice to people with herpes. Call the Herpes Hotline at (415) 328-7710, Monday through Friday, 12:00 to 4:30 P.M. (Pacific time); or the STD Hotline at 1-800-227-8922, Monday through Friday, 5:00 A.M. to 8:00 P.M. (Pacific time).

Write for help. You can also subscribe to *The Helper,* A.S.H.A.'s quarterly publication on all aspects of herpes, by writing to Subscriptions, H.R.C./A.S.H.A., P.O. Box 13827, Research Triangle Park, NC 27709. (Moy ensures that all literature from the Herpes Resource Center comes in plain, unmarked envelopes.)

Don't do unto others. Remember how you got herpes. You now have a responsibility to protect others. When you have sores, you are highly contagious—avoid sex. When sores are not present, you probably will not pass the virus, but you may wish to use a condom for further protection and peace of mind. Incidentally, because you already have herpes doesn't mean you can't catch another form of it. Although this doesn't happen often, genital herpes can recur with more than one strain of virus, says Dr. Sacks.

PANEL OF ADVISERS

Judith M. Hurst, R.N., is coordinator and medical adviser to Toledo HELP, a support group for people with herpes in the Toledo, Ohio, area. She is also an obstetric nurse at Toledo Hospital.

Sandy Moy is coordinator of the Herpes Resource Center at the American Social Health Association (A.S.H.A.), a nonprofit organization that aims to educate the public about sexually transmitted diseases. She has a master's degree in social work.

Stephen L. Sacks, M.D., is an associate professor of medicine at the University of British Columbia in Vancouver, and the founder and director of the UBC Herpes Clinic. A renowned expert on the management of genital herpes, he is the author of a respected book on the subject, *The Truth about Herpes.*

C. Norman Shealy, M.D., Ph.D., heads the Shealy Institute for Comprehensive Pain and Health Care in Springfield, Missouri. He is also a clinical and research professor at the Forest Institute of Professional Psychology, the founding president of the American Holistic Medical Association, and the author of such books as *The Pain Game* and *The Creation of Health.*

Christopher W. Stout, Ph.D., is in private practice in the Denver, Colorado, area and a clinical psychologist specializing in psychoneuroimmunology (the study of the connection between the immune system and human emotions). He is also an industrial consultant.

Will Whittington, M.D., is a research investigator with the Division of Sexually Transmitted Diseases at the Centers for Disease Control in Atlanta, Georgia.

Gingivitis

21 Remedies to Stop Gum Disease

Once upon a time, maybe just last year, plaque was one of those medical terms the dentist threw around and you ignored.

The dentist would say, "Gotta brush and floss these teeth a little better. Lotta plaque on them."

You would say, "Uh huh. Sure. You're right." Then you would go home and brush and floss faithfully for a couple of days. But in a week or so the brushing and flossing would fall back to a lick-and-a-promise schedule that would last until your next dental appointment.

Today was different.

The dentist said, "Your gums are swollen and red. Today's cleaning made them bleed. You have gingivitis. And if you don't do something about it, you're going to lose your teeth."

Ooops. That 30-second lick-and-a-promise has caught up with you.

You aren't alone. A survey reported in the *Journal of the American Dental Association* showed a majority of adults has early signs of periodontal disease. Gingivitis is the *first* sign of periodontal disease. And gum disease is the major reason adults lose their teeth.

But don't despair. There's some good news in that terrible message your dentist just gave you. *You* are the one who can save your teeth. And the treatments aren't so hard. Here's what to do.

Don't just take 30 seconds anymore. If you want to get rid of gingivitis, you have to take time to floss and brush correctly. You're going to have to block out 3 to 5 minutes twice or three times a day for good oral hygiene, says Robert Schallhorn, D.D.S., Aurora, Colorado, dentist and past president of the American Academy of Periodontology.

Brush at the gumline. The plaque-catching area around the gumline is where gingivitis starts, and it is the most neglected area when we brush, says Vincent Cali, D.D.S., a New York city dentist and author of *The New, Lower-Cost Way to End Gum Trouble without Surgery.* Place your brush at a 45-degree angle to your teeth so half of your brush cleans your gums while the other half cleans your teeth. Then, shimmy your brush, don't scrape.

Have two toothbrushes. Alternate between them, advises Dr. Cali. Allow one to dry and air out while using the other.

Get a power tool. Studies show an electric rotary toothbrush typically removes 98.2 percent of plaque, versus 48.6 percent removed by hand brushing.

Bank some bone. Gingivitis is the beginning of what Dr. Cali calls peridontal osteoporosis. Just like the bones in the rest of your skeleton can shrink and get brittle, so, too, can your jawbone. Bolster your bones with plenty of calcium (found in dairy products, salmon, almonds, and dark greens), exercise, and a no-smoking policy.

Try a gum massage. Grip your gums between your thumb and index finger (index on the outside) and rub, suggests Richard Shepard, D.D.S., a retired dentist in Durango, Colorado. He says this will increase healthy blood circulation to your gums.

Stock up on vitamin C. Vitamin C won't cure gingivitis, but it can help check bleeding gums, according to a study at the U.S. Department of Agriculture's Western Nutrition Research Center in San Francisco, California.

MEDICAL ALERT

Ignore Them
and They Will Go Away

What happens if you ignore the sore, bleeding gums that are a sign of gingivitis? You risk more serious periodontal disease and the possible loss of your teeth.

Here are the signs that warn you your gingivitis is getting more serious. If you have any of them, see your dentist.

- You have bad breath that doesn't go away within 24 hours.
- Your teeth look longer—a result of your gums shrinking away from your teeth.
- Your mouth feels out of alignment when you shut it because your teeth come together differently.
- Your partial dentures fit differently.
- Pus pockets form between your teeth and gums.
- Your teeth are loose or fall out.

Also, if your gums still bleed when you brush your teeth and continue to be sore and swollen despite your efforts at good oral hygiene, you need to see your dentist again.

Brandish a proxa brush. A proxa brush is a specially designed brush (available at most drugstores) that's shaped like a tiny bottle brush. It slides between your teeth or under your crown or bridge to reach those hard-to-reach places, says Roger P. Levin, D.D.S., president of the Baltimore Academy of General Dentistry.

Use Listerine. In a study reported in the *Journal of Clinical Periodontology,* Listerine mouthwash was proven to be effective in inhibiting the development of plaque and in reducing gingivitis.

Look at the label. When buying generic mouthwash, look for the chemicals cetylpridinium chloride or domiphen bromide on the label. Research shows these are the active ingredients in mouthwash that reduces dental plaque.

Examine your lifestyle. Too much stress? Too little relaxation? Do you work around toxic chemicals? Any of those factors can adversely affect your gums. Dr. Cali says people need to examine every aspect of their lifestyles to see what they might change to make living more healthy.

Cut your vices. Excessive smoking and drinking can drain your body of vitamins and minerals vital to a healthy mouth, says Dr. Cali.

Scrape your tongue. Remove the bacteria and toxins hiding there. Dr. Cali says it doesn't matter what you use to scrape with, as long as it isn't sharp. He recommends a demitasse spoon, a washed poker chip, a Popsicle stick, a tongue depressor, or your toothbrush. Scrape from back to front 10 to 15 times.

Take an intermission. Don't try to perform all these oral ablutions in one day. Massage your gums one day, scrape your tongue the next, says Dr. Cali. If you do something different after you brush and floss, you won't bore yourself to death.

Snuff it with H_2O_2. Buy a 3 percent solution of hydrogen peroxide, mix it half-and-half with water, and swish it around your mouth for 30 seconds. Don't swallow. Use this wash three times a week to inhibit bacteria, says Dr. Cali.

Wash with an oral irrigation unit. Use an oral irrigation device to flush water around your teeth and gums, says Dr. Cali. To use it correctly, direct the stream of water between your teeth, not down into your gums.

Pack a portable irrigator. When you travel, carry an ear syringe (a rubber bulb with a long nose). Fill it with water, then flush your teeth, says Dr. Cali.

Use a gum stimulator. A rubber or specially designed triangular gum stimulator is better than a toothpick for massaging the gums, says Dr. Cali. It also cleans the surfaces between the teeth. Place the rubber point so it rests between two teeth. Point the tip in the direction of the biting surface until the stimulator is at a 45-degree angle to the gumline. Apply a circular motion for 10 seconds, then move on to the next tooth.

Eat a raw vegetable a day. It will keep gingivitis away, says Dr. Cali. Hard and fibrous foods clean and stimulate teeth and gums.

Try the baking soda and water solution. Take plain baking soda, mix it with a little bit of water, and apply it with your fingers along the gumline in a small section of your mouth. Then brush. You'll clean, polish, neutralize acidic bacterial wastes, and deodorize, all in one swoop, says Dr. Cali.

Say aloe to your druggist. Some people brush their gums with aloe gel, says Eric Shapira, D.D.S., a dentist in private practice in El Granada, California, and assistant clinical professor at the University of the Pacific School of Dentistry. "It's a healing agent and it will reduce some of the plaque in your mouth," he says.

PANEL OF ADVISERS

Vincent Cali, D.D.S., is a New York City dentist and author of *The New, Lower-Cost Way to End Gum Trouble without Surgery.* He also has a postgraduate degree in clinical nutrition from the Fordham Page Institute at the University of Pennsylvania in Philadelphia.

Roger P. Levin, D.D.S., is president of the Baltimore Academy of General Dentistry and a guest lecturer at the University of Maryland in Baltimore.

Robert Schallhorn, D.D.S., has a private practice in Aurora, Colorado, and is past president of the American Academy of Periodontology.

Eric Shapira, D.D.S., is in private practice in El Granada, California. He is an assistant clinical professor and lecturer at the University of the Pacific School of Dentistry in San Francisco, California, and has a master's degree in science and biochemistry.

Richard Shepard, D.D.S., is a retired dentist in Durango, Colorado. He edits the newsletter of the Holistic Dental Association.

Gout

17 Coping Ideas

Gout is a type of arthritis that strikes like a bolt from the blue. Its excruciating, throbbing pain often hits at night, turning the skin red-hot and leaving the affected joint swollen and tender. Worse, an attack can last for *days*.

Once considered the domain of royalty, gout is caused by very plebeian uric acid. We all have it in our bloodstreams. But if you suffer from gout, "either you produce too much or you produce a normal amount and don't excrete enough," says Branton Lachman, Pharm.D., a clinical assistant professor of pharmacy at the University of Southern California School of Pharmacy. Either way, the excess turns into tiny, troublemaking crystals that inflame your joints.

Often the big toe is the prime target, but almost any joint can become a sore point. And while anyone can fall prey to gout, the typical victim is a middle-aged male, who may be overweight and may have a family history of the disease. If you're a current—or potential—sufferer, heed these dos and don'ts from the experts:

Get some R and R. During an acute attack, keep the affected joint elevated and at rest, says Alabama pathologist Agatha Thrash, M.D., co-founder of Uchee Pines Institute, a nonprofit health-training center in Seale, Alabama. You'll probably have little trouble following this advice because the pain will be so intense. During this phase, say doctors, most patients can't bear even the weight of a bed sheet on the tender joint.

Reach for ibuprofen. It is the tremendous inflammation around an affected joint that causes the pain. So when you need a painkiller, says Jeffrey R. Lisse, M.D., an assistant professor of rheumatology at the University of Texas Medical School at Galveston, make sure it's one that can reduce inflammation—namely ibuprofen. Follow bottle directions. But if those dosages don't give relief, he says, consult your doctor before increasing them.

The Alternate Route

The Power of Cherries and Charcoal

Cherries. Although there is no hard scientific evidence that cherries help relieve gout, many people find them beneficial. It doesn't seem to matter whether they use sweet or sour varieties or whether the cherries are canned or fresh. Reported amounts vary from a handful (about ten cherries) a day up to ½ pound. People have also reported success with 1 tablespoon of cherry concentrate a day, says Agatha Thrash, M.D.

Charcoal poultice. Dr. Thrash recommends charcoal poultices. Charcoal has the ability to draw toxins from the body. Mix ½ cup of powdered activated charcoal with a few tablespoons flaxseed (ground to a meal in a blender) and enough very warm water to make a paste. Apply to the affected joint. Cover with a cloth or plastic to hold in place. Change every 4 hours or leave on overnight. Charcoal produces stains, so be careful not to get any on clothes or bed linens.

Charcoal bath. You may also mix charcoal into a bath for soaking your foot, says Dr. Thrash. Use an old basin that you don't mind staining. Mix ½ cup of charcoal powder with water to make a paste. Then gradually add enough hot water so your foot will be submerged. Soak for 30 to 60 minutes.

Charcoal by mouth. Activated charcoal taken by mouth can help reduce uric acid levels in the blood, says Dr. Thrash. Take ½ to 1 teaspoon four times a day at the following times: upon rising, at midmorning, midafternoon, and at bedtime.

Avoid aspirin or acetaminophen. All pain relievers are not created equal. Aspirin can actually make gout worse by inhibiting excretion of uric acid, says Dr. Lisse. And acetaminophen doesn't have enough inflammation-fighting capability to do much good.

Apply ice. If the affected joint is not too tender to touch, try applying a crushed-ice pack, says John Abruzzo, M.D., director of the Division of Rheumatology at Thomas Jefferson University. The ice will have a soothing, numbing effect. Place the pack on the painful joint and leave it for about 10 minutes. Cushion it with a towel or sponge. Reapply as needed.

Avoid high-purine foods. "Foods that are high in a substance called purine contribute to higher levels of uric acid," says Robert Wortmann, M.D., an associate professor of medicine and co-chief of the Rheumatology Division at the Medical College of Wisconsin. So avoiding such foods is prudent.

Those foods most likely to *induce* gout contain anywhere from 150 to 1,000 milligrams of purine in each 3½-ounce serving. They include high-protein animal products such as anchovies, brains, consommé, gravy, heart, herring, kidney, liver, meat extracts, meat-containing mincemeat, mussels, sardines, and sweetbreads.

Limit other purine-containing foods. Foods that may *contribute* to gout have a moderate amount of purines (from 50 to 150 milligrams in 3½ ounces). Limiting them to one serving daily is necessary for those who suffer severe cases. These foods include asparagus, dry beans, cauliflower, lentils, mushrooms, oatmeal, dry peas, shellfish, spinach, whole-grain cereals, whole-grain breads, and yeast.

In the same category are fish, meat, and poultry. Limit them to one 3-ounce serving five days a week.

Drink lots of water. Large amounts of fluid can help flush excess uric acid from your system before it can do any harm. Robert H. Davis, Ph.D., a professor of physiology at the Pennsylvania College of Podiatric Medicine, recommends plain old H_2O. "Most people just don't drink enough water," he says. "For best results have five or six glasses a day."

As a bonus, lots of water may also help discourage the kidney stones that gout patients are prone to.

Consider herb teas. Another good way to take in sufficient liquid is with herb teas. They're free of both caffeine and calories, so large amounts won't make you jittery or pile on unwanted pounds. Colorado nutrition counselor Eleonore Blaurock-Busch, Ph.D., president and director of Trace Minerals International, especially recommends sarsaparilla, yarrow (milfoil), rosehip, and peppermint. Brew as usual and drink often.

Don't drink alcohol. "Avoid alcohol if you have a history of gout," says Gary Stoehr, Pharm.D., an associate professor of pharmacy at the University of Pittsburgh School of Pharmacy. Alcohol seems to increase uric acid production and inhibit its secretion, which can lead to gout attacks in some people. Beer may be particularly undesirable because it has a higher purine content than wine or other spirits, says Dr. Blaurock-Busch.

If you do tipple on special occasions, minimize your risk of a reaction by following this tip from Felix O. Kolb, M.D., a clinical professor of medicine at the University of California, San Francisco, School of Medicine. "Drink slowly and buffer wine with readily absorbed carbohydrates such as crackers, fruit, and cheeses."

Control your blood pressure. If you have high blood pressure in addition to gout, you have double trouble. That's because certain drugs prescribed to lower blood pressure—such as diuretics—actually raise uric acid levels, says Dr. Lachman. So taking steps to lower your blood pressure naturally would be wise. Try decreasing your sodium intake, losing excess weight, and exercising. But never discontinue any prescribed medication without consulting your doctor.

Beware of fad diets. If you are overweight, slimming down is imperative. Heavier people tend to have high uric acid levels. But stay away from fad diets, which are notorious for triggering gout attacks, says Dr. Lisse. Such diets—including fasting—cause cells to break down and release uric acid. So work with your doctor to devise a gradual weight-loss program.

Consult your doctor about supplements. Be careful when taking vitamins, says Dr. Blaurock-Busch, because too much of certain nutrients can make gout worse. Excess niacin and vitamin A, in particular, may bring on an attack, she says. So always consult a physician before increasing your vitamin intake.

Don't hurt yourself. For some unknown reason, gout often strikes a joint that's been previously traumatized. "So try not to stub your toe or otherwise injure yourself," says Dr. Abruzzo. "And don't wear tight shoes, which can also predispose your joints to minor injury."

PANEL OF ADVISERS

John Abruzzo, M.D., is director of the Division of Rheumatology and a professor of medicine at Thomas Jefferson University in Philadelphia, Pennsylvania.

Eleonore Blaurock-Busch, Ph.D., is president and director of Trace Minerals International, Inc., a clinical chemistry laboratory in Boulder, Colorado. She is also a nutrition counselor specializing in the treatment of allergy and chronic diseases at the Alpine Chiropractic Center there, and is the author of *The No-Drugs Guide to Better Health.*

Robert H. Davis, Ph.D., is professor of physiology at the Pennsylvania College of Podiatric Medicine in Philadelphia.

Felix O. Kolb, M.D., is clinical professor of medicine at the University of California, San Francisco, School of Medicine.

Branton Lachman, Pharm.D., is clinical assistant professor of pharmacy at the University of Southern California School of Pharmacy in Los Angeles. He is also vice president of clinical services of Lachman Medical in Corona, California.

Jeffrey R. Lisse, M.D., is assistant professor of rheumatology at the University of Texas Medical School at Galveston.

Gary Stoehr, Pharm.D., is associate professor of pharmacy at the University of Pittsburgh School of Pharmacy in Pennsylvania.

Agatha Thrash, M.D., is a pathologist who lectures worldwide. She is also co-founder of Uchee Pines Institute, a nonprofit health-training center in Seale, Alabama, and author of *Charcoal.*

Robert Wortmann, M.D., is associate professor of medicine and co-chief of the Rheumatology Division at the Medical College of Wisconsin in Milwaukee. He is also chief of medicine at the Clement J. Zablocki Veterans Medical Center there.

Hangnails

7 Tips to a Trim Finger

They're no big deal. Until you catch them on something. Trouble is, you catch them on *everything.* Your hair, your clothes, the newspaper, your cat. Every time you use your hands, little jabs of pain remind you of their presence.

Where do hangnails come from? Those annoying little triangular splits of skin around the fingernails are nothing more than dead skin. The skin in that area, which does not contain a good supply of oil to begin with, simply dries out.

Who gets them? They're particularly common among women who have their hands in water a lot or who bite their nails. But, says Rodney Basler, M.D., an assistant professor of internal medicine at the University of Nebraska College of Medicine, anyone involved in an occupation that dries out the hands is at risk. "The worst cases of hangnails [as well as chapped hands and hand eczema] occur in letter sorters. People who work with paper all the time get terribly dry hands because the paper actually absorbs oil from their hands. Often they think they're allergic to ink on the paper, but it's just the physical effect of oil being removed from their skin."

If your hangnails are giving you nightmares, try these tips.

Get a clip job. "If you get a hangnail, clip it short and clip it early," advises Joseph Bark, M.D., a Lexington, Kentucky, dermatologist. "That'll keep it from getting worse. Don't do major surgery on yourself; just clip off the little tags of skin with small, sharp, sterilized scissors."

Adds Trisha Webster, a top New York City hand model whose livelihood depends on perfectly groomed hands, "Before you clip a hangnail, soak it in a little water or a water and oil solution to soften it. A lot of people make the mistake of clipping a hangnail when it's still hard and end up ripping the skin more."

Take Mom's advice. "I advise the same thing your mother told you: Don't bite hangnails," says Dr. Basler. "If you bite them, you end up with fairly deep cuts around your fingers. And those can get infected."

Go soak. "Soaking in an oil-and-water solution, as you would when getting a manicure, is very helpful," advises Dr. Basler. "I tell my patients to mix 4 capfuls of bath oil such as Alpha-Keri with 1 pint of warm water and to soak their fingertips in it for maybe 10 to 15 minutes."

Wrap up the problem. "If you're having a lot of problems with hangnails, rub an emollient cream or ointment on the affected finger at bedtime and wrap it in a piece of plastic wrap. Secure the end with a bit of tape. The plastic will keep the moisture in overnight. Just be sure to remove the plastic in the morning. You wouldn't want to keep it on too long," says Dr. Basler.

Don't pick on yourself. "If you have a tendency to pick at hangnails when you're nervous, be sure to wear clothes with pockets," advises Diana Bihova, M.D., a dermatologist and clinical instructor of dermatology at the New York University Medical Center in New York City. "Put one hand in each pocket and leave them there until the urge passes."

Make moisturizing a habit. To prevent hangnails in the first place, "moisturize your cuticles every day. Make it a habit, not something you do just when you get a manicure," says Dr. Bihova. "Rub hand lotion into the flesh surrounding your nails to keep the area soft. For a more soothing feeling, warm the moisturizer over a pan of warm water, using a double boiler. Every time you apply moisturizer to your hands, take extra time to rub some into the cuticles."

Webster says, "I make it a point to rub olive oil or safflower oil into my cuticles" to help prevent hangnails.

Cuticle cautions. Because hangnails often form around the cuticle, many people try to avoid them by using cuticle-removing solutions. That's not a good idea, says Dr. Bihova.

"Many of these products, which are designed to tame excess or ragged cuticles, contain sodium hydroxide," she explains. "This caustic chemical can destroy skin tissue, so products containing it can cause irritation if left on too long. Use such products sparingly and always follow package instructions carefully. It's the cuticle, after all, that provides the vital function of protecting your nails from harmful bacteria and fungi.

"Hangnails sound very innocent," she warns, "but if they get infected, they can lead to serious inflammation of the cuticles and other tissues surrounding the nails."

PANEL OF ADVISERS

Joseph Bark, M.D., is a dermatologist in private practice in Lexington, Kentucky, and author of *Retin-A and Other Youth Miracles* and *Skin Secrets: A Complete Guide to Skin Care for the Entire Family.*

Rodney Basler, M.D., is a dermatologist and assistant professor of internal medicine at the University of Nebraska College of Medicine in Lincoln.

Diana Bihova, M.D., is a dermatologist in private practice and clinical instructor of dermatology at the New York University Medical Center in New York City. She is coauthor of *Beauty from the Inside Out.*

Trisha Webster is a top New York City hand model with the Wilhelmina Inc. modeling agency. She has almost 20 years' experience in the business.

Hangover

18 Ways to Deal with the Day After

It's a beautiful morning, and you just can't take it anymore.

The sparrows singing outside the window sound like nuclear-powered vultures cawing through loudspeakers, and all that golden sunlight streaming through the skylight feels like acid on your eyes—you're *sure* they're melting.

You are—regrettably, maybe immorally, definitely avoidably, but absolutely certainly—hung over. And the big question is: What can you do about it?

Unfortunately, not a whole lot. There is no one thing that cures a hangover except time. But there are a few things you can do to relieve the symptoms—the headache, nausea, and fatigue—so you can get through the day after as painlessly as possible.

Drink fruit juice. "Fruit juice contains a form of sugar called fructose, which helps the body burn alcohol faster," explains Seymour Diamond, M.D., director of the Diamond Headache Clinic in Chicago, Illinois. A large glass of orange juice or tomato juice, in other words, will help accelerate removal of the alcohol still in your system the morning after.

Eat crackers and honey. Honey is a very concentrated source of fructose, and eating a little the morning after is another way to help your body flush out whatever alcohol remains, says Dr. Diamond.

Get some pain relief. A headache is invariably a part of the package that goes with a hangover. "You can take aspirin, acetaminophen, or ibuprofen but you don't want anything stronger," Dr. Diamond says. "With more potent pain relievers, you run the risk of habituation, and you don't want the first problem to start another problem."

Drinking Affects Next-Day Performance

You're a hearty party person, but it's no problem—it doesn't matter how much you drink, you always wake up feeling just fine.

If you agree with this self-assessment, beware. Feeling fine doesn't mean you're really fine, according to a study performed at Stanford University in cooperation with the U.S. Navy.

The Stanford team took a close look at Navy pilots who fly P-3 subchasers. Using P-3 simulators, they evaluated the pilots' flying skills when stone-cold sober and 14 hours after drinking enough to get legally drunk.

The result: "Pilots who said they felt absolutely fine and in whom we couldn't find even a trace of alcohol still couldn't fly as well as they did during times they were off alcohol completely," says Von Lierer, Ph.D., director of research and owner of Decision Systems, a research and development firm in Stanford, California.

The meaning for *your* life? Sand in the system is still sand in the system, even when you don't know it's there.

"If you've got an important business meeting the next day, a key presentation you've got to give—*any* situation where you need peak performance—I wouldn't drink the night before," Dr. Lierer says.

But pilots aren't the only ones in peril from hangover aftereffects. Ground-bound drivers suffer the same deterioration of performance, according to a Swedish study reported in the *Journal of the American Medical Association*.

Swedish researchers tested 22 volunteers on a pylon-marked test course using—what else?—a Volvo station wagon. At unpredictable intervals, they received a signal that meant they were to swerve the car right and left around the pylons. Braking time and number of pylons hit were used as measures of driving ability.

Nineteen of the 22 volunteers scored significantly worse as a result of being hung over.

Bark back. Willow bark is a natural alternative if you'd like an organic pain reliever, according to Kenneth Blum, Ph.D., chief of the Addictive Diseases Division at the University of Texas Health Sciences Center at San Antonio. "It contains a natural form of salicylate, the active ingredient in aspirin, which is released as you chew it," Dr. Blum says.

Drink bouillon. Broth made from bouillon cubes or any home-made soup broth will help replace the salt and potassium your body loses when you drink, Dr. Diamond says.

How to Avoid a Hangover

A hangover once is a hangover never wanted again. But it doesn't mean that you have to give up alcohol altogether to have a fun night out turn into a feel-good day after.

"There's good evidence emerging that the chief cause of hangover is acute withdrawal from alcohol," says Mack Mitchell, M.D., vice president of the Alcoholic Beverage Medical Research Foundation in Baltimore, Maryland, and assistant professor of medicine at Johns Hopkins University. "The cells in your brain physically change in response to the alcohol's presence, and when the alcohol's gone—when your body's burned it up—you go through withdrawal until those cells get used to doing without the alcohol."

Couple that with the effects alcohol has on the blood vessels in your head (they can swell significantly depending on the amount you drink), and you end up living through a day after that you'd rather forget. So how do you avoid it all?

Drink slowly. The more slowly you drink, the less alcohol actually reaches the brain—even though you may actually drink more over the long haul. The reason, according to Dr. Mitchell, is simple math: Your body burns alcohol at a fixed pace—about an ounce an hour. Give it more time to burn that alcohol, and less reaches your blood and brain.

Drink on a full stomach. "This is probably the single best thing you can do besides drinking less to reduce the severity of a hangover," Dr. Mitchell says. "Food slows the absorption of alcohol, and the slower you absorb it, the less alcohol actually reaches the brain." The kind of food you eat doesn't matter much.

Drink the right drinks. What you drink can play a major role in what your head feels like the next morning, according to Kenneth Blum, Ph.D. The chief villains are congeners.

Replenish your water supply. "Alcohol causes dehydration of your body cells," says John Brick, Ph.D., chief of research at the Center of Alcohol Studies of Rutgers State University of New Jersey. "Drinking plenty of water before you go to bed and again when you get up the morning after may help relieve discomfort caused by dehydration."

Take B-complex vitamins. Drinking drains the body of these valuable vitamins. Research shows your system turns to B vitamins when it is under stress—and overtaxing the body with too much booze,

"Congeners are other kinds of alcohols (ethanol is what gets you drunk) found in essentially all alcoholic beverages," Dr. Blum says. "How they work isn't known, but they're closely related to the amount of pain you experience after drinking."

The least perilous concoction is vodka. The most perilous are cognacs, brandies, whiskies, and champagnes of all kinds. Red wine is also bad, but for a different reason. It contains tyramine, a histamine-like substance that produces a killer headache. Anyone who's spent an evening entertained by a bottle of red wine knows what we're talking about.

Avoid the bubbly. And that doesn't mean just champagne. Dr. Mitchell and Dr. Blum agree. Anything with bubbles in it (and a rum and Coke is just as bad as champagne) is a special hazard. The bubbles put the booze into your bloodstream much more quickly. Your liver tries to keep up but can't, and the overflow of alcohol pours into your bloodstream. You'll know exactly how much the morning after.

Be size sensitive. With few exceptions, there's no way a 110-pounder can go one-on-one with a 250-pound drinker and wake up the winner. So scale down your drinks. To come out even, the 110-pounder can handle about half the alcohol of the 250-pounder.

Have an Alka-Seltzer cocktail at bedtime. "There's no hard scientific data on this, but my own clinical experience and that of a lot of others says that water and Alka-Seltzer before going to bed can make your hangover much less of a problem," says John Brick, Ph.D. Others claim that two aspirin tablets (which is really Alka-Seltzer without the fizz) can also help.

beer, or wine definitely qualifies as stress, says Dr. Blum. Replenishing your body with a B-complex vitamin capsule can help shorten the duration of your hangover.

Eat amino acids. Amino acids are the building blocks of protein. Like vitamins and minerals, they can also be depleted by use of alcohol. Dr. Blum says that replenishing amino acids plays a role in repairing the ravages of a hangover. Eating a small amount of carbohydrates will help get amino acids back in the bloodstream. Amino acids are also available in capsule form at most health food stores.

Have two cups of coffee. "The coffee acts as a vasoconstrictor —something that reduces the swelling of blood vessels that causes headache," Dr. Diamond says. "A couple of cups can do a great deal to relieve the headaches associated with hangovers." But don't drink too much. You don't need coffee jitters on top of the alcohol jitters.

Eat a good meal. If you can tolerate it, that is. A balanced meal will replace the loss of essential nutrients, explains Dr. Blum. But keep the meal light; no fats or fried foods.

Let time heal. The best and only foolproof cure for a hangover, of course, is 24 hours. Treat your symptoms as best you can. Get a good night's sleep and the next day—hopefully—all will be forgotten.

PANEL OF ADVISERS

Kenneth Blum, Ph.D., is chief of the Addictive Diseases Division of the University of Texas Health Sciences Center at San Antonio.

John Brick, Ph.D., is chief of research in the Division of Education and Training at Rutgers State University of New Jersey's Center of Alcohol Studies in Piscataway, New Jersey.

Seymour Diamond, M.D., is director of the Diamond Headache Clinic and the inpatient headache unit at Louis A. Weiss Memorial Hospital in Chicago, Illinois. He also is executive director of the National Headache Foundation. He has co-written several books on headaches.

Von Lierer, Ph.D., is director of research and owner of Decision Systems, a research and development firm in Stanford, California. He is a former cognitive psychologist at Stanford University.

Mack Mitchell, M.D., is a vice president of the Alcoholic Beverage Medical Research Foundation in Baltimore, Maryland, and assistant professor of medicine at Johns Hopkins University there.

Headaches

40 Hints to Head Off the Pain

"Not tonight, dear, I have a headache."

That line has become the universal stop sign for bedroom romance. Sure, sometimes it's a lie. But many times the headache is real. And notice that husbands and wives don't say, "Not tonight, dear, I've got a toeache." Headaches have earned mutual, painful respect.

"It's a very rare person indeed who has never experienced a headache," says Seymour Solomon, M.D., director of the Headache Unit at Montefiore Medical Center in the Bronx, New York, and a professor of medicine at Albert Einstein College of Medicine at Yeshiva University.

About 90 percent of all headaches are classified as muscle contraction, or more commonly, "tension headaches," according to the National Headache Foundation. These are the head knockers most of us blame on work, bills, and arguments.

The pain is typically generalized all over the head. You may feel a dull ache or a sense of tightness and perhaps experience "a sense of not being clearheaded," says Fred Sheftell, M.D., director of the New England Headache Treatment Program in Stamford, Connecticut. "Most people will describe it as feeling like a band is wrapped around their head." However, Dr. Sheftell adds, "We're not sure muscle contraction is always the real cause of what we call tension headache."

"Some people are born with biology that makes them headache prone," explains Joel Saper, M.D., director of the Michigan Headache and Neurological Institute in Ann Arbor. "Not everybody under stress gets headaches."

But more than 45 million Americans not only get headaches, they get them time and time again. Headaches, for these people, are a chronic problem. Further, an estimated 16 to 18 million of them suffer migraines, which rightfully have an even uglier reputation than tension headaches.

Migraines are part of the vascular headache family and most often strike women. Seventy percent of migraine sufferers are female.

"Migraines can be crippling," says Patricia Solbach, Ph.D., director of the Headache and Internal Medicine Research Center at the Menninger Clinic in Topeka, Kansas. So much so that migraine sufferers lose more than 157 million workdays each year.

Typically, migraines bring severe, one-sided throbbing pain (in 40 percent of cases, however, the pain occurs on both sides). Often this is accompanied by nausea and vomiting and perhaps tremor and dizziness. Some people also experience premigraine warning symptoms, including blurred vision, "floating" visual images, and numbness in an arm or leg.

Unfortunately, even the doctors who operate headache clinics can't guarantee that they can diagnose which kind of headache a patient has.

Give Your Face a Workout

All you need is your own handsome face and a mirror and you're ready to do some face and scalp calisthenics, courtesy of Harry C. Ehrmantrout, Ph.D., author of *Headaches: The Drugless Way to Lasting Relief*. The exercises are designed to relax the muscles of the face and scalp and teach you conscious control over these muscles so you can go into action at the first sign of a headache.

Here in summary are 11 face and scalp calisthenics Dr. Ehrmantrout recommends.

- Eyebrows up and return: Lift both eyebrows up quickly, then relax and let them drop down.
- Right eyebrow up and return: This move could be tough to do. Start by holding the other eyebrow in place and then move the right eyebrow up, as you did before.
- Left eyebrow up and return.
- Squint both eyes closed and release: Do this quickly, hold briefly, then relax.
- Squint right eye hard and release: Squeeze the right side of your face hard enough to raise the corner of your mouth.
- Squint left eye hard and release.
- Frown deeply and release: Squeeze eyebrows down and in toward the bridge of your nose.
- Yawn wide and close: Slowly open your mouth by lowering your jaw gradually to a wide position. Then close slowly.
- Open jaw, move right and left: Open mouth slightly and slide jaw from right to left, and then from left to right.
- Wrinkle nose: Squeeze nose upward, as if smelling a foul odor.
- Make faces: Ad-lib this one, just like when you were a kid. And don't worry, your face won't get stuck.

"There's no laboratory test that can tell you this patient has migraine, this one has tension," says Jerome Goldstein, M.D., a private practitioner and director of the San Francisco Headache Clinic in California. Diagnosis is usually based on the patient's history.

Thus, regardless of the name you give your headaches—tension, migraines, various obscenities—you are the one in the best position to recognize what habits and factors bring on your headaches. And it's up to you to do everything within your control to prevent or treat them. So for a better chance of heading off pain tomorrow, read this today.

Take two, not ten. For that once-or-twice-a-month tension headache, aspirin or one of the many over-the-counter anti-inflammatory drugs may work well. Certainly a lot of us think so—we spend more than $4 billion annually on these pills.

But overuse of these drugs will just cause more pain. "It's like scratching a rash," Dr. Saper says. "The more you scratch, the more it itches."

Don't delay. If you do decide to use aspirin for a headache, "take it right away—at the beginning of the headache," Dr. Solbach says. Otherwise, it may not do you much good.

Exercise to prevent. "Exercise is useful as a preventive measure," says Dr. Solomon. "You're releasing stress."

Cluster, Cluster Go Away

But please don't come back another day. Unfortunately, cluster headaches do tend to come back, even after long periods of remission. These headaches, which afflict about one million people—90 percent of whom are men—hit the unfortunate sufferer with heavy-duty pain, typically around or behind one eye.

Cluster attacks may occur every day for weeks, or even months. The cause is unknown, but "it's probably either hormonal or genetic," says Seymour Solomon, M.D. The male hormone testosterone is currently being studied for possible connections to cluster headaches.

Meanwhile, doctors have noticed a common denominator. "For reasons we don't completely understand, men who have cluster headaches are typically heavy smokers," says Dr. Solomon.

So quit smoking, or at least cut back drastically. And don't nap, advises Joel Saper, M.D. Then, maybe when the cluster headaches go away, they'll stay away.

MEDICAL ALERT

When Headaches Can Mean Real Trouble

"The average person" says Seymour Diamond, M.D., "typically has a tension headache." No big deal, no danger. But occasionally headaches are warning symptoms for serious disease. Here are the red flags.

- You are over 40 and never had recurring headaches before.
- The headaches have changed locations.
- The headaches are getting stronger.
- The headaches are coming more frequently.
- The headaches do not fit a recognizable pattern; that is, there seems to be nothing in particular that triggers them.
- Headaches have begun to disrupt your life; you've missed work on several occasions.
- The headaches are accompanied by neurological symptoms, such as numbness, dizziness, blurred vision, or memory loss.
- The headaches coincide with other medical problems or pain.

If you experience these symptoms, see your doctor.

Exercise during. If the headache isn't too severe, "I think exercise will work to make it better," Dr. Solbach says. "If you have a slight tension headache, I think you can probably end it if you exercise."

But don't exercise if it's severe. You'll just make your head hurt more, especially if you're suffering a migraine.

Sleep. A lot of people sleep a headache off, says Ninan T. Mathew, M.D., director of the Houston Headache Clinic and president of the American Association for the Study of Headache.

But don't oversleep. It's tempting, but "avoid sleeping in on the weekend," Dr. Mathew advises. "You're more likely to wake up with a headache."

Don't nap. While a nap may rid you of an existing headache, you don't want to nap if you're headache-free. "Napping can cause migraines," says Seymour Diamond, M.D., director of the Diamond Headache Clinic and the inpatient headache unit at Louis A. Weiss Memorial Hospital in Chicago, Illinois.

Sleep straight. Sleeping in an awkward position, or even on your stomach, can cause the muscles in your neck to contract and trigger a headache. "Sleeping on your back helps," says Dr. Diamond.

Stand tall, sit straight. The same principle applies here. "Also," adds Dr. Diamond, "avoid leaning or pushing your head in one direction."

Go cold. "Some people like the feeling of cold against their foreheads or necks and for them it seems to help," says Dr. Solbach.

Heat up. "But others," adds Dr. Solbach, "prefer hot showers or putting heat on their necks."

Breathe deeply. Deep breathing is a great tension reliever. "You're doing it right," Dr. Sheftell says, "if your stomach is moving more than your chest."

Do the body scan. Dr. Sheftell suggests checking yourself for signs that you are tensing up and inviting headache—clenched teeth, clenched fists, hunched shoulders.

Learn biofeedback. Studies have proven it effective for both tension headaches and migraines, Dr. Solbach says. And learning this technique doesn't have to shift pain from your head to your wallet. "There are all kinds of free courses given at community centers or maybe even where you work," she says.

Use your hands. Both self-massage and acupressure can help, according to Dr. Sheftell. Two key points for reducing pain with acupressure are the web between the forefinger and thumb (squeeze there until you feel pain) and under the bony ridges at the back of the neck (use both thumbs to apply pressure there).

Pretend it's a rose. "Put a pencil between your teeth, but don't bite," says Dr. Sheftell. "You *have* to relax to do that."

Wear a headband. "This old business of Grandmother tying a tight cloth around her head has some merit to it," Dr. Solomon says. "It will decrease blood flow to the scalp and lessen the throbbing and pounding of a migraine."

Say "no de cologne." "Strong perfume can set off migraine," says Dr. Solbach.

Be gentle. Believe it or not, if you're headache-free and "in the mood," you might develop a headache during sex. "It's considered an 'exertional' type headache," says Robert Kunkel, M.D., head of the Section of Headache in the Department of Internal Medicine at the Cleveland Clinic in Ohio. "It's more common in people with migraines than in those who just have tension headaches."

Seek quiet. Excessive noise is a common trigger for tension headaches.

Protect your eyes. Bright light—be it from the sun, fluorescent lighting, television, or a video display terminal—can lead to squinting, eyestrain, and, finally, headache. Sunglasses are a good idea if you're going to be outside. If you're working inside, "take some rest breaks from the computer screen and also wear some type of tinted glasses," Dr. Diamond suggests.

Watch your caffeine intake. "If you don't get your daily dosage of caffeine, your blood vessels will dilate," possibly giving you a headache, says Dr. Solbach. Too much caffeine will also give you a headache, so try to limit yourself to two cups (or one mug) of coffee a day.

Don't chew gum. The repetitive chewing motion can tighten muscles and bring on a tension headache, says Dr. Sheftell.

Go easy on the salt. High salt intake can trigger migraines in some people.

Eat on time. Skipping or delaying meals can cause headaches two ways. A missed meal can cause muscle tension, and, when blood sugar drops from lack of food, the blood vessels of the brain tighten. When you eat again, they expand, leading to headache.

Nan Finkenaur, once a chronic headache sufferer, says, "I noticed I got headaches if I didn't eat frequently. Now I eat a lot of small meals and it seems to help."

Know your danger foods. For Finkenaur, milk was a culprit. She cut back and the headaches decreased. But there are other headache foods.

Pass on the mustard—and the hot dog. You're certainly not losing out on nutrition and you may spare yourself a headache. Hot dogs, like luncheon and other cured meats, contain nitrates. And nitrates dilate blood vessels, which can mean big-time head pain, says Dr. Mathew.

Read the fortune, Cookie. Confucius never said anything about the wise not eating monosodium glutamate (MSG). But some people who don't absorb it well say they get a throbbing headache from it. Many Chinese dishes are loaded with it.

Say no to chocolate. Hey, it's fattening anyway. It also contains tyramine, a chief suspect in causing headaches. The good news is that many young people outgrow this chemical reaction. "The body appears to build up a tolerance," says Dr. Diamond.

Don't go nuts. And go easy on aged cheeses, too. Both contain tyramine.

Don't smoke and drive. You shouldn't smoke, period. But smoking with the car windows down when you're driving in heavy traffic gives you a double dip of carbon monoxide. This gas appears to adversely affect brain blood flow, according to Dr. Saper.

Curtail the cocktails. One alcoholic drink probably won't hurt, but don't hit your head on the rocks too many times. Also, some liquors contain tyramine.

Don't be a conehead. You probably can remember more than one occasion when you ate a big bite of ice cream and seconds later felt an intense rush of pain to your head.

Eat the ice cream slowly, Dr. Saper advises, "so that your palate will cool gradually instead of receiving a shock of cold."

Go with the flow. Maybe older people are better at this. "We see more headaches in younger individuals," Dr. Diamond says. "And they're under more stress—trying to make a living, supporting a family. But it's important to not overdo."

Decreasing your expectations, both of yourself and others, wouldn't hurt either, adds Dr. Sheftell.

Relax with imagery. "Imagine the muscle fibers in your neck and head to be all scrunched up," says Dr. Sheftell. "Then begin to *smooth* them out in your mind."

Have a sense of humor. "If you take life too seriously," says Dr. Sheftell, "you can see who those people are—they're walking around with their faces all scrunched up." And probably wondering why they have another headache.

For high altitudes, take vitamin C and aspirin. High altitudes can trigger a headache. But taking vitamin C and aspirin before and during that next ski trip can help you adjust, says Dr. Solomon.

He advises taking 3,000 to 5,000 milligrams of vitamin C the day before the trip and each day during the trip. Also, take two aspirin tablets per day beginning one day before the trip. (But check with your doctor first. You should get your doctor's approval before taking large doses of any vitamin.)

PANEL OF ADVISERS

Seymour Diamond, M.D., is director of the Diamond Headache Clinic and the inpatient headache unit at Louis A. Weiss Memorial Hospital in Chicago, Illinois. He also is executive director of the National Headache Foundation. He has co-written several books on headaches.

Harry C. Ehrmantrout, Ph.D., is author of *Headaches: The Drugless Way to Lasting Relief.*

Jerome Goldstein, M.D., is a private practitioner and director of the San Francisco Headache Clinic in California.

Robert Kunkel, M.D., is head of the Section of Headache in the Department of Internal Medicine at the Cleveland Clinic in Ohio. He also is vice president of the National Headache Foundation.

Ninan T. Mathew, M.D., is director of the Houston Headache Clinic in Texas. He also is president of the American Association for the Study of Headache.

Joel Saper, M.D., is director of the Michigan Headache and Neurological Institute in Ann Arbor. He also is author of *Help for Headaches.*

Fred Sheftell, M.D., is director of the New England Headache Treatment Program in Stamford, Connecticut.

Patricia Solbach, Ph.D., is director of the Headache and Internal Medicine Research Center at the Menninger Clinic in Topeka, Kansas.

Seymour Solomon, M.D., is director of the Headache Unit at Montefiore Medical Center in the Bronx, New York. He also is a professor of medicine at Albert Einstein College of Medicine at Yeshiva University in New York City.

Heartburn

23 Ways to Put Out the Fire

Drop this book. Run to the fridge. Prepare two bologna sandwiches with gobs of mayonnaise, and tomatoes, and peppers. Have some beer. Pull out that cold pizza from Friday night. Yum yum. Help yourself to some ice cream with chocolate sauce. Don't forget the coffee, extra cream. Now down it all as fast as you can—then hurry back!

All done?

Good. Now we're ready to talk heartburn.

What's heartburn? Just hold on a couple of minutes and you'll know.

What causes it? It could be a number of things, but in most cases, it's *acid reflux*. That is, some of the digestive juices normally found in your stomach back up out of your stomach into your esophagus, the pipe between your stomach and your mouth. These juices include hydrochloric acid, the corrosive substance used in industry to clean metal.

Whereas the stomach has a protective lining so that it doesn't succumb to the acid, the esophagus has no such lining. That's why upwardly mobile stomach acid burns, sometimes so badly that you may think you're suffering a heart attack.

What causes stomach juices to rise? You guessed it—that sharklike attack on the refrigerator is the most common cause. But it's not the only one.

Unfortunately, some people suffer from heartburn even without overindulging. For all of you sufferers who need to understand a little bit more about how heartburn works—and how to squelch the fire—we turn to the experts.

Don't overdo it. Stomach acids can be forced up into the esophagus when there's too much food in the belly. Fill the belly more, and you'll force up more acid. There can be many reasons for heartburn, but

329

Antacids Do Help

Over-the-counter digestive aids are generally effective and safe. One would hope so; Americans pay billions of dollars a year for these medications. The antacids that got the highest marks from our experts were many of the most common names—all those whose labels say they're made from a mixture of magnesium hydroxide and aluminum hydroxide. (One constipates and the other tends to produce diarrhea; combined, they counter each other's side effects.)

Although the mix may be relatively free of side effects, it still is not a good idea to stay on these antacids for more than a month or possibly two, says Francis S. Kleckner, M.D. They are so effective that they could be masking a serious problem that warrants a physician's care, he says. Our experts agree that liquid antacids, although not as convenient as tablets, are generally more effective.

for the occasional sufferer, it's usually eating too much food too fast, says Samuel Klein, M.D., assistant professor of gastroenterology and human nutrition at the University of Texas Medical School at Galveston.

Don't lie flat. Yes, you feel miserable, and you're inclined to recline. Don't! If you do, you'll have gravity working against you. Stay upright and the acid in your stomach is more likely to stay in your stomach. "Water doesn't travel uphill and acid doesn't either," says Francis S. Kleckner, M.D., a gastroenterologist in Allentown, Pennsylvania.

When you finally do lie down, elevate the head of your bed 4 to 6 inches. You can do this by putting blocks under the legs of the bed itself or by slipping a wedge under the mattress at the head of the bed. (Extra pillows, however, cannot be expected to do the trick.) Keeping the bed on a slant will discourage the heartburn from returning.

Take an antacid. "An over-the-counter antacid such as Maalox or WinGel will generally bring fast relief from occasional heartburn," says Dr. Klein. (For more on antacids, see "Antacids Do Help" above.)

Don't make your problem worse with bad advice. You might have heard that some things, like milk or mints, are good for heartburn. Make sure the guy who gave you this advice doesn't try to sell you a bridge somewhere. What's wrong with milk and mints? Mints are one of several foods that tend to relax your lower esophageal sphincter, or LES, the little valve whose job it is to keep acid in your stomach—and the little lid that can often protect you even when you do overindulge.

MEDICAL ALERT

It Could Be an Ulcer

If you're experiencing heartburn regularly for no apparent reason, it's time to call your doctor, says Samuel Klein, M.D.

How regularly? As a rule of thumb, "two or three times a week for more than four weeks," says Francis S. Kleckner, M.D. Although heartburn is most usually caused by simple acid reflux, he cautions that it can also be a sign of an ulcer.

Heartburn accompanied by any of the following symptoms, says Dr. Klein, should be checked out by a physician *fast*. It could mean you're having a heart attack.

- Difficulty or pain when swallowing
- Vomiting with blood
- Bloody or black stool
- Shortness of breath
- Dizziness or light-headedness
- Pain radiating into your neck and shoulder

In addition, know that heartburn caused by simple acid reflux is normally worse *after* meals. If your heartburn worsens *before* meals, it may be a sign of an ulcer.

And what's wrong with milk? It's this: Fats, proteins, and calcium in milk can stimulate the stomach to secrete acid. "Some people recommend milk for heartburn—but there's a problem with it," says Dr. Klein. "It feels good going down, but it does stimulate acid secretion in the stomach."

Other foods that can relax your sphincter, and should be avoided to alleviate or prevent heartburn, include beer, wine, and other alcoholic beverages, and tomatoes.

Go easy on the caffeine. Caffeinated drinks such as coffee, tea, and cola may irritate an already inflamed esophagus. Caffeine also relaxes the sphincter.

Shun the world's worst-for-you dessert. What's the number one food to avoid when you're suffering from heartburn? Chocolate. The sweet confection deals heartburn sufferers a double whammy. It is

---

The Alternate Route

Remedies from the Garden

Walk into your favorite health food store and chances are you'll find a number of herbs that are reputed to fight heartburn. Daniel B. Mowrey, Ph.D., a psychologist and psychopharmacologist who has been researching herb use in medicine for 15 years, has looked at the evidence thoroughly and has come to the conclusion, that, yes, *some* herbal remedies do relieve and prevent heartburn.

Gingerroot. This, says Dr. Mowrey, is the most helpful. "I've seen it work often enough that I'm convinced," he says. "We're not sure how it works, but it seems to absorb the acid and have the secondary effect of calming the nerves," he says. Take it in capsule form just after you eat. Start with two capsules and increase the dosage as needed. You know you've taken enough, says Dr. Mowrey, when you start to taste ginger in your throat.

Bitters. A class of herbs called bitters, used for many years in parts of Europe, is also helpful, Dr. Mowrey says. Examples of common bitters are gentian root, wormwood, and goldenseal. "I can vouch that they work," says Dr. Mowrey. Bitters can be taken in capsule form or as a liquid extract, just before you eat.

Aromatics. The aromatic herbs, such as catnip and fennel, are also reputed to be good for heartburn, "but the research on these is sporadic," says Dr. Mowrey.

Some you should forget about. A group of herbs that includes Irish moss, plantain, and slippery elm is often recommended, but "I have the least confidence in these," he says.

Apple cider vinegar. Outside the herb family, an oft-touted remedy for heartburn is 1 teaspoon of apple cider vinegar in ½ glass of water sipped during a meal. "I've used it many times—it definitely works," says Betty Shaver, a lecturer on herbal and home remedies at the New Age Health Spa in Neversink, New York. It may sound bizarre to ingest an acid when you have an acid problem, admits Shaver, but "there are good acids and bad acids," she says.

---

nearly all fat, *and* it contains caffeine. (For chocolate addicts, however, here's good news: White chocolate, while just as fatty, has little caffeine.)

Clear the air. "It doesn't matter whether it's yours or someone else's tobacco smoke—avoid it," says Dr. Kleckner. It will relax your sphincter and increase acid production.

Swear off fizzy drinks. All those little bubbles can expand your stomach, having the same effect on the sphincter as overeating, says Larry I. Good, M.D., a gastroenterologist in Merrick, New York, and an assistant professor of medicine at the State University of New York at Stony Brook.

Feed that hamburger to the dog. If you've just knocked off a triple cheeseburger with fries and a double milkshake, that probably explains your pain. Greasy, fried, and fatty foods tend to sit in the stomach for a long time and foster surplus acid production. Avoidance of fatty meats and dairy products will almost certainly discourage repeated attacks, says Dr. Good.

Check your waistline. The stomach may be compared to a tube of toothpaste, says Dr. Kleckner. If you squeeze the tube in the middle, he says, something's going to come out of the top. A roll of fat around the gut squeezes the stomach much as a hand would squeeze a tube of toothpaste. But what you get is stomach acid.

Loosen your belt. Think again of the toothpaste analogy, says Dr. Kleckner. "Many people can get relief from heartburn simply by wearing suspenders instead of a belt," he says.

If you're lifting, bend at the knees. If you bend at the stomach, you'll be compressing it, forcing acid upward. "Bend at the knees," says Dr. Kleckner. "It's not only a way to control acid, it's also better for your back."

Check your medicine cabinet. You may find the source of your grief lurking within it. A number of prescription drugs, including some antidepressants and sedatives, may aggravate heartburn. If you're suffering heartburn and are on any prescription drug, "review it with your physician," says Dr. Kleckner.

Think mild, for spice isn't always nice. Chili peppers and their spicy cousins may seem like the most likely heartburn culprits, but they're not. Many heartburn sufferers can eat spicy foods without added pain, says Dr. Klein. Then again, some can't.

Be cautious about, but not afraid of, the Florida sunshine tree. Acidic foods like oranges and lemons may seem like trouble, but the acid they contain is kid stuff compared to what your stomach produces, says Dr. Kleckner. He suggests you let your tummy decide on these foods.

Vow to eat dinner earlier tomorrow night. "Never eat within 2½ hours before bedtime," says Dr. Kleckner. A bulging stomach and gravity working together are a sure way to force stomach acid upward into the esophagus.

Take life a little easier. "Stress," says Dr. Klein, "may cause an increase in acid production in the stomach. Some good relaxation techniques might be of help in reducing your level of tension, allowing you to rebalance your unbalanced body chemistry."

PANEL OF ADVISERS

Larry I. Good, M.D., is a member of the Long Island Gastrointestinal Disease Group in Merrick, New York. He is also an assistant professor of medicine at the State University of New York at Stony Brook.

Francis S. Kleckner, M.D., is a gastroenterologist who practices in Allentown, Pennsylvania.

Samuel Klein, M.D., is assistant professor of gastroenterology and human nutrition at the University of Texas Medical School at Galveston. He is also an editorial adviser to *Prevention* magazine.

Daniel B. Mowrey, Ph.D., of Lehi, Utah, is a psychologist and psychopharmacologist who has been researching the use of herbs in medicine for 15 years. He is author of *The Scientific Validation of Herbal Medicine* and *Next Generation Herbal Medicine.*

Betty Shaver is a lecturer on herbal and other home remedies at the New Age Health Spa in Neversink, New York.

Heat Exhaustion

27 Ways to Stave Off Trouble

Each summer, with everything from garden hoes to golf clubs in hand, the same people who are cautious enough to carry umbrellas when rain is predicted push themselves beyond safe limits in the sun.

The not uncommon result: heat exhaustion, a condition in which excessive loss of body fluid results in a rise in body temperature.

It's important to understand that no one is immune to heat exhaustion, not even the most finely conditioned athlete, says Richard Keller, M.D., an emergency room physician at St. Therese Hospital in Waukegan, Illinois. That's because the hotter we get, the more we perspire, and if we sweat *too* much, we start to run low on water.

Heat exhaustion is caused by water depletion (dehydration), or in rare cases—rare because of Americans' typically high-salt diets—by salt depletion. (We lose salt along with our sweat.)

Thirst is likely to be the first symptom, followed by loss of appetite, headache, pallor, dizziness, and a general flulike feeling that may include nausea and even vomiting. In more extreme cases, the heart may race and concentration may become more difficult.

Hopefully, you won't find yourself in that situation. Here's how to avoid it, and if necessary, how to cope with it.

Get out of the sun. This is as critical as it is obvious, especially for the person already suffering heat exhaustion. Otherwise body temperature could continue to rise, even if the person is resting and drinking water, Dr. Keller says. He adds that returning to the sun for very long, even if many hours later, could cause a relapse in some cases.

Drink water. It's still the best beverage to turn to for hydration, says Dr. Keller. It should be taken a little at a time—not gulped down. The doctor adds, "Ideally, you would have loaded up on water ahead of time—*before* going out into the sun."

Eat more fruit and vegetables. "They have a fairly high water content and good salt balance," Dr. Keller says.

Drink diluted electrolyte drinks. Gatorade is the best-known example and is widely used by professional sports teams. Football teams, for instance, often have twice daily practices in July and August, and players who sweat heavily can lose a lot of potassium and sodium, says Bob Reese, head trainer for the New York Jets and president of the Professional Football Athletic Trainers Society. "We have Gatorade and water available on the field at all times," he says.

Avoid salt tablets. Once routinely handed out to athletes and anyone else who wanted them, these pills now are considered bad medicine by most doctors. "They do the opposite of what they're supposed to do," says Larry Kenney, Ph.D., an assistant professor of applied physiol-

MEDICAL ALERT

First Aid for Heatstroke

Heatstroke kills. A large number of well-documented cases proved fatal, says Larry Kenney, Ph.D.

Of course, no one goes directly from feeling fine to the brink of death—no matter how hot it is. Rather, heatstroke turns lethal when signs of heat exhaustion, and later, heatstroke itself, are ignored or recognized too late, says Richard Keller, M.D.

"And it's sometimes difficult to distinguish between heat exhaustion and heatstroke," he says. For this reason, a person who does not respond to self-help measures for heat exhaustion within 30 minutes should be taken to the doctor. "If you have heat exhaustion, the worst you'll get is confused. If you have trouble walking, or become unconscious, then you're getting into heatstroke."

Heatstroke is a major malfunction of the body's thermoregulatory system—internal temperature is allowed to rise dangerously high. Symptoms can be similar to those of heat exhaustion—dizziness and nausea, for example. In addition, the person may become very disoriented and even agitated. And when the body quits regulating temperature, the heatstroke victim typically ceases sweating. But not always.

"Young people [30 and under] can sweat the whole way through," Dr. Keller says, "provided they're in pretty good shape."

Fainting may or may not signal heatstroke. "If they revive quickly—say in 2 to 5 minutes—that's more likely heat exhaustion," says Dr. Keller, adding that seizure and coma are additional possibilities with heatstroke.

It's important to get the person to a doctor as soon as possible for emergency care and observation, says Dr. Kenney, noting that complications such as shock and kidney shutdown could develop.

ogy in the Laboratory for Human Performance Research at Pennsylvania State University. "The increased salt in the stomach keeps fluids there longer, which leaves less fluid available for necessary sweat production."

Avoid alcohol. Booze fast forwards dehydration, says Danny Wheat, an assistant trainer for the Texas Rangers baseball club. The team often plays in 100-degree-plus conditions in Arlington, Texas. "We stress to players that the night before a day game, they should limit their alcohol consumption," he says.

And unless heatstroke strikes in a hospital parking lot, you'll need to administer some fast first aid. So here are recommendations on how to treat heatstroke until you can get to a doctor.

Cool with water. "Splash the person with water instead of immersing them in cold water, if possible," Dr. Keller says. "The water will evaporate on the skin more quickly and have a cooling effect."

Take advantage of technology. If possible, move the person into an air-conditioned setting.

Force fluids. Water is best, provided the person is conscious, Dr. Keller says.

Apply cool towels. Again, this is a better choice than immersing the person in ice cold water.

Take charge. Some of those afflicted let pride get in the way of treatment. Roofing, for example, can be intensely hot work. "The hot tar is 325°F when you're putting it down," says roofing safety director David Tanner. Add the sun's heat and the humidity and, "We've had people wait too long, become delirious, and just start running across the roof and almost fall off."

Know who is at increased risk and exercise caution. Infants are more vulnerable, according to Dr. Kenney, because their sweat glands are not fully developed. "Older people, in general, don't hydrate as well," adds Dr. Keller. "And certain medications, such as those for high blood pressure, can interfere with hydration."

Avoid caffeine. Like alcohol, it speeds dehydration and "can make you sweat more than normal," says Dr. Keller.

Don't smoke. Smoking can constrict blood vessels, Dr. Keller says, and impair the smoker's ability to acclimate to heat.

Acclimate slowly. "You can't work and live in air conditioning all the time and then go out and be a weekend warrior," says Dr. Keller. "Starting early in the season, you should get some outdoor time every day and slowly build from there."

Go slower. Whatever you're doing outside, you should do it more slowly than usual when it's extremely hot, Dr. Keller suggests.

Pour a cold one—on yourself. Dousing your head and neck with cold water will help if it's hot and dry, says Dr. Kenney, because the water will evaporate and then cool you off. "In humid conditions," he says, "there's probably no benefit."

Be your own fan. Use a newspaper, a picnic tablecloth—whatever you have—to keep yourself in a cool breeze.

Cheat the sun. You can't beat the sun, so do what you have to do outdoors early and late. "On hot days we start work at daylight," says David Tanner, safety director and project manager for Tip Top Roofers in Atlanta, Georgia. "Then we knock off about 2 or 3 o'clock in the afternoon."

Hit the scales. Heat exhaustion isn't necessarily built in a day. You could be dehydrating gradually over several days. "During training camp we check players' weights every day to make sure the water they sweat off in practice is getting put back," Reese says.

Drink like a baby. Pedialyte and other rehydrant formulas for infants are effective enough that the Texas Rangers give them to their players in extremely hot weather, Wheat says. The primary ingredients are sugar, sodium, and potassium. Drinking 1 quart before a race or tennis match and 1 quart during or after the workout "might not be a bad idea," says Dr. Keller.

Give the weatherman a little credit. Granted, in the winter, predicted 2-inch snowfalls sometimes turn into 10-inch snowfalls. But when it comes to summertime heat and humidity, the forecast is usually accurate. When they say it is going to be hot enough to fry an egg on Main Street, don't make that the day to begin painting your house.

Wear a hat. Preferably one that also shades the neck and is well-ventilated. A wide-brimmed hat with lots of tiny holes, for example, would be a good choice. "The blood vessels in your head and neck are very close to the skin surface, so you tend to gain or lose heat there very quickly," says Dr. Kenney. "And the top of the head is especially sensitive in people who are bald or balding."

Don't bare your chest. "You pick up more radiant heat exposure with your shirt off," says Lanny Nalder, Ph.D., director of the Human Performance Research Center and the Wellness Center at Utah State University.

"Once you start perspiring, a shirt can act like a cooling device when the wind goes through," he adds.

Carry a spare. If your shirt gets wet with perspiration, take it off and wash it as soon as possible. "The dried salt from your sweat impairs the 'breathing' quality of the shirt," Dr. Nalder says. Change it and wash it as soon as possible.

Wear cotton/polyester blends. They breathe better than shirts that are 100 percent cotton or 100 percent tightly woven nylon.

Wear light colors. They reflect the heat, says Dr. Nalder, while dark colors absorb it.

PANEL OF ADVISERS

Richard Keller, M.D., is an emergency room physician at St. Therese Hospital in Waukegan, Illinois.

Larry Kenney, Ph.D., is an assistant professor of applied physiology in the Laboratory for Human Performance Research at Pennsylvania State University in University Park.

Lanny Nalder, Ph.D., is director of the Human Performance Research Center and the Wellness Center at Utah State University in Logan.

Bob Reese is head trainer for the New York Jets and president of the Professional Football Athletic Trainers Society.

David Tanner is safety director and project manager for Tip Top Roofers in Atlanta, Georgia.

Danny Wheat is an assistant trainer for the Texas Rangers baseball club in Arlington, Texas.

Hemorrhoids

18 Coping Remedies

How do you locate the hemorrhoid creams in your local supermarket or pharmacy? It's easy. Look for all the shoppers in trenchcoats, dark sunglasses, and fake moustaches.

For many, hemorrhoids are an enormous embarrassment. But they really needn't be. Hemorrhoids are among the most common of all health ailments, striking an estimated eight out of ten of us throughout our lifetimes. Even Napoleon suffered hemorrhoids. It is said that the distracting pain of the emperor's hemorrhoids contributed to his crushing defeat at Waterloo.

But hemorrhoids don't have to be *your* Waterloo. Much like varicose veins, these swollen veins in the anus are partially hereditary, but they can also be caused by—and be remedied by—such things as diet and toilet habits.

So stop blushing, sit yourself down on a comfortable pillow, and read what the experts say about this common problem.

Strive for soft and easy bowel movements. The most effective strategy against hemorrhoids is to go right to the source of the problem. More often than not, on top of every rear end with hemorrhoids sits a person grunting and groaning. If it's news to you that passing one's stools is not supposed to be a long and arduous affair, you've likely got hemorrhoids. Huffing and puffing on the toilet provides just the kind of strain needed to engorge and swell the veins in your rectum. Hard stools then make matters worse by scraping the already troubled area. Solution? Drink lots of fluids, eat lots of fiber, and refer often to the following remedies.

Oil your inner workings. Once you've increased the fiber and fluids in your diet, your stool should become softer and pass with less effort. You may help your bowels to move even more smoothly by lubricat-

---

MEDICAL ALERT

Hemorrhoids That Need Help

If you've always had a healthy bottom and all of a sudden you experience discomfort, it may well be hemorrhoids. It could also be something else. If discomfort is accompanied by itching and you've recently returned from a trip abroad, for example, you might have parasites. You will need medical treatment to get rid of them.

Bleeding from the rectum should always warrant a trip to the doctor, says Edmund Leff, M.D. "Hemorrhoids can never become cancer, but hemorrhoids can bleed and cancer can bleed," explains Dr. Leff.

Other times an enlarged vein in your anus can clot, creating "a big, blue, swollen, hard area that's very painful," says John O. Lawder, M.D. In most cases, the clot can be easily extracted by your doctor.

---

ing your anus with a dab of petroleum jelly, says Edmund Leff, M.D., a colon and rectal surgeon in private practice in Phoenix and Scottsdale, Arizona. Using a cotton swab or your finger, apply the jelly about ½ inch into the rectum.

Clean yourself tenderly. Your responsibility to your hemorrhoids shouldn't end when you're through moving your bowels. It's extremely important to clean yourself properly and gently, says John O. Lawder, M.D., a family practitioner specializing in preventive medicine and nutrition in Torrance, California. Toilet paper can be scratchy, and some types contain chemical irritants. Purchase only nonperfumed, noncolored (white) toilet paper, and dampen it under the faucet before each wipe.

Elect a kinder, gentler toilet paper. If you've never heard of lubricated toilet paper, that's because it isn't sold yet. But you can find facial tissues coated with moisturizing cream—and these, says Dr. Lawder, offer the most hemorrhoid-friendly backside wipe on the market.

Don't scratch. Hemorrhoids can itch, and scratching can make them feel better. But *don't* give in to the urge to scratch. "You can damage the walls of these delicate veins," and make matters much worse for yourself, says Dr. Lawder.

Don't lift any pianos today. Heavy lifting and strenuous exercise can act much like straining on the toilet, says Dr. Leff. If you're prone to hemorrhoids, get a friend to help or hire someone to help you move that piano or dresser.

Go soak yourself. The sitz bath—sitting with your knees raised in 3 or 4 inches of warm water in a bathtub—is a remedy that still tops the list of most experts as a way to deal with hemorrhoids. The warm water helps to kill the pain while increasing the flow of blood to the area, which can help shrink the swollen veins, says J. Byron Gathright, Jr., M.D., chairman of the Department of Colon and Rectal Surgery at the Ochsner Clinic in New Orleans, Louisiana, and an associate professor of surgery at Tulane University.

Apply a hemorrhoid medication. There are many hemorrhoid creams and suppositories on the market, and while they generally will *not* make your problem disappear (contrary to what the ads may say), most are designed as local painkillers and can relieve some of the discomfort, says Dr. Gathright.

Choose a cream. Choose a hemorrhoid cream over a suppository any day, says Dr. Leff. Suppositories are "absolutely useless," for external hemorrhoids, and even for internal hemorrhoids, suppositories tend to float too far up the rectum to do much good, he says.

Work wonders with witch hazel. A dab of witch hazel applied to the rectum with a cotton ball is one of the very best remedies available for external hemorrhoids, especially if there's bleeding, says Marvin Schuster, M.D., chief of the Department of Digestive Diseases at Francis Scott Key Medical Center in Baltimore, Maryland, and a professor of medicine and psychiatry at the Johns Hopkins University School of Medicine. "Barbers use witch hazel when they cut you—because it causes the blood vessels to shrink down and contract," he says.

While anything cold, even water, can help kill the pain of hemorrhoids, give your hemorrhoids a special treat by putting a bottle of witch hazel into a bucket of ice, just as you would a champagne bottle. Then take a cotton ball, soak it in the witch hazel and apply it against your hemorrhoids until it's no longer cold, then repeat, suggests Dr. Schuster.

Watch your weight. Because they have more pressure on the lower extremities, overweight people tend to have more problems with hemorrhoids, just as they do with varicose veins, explains Dr. Lawder.

Control your salt intake. Sure, you like your french fries covered with salt, but it can make your hemorrhoids worse. Excess salt retains fluids in the circulatory system that can cause bulging of the veins in the anus and elsewhere, says Dr. Lawder.

Avoid certain foods and drinks. Some foods, while they won't make your hemorrhoids worse, can contribute to your anal misery by creating further itching as they pass through the bowels. Watch out for excessive coffee, strong spices, beer, and cola, says Dr. Leff.

Pregnant? Take the pressure off. Pregnant women are particularly prone to hemorrhoids, in part because the uterus sits directly on the blood vessels that drain the hemorrhoidal veins, says Lewis R. Townsend, M.D., a clinical instructor of obstetrics and gynecology at Georgetown University Hospital in Washington, D.C. A special hemorrhoid remedy if you are pregnant is to lie on your *left* side for about 20 minutes every 4 to 6 hours, says Dr. Townsend. By doing so, you decrease pressure on the main vein draining the lower half of the body.

The Alternate Route

Stoneroot, the Herbal Solution?

"I have one patient who has found that collinsonia is the only thing that will control his hemorrhoids," says Grady Deal, D.C., Ph.D., a nutritional chiropractor and psychotherapist in Koloa, Kauai, Hawaii. Collinsonia, also known as stoneroot, is an old-fashioned herbal remedy, popular in the last century, although it can still be found in some health food stores today.

In the *New Age Herbalist* by Richard Mabey, *Collinsonia canadensis,* or stoneroot, is described as an herb whose "main use is to strengthen the structure and function of the veins. It is particularly good for the treatment of hemorrhoids." Dr. Deal says it acts as an astringent that may be helpful for hemorrhoids.

"Take two capsules [375 milligrams each] twice a day with a full glass of water between meals for acute problems. Some people need to take a maintenance dose of two tablets daily indefinitely to control symptoms," says Dr. Deal. (But check with your doctor first.) "I keep them on hand all the time for hemorrhoid patients."

Give it a little shove. Sometimes the word hemorrhoid refers not to a swollen vein but to a downward displacement of the anal canal lining. If you have such a protruding hemorrhoid, try shoving it back into the anal canal, says Dr. Townsend. Hemorrhoids left hanging are prime candidates to develop into clots.

Sit on a doughnut. We're talking about a doughnut-shaped cushion here. They are available in pharmacies and medical supply stores and can be useful to hemorrhoid sufferers who do a lot of sitting, says Dr. Townsend.

Try the ClenZone. This little appliance attaches to your toilet seat and squirts a thin stream of water into your rectum after every bowel movement. It gets you superclean and serves as a soothing mini-sitz bath at the same time.

ClenZone is available from Hepp Industries, Inc., 687 Kildare Crescent, Seaford, NY 11783. The cost is about $22.

PANEL OF ADVISERS

Grady Deal, D.C., Ph.D., is a nutritional chiropractor and psychotherapist in Koloa, Kauai, Hawaii. He is also the founder and owner of Dr. Deal's Hawaiian Fitness Holiday health spa in Koloa.

J. Byron Gathright, Jr., M.D., is chairman of the Department of Colon and Rectal Surgery at the Ochsner Clinic in New Orleans, Louisiana, and an associate professor of surgery at Tulane University in New Orleans. He is also president of the American Society of Colon and Rectal Surgeons.

John O. Lawder, M.D., is a family practitioner specializing in nutrition and preventive medicine in Torrance, California.

Edmund Leff, M.D., has a private practice in colon and rectal surgery in Phoenix and Scottsdale, Arizona.

Marvin Schuster, M.D., is chief of the Department of Digestive Diseases at Francis Scott Key Medical Center in Baltimore, Maryland, and professor of medicine and psychiatry at Johns Hopkins University School of Medicine in Baltimore.

Lewis R. Townsend, M.D., is in private practice in Bethesda, Maryland, and is a clinical instructor of obstetrics and gynecology at Georgetown University Hospital and director of the physician's group at the Columbia Hospital for Women Medical Center, both in Washington, D.C.

Hiccups

17 Home-Tested Cures

Hiccuping is a truly useless experience, but most of us did it before we were born and will keep on doing it every now and then for the rest of our lives.

Why? Nobody is really sure. Some scientists believe hiccuping is the last vestige of a primitive reflex that at one time served some useful purpose, but not anymore. What causes it? The explanations are nearly endless, but most experts start their lists of hiccup sins with eating too fast and swallowing too much air. It seems a good place to start.

You probably remember that time you were hiccuping for several minutes and even felt kind of queasy. You think you had it bad? You didn't have it bad. Charles Osborne of Anthon, Iowa, had it bad. Osborne started hiccuping in 1922 and hiccuped for the next 65 years. That's 430 million times!

Hiccup cures date to antiquity and number in the hundreds, perhaps thousands. The general goal of all hiccup cures is to either increase carbon dioxide levels in the blood or to disrupt or overwhelm the nerve impulses causing the hiccups. Do they work? Some physicians say it doesn't really matter—most hiccups stop on their own after a few minutes anyway. Then again, that's probably what they told Charles Osborne. Read on. Maybe one or more of the following will be your sure cure.

Doctor Dubois' surefire sugar cure. "One cure that I find effective is a teaspoon of sugar, swallowed dry," says André Dubois, M.D., a gastroenterologist in Bethesda, Maryland. "That quite often stops the hiccups in minutes. The sugar is probably acting in the mouth to modify the nervous impulses that would otherwise tell the muscles in the diaphragm to contract spasmodically," he says.

"I've been using that cure since I was little," says Steve Lally, associate editor for *Prevention* magazine. "It's never failed me yet." Lally, how-

The Laundry List

The truth must be told. Doctors approach nonpersistent hiccups exactly the same way you do—by running through a list of favorite treatments until they find one that works.

Thoughtfully, the *Journal of Clinical Gastroenterology* published a list of suggested hiccup cures to help those doctors whose personal lists were a little weak. Here are the journal's recommendations.

- Yank forcefully on the tongue.
- Lift the uvula (that little boxing bag at the back of your mouth) with a spoon.
- Tickle the roof of your mouth with a cotton swab at the point where the hard and soft palate meet.
- Chew and swallow dry bread.
- Suck a lemon wedge soaked with Angostura bitters.
- Compress the chest by pulling the knees up or leaning forward.
- Gargle with water.
- Hold your breath.

Two other treatments that the journal didn't list but that may warrant a try include:

- Suck on crushed ice.
- Place an ice bag on the diaphragm just below the rib cage.

ever, recommends a tablespoon of sugar, but that may be a matter of personal taste. Either way, some doctors seem to think sugar is a surefire cure. (Parents take note: One-half teaspoon of sugar dissolved in 4 ounces of water may work wonders on baby's hiccups.)

"Mac" McCallum's guaranteed gulp. "I cure my hiccups by filling a glass of water, bending over forward, and drinking the water upside down," says Richard McCallum, M.D., professor of medicine and chief of the Gastroenterology Division at the University of Virginia Health Sciences Center. That always works and I firmly recommend it for my normally healthy patients."

That cure came through for musician Mark Golin, who found himself beset with hiccups after a late-night gig in New York City. "A woman told me to bend over and drink the water from the opposite side of the glass," he says. "It worked then and has worked dozens of times since then."

The Dreisbach deflator. As a hard-driving researcher for a major northeastern publishing company, Christine Dreisbach knows what it's like to work through lunch and sometimes suffer the con-sequences—a bad bout of hiccups. "I used to try holding my breath," she says, "but lately, I've been blowing air out of my body in a slow, steady stream." Simple as it sounds, "that seems to work for me," she says.

Betty Shaver's sensation swallower. "When you're eating, just be quiet and eat," says Betty Shaver, a lecturer on herbal and other home remedies at the New Age Health Spa in Neversink, New York. "Then you won't get hiccups."

That's probably sage advice, but for those who are already afflicted, Shaver offers this remedy: "Hold your breath for as long as possible and swallow at the time you feel the hiccup sensation coming. Do that two or three times, then take a deep breath and repeat again. That should do it," she says.

That cure has worked wonders for one well-known author who used to get hiccups when forced to read aloud before her elementary school classmates, and who has suffered ceaselessly since then when making public appearances. "I always needed something that would work quickly, because I wouldn't start hiccuping until the kid ahead of me got up to read," she says. "Swallowing is the only thing that got me through the *Dick and Jane* series."

The half-minute hiccup helper. Dawn Horvath can diagnose digestive disturbances with great dexterity. She's a researcher just like Dreisbach, and that profession seems to know no end of alimentary ailments.

Horvath's helper goes like this: "Fill a Dixie cup with water and place it on a counter, then press your index fingers in your ears. Bend over at the waist and pick up the cup with the pinky finger and thumb of each hand and, while holding your breath, drink the water down in one or two gulps."

The tot tickler. When you have a roomful of active kids running around giggling and laughing at the day-care center, you can bet some will end up with hiccups before the day is done.

"I tickle them while they hold their breath, and they try real hard not to laugh," says Ronnie Fern, director of the ACJC Day-Care Center in Easton, Pennsylvania. "It works, too," says she. "I suppose it makes you gasp for breath and makes your diaphragm go back to doing what it's supposed to do." Maybe, but it sounds like fun either way.

Pat's brown bagger. We were going to leave out the old tip about breathing into a brown paper bag, figuring everybody probably knew it already and—worse yet—that it never worked very well anyway. But then we started hearing tales about Pat Leayman, a mail clerk for a major firm located in the industrial heartland. Seems she's cured large numbers of hiccuping mail workers (must be something in the stamps) using nothing more than that old brown paper bag!

"It's in the technique," Leayman says, sensing our skepticism. "You have to blow in and out exactly ten times, and you have to do it really hard until you're red in the face. You also have to do it fast, and you have to form a good seal around your mouth with the bag so that no air gets in. If you follow those directions exactly," she says, "the bag will work every time."

PANEL OF ADVISERS

André Dubois, M.D., is a gastroenterologist in Bethesda, Maryland.

Ronnie Fern is director of the ACJC Day-Care Center in Easton, Pennsylvania.

Richard McCallum, M.D., is a professor of medicine and chief of the Gastroenterology Division at the University of Virginia Health Sciences Center in Charlottesville. He does research on gastrointestinal problems.

Betty Shaver is a lecturer on herbal and other home remedies at the New Age Health Spa in Neversink, New York.

Hives

10 Hints to Stop the Itch

Hives are the way the skin sometimes reacts to allergies, physical irritation, stress, or emotions. Special cells start releasing histamine, which makes blood vessels leak fluid into the deepest layers of skin. The often intensely itchy wheals that result may disappear in minutes or hours, and usually within a couple of days. But while you have them, you may not want to appear all swollen and scratching in public. Here are a

---

A Touch of the Natural

For those who are willing to try something different, here are a few alternatives.

Take tea and see. If you suspect emotional times cause your hives and if you want to stay away from synthetic internal medication like antihistamines, you may want to try a nerve-calming herb tea, says SFC Thomas Squier, an instructor in survival training for the U.S. Army Special Forces at Fort Bragg, North Carolina, and an herbologist. He recommends peppermint or passion flower teas. Chamomile, valerian, and catnip are other common sedative herb teas.

Make a poultice or paste. Herbal manuals often list a poultice of the crushed leaves of chickweed as a remedy for itchy skin. Some people make a paste of water and cream of tartar and apply it to the hives, replacing it when the paste dries and gets crumbly.

Put on pressure. Finally, Michael Blate, founder and executive director of G-Jo Institute in Hollywood, Florida, says he's had quick success in getting rid of hives with acupressure. Deeply massage the point on your trapezius muscle (running between your neck and shoulder) located midway on the muscle and just an inch or so over the backside of the ridge. "If it doesn't hurt somewhat, you haven't found exactly the right point," he says.

---

few things you can do that may relieve the itch and swelling. Like many remedies, what works for some won't work for others, so experimentation is in order.

Send antihistamines to the rescue. Over-the-counter antihistamines are about the best thing you can do without a prescription, says allergist Leonard Grayson, M.D., clinical associate allergist and dermatologist at Southern Illinois University School of Medicine. Benadryl (diphenhydramine) and Chlor-Trimeton (chlorpheniramine) are the most commonly used and are often found in cold and hay fever medications. Caution: Most antihistamines can make you drowsy.

Cool down. Cold compresses or baths are about the best, and only, topical treatment for hives, Dr. Grayson says. Another cool way: Rub an ice cube over the hives. The cold shrinks the blood vessels and keeps

---

MEDICAL ALERT

The Danger Zone

Hives can kill by blocking breathing passages. If you get hives in your mouth or throat, call your emergency number immediately. If you know you're subject to this kind of reaction, you should be under a doctor's care and have a readily available supply of epinephrine. People with chronic hives (longer than six weeks) or with severe acute hives should also see a doctor.

---

them from opening, swelling, and allowing too much histamine to be released. "But it's only temporary," he says. "And if you get hives from cold weather or water, you're out of luck." Hot water only makes the itching worse.

Use calamine lotion to relieve the itch. This astringent is famous for its effects on poison ivy rash, but it may help temporarily soothe the itch of your hives as well. Since astringents reduce discharge, they may keep the blood vessels from leaking fluid and histamine. Other astringents that may help hives include witch hazel (especially chilled) and zinc oxide.

Try the alkaline answer. "Anything that's alkaline usually helps relieve the itch," Dr. Grayson says. So try dabbing milk of magnesia on your hives. "It's thinner than calamine, so I think it works better," he says.

Help with hydrocortisone? If you have just a small number of small hives, a hydrocortisone cream like Cortaid applied directly on the hives may relieve the itching for a while, says Beachwood, Ohio, dermatologist Jerome Z. Litt, M.D.

Call in the vegetation vigilantes. The leaves and bark of red alder, brewed into a strong tea, will help hives, says Varro E. Tyler, Ph.D., a professor of pharmacognosy at Purdue University and author of *The Honest Herbal*. "Apply it locally to the affected area, and you can also take a couple of tablespoonfuls internally." Repeat it until the hives are relieved. Red alder contains the astringent tannin. The leaves of the black nightshade may help also, he says. Wash and boil the leaves in water, put them on a cloth, and apply the leaves as a poultice on the hives.

Remember that an ounce of prevention is worth a pound of hives. "There are myriad causes of hives," says Dr. Litt. "You have to be a detective to find out what causes them." Some of the more common causes are medications, foods, cold, insect bites, plants, and emotions. Once you find out, of course, try to avoid exposure. "If you know you're going to get hives for whatever reason," he suggests, "take an antihistamine beforehand, and it may prevent them."

PANEL OF ADVISERS

Michael Blate is founder and executive director of the G-Jo Institute of Hollywood, Florida, a national health organization that promotes acupressure and oriental traditional medicine.

Leonard Grayson, M.D., is a skin allergy specialist and clinical associate allergist and dermatologist at Southern Illinois University School of Medicine in Springfield.

Jerome Z. Litt, M.D., is a dermatologist in private practice in Beachwood, Ohio, and is author of *Your Skin: From Acne to Zits.*

SFC Thomas Squier, of the U.S. Army Special Forces, is an instructor at the JFK Special Warfare Center and School, Survival-Evasion-Resistance-Escape/Terrorist Counteraction Department in Fort Bragg, North Carolina. He is a Cherokee herbologist and grandson of a medicine man. He also writes a newspaper column called "Living off the Land".

Varro E. Tyler, Ph.D., is a professor of pharmacognosy at Purdue University in West Lafayette, Indiana, and author of *The Honest Herbal.* He also serves as a *Prevention* magazine adviser.

Hyperventilation

8 Tactics to Overcome It

The first time it happened, Gary Varner thought he was having a heart attack. "My heart was racing and it just felt like everything inside my body—my chest—was vibrating. And I felt some tingling."

Understandably, he was scared. But at a hospital, emergency room doctors said his heart was fine. Their diagnosis: hyperventilation.

MEDICAL ALERT

Let Your Doctor Diagnose

One moment you're breathing normally—then suddenly you are breathing fast—out of control—your heart is pounding, your fingers are tingling, and your palms are sweating. You feel as if you're going to die, but in all probability you'll live to pay next year's taxes.

Hyperventilation, in most cases, is caused by anxiety. But if you've never experienced hyperventilation before, "you probably should be seen by a doctor," says Stephen J. Harrison, M.D.

Though it is uncommon, hyperventilation could be connected to a lung disease, a blood infection, pneumonia—even poisoning. Also, it's possible that what feels like a heart attack *is* a heart attack.

Of course, it's probably nothing that serious—but leave the official diagnosis to a doctor.

Simply put, hyperventilation is "breathing fast," or overbreathing, says Stephen J. Harrison, M.D., senior emergency medical resident at the Medical Center of Delaware in Wilmington.

"Anxiety is a common cause," says Gabe Mirkin, M.D., a sports medicine expert from Silver Spring, Maryland, and an associate clinical professor at Georgetown University School of Medicine. "When some people are frightened, they breathe rapidly and deeply, even though they don't need the extra oxygen. This causes them to breathe out a large amount of carbon dioxide, and excessive loss of carbon dioxide causes the blood to become alkaline. This in turn causes the symptoms of a panic attack."

Episodes of hyperventilation can last for hours but typically last 20 to 30 minutes. But to the heavy-breathing sufferer it can seem like hours.

Of course Varner was relieved to learn he had not suffered a heart attack. But his experience with hyperventilation was just beginning—repeat attacks are not uncommon. But Varner learned there are things you can do to stop attacks and to prevent them.

Breathe into a paper bag. This has long been the primary treatment for hyperventilation. The theory is that rebreathing into a paper bag will allow the person to replace the carbon dioxide "blown off" while hyperventilating.

"Blowing into a paper bag is fine," Dr. Harrison says, "if you've hyperventilated before, been evaluated by a doctor, and are sure there is nothing seriously wrong." Most people who hyperventilate meet that criteria, but a few may have more severe problems. (See "Let Your Doctor Diagnose" on the opposite page.)

Varner says using a paper bag not only helped him halt attacks, but it may have prevented some, too. "When I was battling this problem daily, I would carry a paper bag with me all the time," he says. "And just knowing I had that sack with me was a big help."

Sit down, be calm, and relax. You need to slow your breathing, says Dr. Mirkin. The more tense you are, the faster you'll breathe.

Practice breathing naturally. Don't take exaggerated breaths and don't take very shallow breaths—take normal breaths. That's one breath every 6 seconds or ten breaths a minute. Do this twice a day, 10 minutes per session, Dr. Mirkin advises.

Think beyond yourself. "Once I had that first hyperventilation experience, I became consumed with thoughts of having another one. And I did have several more," Varner says. So while you want to focus on your breathing in the practice sessions, Dr. Mirkin suggests you don't want to spend all your time thinking about your breathing and the possibility of hyperventilating.

"After all," says Dr. Harrison, "breathing is a natural thing."

Exercise. "It decreases anxiety and helps people cope better," Dr. Harrison says. "Especially if you get your heart rate up." And when exercising, breathing a little faster is fine.

Avoid uncomfortable situations. For Varner, that means not trapping himself in a crowd where he has to sit or stand still for long periods of time. Identify situations in your life that trigger hyperventilation and eliminate or reduce them. "If your fear of black cats, for example, makes you hyperventilate, then steer clear of black cats," says Dr. Mirkin.

Cut caffeine. It's a stimulant, and therefore, a potential trigger for hyperventilation, says Dr. Harrison. Watch out for coffee, tea, colas, and chocolate.

Don't smoke. Nicotine is also a stimulant.

PANEL OF ADVISERS

Stephen J. Harrison, M.D., is senior emergency medical resident at the Medical Center of Delaware in Wilmington.

Gabe Mirkin, M.D., is in private practice at the Sportsmedicine Institute in Silver Spring, Maryland. He is also associate clinical professor of pediatrics at Georgetown University School of Medicine in Washington, D.C. He is the author of several sports medicine books, including *Dr. Gabe Mirkin's Fitness Clinic,* and is a syndicated newspaper columnist and radio broadcaster.

Impotence

14 Secrets for Success

Sure it's a night you'll remember. For all the wrong reasons.

It had been a hectic week. You'd been working hard on that proposal, and never once made it home before midnight. Tonight, you were going to make it up to your wife.

You brought roses. She uncorked your favorite wine. After dinner, when you took the phone off the hook, she slipped behind you, kissing your neck in that way of hers that always drives you crazy. Everything seemed to unfold according to plan.

Everything, that is, except a certain part of your anatomy. A certain crucial part.

And that left you to wonder: What in tarnation is going on? Is this going to happen the next time? What the heck can I do about it?

Plenty. Realize, first, that you're not the only man in the world who's had this happen. "If men are honest, every one of them will tell you they've sustained an impotence episode at one time in their lives," says Neil Baum, M.D., director of the New Orleans chapter of the Male Infertility Clinic and an assistant professor of urology at Tulane University School of Medicine. "Not every incident is a ten."

"It can be devastating when it occurs," he says. "A man's whole concept of his masculinity may be undermined."

Experts say an estimated ten million men suffer from impotence, the term used when a man is unable to achieve and maintain penetration until he ejaculates.

Until the early 1970s, experts thought that most erection problems pointed to underlying problems in the psyche. Today, the medical community recognizes that almost half of all impotent men have a physical or structural problem that's at least partly responsible.

What can you do to keep erection problems at bay? Here's what our experts advise.

Give yourself time. "As a man gets older, it may take a longer period of genital stimulation to get an erection," says Dr. Baum. "For men aged 18 to 20, an erection may take a few seconds. In your thirties and forties, maybe a minute or two. But if a 60-year-old doesn't get an erection after a minute or two, that doesn't mean he's impotent. It just takes longer."

The time period between ejaculation and your next erection also tends to increase with age. In some men aged 60 to 70, it may take a whole day or longer to regain an erection. "It's a normal consequence of aging," says Dr. Baum.

Consider your medication. Drugs your doctor has prescribed might be at the root of the problem. Or it might be those over-the-counter antihistamines, diuretics, or sedatives you're using. Realize, of course, that what affects your neighbor may have no effect on you.

More than 200 drugs have been identified as problematic. Drug-induced impotence is most common in men over 50, says Dr. Baum. In fact, in an *American Medical Journal* study of 188 men, drugs were the problem 25 percent of the time.

If you suspect your medication, consult your doctor or pharmacist. He may be able to change the dosage or switch you to a different drug. Do not, however, attempt to do this on your own.

Beware of recreational drugs. Troublemakers that Richard E. Berger, M.D., a urologist with Harborview Medical Center in Seattle, Washington, lists in his book *BioPotency: A Guide to Sexual Success*, include cocaine, marijuana, opiates, heroin, morphine, amphetamines, and barbiturates.

Go easy on the alcohol. Shakespeare hit it on the head when he said in *MacBeth* that alcohol provokes desire but it takes away the performance. That happens because alcohol is a nervous-system depressant. It inhibits your reflexes, creating a state that's the opposite of arousal, says Dr. Berger. Even two drinks during cocktail hour can be a cause for concern, he says.

Over time, too much alcohol can cause hormonal imbalances.

"Chronic alcohol abuse can cause nerve and liver damage," says Dr. Baum. "When you have liver damage, you cause a dynamic where the man has an excess amount of female hormones in his body." You need to have the right proportion of testosterone for everything to work properly.

Know that what's good for the arteries is good for the penis. "In the last five years, it's become quite evident that the penis is a vascular organ," says Irwin Goldstein, M.D., co-director of the New England Male Reproductive Center at Boston University Medical Center in Massachusetts. The very things that clog your arteries—dietary cholesterol and saturated fat—also affect blood flow to the penis. In fact, says Dr. Goldstein, all men over age 38 have some narrowing of the arteries to the penis.

So watch what you eat. "High cholesterol is probably one of the leading causes of impotence in this country," says Dr. Goldstein. "It appears to affect erectile tissue."

Don't smoke. Studies show that nicotine can be a blood vessel constrictor, says Dr. Baum. A study of healthy adult mongrel dogs at the University of California at San Francisco showed that the inhalation of smoke from just two cigarettes was enough to prevent five dogs from getting a full erection and a sixth dog from maintaining one. The researchers believe that inhalation of cigarette smoke blocks erection by inhibiting the smooth muscle relaxation of the erectile tissue.

Do what you need to feel good about your body. Are you thinking about taking off a few pounds? Studying karate? Starting a weight-training program? Do it. "Sex is body contact," says James Goldberg, Ph.D., research director of San Diego's Crenshaw Clinic in California. "The more a person feels good about his body, the better he'll feel going into the event."

Don't overdo it on the exercise. If you exercise excessively, you'll stimulate the body's natural opiates, the endorphins. "We're not sure how they work, but they tend to lessen sensation," says Dr. Goldberg. "Over the short run, exercise is good for you. Beyond a certain point, though, the body gets into the habit of protecting itself."

Wait out pain. Your body also produces its own opiates when you're in pain, says Dr. Goldberg. These opiates can turn off any sexual stimuli. "There's not much you can do," he says, except wait for a better time.

Relax. Being in a relaxed frame of mind is crucial. Here's why. Your nervous system operates in two modes. When the sympathetic nerve network is dominant, your body is literally "on alert." Adrenal hormones prepare you to fight or take flight. Nerves shuttle your blood away from your digestive system and penis and into your muscles.

You can turn on your sympathetic nervous system just by being too anxious, says Dr. Baum. "For some men, the fear of failure is so overwhelming that it floods the body with norepinephrine, an adrenal hormone. That's the opposite of what you need to have an erection."

The key here is to relax and let your parasympathetic nervous system take over. Signals that travel along this network will direct the arteries and sinuses of the penis to expand and let more blood flow in.

Avoid whole-body stimulants. That means caffeine and certain questionable substances touted as potency enhancers. "The main thing during sex is to be relaxed," says Dr. Goldberg. "Stimulants tend to have an overall effect. They constrict the smooth muscle that must dilate before an erection can occur."

Refocus your attention. One way to relax is to focus with your partner on the more sensual aspects of intimacy. Play with and enjoy each other without worrying about that erection.

"The skin is the largest sexual organ in the body," says Goldberg, "not the penis. So don't be led by your penis. The whole body has to react."

Plan ahead. Dr. Berger thinks it is a good idea to decide in advance what you'll do if you don't get an erection. "What are your alternatives?" If you're not so focused on the erection itself, it will make it easier for the erection to come back, he says.

Talk to your partner. Don't risk increasing the tension in the bedroom by maintaining a sullen silence. Together, you can play detective and figure out what's going on. Pressure at work? Strain over a child's illness? A touchy issue you two haven't resolved yet?

"If you understand some of the things that can cause impotence, you can find a way to explain it without attributing it to something that's not there," says Dr. Berger. "And you should talk about what your alternatives are. Will you continue your lovemaking in a different way? Don't let the erection, or lack of it, interfere with your intimacy."

PANEL OF ADVISERS

Neil Baum, M.D., is director of the New Orleans Male Infertility Clinic, a clinical assistant professor of urology at Tulane University School of Medicine, and a staff urologist with Touro Infirmary in New Orleans, Louisiana.

Richard E. Berger, M.D., is a urologist with Harborview Medical Center in Seattle, Washington. He is the author of *Biopotency: A Guide to Sexual Success.*

James Goldberg, Ph.D., is research director of the Crenshaw Clinic in San Diego, California, and a clinical research pharmacologist.

Irwin Goldstein, M.D., is co-director of the New England Male Reproductive Center at the Boston University Medical Center in Massachusetts and is an assistant professor of urology at Boston University School of Medicine.

Incontinence

20 Coping Tips

Urinary incontinence is a symptom, not a disease. But the consequences of involuntary loss of urine can be debilitating to a person's self-esteem, social life, and job.

"I call incontinence a social disease," says Robert Schlesinger, M.D., an assistant professor of surgery at Harvard Medical School and co-director of the Center for the Treatment of Incontinence of Faulkner Hospital in Boston, Massachusetts. "People will go to almost any extent to adjust their lives to it. We had one woman who didn't go out of her house for three years because she was so ashamed."

Notice Dr. Schlesinger said that people "adjust their lives to it." It doesn't have to be that way. He and other experts are putting out a clear message that people should not be stigmatized by incontinence, says Katherine Jeter, Ed.D., who founded Help for Incontinent People (HIP) and is a clinical assistant professor of urology at the Medical University of South Carolina College of Medicine. "Nearly everybody can be made better or cured." That's saying something, when you consider there are ten million adult Americans who are incontinent.

In most cases, incontinence is a matter of degree. And reject the notion that it is a normal part of aging, says Neil Resnick, M.D., chief of geriatric service and director of the Continence Center at Brigham and Women's Hospital in Boston, Massachusetts, and an assistant professor of medicine at Harvard Medical School. "It's not inevitable and it's not irreversible." Sometimes only minimal effort can reduce, even prevent, the problem. You can adjust your incontinence to your life, not the other way around. Here are some ways you can help yourself.

Keep a bladder diary. For a week, write down, "what did I eat, what did I drink, when did I go to the bathroom, and how often did I leak?" Dr. Jeter suggests. The diary will help you and your doctor track down the cause.

Go easy on fluids. Your bladder diary may reveal you've been downing gallons of water a day, Dr. Jeter says. "Usually it's because a person is on a diet that requires forcing liquids. If you drink a little less, your incontinence problem would ease up." A good time to ease up is before bedtime.

But not too easy. Cutting your fluid intake to below-normal levels without your doctor's approval can lead to dehydration, worsening urinary problems and possibly causing serious illness.

Avoid alcohol. Booze is a great stimulus for trotting to the bathroom.

Avoid caffeine. Caffeine is another well-known diuretic. Like alcohol, it's found not just in beverages but in medications. Your diary will help you notice whether the beverages you drink provoke incontinence.

Avoid grapefruit juice. Grapefruit juice is also a famous diuretic, which is why it formed the basis for a once-popular diet.

Substitute cranberry juice. Cranberry juice is acidic and low in ash, and well-known as beneficial to the bladder.

Stay loose. Constipation can contribute to incontinence. So eat a high-fiber diet, and be sure to drink adequate amounts of fluid. One incontinence clinic's prescription: daily helpings of popcorn!

Don't smoke. Nicotine irritates the bladder surface. And if you have stress incontinence, coughing can trigger leaking.

Lose excess weight. Letters to the Simon Foundation for Continence in Wilmette, Illinois, says foundation president Cheryle Gartley, show that people who lose even a few pounds can lessen their incontinence.

Try "double voiding." When you urinate, stay on the toilet until you feel your bladder is empty. Then, stand up and sit down again, lean forward slightly at the knees and try again.

Go when you have to. "It's a real sensible idea to empty your bladder on a regular basis," Dr. Jeter says. For example, don't, out of embarrassment, sit at the dinner table and hold it until dinner's over. Holding it too long may lead to bladder infection and an overstretched bladder. Also, if you have a too-full bladder and a weak sphincter muscle, she says, you're likely to leak when all you really want to do is cough, sneeze, or laugh. Best bet: Empty your bladder before and after meals, and at bedtime.

Get in the habit. First, void at regular short intervals—hourly is a good place to start—and gradually increase the interval. In certain types of incontinence, this method can be highly effective, but no one knows why. "We don't know whether it truly retrains the bladder to function normally," Dr. Resnick says, "or whether it trains the brain to cope with a persistent bladder dysfunction."

Aim for 3 to 6 hours. An average interval between trips to the bathroom is 3 to 6 hours, Dr. Jeter says. Try to work up to this interval range over a period of weeks.

Compensate for your age. "Normal is what you have always done plus extra time to compensate for the weaknesses you get as you age," says Dr. Jeter. "Because you're older, it's longer between the time your bladder says you have to go and the time you arrive at the bathroom." In other words, try to sleep and spend your time closer to a bathroom than you did when you could still sprint.

Be ready for emergencies. Keep a bedpan or commode within reach of your bed.

Do special exercises. These are the Kegel exercises, developed in the late 1940s by Arnold Kegel, M.D., to help women with stress incontinence during and after pregnancy. The experts say they can reduce and maybe prevent some forms of incontinence in both sexes and at all ages. Here are HIP's guidelines.

Without tensing the muscles of your legs, buttocks, or abdomen, imagine you're trying to hold back a bowel movement by tightening the ring of muscles (the sphincter) around the anus. This exercise identifies the back part of the pelvic muscles.

Next, when you're urinating, try to stop the flow, and then restart it. This identifies the front part of the pelvic muscles. (For women: Imagine you're trying to grip a slipping tampon.)

You're now ready for the complete exercise. Working from back to front, tighten the muscles while counting to four slowly, then release them. Do this for 2 minutes, at least three times a day—this means at least 100 repetitions.

Anticipate accidents. If you know you're going to sneeze, cough, lift, or bounce up and down—squeeze that sphincter ahead of time and ward off an accident.

Don't panic if you have no warning. If you have urge incontinence, you have almost no warning of the need to go. Don't panic. Instead, at first notice, relax. Then tighten your sphincter. Then, relax your abdominal muscles. When the urge sensation passes, walk slowly, without panic, to the nearest restroom.

Buy special supplies. There are several brands of absorbent products in the form of underpants or pads and shields. The new products absorb 50 to 500 times their weight in water, neutralize odor, and congeal fluid to prevent leakage. The kind you need depends on your individual anatomy and the kind and degree of incontinence you have. It's understandable to be embarrassed to buy them. Find an understanding pharmacist and ask to have your purchase waiting for you when you arrive.

PANEL OF ADVISERS

Cheryle Gartley is president of the Simon Foundation for Continence in Wilmette, Illinois, and editor of *Managing Incontinence*.

Katherine Jeter, Ed.D., is founder and director of Help for Incontinent People (HIP). She is a clinical assistant professor of urology at the Medical University of South Carolina College of Medicine in Charleston and an affiliate in enterostomal therapy at the Spartanburg, South Carolina, Regional Medical Center.

Neil Resnick, M.D., is chief of geriatric service and director of the Continence Center at Brigham and Women's Hospital in Boston, Massachusetts, and an assistant professor of medicine at Harvard Medical School there.

Robert Schlesinger, M.D., is an assistant professor of surgery at Harvard Medical School in Boston, Massachusetts, and co-director of the Center for the Treatment of Incontinence at Faulkner Hospital there.

Infertility

18 Pointers to Aid Conception

You've decided to become parents. In a celebratory mood several months ago, you destroyed your last few condoms in a water balloon fight, dumped your spermicide stash into the trash, and retired the old diaphragm. Ever since, you've been having glorious, unprotected sex.

Small problem, though. Your lovemaking isn't making any babies. And that's beginning to worry you. Just how long does this conception business take? What can you do to help nature along?

FOR COUPLES

Here is what experts advise couples who are beginning to worry about their lack of success at conception.

Give it a year. If you're under 28, your sex life is wonderful, and there's nothing in your medical history that points to a possible reproductive problem, our experts say keep trying for a year.

"About 60 percent of couples conceive within six months and 90 percent within the year," says Mitchell Levine, M.D., an obstetrician/gynecologist with Women-Care in Cambridge, Massachusetts. "When you get older, naturally, fertility decreases a bit."

MEDICAL ALERT

When the Stork Needs More Than a Nudge

You'd like to have a child. But your body isn't cooperating. Should you give it a little longer? Or is it time to consult a fertility specialist?

According to our experts, seek medical counsel if:

- Your menstrual periods are scant or irregular, and your cervical mucus doesn't change. You may not be ovulating.
- You've used an over-the-counter ovulation kit for three cycles now, but it's never given you any indication you're ovulating.
- You are under 35 and have been unable to conceive despite a year of unprotected intercourse, or over 35 and have been unable to conceive after six months.
- You're producing milk, or you have male-pattern hair growth on your breasts, upper lip, or chin. You may have a hormonal imbalance.
- You or your partner have suffered from chlamydia, a sexually transmitted disease that can destroy the fallopian tubes in women and inflame and scar the ductal system in men.
- Your medical history includes pelvic infections, endometriosis, polycystic ovary disease, abdominal or urinary tract surgery, injuries to the perineum, excessively high fevers, or the mumps or measles.
- You've used an intrauterine device (IUD).
- You or your mate suspect exposure to some substance like lead that is known to impair fertility.

Even women in their twenties don't ovulate every month, adds Joseph H. Bellina, M.D., Ph.D., director of Omega International Institute, a fertility clinic in New Orleans, Louisiana. In the thirties, the likelihood of monthly ovulation begins to lessen. That's why the older you are, the sooner you'll want to consult a specialist.

Talk it out. Are you both sure you want that baby, or is one of you ambivalent? Our experts have had plenty of stories about couples who try half-heartedly for years but don't conceive until after one partner's uncertainty is resolved.

"I had a couple where the man was older, he had children from another marriage, and he wasn't sure he wanted to be a father at this point in his life," says Dr. Levine. "After a couple of sessions of really talking it out, he got really excited about becoming a father again. And that's when they conceived."

"It's eerie," adds Marilyn Milkman, M.D., a San Francisco obstetrician/gynecologist and clinic faculty member at the University of California, San Francisco. "I've had four patients come in for infertility evaluations, walk out the door, and become pregnant within the month."

Let the passion take you. Forget about ovulatory charts, mucus charts, and scheduled sex until you absolutely have to worry about them. If you've got time, "let the passion take you," says Dr. Milkman. "Often that does better."

The Alternate Route

Goodbye K-Y Jelly, Hello Egg White

Heads turned when Emory University fertility specialist Andrew Toledo, M.D., an assistant professor in the Department of Gynecology and Obstetrics, suggested that couples use egg white as a vaginal lubricant to induce conception.

"This is not some magic bullet," cautions Dr. Toledo. "It's only useful as a lubricant for those couples who find dryness a problem."

He advises couples to use egg white only during the few days each month when a woman is fertile. The rest of the month they should use whatever lubricant they prefer.

Why egg white?

Dr. Toledo says he was intrigued by the results of a study in Canada that found egg white had the least effect on sperm motility and survival.

It makes sense, he says. Egg white is pure protein. And the vast amount of sperm is pure protein in nature. "Sperm does not do well in a carrier different from its structure."

"For the six, seven, or eight couples who told me they needed to use some kind of lubricant, this helped." Several couples who tried this did conceive.

But don't use egg white if you're allergic to it, he cautions. Take the egg out of the refrigerator ahead of time, so that it's not cold, and separate the white from the yolk. It makes no difference whether you apply the substance to the glans of the penis or the vagina.

Ease up on your work schedule. Workaholism and constant pressure can put the squeeze on fertility, says Dr. Levine. "I see a lot of career people and I say to them 'take a look at what message you're giving to your body.' " For Dr. Levine, it makes sense from an evolutionary standpoint. Your body knows that a period of extreme stress is not an ideal time to get pregnant.

Use the standard missionary position on days when you suspect the woman is fertile. The man-on-top style of intercourse is best for conception, says Dr. Bellina. The woman should remain lying down for 20 minutes after her partner ejaculates.

"I advise couples to have intercourse on those nights and then fall asleep," he says.

Stop smoking. Cigarettes can impair fertility in men and women. Studies of men have shown that smokers are more likely than nonsmokers to have sperm counts below the normal range, and to have less sperm motility. An English study of 17,032 women showed that the more cigarettes a woman smoked per day, the less fertile she was likely to be. Researchers suspect that smoking may alter hormone levels in a woman's body.

FOR WOMEN ONLY

Here are some helpful measures that women can take to help increase the chances of pregnancy.

Make sure you're ovulating. Are you having regular periods? If not, you may not ovulate.

"One key to ovulation is noticeable changes in cervical mucus midway through the cycle," says Dr. Milkman. "The mucus will be thin, watery, and clear." Other signs include premenstrual breast tenderness, cramps, and what the Germans call mittelschmerz — ovulation pain, she says.

Another way to test ovulation is with a kit you buy at the drugstore. The kit, which reads levels of the ovulation release hormone in your urine, is only about 50 percent effective when you use it morning and night, says Dr. Bellina. Kits available only through your doctor's office tend to be more accurate. The best time to test is between 10:00 A.M. and noon.

If you get a positive result the first month you use it, great. If three cycles pass without giving you a positive result, it could mean that either the kit isn't sensitive enough for you or you're not ovulating. Either way, consult your doctor.

If you want to be a fertility goddess, try to look like one. Some women can induce ovulation by putting on a few pounds or taking off a few. In general, the closer your actual weight is to the ideal weight listed in the Metropolitan Life statistical tables, the better. You want to be within 95 percent of that ideal but below 120 percent.

Researchers have found that body fat can actually produce and store estrogen, a hormone that primes the body for pregnancy. When total body estrogen is too high or too low, the system can be thrown off balance. The more fat, the more estrogen produced.

In one study by reproductive endocrinologist G. William Bates, M.D., a professor of obstetrics and gynecology and dean of the Medical University of South Carolina College of Medicine, 29 slim and nonovulatory women attained ovulation when they gained enough weight to put them within 95 percent of the ideal. Within three years of entering the program, 24 of the 29 became pregnant. In another study by Bates, 11 of 13 overweight and nonovulatory women regained ovulation after they lost weight; 10 conceived.

Go easy on the exercise. There are two reasons for this. If exercise causes you to lose too much body fat, you can stop ovulating. But even if you maintain normal body weight, you may still put yourself at risk if you spend more than an hour a day working hard at activities like running, cross-country skiing, or swimming.

In a study of 346 women with ovulatory dysfunction, Beverly Green, M.D., a maternal and infant health specialist in Silverdale, Washington, found some evidence that women who had never been pregnant and who exercised vigorously for more than an hour a day increased their risk of infertility. The study found that exercise exerted its effect on fertility through a means independent of its ability to promote weight loss.

What's going on here? Dr. Green is not sure. Dr. Bellina suspects the endorphins, brain chemicals released during vigorous exercise, may, like morphine, affect a woman's prolactin levels. Elevated prolactin levels may interfere with ovulation.

At any rate, Dr. Green, a marathon runner who had no difficulty bearing children, cautions against overinterpreting her study. Her advice to dedicated athletes? "Try to cut back and see if it makes a difference."

Time it just right. If ovulation is occurring normally, maybe you're just not making love when you're fertile. It could be that simple, says Dr. Levine.

"Sometimes you've got two career people, they're having intercourse maybe once or twice a week, and they're just not hitting it," he says.

How do you remedy this? Try to predict ovulation. If you don't want to fuss much, you can predict the date of your next period and count back 14 days. Then make love every night from day 11 through day 16. Or you can buy an over-the-counter ovulation test kit, which will give you about 24 to 36 hours advance warning of ovulation. When the test indicates ovulation, make love that night and the night after, advises Dr. Bellina.

Thou shalt not douche. Anything that interferes with the pH level of the vagina can make life unfriendly for sperm. That includes douches, lubrication agents, and jellies.

"I tell people never to douche," says Dr. Milkman. "If you leave the vagina alone, it will do just fine at cleaning itself."

Go easy on caffeine. More than a cup of coffee a day can hurt your chances of becoming pregnant. The same holds true if you ingest the equivalent amount of caffeine from chocolate, soft drinks, or other caffeinated beverages.

In a study of 104 women who were attempting to become pregnant, researchers at the National Institute of Environmental Health Sciences found that those who drank more than the caffeine equivalent of a cup of coffee a day were half as likely to conceive as those who consumed less.

FOR MEN ONLY

And on the male side of the equation, there is more advice.

Give your sperm time to bounce back. Any viral illness associated with fever can depress sperm count for up to three months, says Neil Baum, M.D., director of the Male Infertility Clinic in New Orleans, Louisiana, and a clinical assistant professor of urology at Tulane University School of Medicine. Bad colds can have the same effect.

Why is the effect so long-lasting? According to Dr. Baum, the normal cycle to produce a sperm is 78 days. It takes another 12 days for the sperm to mature. Healthy semen, by the way, contains in excess of 20 million sperm per teaspoon. If you looked at the sample under a microscope, more than 60 percent would appear to be swimming forward.

If your sperm count is healthy, a cold or flu probably won't knock it out of the fertility range. But if it's borderline, an illness may.

Say no to steroids. Anabolic steriods can shut off the pituitary gland and alter the body's natural hormone balance, says Dr. Baum. "It's not uncommon for athletes to have infertility problems," he adds. "Long-time use of steroids can permanently damage the testicles."

Be wary of drugs and alcohol. Various over-the-counter and prescription drugs can depress sperm count. If you're not sure about the medications you use, consult your pharmacist or doctor. Tagamet, an ulcer medication, is one to watch out for. Others include chemotherapeutic agents and certain antibiotics. And various studies over the years show that chronic drinking and habitual marijuana use can be at fault, too.

Keep 'em cool. Nature's way of keeping your testicles a half-degree cooler than your core body temperature is to house them outside the body. But if you heat the core temperature too much, or heat the testes themselves, you can affect sperm production.

Dr. Baum advises you to be careful about excessive physical activity, temperature extremes, hot tubs, and close-fitting underwear if you want to father a child.

Remember that abstinence makes the sperm grow stronger. If a baby is what you're after, daily intercourse can be too much of a good thing because it can decrease your sperm count.

"For the average couple, this doesn't matter," says Dr. Levine. "But in a borderline case, this may do it." Most experts recommend you abstain for two days prior to the woman's fertile period to let the sperm build up, then make love every other day.

PANEL OF ADVISERS

G. William Bates, M.D., is a reproductive endocrinologist, professor of obstetrics and gynecology, and dean of the College of Medicine at the Medical University of South Carolina in Charleston.

Neil Baum, M.D., is director of the New Orleans Male Infertility Clinic, a clinical assistant professor of urology at Tulane University School of Medicine, and a staff urologist with Touro Infirmary in New Orleans, Louisiana.

Joseph H. Bellina, M.D., Ph.D., directs the New Orleans–based Omega International Institute, a fertility clinic in Louisiana. He is a national adviser of the Child and Human Development Council of the National Institutes of Health.

Beverly Green, M.D., works in infant preventive health and family medicine with Group Health Cooperative of Puget Sound in Silverdale, Washington. She specializes in maternal and infant health.

Mitchell Levine, M.D., is an obstetrician/gynecologist with Women-Care in Cambridge, Massachusetts.

Marilyn Milkman, M.D., practices obstetrics and gynecology in San Francisco, California. She is on the clinic faculty of the University of California, San Francisco.

Andrew Toledo, M.D., is a reproductive endocrinologist and an assistant professor in the Department of Gynecology and Obstetrics at Emory University in Atlanta, Georgia.

Ingrown Hair

10 Ways to Get a Clean Shave

The Ballad of Iggy, the Ingrown Hair

Well, early one mornin', 'bout the break of dawn,
> (duh-doo-whisker-whisker-whisk, duh-doo-whisk-whisk)

Iggy, he woke up to a terrible sound.
> (duh-doo-whisker-whisker-whisk, duh-doo-whisk-whisk)

A-screechin' and a-scrapin' and a-makin' a moan,
> (duh-doo-whisker-whisker-whisk, duh-doo-whisk-whisk)

Closer and a-closer, like to shiver his bones.
> (duh-doo-whisker-whisker-whisk, duh-doo-whisk-whisk)

Yeah, the blades caught his eye,
Yeah, they really made him cry,
Yeah, he ducked his head inside,
> (duh-doo-whisker-whisker-whisk, duh-doo-whisk-whisk).

But that wasn't the end of Ingrown Iggy, folks. No sir. He burrowed his hairy little head under the skin like an ostrich in the sand and stayed there warm and snug in his little blanket of infection. He and his buddies in the Great Neck Desert thought they were safe, but one day Mr. Tweezers arrived and started plucking them out like a robin does earthworms. Mr. Tweezers seized Iggy with big steel jaws and a viselike grip and yanked him out by his roots. "You can wash me down the drain," Iggy shrieked defiantly at Mr. Tweezers, "but I'll be back, I swear, *I'll be back!*"

Mr. Tweezers is about the only way to get rid of Iggy the Ingrown Hair, dermatologists say, but there are ways to make him stay gone.

Send Mr. Tweezers to the rescue. If you can see little Iggy hiding beneath the skin, says University of Nebraska College of Medicine dermatologist and assistant professor of internal medicine Rodney Basler,

M.D., apply a warm, damp compress for a couple of minutes to soften the skin. Then sterilize a needle or tweezers and pluck him out. Follow with an antiseptic like hydrogen peroxide or rubbing alcohol.

Bring Iggy to the surface. If you *can't* see the ingrown hair, don't go fishing for it, Dr. Basler warns, "because it might not be an ingrown hair at all." Instead, treat it with the compress until you can see a hair lurking there. *Then* use the sterilized needle or tweezers, followed by an antiseptic.

Think about growing a beard. "The curlier your hair is, the more likely you are to get ingrown hairs," says Dr. Basler. "If it's a real problem, seriously consider growing a beard. It's a legitimate alternative." If beards are frowned upon in your job, ask your doctor to tell your boss a beard is a medical necessity for you.

Make your whiskers April soft. If there's no way you can have a beard, properly preparing your whiskers for shaving will help avoid lots of little Iggys. "Wash your face thoroughly with soap and water for 2 minutes," recommends Ohio dermatologist Jerome Z. Litt, M.D. That softens the hair. "Rinse well, apply shaving cream or gel, and leave it on for 2 minutes to further soften the hair."

Hide behind your shadow. Reconcile yourself to "having a continual five o'clock shadow," Dr. Basler says. Don't shave close. The best way to do this, he says, is to use an electric razor.

Don't double up. You may not care for electric razors, but double-track razors are double trouble. The first blade cuts and sharpens the hair; the second blade cuts below the skin level, Dr. Litt says. The result: The sharpened hair curls around and grows back into the skin. Instead, use a single-track razor and settle for a shave that is not as close.

Train your whiskers. Does your beard grow in eleventy-four different directions? Dr. Litt advises you to "train it to grow out straight." Do this by shaving in two directions: down on the face, and up on the neck (to prevent neck nicks). Don't shave in all kinds of different directions or back and forth. "You won't get as great a shave at first," he says, "but if you keep shaving down on the face and up on the neck, your beard should start growing out straight in a matter of months."

Try the aftershave special. "It's a good idea to put a damp towel on your face for a few minutes after shaving," Dr. Basler says. "It softens the whiskers so they're less able to repenetrate the skin." Use a creamy aftershave lotion, not the typical alcohol-loaded aftershave splash. "It's soothing and keeps the hair moisturized," he says.

Fight infection. If, despite your best efforts, a whisker does manage to burrow inside, you can cut down on the amount of bacteria it carries with it. A 10 percent benzoyl peroxide solution has some antibiotic effect, Dr. Basler says, "and probably will help if used as an aftershave." Typical aftershaves contain lots of alcohol and may also help decrease the bacterial load.

Ladies, shave down instead of up. "Women typically shave their legs up from ankle to knee," Dr. Litt says. This is against the grain and can cause ingrown hairs. Instead, shave down, from knee to ankle.

PANEL OF ADVISERS

Rodney Basler, M.D., is a dermatologist and assistant professor of internal medicine at the University of Nebraska College of Medicine in Lincoln.

Jerome Z. Litt, M.D., is a dermatologist in private practice in Beachwood, Ohio, and is author of *Your Skin: From Acne to Zits.*

Ingrown Nails

7 Treatment Methods

If you have an ingrown nail, you *know* how it feels—sort of like an elephant stomped on your toe and then a lobster grabbed hold of it—for keeps. The problem occurs when a nail—usually on the big toe—grows or is pushed into the soft tissue alongside it. People whose toenails are somewhat convex are more susceptible, but literally anyone can fall victim.

Watch What You're Doing!

While ingrown nails come mostly from improper cutting, says Frederick Hass, M.D., they can also result from any number of accidents. Stubbing your toe at home can be just as much at fault as dropping a heavy object on your foot at work.

"I'd recommend stout, comfortable shoes for housework," he says. "If you constantly handle heavy objects such as machinery and crates at work, I'd definitely advise work shoes with steel toe boxes. They can protect your toes in all but the most serious accidents."

And at this point you couldn't care less how the situation developed; you want to know how to wrest yourself free of it. Although your long-term goal is to prevent a return engagement, your immediate aim is to soothe the pain. Here's how to accomplish both.

Try an OTC. There are a variety of nonprescription over-the-counter products that may soften the nail and the skin around it, thereby relieving pain, says Suzanne M. Levine, D.P.M., clinical assistant podiatrist at Mount Sinai Hospital in New York City. Dr. Scholl's Ingrown Toenail Reliever and Outgro Solution are two that have helped some people. But make sure you follow directions to the letter. And *don't* use them if you have diabetes or impaired circulation.

Get a wisp of relief. Your mission is to help that embedded toenail grow out over the skin folds at its side. Start by soaking your foot in warm water to soften the nail, says California practitioner Frederick Hass, M.D., author of *The Foot Book* and a staff member of Marin General Hospital in Greenbrae. Dry carefully, then gently insert a *wisp* (not a wad) of sterile cotton beneath the burrowing edge of the nail. The cotton will slightly lift the nail so it can grow past the tissue it is digging into. Apply an antiseptic as a safeguard against infection. Change the cotton insert daily until the nail has grown past the trouble spot.

V is *not* for victory. Whatever you do, says podiatrist Glenn Copeland, D.P.M., of Women's College Hospital in Toronto, don't fall for that old wives' tale about cutting a V-shaped wedge out of the center of the nail. "People think that an ingrown nail is too big and that if you take a wedge from the middle, the sides will grow toward the center and away from the ingrown edge. That's utter nonsense. All nails grow from back to front only."

Let your toes breathe. Simply put, ill-fitting footwear can cause an ingrown nail, especially if your nails tend to curve. That's why you should avoid pointed or tight shoes that press on toenails, says Dr. Levine. Opt instead for sandals where appropriate, or wide-toed shoes. If necessary, she says, modify offending shoes by cutting out the portion that presses on your toe. That may seem a little drastic, but a badly ingrown nail will put you in a drastic mood. Likewise, stay away from tight socks and panty hose.

Cut nails with precision. Never cut your nails too short, says Dr. Hass. Soften them first in warm water to reduce possible splitting, then cut straight across with a substantial, sharp, straight-edged clipper. Never cut a nail in an oval shape so that the leading edge curves down into the skin at the sides. Always leave the outside edges parallel to the skin. And don't trim the nail any deeper than the tip of the toe; you want it long enough to protect the toe from pressure and friction.

Fix mistakes properly. If you accidentally cut or break a nail too short, carefully smooth it at the edges so that no sharp points are left to penetrate the skin, says Dr. Hass. Do the smoothing with an emery

---

MEDICAL ALERT

Beware of an Infection

If your toe becomes infected, says Suzanne M. Levine, D.P.M., you should definitely see a physician. To reduce inflammation until your appointment, periodically soak your foot in an iodine solution, then apply an antibiotic cream.

"If you let an ingrown nail become seriously infected," she cautions, "you can end up in big trouble. Several patients have come to me only after their toes became red and swollen with pus. If your circulation is poor, you run the risk of gangrene. Sometimes a bloody growth, called proud flesh, builds up on the side of the nail. This inflamed soft tissue can become quite sensitive when it extends into the nail groove."

board or a nail file. "Don't be tempted to use scissors, no matter how small they are. There is simply not enough space for you to work them properly, and they often leave a sharp edge."

PANEL OF ADVISERS

Glenn Copeland, D.P.M., is a podiatrist with a private practice at Toronto's Women's College Hospital. He is also consulting podiatrist for the Canadian Back Institute, podiatrist for the Toronto Blue Jays baseball team, and author of *The Foot Doctor.*

Frederick Hass, M.D., is a general practitioner in San Rafael, California. He is on the staff of Marin General Hospital in Greenbrae. He is the author of *The Foot Book* and *What You Can Do about Your Headaches.*

Suzanne M. Levine, D.P.M., is a podiatrist in private practice and clinical assistant podiatrist at Mount Sinai Hospital in New York City. She is author of *My Feet Are Killing Me* and *Walk It Off.*

Insomnia

19 Steps to a Good Night's Sleep

It's been a long day that has left you dead tired, downright bushed. Yet it's happening again. You lie in bed, wide awake in the middle of the night. You hit the hay 3 hours ago, but try as you might, there's no way you can catch the dreamland express.

Your mind is racing a mile a minute, but the alarm clock next to the bed keeps ticking—ticking—ticking, and the minutes pass by like hours. You'd do anything for a good night's sleep—and so would millions of others.

Insomnia ranks right behind the common cold, stomach disorders, and headaches as a reason why people seek a doctor's help. In a Gallup poll of more than 1,000 adults, one-third of them complained that they woke up in the middle of the night and couldn't get back to sleep.

MEDICAL ALERT

Some Insomniacs Need Help

Serious sleeping troubles sometimes can result in what experts call chronic insomnia, which could have profound underpinnings, such as psychiatric disturbance, breathing problems, or unexplained leg movements during the middle of the night. Experts agree that if you can't easily fall asleep or stay asleep throughout the night for a month or so at a time, it may be time to consult an expert.

According to the American Sleep Disorders Association, you should first explain your problems to your personal physician. If your doctor can't offer any advice, have him or her recommend a sleep-disorders specialist.

At one time, doctors might have automatically prescribed a pill or two to ease you into the arms of Morpheus, but that isn't always the case today. Researchers and doctors are learning more about sleep each year, and that has broadened their knowledge of how to deal with its related problems.

Indeed, there are quite a few commonsense approaches you can use to try to correct the problem yourself. It may take just one therapy; it may take a combination. In any case, the key to success is discipline. As Michael Stevenson, Ph.D., psychologist and clinical director of the North Valley Sleep Disorders Center in Mission Hills, California, says, "Sleep is a natural physiological phenomenon, but it's also a learned behavior."

Set a rigid sleep schedule seven days a week. "Sleep is an unavoidable interval in the 24-hour day," says Merrill M. Mitler, Ph.D., director of research for the Division of Chest, Critical Care and Sleep Medicine at the Scripps Clinic and Research Foundation in La Jolla, California. "We insist on people trying to be as regular with their habits as possible."

The key is to get enough sleep so you can make it through your day without drowsiness. To help achieve that goal, try to get to bed at the same time each night so you can set your system's circadian rhythm, the so-called body clock that regulates most internal functions. Just as important is arising at the same time each morning.

Set a sleeping time of, say, 1:00 to 6:00 A.M. If you're sleeping soundly through that 5-hour period, add 15 minutes each week until you get aroused in the middle of the night. Work on getting through that arousal before adding another 15 minutes. You'll know when you reach the point where you've had enough sleep — you'll wake up refreshed, energetic, and ready to take on the day.

If you wake up during the night and can't get back to sleep in 15 minutes, don't fight it, says Dr. Mitler. Stay in bed and listen to the radio until you're drowsy again.

Again, be sure to wake up at the appointed hour in the morning; don't *sleep in* trying to pick up on "lost" sleep. That goes for the weekends as well. Don't sleep late on Saturday and Sunday mornings. If you do, you may have trouble falling asleep Sunday night, which can leave you feeling washed out on Monday morning.

Don't waste your time in bed. As you grow older, your body needs less sleep. Most newborn babies sleep up to 18 hours a day. By the time they're 10 years old, that usually drops to 9 or 10 hours.

Experts agree that there is no "normal" amount of sleep for an adult. The average is from 7 to 8 hours, but some people operate well on as few as 5 hours; others need up to 10 hours. The key is to become what experts call an efficient sleeper.

Go to bed only when you're sleepy, advises Edward Stepanski, Ph.D., director of the Insomnia Clinic at the Henry Ford Hospital's Sleep Disorders and Research Center in Detroit, Michigan. If you can't fall asleep in 15 minutes or so, get up and do something pleasantly monotonous. Read a magazine article, not a book that may engross you. Knit, watch television, or balance the checkbook. Don't play computer games that can excite you or perform goal-oriented tasks such as the laundry or housework.

When you feel drowsy, go back to bed. If you can't fall asleep, repeat the procedure until you can. But remember: Always wake up at the same time in the morning.

Set aside some "quiet time" before bed. "Some people are so busy that when they lie down to go to sleep, it's the first time all day that they've had the chance to think about what happened that day," says psychiatrist David Neubauer, M.D., of the Johns Hopkins University Sleep Disorders Center at the Francis Scott Key Medical Center in Baltimore, Maryland.

An hour or two before going to bed, sit down for at least 10 minutes or so. Reflect on the day's activities and try to put them into some perspective. Review your stresses and strains, as well as your problems. Try to work out solutions. Plan tomorrow's activities.

This exercise will help clear your mind of the annoyances and problems that might keep you awake once you pull up the covers. With all that out of the way, you'll be able to program your mind with pleasant thoughts and images as you try to drift off to sleep. If, for some reason, cold reality begins to seep into your conscience, shut it out by saying, "Oh, I've already dealt with that and I know what I'm going to do about it."

Don't turn your bed into an office or a den. "If you want to go to bed, you should be prepared to sleep," says Magdi Soliman, Ph.D., a professor of neuropharmacology at Florida A&M University College of Pharmacy. "If there's something else to do, you won't be able to concentrate on sleep."

The Alternate Route

Light Up Your Life

Researchers at the National Institute of Mental Health (NIMH) are using bright lights in the morning to help chronically poor sleepers set their circadian rhythms, or "body clocks," on a more regular pattern.

According to Jean R. Joseph-Vanderpool, M.D., a psychiatrist in the NIMH's clinical psychobiology branch, many people suffer from what he calls delayed sleep phase syndrome. In plainer terms, they just can't get started in the morning.

That's why when they get up, say around 8:00 A.M., they're being placed in front of high-intensity, full-spectrum fluorescent lights for 2 hours— strong light that resembles what someone would encounter on a summer morning in Washington, D.C. Those lights, in turn, tell the body that it's morning and that it's time to get moving. Then, in the evening, they wear dark glasses so that the body knows it's time to begin to wind down.

So far, Dr. Joseph-Vanderpool has gotten good results from his patients, who report more alertness in the morning and better sleep at night after several weeks of the therapy.

At home, he says the same effect can be accomplished by walking around the neighborhood, sitting in the sun, or doing some yardwork as soon as you arise. During the winter, it might be worth consulting your doctor about the best type of artificial light to use.

Don't watch TV, talk on the phone, argue with your spouse, read, eat, or perform mundane tasks in bed. Use your bedroom only for sleep and sex.

Avoid stimulants after twilight. Coffee, colas, and even chocolate contain caffeine, the powerful stimulant that can keep you up, so try not to consume them past 4:00 P.M., says Dr. Mitler. Don't smoke either; nicotine is a stimulant, too.

Say no to the nightcap. Avoid alcohol at dinner and through-out the rest of the evening, suggests Dr. Stevenson. And don't fix a so-called nightcap to relax you before bed. Alcohol does depress the central nervous system, but it also will disrupt your sleep. In a few hours, usually during the middle of the night, its effects will wear off, your body will slide into withdrawal, and you'll wake up.

Question your medication. Certain medications, such as asthma sprays can disrupt sleep. If you take prescription medication routinely, ask your doctor about the side effects. If he suspects the drug could be interfering with your sleep, he may be able to substitute another medication or adjust the time of day you take it.

Examine your work schedule. Research has shown that people who work on "swing" shifts—irregular schedules that frequently alternate from day to night—have problems sleeping, says Mortimer Mamelak, M.D., director of the sleep laboratory at Sunnybrook Hospital, University of Toronto Clinic. The stress of an up-and-down schedule may create jet lag–like tiredness all the time, and sleep mechanisms can break down altogether. The solution: Try to get a steady shift, even if it's at night.

Eat a light snack before bedtime. Bread and fruit will do nicely an hour or two before you hit the hay, says Sonia Ancoli-Israel, Ph.D., a psychologist and associate adjunct professor of psychiatry at the University of California, San Diego, School of Medicine. So will a glass of warm milk. Avoid sugary snacks that can excite your system or heavy meals that can stress your body.

A caution: If you're older, don't drink a lot of fluids before bed; you might wake up later in the night when bathroom duty calls.

Create a comfortable sleep setting. "Insomnia can often be caused by stress," says Dr. Stevenson. "You get into bed and you're nervous and anxious and the nervous system is aroused and that impairs your ability to sleep. Soon, the bedroom becomes associated with sleeplessness, and that triggers a phobic response."

You can help change that by making the bedroom as comfortable a setting as possible. Redecorate with your favorite colors. Soundproof the room and hang dark curtains to keep out the light.

Buy a comfortable bed. It doesn't matter whether it's a coiled-spring mattress, a waterbed, a vibrating bed, or a mat on the floor. If it feels good, use it. Wear loose-fitting sleeping clothes. Make sure the bedroom's temperature is just right—not too hot, not too cold. Be sure there's no clock within view that can distract you throughout the night.

Turn off your mind. Keep yourself from rehashing a stressful day of worries by focusing your thoughts on something peaceful and nonthreatening, says Dr. Stevenson. Play some soft, soothing music as you drift off, or some environmental noise, such as the sound of a waterfall, waves crashing on a beach, or the sound of rain in a jungle. The only rule: Be sure that it's not intrusive and distracting.

Use mechanical aids. Earplugs can help block out unwanted noise, especially if you live on a busy street or near an airport, says Dr. Ancoli-Israel. Eyeshades will screen out unwanted light. An electric blanket can help warm you, especially if you're a person who always seems to be on the brink of a chill.

Learn and practice relaxation techniques. The harder you try to sleep, the greater the chances are that you'll end up gnashing your teeth all night rather than stacking some zs. That's why it is important to relax once you're in bed.

"The one problem with insomnia is that people often concentrate too much on their sleep, and they press too hard," Dr. Stevenson says. "The key to successfully falling asleep is to reduce your focus and avoid working yourself into a frenzy."

Biofeedback exercises, deep breathing, muscle stretches, or yoga may help. Special audiotapes can teach you how to progressively relax your muscles.

It may not come easy at first, but as Dr. Neubauer says, "It's like dieting; you must work on it all the time. It will take time to get results, but if you stick with it, it will pay off."

Here are two techniques doctors have found particularly successful.

- Slow down your breathing and imagine the air moving slowly in and out of your body while you breathe from your diaphragm. Practice this during the day so it's easy to do before you go to bed.
- Program yourself to turn off unpleasant thoughts as they creep into your mind. To do that, think about enjoyable experiences that you've had. Reminisce about good times, fantasize, or play some mental games. Try counting sheep or counting backward from 1,000 by 7s.

Take a hike. Get some exercise late in the afternoon or early in the evening, suggest Dr. Neubauer and Dr. Soliman. It shouldn't be too strenuous—a walk around the block will do just fine. Not only will it fatigue your muscles, but it will raise your body temperature. When that begins to fall, it may help induce sleepiness. Exercise also may help trigger the deep, nourishing sleep that the body craves the most for replenishment.

Try sex before bedtime. For many, it's a pleasurable and mentally and physically relaxing way to let loose before settling down to sleep. Indeed some researchers have found that hormonal mechanisms triggered during sexual activity help enhance sleep.

But again, it depends on the person, according to James K. Walsh, Ph.D., a clinical polysomnographer who runs the Sleep Disorders Center at Deaconess Hospital in St. Louis, Missouri.

"If sex causes anxiety and creates problems, it's not such a good idea," he says. "But if you find it enjoyable, it can do a lot for you."

Take a warm bath. One theory held by sleep experts has it that normal body temperatures play off the body's circadian rhythm. Those temperatures are low during sleep and at their highest point during the day.

Along those lines, it's thought that the body begins to get drowsy as its temperature drops. Therefore, a warm bath taken about 4 or 5 hours before bedtime will raise that temperature. Then, as it begins to fall, you'll feel more tired, which will make it easier to fall asleep.

PANEL OF ADVISERS

Sonia Ancoli-Israel, Ph.D., is a psychologist and an associate adjunct professor in the Department of Psychiatry at the University of California, San Diego, School of Medicine.

Jean R. Joseph-Vanderpool, M.D., is a psychiatrist in the clinical psychobiology branch at the National Institute of Mental Health in Bethesda, Maryland.

Mortimer Mamelak, M.D., is director of the sleep laboratory at the Sunnybrook Hospital, University of Toronto Clinic. He is also the author of the booklet *Insomnia*.

Merrill M. Mitler, Ph.D., is the director of research for the Division of Chest, Critical Care and Sleep Medicine at the Scripps Clinic and Research Foundation in La Jolla, California. He is also clinical professor of psychiatry at the University of California, San Diego.

David Neubauer, M.D., is a general psychiatrist in the Johns Hopkins University Department of Psychiatry in Baltimore, Maryland. He's also associated with the Johns Hopkins University Sleep Disorders Center at the Francis Scott Key Medical Center in Baltimore.

Magdi Soliman, Ph.D., is a professor of neuropharmacology at Florida A&M University College of Pharmacy in Tallahassee, Florida.

Edward Stepanski, Ph.D., is the director of the Insomnia Clinic at Henry Ford Hospital's Sleep Disorders and Research Center in Detroit, Michigan.

Michael Stevenson, Ph.D., is a psychologist and clinical director of the North Valley Sleep Disorders Center in Mission Hills, California.

James K. Walsh, Ph.D., is a clinical polysomnographer accredited by the American Sleep Disorders Association. He is also director of the Sleep Disorders Center at Deaconess Hospital in St. Louis, Missouri.

Intermittent Claudication

8 Ways to Ease the Pain

Intermittent claudication, a chronic pain experienced in the calf when walking, afflicts more than one million people over the age of 50 in the United States every year. Though a painful and serious condition in its own right, intermittent claudication is really the *symptom* of a larger, more serious problem — peripheral vascular disease.

Just as clogged blood vessels in the heart lead to angina (chest pains), intermittent claudication signals the onset of restricted blood flow in the "periphery," that is, the area furthermost from the heart — the arms and legs.

"We're talking about the symptom phase of arterial disease," says Jess R. Young, M.D., chairman of the Department of Vascular Medicine at the Cleveland Clinic Foundation in Ohio. "If you get arterial disease in the heart, you get angina and heart attacks. If you get it in the head circulation, you get strokes. Intermittent claudication's the same process, but in the legs and arms."

For that reason, intermittent claudication should not be taken lightly. If you've been diagnosed as having this condition, you should continue seeing your doctor so he can monitor the underlying disease that has resulted in the pain you now feel in your legs. The pain, after all, is only a symptom. The real disease is a killer.

On the up side, there are a number of things you can do at home to rid yourself of claudication's pain and help slow the progression of peripheral vascular disease.

Stop smoking. "The number one thing on everyone's list with this affliction should be to stop smoking," says Dr. Young. "About 75 to 90 percent of all claudicators are smokers."

Stopping smoking is so important, in fact, that our experts say you must quit before any other remedy listed below will work. Is it worth it? Consider the following: Cigarette smoking increases the damage the disease can do by substituting carbon monoxide for oxygen in the already oxygen-starved muscles of your legs. Nicotine also causes constriction of the arteries, which further restricts blood flow, possibly damaging the arteries themselves and leading to blood clots. Such clots can result in gangrene and make amputation necessary.

"Stopping smoking is the most important thing, period," notes Robert Ginsburg, M.D., director of the Center for Interventional Vascular Therapy at Stanford University Hospital in California.

Start walking. "Next to stopping smoking, exercise is most important," says Dr. Young. The type of exercise he's talking about, and the type our experts overwhelmingly recommend, is the simplest of all—walking.

"Get out every day for at least an hour of walking exercise," says Dr. Young. "You can break that up any way you want, but you have to bring on the discomfort of intermittent claudication to have the walking do any good." Walk until you bring on the pain, he says, but don't stop at the first sign of pain. "Wait until it gets moderately severe. Then stop and rest a minute or two until it goes away, then start up walking again." Repeat that pain/walk cycle as often as you can during your 60 minutes of daily walking.

Be warned, however, that improvement won't happen overnight. "It will be two or three months, minimum, before you see results," says Dr. Young. So don't get discouraged.

Don't let foul weather stop you. "Walking is the best *singular* exercise," says Dr. Ginsburg, "but bicycling on a stationary bike can also help if it works the calves." In fact, any indoor exercise that works the calves enough to bring on the pain of claudication can help. Some exercises to try include toe raises, stair climbing, running in place, jumping rope, and dancing (get your doctor's okay before trying these more strenuous exercises.)

"Indoor exercises are better than trudging out through a foot of snow in the middle of winter and getting the feet wet," Dr. Ginsburg notes. But, he adds, walking is still the best exercise whenever weather permits.

Take care of your feet. "Anytime there's a break in the skin on the feet, you have to be on guard that it heals up in short order," says Michael D. Dake, M.D., a vascular specialist at the Miami Vascular Insti-

---

MEDICAL ALERT

The Danger of Infection

Chronic foot problems that get infected are a leading cause of amputation in people who suffer with intermittent claudication. If you have a cut, scrape, blister, or other foot problem that develops the redness, swelling, heat, and pain of infection, seek immediate medical help.

---

tute in Florida. "Nonhealing foot problems that get infected are probably the leading cause of amputation."

Foot problems that are minor inconveniences for people with healthy circulation can become major infections for those with impaired blood flow to the limbs.

Many problems can be avoided, however, with proper care of the toenails, treatment of athlete's foot, and avoidance of extremely hot or cold temperatures. The feet should be carefully inspected every day, and you should get prompt medical attention for any signs of injury or infection.

Take a load off. Obesity can be a major problem for those with claudication, not only because of the strain it places on circulation, but because of the damage it inflicts on the feet.

"You're traumatizing tissue in the feet that just doesn't have a good enough blood supply to take that abuse and heal," notes Dr. Young.

Avoid heating pads. Because of the restricted blood flow in the legs, people who suffer from intermittent claudication often suffer from cold feet, too. But regardless of how cold your feet may be, they should never be warmed with a heating pad or hot-water bottle. "You need increased blood flow to help dissipate that heat," Dr. Young explains. "If the blood flow is limited, however, it can't get down to where you're putting the heat and you'll burn the skin." Try loose wool stockings to warm your feet instead.

Know your blood pressure and cholesterol level. "If you suffer with intermittent claudication, you should also be checked for hypertension and hyperlipidemia," says Dr. Young. "These are important risk factors that tend to markedly increase the severity of the underlying disease, and it's very important to keep both of those conditions tightly controlled."

Get to know your cardiologist. "If you have intermittent claudication and haven't seen a cardiologist," warns Dr. Ginsburg, "make an appointment to see one." The reason for that warning becomes apparent when you examine the statistics. The incidence of coronary artery disease in people with peripheral vascular disease is about 75 to 80 percent. Intermittent claudication is a symptom of peripheral vascular disease.

"If a person comes in and has symptoms of a lack of blood flow in the legs," Dr. Ginsburg says, "there's a strong possibility that he or she already has blockages in the heart, or in the carotid arteries going to the brain. So it's very important that this person be evaluated not only for problems with the vessels, but with the organs those vessels are feeding."

PANEL OF ADVISERS

Michael D. Dake, M.D., is a vascular specialist at the Miami Vascular Institute in Florida.

Robert Ginsburg, M.D., is director of the Center for Interventional Vascular Therapy at Stanford University Hospital in California.

Jess R. Young, M.D., is chairman of the Department of Vascular Medicine at the Cleveland Clinic Foundation in Ohio.

Irritable Bowel Syndrome

22 Coping Suggestions

Just as some people are the grumpy and irritable type, so, too, are some bowels. What exactly does it mean to have an irritable bowel? It means that certain foods and drinks and stressful events in your life— things that don't normally wreak havoc on other people —give you alternating bouts of diarrhea, constipation, and abdominal pain. Sometimes, you get all three at the same time.

Some doctors think that irritable bowel syndrome (also known as spastic colon) may be second only to the common cold as America's most widespread medical complaint. And your doctor now says that irritable bowel syndrome (IBS) is the source of *your* complaint. Well, rest assured that there are lots of things you can do to take the irritability out of your bowel.

Take the news in stride. "There's a very good connection between stress and an irritable bowel," says Douglas A. Drossman, M.D., a gastroenterologist and psychiatrist at the University of North Carolina at Chapel Hill School of Medicine. What you don't want to do is get stressed *because* you have an irritable bowel, and thereby create a "vicious cycle," he says. Especially during flare-ups of abdominal pain, it is important to "take a deep breath. Think about what's happening. Recognize that it's happened before and it will pass. Know that you're *not* going to die—because people don't die from an irritable bowel," he says.

Become a more relaxed person. Anything you can do to help yourself unwind should help to alleviate your symptoms, says Dr. Drossman. You may benefit from relaxation techniques, such as meditation,

The Alternate Route

See Yourself Pain-Free

Remember the last time your irritable bowel gave you an attack of abdominal pain? You panicked. You got all stressed up inside. Didn't you? And—ironically—by getting stressed, you tensed your bowel, and probably helped to bring on more pain.

How can you break this nasty cycle?

With visualization, says Donna Copeland, Ph.D., a clinical psychologist and president of the American Psychological Association's Division of Psychological Hypnosis. It's "a very effective tool for dealing with pain and anxiety." Learning visualization techniques with a professional is probably the best route. But there's nothing wrong with trying a few on your own.

Dr. Copeland suggests the following: If you feel pain, stop what you're doing, find a comfortable place to sit or lie down, close your eyes, and—instead of focusing on your pain—see yourself instead:

- Diving expertly into the warm ocean surf off a beautiful, white-sanded, tropical island beach.
- Standing atop a tall, snow-crested mountain, breathing the cool air, and listening to the crunch of snow under your feet.
- Sitting in a large wooden hot tub, chatting idly with several of your closest friends.
- Walking through a lush garden in a far-off, exotic land.

self-hypnosis, or biofeedback. If the stress in your life is particularly problematic, you may want to consider psychological counseling. The key is to find what works for you.

Keep a stress diary. Persons with an irritable bowel have an intestinal system that overreacts to food, stress, and hormonal changes. "Think of your irritable bowel as a built-in barometer, and use it to help you determine what things in your life are most stressful," says Dr. Drossman. If, for instance, you have stomach pain every time you talk to your boss, see it as a sign that you need to work on that relationship (perhaps by talking it over with your boss, a friend or family member, or a therapist).

Log in your food and beverage intake, too. Certain foods and beverages, just like stress, can activate an irritable bowel, so it's also helpful to record in your diary the foods and beverages that give you the most trouble, says Dr. Drossman. Although there are some things that are likely to disturb most people, everyone is different.

Add fiber to your diet. Many people with IBS do much better simply by adding fiber to their diets, says James B. Rhodes, M.D., a professor of medicine with the Division of Gastroenterology at the University of Kansas Medical Center in Kansas City. Fiber tends to be most effective with people who tend toward constipation and small, hard stools, but it may also help you if you're suffering from diarrhea. The best fiber to add to your diet is the nonsoluble type—found in bran, whole grains, fruit, and vegetables.

Call psyllium seed to the rescue. An easy way to increase your fiber intake is with crushed psyllium seed, says Dr. Drossman. It's a natural laxative sold in pharmacies, supermarkets, and health food stores. Unlike chemical laxatives often found on the same shelves, psyllium-based laxatives such as Metamucil are nonaddictive and generally safe, even when taken over long periods.

Drink lots of fluid. To keep your bowels moving smoothly, you need not only fiber, but fluids as well. You'll need more on August days spent playing tennis than on December days spent at the movies, but in general, "you should drink between six and eight glasses of fluid a day," says Dr. Rhodes.

Reconsider dairy products. One fluid you may do better without is milk. "A large number of people who say they have IBS are really lactose intolerant," says William J. Snape, Jr., M.D., a professor of medicine, chief of the Gastroenterology Unit, and director of the Inflammatory Bowel Disease Center at the Harbor-UCLA Medical Center in Torrance, California. It means your body has difficulty absorbing lactose, an enzyme found in milk. Your doctor can test you for lactose intolerance, or you can give up dairy products for a couple of days and see how you do. In either case, you may find this one dietary change can clear up all your problems. (For more on lactose intolerance, see page 407.)

Cut out the fat. There are lots of good reasons to eat a low-fat diet—and now you have one more. "Fat is a major stimulus to colonic contractions," says Dr. Snape. In other words, it can worsen your IBS. A good place to begin to cut fat out of your diet is by eliminating heavy sauces, fried foods, and salad oils, says Dr. Snape.

Pass on the gas. Some people with IBS are particularly sensitive to gas-producing foods, says Dr. Rhodes. If you fall into this group, you may find relief by avoiding such flatulence champs as beans, cabbage, brussels sprouts, broccoli, cauliflower, and onions.

Go easy on the bran. If you are adding fiber such as bran to your diet, add it slowly to give your body time to adjust. Too much fiber, too fast, can produce gas, says Dr. Rhodes.

Beware of spicy foods. Some people with IBS are sensitive to foods laden with peppers and other spices, says Dr. Rhodes. Try eating a lot of spicy foods for one week and a lot of bland foods the next week, and note if your condition changes, he suggests.

Be careful of acids. Acidic foods tend to bother some people with IBS, says Dr. Rhodes. Here again, you may wish to experiment by laying off such things as oranges, grapefruits, tomatoes, and vinegary salad dressings for a while, to see if things get better.

Don't brew trouble with coffee. Coffee is a major cause of woes among people with IBS, says Dr. Snape. To some extent, the culprit may be caffeine, but it may also be the resins in the coffee bean itself. You may get some relief if you switch to decaffeinated—if not, try cutting down on all coffee.

Know that some alcoholic beverages are worse than others. Alcoholic beverages can exacerbate your problems, but it's probably not the alcohol itself, says Dr. Snape. Rather, it's the complex carbohydrates in beer and the tannin in red wine that probably cause the most grief. Drinkers with IBS should order anything but these two drinks, he says.

Put out that cigarette. "A large number of people experience IBS problems with smoking," says Dr. Snape. The most probable culprit is the nicotine, so if you're trying to quit with the help of nicotine gum, you may not see any difference in your tummy problems.

Spit out the gum. Nicotine gum is not the only kind of gum that can give you troubles. Gums and candies artificially sweetened with sorbitol are not easily digested and can worsen your IBS, says Dr. Drossman.

While the amount of sorbitol found in one stick of gum or one hard candy isn't likely to affect you greatly, if you gobble up ten or more such sweeties a day, it's time to cut back.

Eat regular meals. It's not only *what* you eat, but *how* you eat that can vex an irritable bowel, says Dr. Snape. Digesting a lot of food eaten all at once overstimulates the digestive system. That is why it's much better to eat frequent smaller meals than infrequent larger ones.

Go for a jog. "Good body tone, good bowel tone," says Dr. Rhodes. Exercise strengthens the body (of which the bowel is a part). It helps relieve stress. And it releases endorphins that help you control pain. All in all, regular exercise will more than likely calm your irritable bowel. Be careful, however, not to overdo it. Too much exercise can lead to diarrhea.

Try a painkiller. Hormonal changes can sometimes pique an irritable bowel. For this reason, women often get attacks during their periods, says Dr. Drossman. Ibuprofen medications such as Advil or Panadol may help to inhibit some of the hormonal releases that are the root of the problem. For the rest of us, these pills can help with the pain.

Call a hot-water bottle to the rescue. If you're experiencing an attack of abdominal pain, the best thing to do is to sit or lie down, take a deep breath, and try to relax. Some people also find it helpful to put a hot-water bottle or a heating pad on the tummy, says Dr. Snape.

PANEL OF ADVISERS

Donna Copeland, Ph.D., is a clinical psychologist and president of the American Psychological Association's Division of Psychological Hypnosis. She is also an associate professor in pediatrics and director of the Mental Health Section at the University of Texas M. D. Anderson Cancer Center in Houston.

Douglas A. Drossman, M.D., is a gastroenterologist and a psychiatrist. He is an associate professor of medicine and psychiatry with the Division of Digestive Diseases and Nutrition at the University of North Carolina at Chapel Hill School of Medicine.

James B. Rhodes, M.D., is a professor of medicine with the Division of Gastroenterology at the University of Kansas Medical Center in Kansas City.

William J. Snape, Jr., M.D., is a professor of medicine, chief of the Gastroenterology Unit, and director of the Inflammatory Bowel Disease Center at the Harbor–UCLA Medical Center in Torrance, California.

Jet Lag

22 Hints for Arriving Alert

Just suppose that instead of setting the clock ahead 1 hour each spring for daylight saving time, we set it ahead *3* hours. What do you think would happen?

Besides creating "endless summer" nights, we would also create a nation of jet-lagged zombies. Adjusting our own inner body clocks isn't as easy as changing the time of the clock on the wall.

Yet when we fly across several time zones, we ask our bodies to adjust to a new time and a new place *right now.* It's a very unrealistic expectation. That's why we suffer jet lag. And the more time zones we cross, the more we suffer.

Typically, each time zone crossed requires about one day of adjustment, says Charles Ehret, Ph.D., author of *Overcoming Jet Lag* and president of General Chronobionics in Hinsdale, Illinois. (Chronobiology, by the way, is the study of time's effect on plants, animals, and people.)

The previously mentioned inner body clock, says Dr. Ehret, is really a whole set of clocks controlled by a master clock. "Every cell in the body is a clock," he explains, "and they're all brought together by a special pacemaker in the brain."

Normally our body clocks operate on cycles approximately 24 to 25 hours long. But rapid time changes disrupt all that. The result is jet lag—fatigue, lethargy, inability to sleep, trouble concentrating and making decisions, irritability, perhaps even diarrhea and a lack of appetite.

Hardly what you envisioned when you wrote out a big fat check to the travel agency for your dream vacation to Europe. But before you ground yourself and settle for that 29th annual driving vacation to the Grand Canyon, read on.

Though you can't make time stand still, there's a lot you *can* do to take some of the zap out of jet lag.

392 The Doctors Book of Home Remedies

Fight Jet Lag with Feast and Fast

The now-famous anti–jet lag diet developed by Charles Ehret, Ph.D., grew out of extensive animal research at the Argonne National Laboratory. In actuality, it is more than a diet. Daylight, social cues, sleeping patterns, and mental and physical exercise all play a role in making the diet work, Dr. Ehret says.

But the core of the plan involves a four-day sequence of feast-fast/feast-fast prior to the day of arrival. For these purposes, feast means to eat as much as you want and fast means to eat lightly.

Here are some sample menus for a fast day. Breakfast: two eggs, any style, and one-half piece of lightly buttered toast—214 calories. Lunch: one chicken breast, skin removed; 1 cup bouillon; ½ cup of low-fat pot cheese or cottage cheese—245 calories. Supper: one small bowl of pasta, lightly buttered with margarine; one piece of bread, lightly buttered; 1 cup cooked vegetables—broccoli, string beans, summer squash, or carrots; one alcoholic beverage (optional)—355 calories.

Caffeine is also a major part of the plan. Experiments with laboratory animals, Dr. Ehret says, have shown that caffeine can be used to reset body clocks.

Now let's examine some additional aspects of Dr. Ehret's plan as applied to a westward flight with a 3-hour time change, for example, a trip from New York to San Francisco in which you arrive in San Francisco at 8:30 A.M. local time.

Change your caffeine habits. Three days before the flight, stop consuming caffeine—except from 3:00 to 4:30 P.M. One day before the flight, caffeine is allowed only between 7:00 and 8:00 A.M. On the day of the flight, drink 2 to 3 cups of black coffee. But do this no later than 11:30 A.M. and have no more caffeine the rest of the day.

Set your watch to the new destination time. Start acclimating yourself to the time change; stay mentally active in the half-hour immediately preceding breakfast time at your destination.

Pass up breakfast with the passengers. Arrange to have breakfast at the breakfast time of your destination. In this situation, it would be soon before landing.

Eat a hearty lunch with the natives. You may arrive in San Francisco in the morning, but you should put off eating until lunchtime. But it's also a feast day, so enjoy.

Live on a schedule. Weeks, or at least days before you leave, you should be maintaining a sensible schedule. "People who have no order in their lives—who stay up late to watch a movie and start doing their laundry at 2:00 A.M.—have more trouble with jet lag," says Dr. Ehret. "Make sure your circadian rhythms [body clock cycles] are in sync."

Get enough sleep. Shortchange yourself on sleep before your trip, Dr. Ehret says, and you can just about count on making jet lag worse. "Give yourself about 15 extra minutes of sleep each of the last few nights before you travel."

Fly by day, arrive at night. "The best plan is to arrive at your destination in midevening, get something light to eat, and go to bed by 11:00 P.M. destination time," says Timothy Monk, Ph.D., an associate professor of psychiatry and director of the Human Chronobiology Research Program at the University of Pittsburgh School of Medicine.

This scenario, Dr. Monk says, gives your body optimal opportunity to adjust to the change in time zones.

Drink plenty of fluids during the flight. Airplane cabins are notoriously dry, Dr. Monk says, and fluids will help combat dehydration. Being dehydrated obviously won't help you beat jet lag.

Avoid alcohol. Ask for juice instead. Alcohol is a diuretic and will further dehydrate you.

Pretend you're not on a plane. Trans World Airlines flight attendant Jonie Nolan does this when she is not working and just traveling as a passenger. "I get a pillow and shut my eyes, but I don't go to sleep, and I pretend I'm not on the flight," she says. "I daydream—thinking pleasant, positive thoughts or just making plans for what I'm going to do next week."

She says she hasn't tried this on really long flights, but finds it effective for trips where she crosses two time zones.

Be quiet and relax. This is Nolan's strategy when she is flying coast-to-coast. Use the flight as an opportunity to enjoy solitude and get some relaxation. That way you aren't overstressed before asking your body to suddenly shift 3 hours.

Do as the Romans do. When you arrive, start adapting to your new environment as quickly as possible. "Get involved—notice the new street names and the language of the people," says Dr. Ehret. "This will help you to adjust."

Socialize. This is especially important if your body is craving sleep, but it's only midafternoon at your destination. "When we're socializing, our bodies assume it's daytime because human beings are, by nature, daytime creatures," says Marijo Readey, Ph.D., a researcher at the Argonne National Laboratory. "That's why many shift workers have symptoms like chronic jet lag."

Don't nap. Or if you do, limit the nap to 1 hour. Napping, Dr. Monk says, will just delay your adjustment to the new time zone.

Soak up some sunshine. "One school of thought, and the one I subscribe to, says get out in the sun at your destination as much as possible," says Dr. Monk. The theory, he adds, is that this exposure will help keep your biological clock in the stimulated and awake state during daylight hours at your destination.

"When light strikes the eye, neurotransmitters are released that send an immediate signal to specific regions of the brain," Dr. Ehret explains. "In turn, these brain regions signal the rest of the body that your awake-and-active phase is about to begin."

Make a date with the sun. Some experts feel the time of day you get out in the sunshine is also important. Light earlier in the day appears to shift the body's clock to an earlier hour, while light later in the day seems to shift the body's clock to a later hour, according to Al Lewy, M.D., Ph.D., a psychiatrist at the Oregon Health Sciences University School of Medicine.

So if you've traveled east, Dr. Lewy suggests getting outside light in the morning. And if you've traveled west, he recommends getting outside light in the afternoon. This only works, however, if you're crossing six or fewer time zones.

Exercise. "It makes sense," Dr. Monk says, "that if you usually go jogging, you should go jogging at your destination. It will get your body pumped up, help alertness, and get you out in the sunlight."

A study at the University of Toronto also suggests that exercise will actually reduce the number of days jet lag affects you. Researchers exposed golden hamsters (nocturnal animals with stable activity rhythms) to artificial light and advanced the onset of darkness 8 hours, simulating the conditions of a long flight east.

After darkness, one group of hamsters exercised on a running wheel. The other group mostly slept. While the nonrunning hamsters took 5.4 days to adjust and to resume normal nocturnal activity, the running hamsters adjusted in just 1.6 days.

The Alternate Route

How Three Famous Globe-Trotters Tried to Cope

Quick, what did Henry Kissinger, Dwight D. Eisenhower, and Lyndon Johnson all have in common?

Each had a personal strategy for trying to beat jet lag. In his book *Overcoming Jet Lag,* Charles Ehret, Ph.D., tells about each method. He also says that none of these methods are very reliable. But here they are, should you want to give them a try.

Take the diplomatic route. Several days before the flight, start going to bed 1 hour earlier and getting up 1 hour later. This was former Secretary of State Henry Kissinger's routine. The problem with this plan, Dr. Ehret says, is the rigidity it demands. Kissinger couldn't always follow it consistently, and most people would probably have the same problem. There's also no proof, Dr. Ehret adds, that this approach measurably reduces jet lag.

Arrive extra early. Former President Eisenhower tried to arrive several days ahead of time before meeting with foreign leaders. The problem with Eisenhower's plan, Dr. Ehret says, is that often he didn't arrive early enough to compensate for the one-time-zone-crossed-equals-one-day-of-adjustment rule.

Live by your home clock. After arriving at a new destination, former President Lyndon Johnson insisted on maintaining his old schedule—eating and sleeping at his usual time. He even arranged meetings at hours that were convenient by Washington, D.C., time, but not so convenient for the foreigners with whom he was meeting.

Perhaps you can get away with this if you're the president of the United States, Dr. Ehret says, but for the average traveler it may be hard to get dinner reservations for 2:00 A.M.—even in Paris.

Think before you react. Put off all important decision-making for 24 hours or at least until you feel well rested, advises Dr. Ehret. You will not be doing your clearest thinking after a long trip.

In business, he says, "People have made bad deals and later identified jet lag as the reason."

Reverse the process. If possible, use these tips to prepare for your return flight home, too. Jet lag is a two-way sky.

PANEL OF ADVISERS

Charles Ehret, Ph.D., is president of General Chronobionics in Hinsdale, Illinois, and author of *Overcoming Jet Lag*. He also is a retired senior scientist from the Argonne National Laboratory, a unit of the U.S. Department of Energy.

Al Lewy, M.D., Ph.D., is a psychiatrist at Oregon Health Sciences University School of Medicine in Portland. He has done studies on the effects of sunlight on the human body clock.

Timothy Monk, Ph.D., is an associate professor of psychiatry and director of the Human Chronobiology Research Program at the University of Pittsburgh School of Medicine in Pennsylvania.

Jonie Nolan has been a flight attendant for Trans World Airlines since 1981. She is based in St. Louis, Missouri.

Marijo Readey, Ph.D., is a researcher at the Argonne National Laboratory, a unit of the U.S. Department of Energy.

Kidney Stones

12 Lines of Defense

"I used to think I could bear any kind of pain; I used to have my teeth drilled without anesthetic—but when I had my kidney stone, I cried," says Major Norman Ellis, a retired Air Force officer living in Colorado Springs, Colorado.

If you have a kidney stone, you might be crying, too. Although doctors aren't always sure why some people form these little crystals of salt and minerals in their kidneys, one thing is crystal clear: They *hurt*.

The Alternate Route

What's This about Cranberry Juice?

Folklore has it that cranberry juice is good for kidney ailments, and even kidney stones. But is there any truth to it?

"I suppose the theory is that cranberries are acidic, so that drinking the juice will acidify your urine and discourage calcium stones from forming. But I doubt you could drink enough to make your urine acidic," says Peter D. Fugelso, M.D.

Is this to say that drinking cranberry juice will have no benefits whatsoever? Not exactly. "To the extent it's another source of fluid, I suppose it could be helpful," says Dr. Fugelso. But plain water, he adds, would serve the same purpose, with fewer calories.

For some people, it can take months of patience (and pain) to pass a stone. Hopefully, you won't be one of them. Doctors today have a number of strategies for ridding you of a stone. What doctors *can't* always do is guarantee that you won't get another.

"Once you've had one stone, you are at a somewhat higher risk of getting another. Once you've had a second stone, your risk is markedly increased," says Leroy Nyberg, M.D., director of the urology program at the National Institute of Diabetes and Digestive and Kidney Diseases at the National Institutes of Health.

Major Ellis suffered six kidney stones before his last, ten years ago. Since then, he's been taking prescription medication to help prevent their reappearance—and he's made several important changes in lifestyle.

Before *you* make any changes in *your* lifestyle, be aware that there are several kinds of kidney stones, and only your doctor can tell one from the other. Once your doctor is acquainted with your particular stone, the following tips will help reduce your chances of forming another.

Drink lots of fluids. Regardless of what kind of stone you've had, "by far the single most important preventive measure is to increase water consumption," says Stevan Streem, M.D., head of the Section of Stone Disease and Endourology at the Cleveland Clinic Foundation in Ohio. Water dilutes the urine and helps to prevent high concentrations of those salts and minerals that clump together to form stones.

How much fluid should you drink? "Enough to pass 2 quarts of urine a day," says Peter D. Fugelso, M.D., medical director of the Kidney Stone Department at St. Joseph's Medical Center in Burbank, California, and a clinical professor of urology at the University of Southern California in Los Angeles. "If you've been working out in the garden all day under the hot sun, that could mean you'll need to drink 2 gallons," he says. "It's the amount of *urine* that matters." He suggests you urinate several times into an empty milk carton to get a gauge on how much you are passing.

Keep a cap on your calcium. "Of all the stones we see, 92 percent are made of calcium or calcium products," says Dr. Fugelso. If your doctor says your last stone was calcium-based, you should be concerned about your intake of calcium. If you're taking supplements, the first thing to do is check with your doctor to see if they are really necessary. The next thing to do is check the amount of calcium-rich foods—milk, cheese, butter, and other dairy foods—you eat on a daily basis. The idea is to limit—not eliminate—calcium-rich food in your diet. "And almost all of the calcium in your diet comes from dairy products," says Dr. Fugelso.

Check your stomach medicine. Certain popular antacids are enormously high in calcium, warns Dr. Fugelso. If you've had a calcium stone, and if you are taking an antacid, check the ingredients on the side of the box to make sure it's not calcium-based. If it is, choose another brand.

Don't eat too many oxalate-rich foods. About 60 percent of all stones are known as calcium oxalate stones, says Brian L. G. Morgan, Ph.D., a research scientist with the Institute of Human Nutrition at Columbia University College of Physicians and Surgeons. If everything in your body were working right, the oxalate you consume when you eat certain fruits and vegetables would be excreted. But if you've had calcium oxalate stones, things obviously aren't working right. So you should restrict your consumption of oxalate-rich foods. These include beans, beets, blueberries, celery, chocolate, grapes, green peppers, parsley, spinach, strawberries, summer squash, and tea.

Try magnesium and B6. Swedish researchers found that a daily supplement of magnesium curtailed stone recurrence by almost 90 percent in a group of patients. Scientists speculate that magnesium works because it—like calcium—can bond with oxalate. But unlike the calcium/oxalate bond, this link-up is less likely to form painful stones. Vitamin B6, meanwhile, may actually lower the amount of oxalate in the urine. In one study, 10 milligrams a day seemed to do the trick.

MEDICAL ALERT

Three Good Reasons to See a Doctor

If you've had a kidney stone and are experiencing pain, chances are you may be getting another. You should see your doctor to be sure.

- Any intense pain and/or blood in your urine calls for a physician's assessment, says Peter D. Fugelso, M.D.
- If you pass a stone, you should take it to your doctor for laboratory analysis. "Finding out what kind of stone it is will help you to prevent future ones," says Leroy Nyberg, M.D.
- A doctor can look at your stone via an x-ray to see how large it is. "Large stones can create significant blockage and even infection," notes Stevan Streem, M.D. That's to say nothing of the pain. With shock wave therapy or other relatively noninvasive procedures, such as laser or ultrasound treatment, your doctor can see to it that you won't suffer. Medication can then be prescribed to prevent recurrences.

Eat vitamin A–rich foods. It doesn't matter which kind of stone you've had, vitamin A is necessary to keep the lining of the urinary tract in shape and help discourage the formation of future stones. "Be sure to get 5,000 international units—the Recommended Dietary Allowance [RDA] for healthy adults—of vitamin A daily," says Dr. Morgan. This is not particularly hard to do. One half cup of canned sweet potatoes, for instance, will give you 7,982 international units, and a similar portion of carrots will give you 10,055. Other foods high in vitamin A include apricots, broccoli, cantaloupes, pumpkins, winter squash, and beef liver. (Vitamin A supplements, however, should not be taken without your doctor's supervision. Vitamin A is toxic in large doses.)

Stay active. "People who are inactive tend to accumulate a lot of calcium in the bloodstream," says Dr. Nyberg. "Activity helps to pull calcium back into the bones, where it belongs." In other words, if you're prone to calcium stones, don't sit around all day and wait for them to form. Get out, take a walk, fly a kite, or ride a bike.

Watch your protein intake. "There is a direct correlation between the incidence of kidney stone disease and the amount of protein eaten," says Dr. Morgan. Protein tends to increase the presence of uric acid, calcium, and phosphorus in the urine, which, in some people, leads to the formation of stones, he says. Be concerned about consuming excessive protein if you've had calcium stones, and especially if you've had uric acid or cystine stones. Limit yourself to 6 ounces of protein-rich food a day, says Dr. Morgan. This includes meat, cheese, poultry, and fish.

Lay off the salt. If you've had calcium stones, it's time to cut down on salt. "You should reduce your salt intake to 2 to 3 grams per day," says Dr. Morgan. This means reducing your consumption of table salt, pickled foods, and salty foods such as luncheon meat, snack chips, and processed cheese.

Take a look at vitamin C. "If you tend to develop calcium oxalate stones, you should restrict your consumption of vitamin C," says Dr. Morgan. "Large amounts—more than 3 to 4 grams a day—can increase oxalate production and increase the risk of stones." It is highly unlikely that you could consume this much vitamin C in your diet (you would need to eat 37 navel oranges a day), so your concern here should be with high-potency supplements. His suggestion: Don't take them.

Don't get too much vitamin D. "Excessive amounts of vitamin D can lead to excess calcium in all parts of the body," says Dr. Morgan. "You should never get more than the RDA of 400 international units," he says.

PANEL OF ADVISERS

Peter D. Fugelso, M.D., is medical director of the Kidney Stone Department at St. Joseph's Medical Center in Burbank, California. He is also a clinical professor of urology at the University of Southern California in Los Angeles.

Brian L. G. Morgan, Ph.D., is a research scientist with the Institute of Human Nutrition at Columbia University College of Physicians and Surgeons in New York City.

Leroy Nyberg, M.D., is director of the urology program at the National Institute of Diabetes and Digestive and Kidney Diseases at the National Institutes of Health in Bethesda, Maryland.

Stevan Streem, M.D., is head of the Section of Stone Disease and Endourology at the Cleveland Clinic Foundation in Ohio.

Knee Pain

16 Ways to Handle the Hurt

Call it God's mistake. Of the 187 joints in your body, probably none brings about more suffering than the knee.

Now that America has become more active, the problem with knees has grown in response. An estimated 50 million people have suffered or are suffering knee pain or injury. But you don't have to be a fitness buff to know about that. One out of every three automobile injuries is an injury to the knee. Other hazardous activities or environments? Look around: climbing stairs, scrubbing floors, slippery sidewalks. The list seems endless.

Part of the problem is design, or rather the inability of knee design to change whenever human beings place new demands on it. "It is, without question, ill-suited for the jobs we ask it to do," says James M. Fox, M.D., director of the Center for the Disorders of the Knee in Van Nuys, California, and author of the book *Save Your Knees*. "It wasn't designed for football, soccer, automobile accidents, being a carpenter or plumber, or squatting and kneeling all day long. It was well designed originally, but there was no way to anticipate all the things we would end up asking it to do." If you're one of the countless felons of knee abuse, here are a few things you can do to make amends.

Take a load off. "Body weight is a major contributor to knee problems," says Dr. Fox. "For every pound you weigh, that's multiplied by about six in stress placed across the knee area." If you're 10 pounds overweight, that's an extra 60 pounds your knee has to carry around. And, as Dr. Fox says, "You don't put a Mack truck on Volkswagen tires."

Save the braces for teeth. Knee braces can be purchased at just about any sporting goods store, but the experts we spoke to say you should leave them on the shelf. "Some braces are truly meant to be preventive, but these are typically very complex and designed just for

---

MEDICAL ALERT

Accidents That Need a Doctor's Care

Yesterday you were out shooting some baskets or maybe playing some touch football when you made this sudden turn and heard a soft "pop." Soft popping sounds don't usually get you excited, but this one came from your knee. The next thing you knew, your hands were wrapped around that rascal and your eyes were filled with tears of pain.

Today you woke up with swelling, tenderness, radiating pain, and perhaps some discoloration and loss of motion.

What kind of damage could have occurred? Well, there are basically three common forms of destruction to choose from: torn cartilage, a torn ligament, or both.

What should you do about it? That's easy. Put it on ice and go to a doctor—today.

---

you; they can cost from $300 to $1,000," says Dr. Fox. "The wraps or braces you buy off the shelf at a sporting goods store shouldn't be used for anything more than to remind you that you have a bad knee."

Marjorie Albohm, a certified athletic trainer and associate director of the International Institute of Sports Science and Medicine at the Indiana University School of Medicine, is a bit more direct. "Forget knee braces or knee wraps you buy off the shelf," she says. "Some of them—by pushing your kneecap into the joint—can do more harm than good."

Try the rub that soothes. "Some wintergreen lotions produce heat, and heat can be a symptom reliever and make you feel more comfortable," says Dr. Fox. Sometimes, by covering the knee in plastic after applying the lotion and then wrapping it, you can make the liniment hotter. "But you need to be careful that you don't burn the skin or cause irritation," Dr. Fox warns. "But as far as being curative, lotions are not."

Reach for an OTC. Ibuprofen (Advil, Medipren, Nuprin, etc.) is the over-the-counter painkiller of choice recommended by our experts. It reduces inflammation and provides pain relief without causing the stomach problems associated with aspirin. Acetaminophen (Tylenol) is a fine painkiller and causes fewer stomach problems, but it does little to reduce inflammation.

Recent studies have also shown ibuprofen can significantly improve joint mobility in those people with acute knee ligament damage. When compared to either aspirin or acetaminophen, "ibuprofen may be the best of both worlds," Albohm concludes.

Strengthen with exercise. "The only things holding the knee together are the muscles and the ligaments," says Dr. Fox. "Building up the muscles is critical, because the muscles are the real supporting structures. If they don't have their power or endurance, you're going to be in trouble with your knees."

That means a certain amount of exercise for knee pain sufferers, even for those who detest it. Stronger muscles provide you with a stronger joint, one that's better able to withstand the considerable strain that even walking or stair climbing places on the knees. As Dr. Fox notes, "You've only got two knees, and the replacement parts that are out there are not that good." So let's get going. The following are not hard to do and hurt a lot less than aching knees.

Isometric knee builder. "The quadriceps and hamstrings are the muscles you need to build," says Dr. Fox. For the former (those thigh muscles in the front), here's one the doctor really recommends.

Sit on the floor with your sore knee straight out in front of you. Place a rolled towel under the small of the knee, then tighten the muscles in your leg without moving the knee. Hold that contraction and work up to where you can keep the muscles taut for at least 30 seconds, then relax. Repeat this tightening and relaxing process up to 25 times.

Sitting leg lifts. Here's the best way to do leg lifts for those who are weak of knee.

Sit with your back against a wall and place a pillow in the small of your back. (Sitting against a wall ensures that the leg muscles do the lifting, and this type of leg lift won't aggravate back pain.) Once you're in position, do the isometric contraction described above for a count of five, then raise your leg a few inches and hold it to a count of five, then lower it and relax for a count of five. Work up to doing three sets of ten lifts each, always using the five-count for pacing.

Hamstring helper. Not only do you have to build the quadriceps, but the hamstring muscles in back of the thighs must be developed for real knee strength. "They have to be in balance," says Dr. Fox. "If just one or the other is developed, then the joint is going to pick up stress."

To build the hamstrings, lie on your stomach with your chin to the floor. With an ankle weight (you can use a purse, or a sock filled with coins and draped over the ankle works fine) and your knee bent, slowly lift the lower leg 6 to 12 inches off the floor, then slowly lower it back down, stopping before you touch the floor. Repeat the movement again, always working slowly and steadily through each repetition. Work up to doing three sets of as many of these as you comfortably can (largely determined by the amount of weight you use).

A word of caution: "The most important thing to understand is that if an exercise causes increasing discomfort or pain, then stop," Dr. Fox advises. "You have to listen to your body and not simply assume that you need to 'work through the pain.' God gave you pain for a reason."

Try to modify. "If you're an athlete and you have a chronic knee problem, you're going to have to modify your level of training or daily activity," says Albohm. But that doesn't mean turning into a couch potato. "If you like racquetball and you've got this chronic knee condition that racquetball gradually made worse, you're probably going to have to get away from that," she says.

Options? Try swimming, biking, or rowing, all activities that are beneficial to health without placing great strain on the knees. The key phrase is "non-weight-bearing" activity. In fact, by helping to strengthen thigh muscles, such non-weight-bearing exercises as biking and rowing can give you better knees without sacrificing aerobic capacity or caloric burn.

Whatever you do, don't give up a healthy lifestyle because of knee pain. "No one should have to stop being active," Albohm says. "What you want to do is simply avoid anything that causes pain in that knee."

Change to a softer running surface. For the dedicated runner, first the bad news: "A lot of runner's pain is caused by tendinitis and results from poor training habits," says Dr. Fox. Now the good: "These are not significant mechanical problems," he says, "and they can usually be minimized by a change in the running shoe or running surface."

We'll deal with shoes in a minute, but for now let's talk running surface. Basically, it comes down to this: Run on grass before asphalt, run on asphalt before concrete. Concrete is the hardest surface of all and should be avoided like the plague. Don't make a habit of jogging on sidewalks, and if you can find a golf course to run on without getting beaned by a wayward duffer, do it. "Remember, when you run a mile, your foot is striking the ground between 600 and 800 times," Dr. Fox adds. Enough said.

Get enough RICE. "Following any activity that causes knee pain," Albohm says, "immediately rest the area and apply ice, compression, and elevation for 20 to 30 minutes." That advice is commonly called RICE, short for rest, ice, compression, and elevation. It's a handy acronym to remember—especially the I part.

"Don't underestimate the power of ice," says Albohm. "If you're conscientious, you might also want to ice later that evening, or the next morning when you get up. Ice is a tremendous anti-inflammatory and will really help the condition."

Keep your icing routine simple, she says. When you return from working out, just prop the leg up, wrap an Ace bandage around it, and plop the ice pack on for 20 to 30 minutes. "That should always be your first try at relieving pain."

Use heat with caution. When there is *no* swelling present, using a heating pad before an activity may let you exercise with less pain. "But," Albohm cautions, "if there's any swelling, or if you have any doubt that there might be swelling, don't use heat."

And, she says, don't use heat after an activity. "We're assuming the area is becoming irritated by activity, and heat is only going to increase any irritation that's there."

Update your shoes. "If your shoes can't take the shock anymore," says Gary M. Gordon, D.P.M., director of the running and jogging programs at the University of Pennsylvania Sports Medicine Center in Philadelphia, "well, that shock has to go someplace."

Where it goes is through your foot, up your shin, and into the knee. Sometimes it keeps on going, up to the hip and back as well.

"I tell runners that if they run 25 miles a week or more, they need new shoes every two to three months," Dr. Gordon says. "If they run less than that, they need new shoes every four to six months. Aerobic dancers and basketball and tennis players who work out twice a week can probably get by on new shoes every four to six months. If they're doing it up to four times or more a week, they also need new shoes every two months. Most people don't want to hear that."

Get into low gear. Many experts like bike riding, either stationary or freewheel, as an alternative to the knee strain and pain that can be caused by running. But biking is only a great way to stay in shape and take a load off your knees if you do it with caution. Cyclists also damage their knees, typically by thinking that the harder it is to pedal, the more exercise you get.

So, depending on the type of biking you do (steep hills are not advised), riding may still be too strenuous. Fast pedaling in gears that feel easy is what you want. "In general, a lower gear [easier to pedal] is a better gear," Albohm says.

Find the trigger point for pain. "There's a trigger point on the inside of the thigh that contributes to what's called weak knee syndrome," says Rich Phaigh, co-director of the American Institute of Sports Massage in New York City and the Institute of Clinical Biomechanics in Eugene, Oregon, and a masseur for the likes of running stars Alberto Salazar and Joan Samuelson. "That trigger point's responsible for a lot of generalized pain on the inside of the knee, too."

To get rid of that pain, move your hand straight up from the kneecap along the front of the thigh for about 3 inches, then move it inward for another 2 to 4 inches. Using the tip of your thumb, press in firmly and hold until you feel the muscle release its tension. "That can be anywhere from 30 to 90 seconds," Phaigh says. "Then release."

First and finally, stretch. Lisa Dobloug is a private fitness consultant based in Washington, D.C. Many of her clients are older individuals who have special needs when it comes to protecting their knees. Her emphasis is on the quality—not quantity—of exercise and the importance of stretching.

"It's very important to warm up and cool down properly," she says. "Take about 10 minutes and do very light stretching before. Not stretching to accomplish flexibility, just light stretching. Perhaps go through the motions of whatever exercise you'll be participating in without really extending it. Then do a little aerobics—jogging in place or walking around. After you're done working out, then you should really stretch. Try to counteract the pounding that the exercise put your knees through."

Here's one stretch that Dobloug likes for post-workout stiffness. "Lie down on your back and pull your knees into your chest, then start to straighten one leg," she says. "Act like you're trying to press your heel toward the ceiling." Hold the stretch for a count of ten, then relax. Repeat with the other leg.

PANEL OF ADVISERS

Marjorie Albohm is a certified athletic trainer and associate director of the International Institute of Sports Science and Medicine at the Indiana University School of Medicine in Mooresville. She served on the medical staff for the 1980 Winter Olympics and the 1987 Pan American Games.

Lisa Dobloug is a private fitness consultant in Washington, D.C. She is president of Scandinavian Fitness Corporation. Many of her clients are older people who wish to remain active and who appreciate her sound advice about warming up, stretching, and cooling down.

James M. Fox, M.D., is director of the Center for the Disorders of the Knee in Van Nuys, California, and author of the book *Save Your Knees.* He was also a member of the medical staff for the 1984 Summer Olympics.

Gary M. Gordon, D.P.M., is director of the running and jogging programs at the University of Pennsylvania Sports Medicine Center in Philadelphia. He specializes in podiatric medicine, foot surgery, and sports medicine.

Rich Phaigh is co-director of the American Institute of Sports Massage in New York City and the Institute of Clinical Biomechanics in Eugene, Oregon. He is also a massage instructor at East-West College of the Healing Arts in Portland. Phaigh is the author of *Athletic Massage* and has worked on the likes of running stars Alberto Salazar and Joan Samuelson.

Lactose Intolerance

15 Soothing Ideas

When you drink a glass of milk, do you bloat up with enough gas to float yourself and Phineas T. Fogg around the world in 80 days? When you eat ice cream, could your subsequent intestinal rumblings substitute for the timpani in the *1812* Overture? Does a cheese pizza in your belly produce diarrhea in quantities worthy of a laxative study?

If so, you probably have lactose intolerance. That is, your small intestine doesn't produce enough lactase, the enzyme you need to digest lactose, the natural sugar found in dairy products. Never fear, it's not dangerous.

Nor are you alone in your intolerance. The majority of humans get some degree of lactose intolerance by the time they're 20, according to gastroenterologist Seymour Sabesin, M.D., director of the Section of Digestive Diseases at Rush–Presbyterian–St. Luke's Medical Center in

Chicago, Illinois. As many as 30 million adult Americans may have some degree of lactose intolerance. But there's good news. You can have your ice cream and eat it, too. Here's how.

Take the tolerance test. Since most everyone's degree of tolerance is different, you'll want to find out how much of a good thing you can have before you stop enjoying it, says Theodore Bayless, M.D., the director of clinical gastroenterology at Johns Hopkins University Hospital in Baltimore, Maryland.

The obvious thing to do is decrease the amount of milk and dairy products you eat until your symptoms go away.

"Some people are bothered by as little as one-fourth of a glass of milk," he says. "About 30 percent of lactose-intolerant people will get symptoms only after a quart, maybe 30 to 40 percent from a glass."

Don't forget your calcium. "Milk products are a major source of calcium," Dr. Bayless cautions. "Most people should get the calcium equivalent of two glasses of milk daily." If milk is your main source of calcium and you cut back on milk, then you should supplement your diet with substitutes "like Tums, or sardines with bones, or spinach or broccoli," he says. Calcium supplements are another option, as are lactase enzymes, pills, or lactase-treated milk.

Never drink milk alone. "Some people find their symptoms disappear if they take their dairy products with meals," Dr. Bayless says.

Inoculate yourself. It may be worth trying to take just a small amount of milk products each day, gradually increasing the dose to build up your tolerance, Dr. Bayless suggests. Back off if your symptoms reappear.

Eat yogurt. The organisms that make yogurt what it is, also produce lactase to digest the lactose contained in yogurt, says Naresh Jain, M.D., a gastroenterologist in private practice in Niagara Falls, New York. "Secondly, the bacteria themselves also probably break down the lactose in the milk. Most people with lactose intolerance don't have it very severely," Dr. Jain says. "Maybe 70 to 80 percent of all otherwise healthy lactose-intolerant people should be able to tolerate yogurt quite well."

Dr. Sabesin notes that "yogurt has only about 75 percent of the lactose content of an equal amount of milk." That difference, Dr. Sabesin says, may be all you need to be able to tolerate lactose. About 4 to 6 ounces a day is about all you need to keep gas away.

Here are some other tips on yogurt.

Choose regular over frozen. The only problem with frozen yogurt would be if it has been repasteurized, Dr. Jain says. Yogurt is made from pasteurized milk. But sometimes manufacturers repasteurize the yogurt before they freeze it. "This would kill the beneficial organisms that produce lactase," he says. So try to find yogurt that has not been repasteurized.

Choose nonfat. "Fat slows gastric emptying," Dr. Jain says. "Yogurt with fat in it sits in the stomach for a longer time. This means stomach acid may have more of a chance to kill the organisms."

And since lactose digestion takes place in the small intestine, you want your organisms to get there as soon as possible, even if your stomach acid doesn't kill them. Although this is still only a theory, Dr. Jain says, it's probably best to stick with nonfat yogurt.

Eat it every day. "We gave study subjects yogurt on a regular basis every day," Dr. Jain says, "and we demonstrated improvements in their digestion."

Eat yogurt before ice cream. "If you eat yogurt 5 to 15 minutes before you eat ice cream [or other milk products], probably any symptoms of lactose-intolerance would be less," Dr. Jain says.

Add your own lactase. Several companies make lactase enzyme and add it to milk. Or you can buy it in liquid form and add it yourself. Lactaid, using research done by Dr. Bayless and David Paige, M.D., at Johns Hopkins University Hospital in Baltimore, Maryland, makes tablets you can take at the same time as you eat lactose-containing foods. A few drops of lactase liquid in a quart of milk renders the milk flatulence-free with a slightly sweeter taste.

"The only problem is whether you add enough lactase," Dr. Sabesin says. "Each person has a different degree of lactose intolerance, so it's a matter of trial and error." The tablets and drops are available OTC in pharmacies, while supermarkets nationwide carry tummy-ready Lactaid milk. Lactase-treated cheese and cottage cheese are available in some areas.

Try buttermilk. "Buttermilk should be pretty much tolerable," Dr. Jain says. (Despite its name, buttermilk also has less fat and less cholesterol than even 2 percent milk.)

And cheese, too. "Cheese has less lactose in it than milk," Dr. Jain says. Hard cheeses are the best, Dr. Bayless says, because they're fermented the most. Adds Dr. Sabesin, "Swiss cheese or extra sharp cheddar cheese contain only a trace amount of lactose and are thus less likely to produce digestive upset."

Know that acidophilus milk doesn't help. Although acidophilus organisms are highly beneficial for digestion, they colonize the *large* intestine, notes Jeffrey Biller, M.D., a gastroenterologist at the Center for Pediatric Gastroenterology and Nutrition in Boston, Massachusetts. Lactose digestion occurs in the *small* intestine, so acidophilus whizzes right on by the lactose.

Beware the fillers. Lactose is a very common filler in many kinds of medication and nutritional supplements. "In some pills and for some people," Dr. Jain warns, there's enough lactose to cause lactose-intolerance symptoms. Read labels carefully. Ask your pharmacist if your medication has a lactose filler.

Call a hotline. Lactaid has a toll-free phone line for questions about lactose intolerance. Phone 1-800-257-8650.

PANEL OF ADVISERS

Theodore Bayless, M.D., is the director of clinical gastroenterology at the Johns Hopkins University Hospital in Baltimore, Maryland.

Jeffrey Biller, M.D., is a gastroenterologist at the Center for Pediatric Gastroenterology and Nutrition in Boston, Massachusetts.

Naresh Jain, M.D., is a gastroenterologist in private practice in Niagara Falls, New York.

Seymour Sabesin, M.D., is a gastroenterologist and director of the Section of Digestive Diseases at Rush–Presbyterian–St. Luke's Medical Center in Chicago, Illinois.

Laryngitis

16 Healing Hints

You had to forgo your usual morning solo in the shower. The song that barely scratched its way out of your throat sounded more like a croak than an aria. You cleared your throat to try again. The sounds coming out of you were anything but musical. If this keeps up, you won't have any voice at all.

Want to know what your problem is?

Bad vibrations.

For you to sound like you, the air you exhale through your larynx — that voice box commonly known as your Adam's apple — has to vibrate through your vocal cords in just the right way. When the cords are scarred or swollen, they don't create the right shaped "container" for that air. That allows breath to escape.

Even a slight change in your vocal cords can render your voice unrecognizable. Your vocal cords contain a central muscle bundle, various layers of connective tissue and a skinlike covering called the mucosa. "An alteration in any one of these layers can disrupt the optimal vibration through the tissue," says Scott Kessler, M.D., an otolaryngologist whose patients include opera stars and rock singers. He is on the staffs of Mount Sinai Hospital and Beth Israel Hospital in New York City.

Damage can occur any number of ways. Misusing your voice can temporarily scar your vocal cords. An upper respiratory infection or an allergic reaction can inflame them. Even dry air can cause mucus to stick between the cords. The result? Laryngitis.

What's the best way to recover your voice? Here's what our experts advise.

Don't talk. No matter what the cause of your laryngitis, the most important thing you can do for your voice is to give it a rest, says Laurence Levine, M.D., D.D.S., an otolaryngologist in Creve Coeur and St.

411

MEDICAL ALERT

When Laryngitis Is Life-Threatening

If your voice loss is accompanied by pain so severe you have trouble swallowing your own saliva, see a physician immediately, says George T. Simpson II, M.D. Swelling in the upper part of your larynx may be blocking your airway.

You should also contact your physician if you find yourself coughing up blood, hear noises in your throat when you breathe, or find that continued voice rest does nothing to alleviate your hoarseness. When laryngitis persists, it may signal the presence of a throat tumor. In any case, consult your doctor if your voice doesn't return to normal within three to five days.

Charles, Missouri, and an associate clinical professor of otolaryngology at Washington University School of Medicine. Try to go a day or two without talking.

Don't even whisper. If you have to communicate, pass notes. "Whispering causes you to bang your vocal cords together as strongly as if you were shouting," explains George T. Simpson II, M.D., chairman of the Department of Otolaryngology at the Boston University School of Medicine, University Hospital, and Boston City Hospital.

Don't take aspirin. If you've lost your voice because you were yelling too loudly last night, you've probably ruptured a capillary, says Dr. Levine. So stay away from aspirin. Aspirin increases clotting time, which can impede the healing process.

Use a cold-air humidifier. The mucosa that blanket your vocal cords need to be kept moist. When they're not, mucus can become sticky and adherent, a virtual flypaper for irritants. Fight back with a cold-air humidifier, says Dr. Kessler.

Steam it away. Steaming can also restore moisture. Robert Feder, M.D., a Los Angeles, California, otolaryngologist and singing coach, suggests hanging your head over a steaming bowl of water for 5 minutes twice a day.

Drink plenty of fluids. Dr. Simpson favors eight to ten glasses a day, preferably water. Dr. Feder recommends juice, and tea with honey or lemon.

Don't use ice. Warm fluids are best, says Dr. Feder. Cold drinks can just aggravate the problem.

Breathe through your nose. "Breathing through your nose is a natural humidifier," says Dr. Kessler. "People who have a deviated nasal septum breathe through the mouth while asleep. That exposes the voice to dry and cold air. Evaluating how you breathe is critical to understanding the nature of hoarseness."

Nix the cigarettes. Smoking is a prime cause of throat dryness, says Dr. Kessler.

Lubricate with slippery elm. "Slippery elm bark tea is a good lubricant for the back of the throat," says Dr. Kessler. "Drinking won't lubricate the vocal cords directly. That's because the epiglottis closes over them like a trapdoor. But drinking will provide more water to assist the mucous glands in the larynx to provide a smooth coating on the cords."

Choose your cough drops wisely. Avoid mint and mentholated products, says Dr. Feder. Stick to honey- or fruit-flavored soft cough drops instead.

Beware of airplane air. Talking on an airplane can sabotage your voice. That's because the pressurized air inside the cabin is so dry. To keep your cords moist, breathe through your nose, says Dr. Kessler. Chew gum or suck on lozenges so that you'll have no choice but to keep your mouth closed. At the same time, it will help increase saliva production.

Check your medication. Certain prescription drugs can be very drying, our experts say. Check with your doctor if you're uncertain. Likely culprits include blood pressure and thyroid medications and antihistamines.

Don't strain, amplify. If your job requires you to raise your voice to be heard, why not use mechanical means to make yourself louder? "Often, we don't make enough use of amplification systems to protect voice function," says Dr. Levine.

Respect your voice. If you have a presentation to do and you find yourself hoarse, it's better to cancel than risk doing long-term damage to your voice, says Dr. Kessler.

Consider voice training. And if you find yourself speaking a lot, consider getting some voice training. In a nontrained voice, the muscles that suspend the larynx strain against each other, says Dr. Levine. Training the voice can get those muscles to work together as a team.

PANEL OF ADVISERS

Robert Feder, M.D., is an otolaryngologist in private practice in the Los Angeles, California, area. He is a professor of drama and a professor of otolaryngology at the University of California, Los Angeles. He is also a professor of singing at the School of Music at the University of Southern California in Los Angeles.

Scott Kessler, M.D., is a New York City otolaryngologist specializing in performing arts medicine. He is the physician for many of the performers at the Metropolitan Opera and the City Opera, as well as for cast members of Broadway plays and cabarets. He is also on the staffs of Mount Sinai and Beth Israel hospitals in New York City.

Laurence Levine, M.D., D.D.S., is an otolaryngologist in Creve Coeur and St. Charles, Missouri. He is also an associate clinical professor of otolaryngology at Washington University School of Medicine in St. Louis.

George T. Simpson II, M.D., is chairman of the Department of Otolaryngology at Boston University School of Medicine, University Hospital, and Boston City Hospital in Massachusetts. He is an attending physician at Children's Hospital Medical Center and the Veterans Administration Hospital. He is also a member of the scientific advisory committee for the Voice Foundation.

Menopause

21 Ways to Stay Symptom-Free

Do you have PMZ?

No, not PMS—that's premenstrual syndrome. When you say PMZ, think liberation, not liability.

PMZ stands for postmenopausal zest, a phrase coined by anthropologist Margaret Mead. And what she meant was that women should seize this stage of life and live it to the fullest. You are now unencumbered by contraception and pregnancy and that once-a-month cycle that used to slow you down. *This,* she says, is freedom.

"It's a time for exploring what it feels like to be a woman in the human sense, not just as someone who raises children," says Irene Simpson, a naturopathic practitioner in Arlington, Washington. "My friends and I are on the verge of menopause and we are finding it very empowering. We are finding personal growth at a time when women used to decline."

Menopause begins when your ovaries no longer function, when estrogen secretion slows, then stops, and monthly menstruation becomes irregular, then ceases. Normally, women reach menopause by age 51.

During the six months to three years of this cycle of your life, you may feel some of the traditional symptoms of menopause, including hot flashes and sudden chills, lowered sexual desire, vaginal dryness, emotional upset, and sleeping problems. Your doctor can advise you on medical help for these problems.

GETTING A BETTER OUTLOOK ON LIFE

The architecture of this cycle of life can be your design. Menopause can be bittersweet. Or, it can be a time of PMZ, with an emphasis on the Zest. Here's how.

Design your own zest! Education about physiological changes and an adventurous outlook can make a big difference in handling the stresses that come with menopause, as well as the life changes (children moving out, parents moving in, for example) that many women are faced with in their late forties and early fifties, says Simpson.

Research shows that today's woman spends a third of her life postmenopausal. So consider menopause a step forward in life and make a change for the better, Simpson says. Go back to school. Find a new hobby. Change careers. Take charge of your own health. Make life an adventure.

Find support. Support groups offer reassurance that menopause is a natural cycle, says Sadja Greenwood, M.D., a family physician in San Francisco, California, and author of *Menopause, Naturally.* Members can offer practical coping techniques that they've discovered, as well as sisterly support for new endeavors. To find a support group, call your local women's center. To start one, place an ad in the newspaper or tack a notice on a bulletin board where women congregate, such as the YWCA.

Exercise daily. Walking, jogging, bicycling, jumping rope, dancing, swimming, or any other daily exercise can relieve a lot of the symptoms of menopause, according to a study at the University of Medicine and Dentistry of New Jersey Robert Wood Johnson Medical School. Exercise can help prevent or lessen symptoms such as hot flashes and night sweats, depression, and other emotional problems, as well as vaginal problems.

Improved physical fitness, of course, is the most obvious result of exercise. But exercise also improves psychological health by boosting brain concentrations of the neurotransmitters norepinephrine and serotonin, according to Gloria A. Bachmann, M.D., an associate professor of medicine in the Department of Obstetrics and Gynecology at University of Medicine and Dentistry of New Jersey Robert Wood Johnson Medical School.

She recommends aerobics and stretching exercises for flexibility, muscle strengthening, and relaxation. Yoga, she reports, also aids flexibility and has an added benefit—it improves diaphragmatic breathing, which induces relaxation and reduces stress.

AWAY WITH HOT FLASHES

Hot flashes are the body's response to lowered estrogen levels, says Dr. Greenwood. "There's a dysfunction in the temperature-regulating portion of the brain until the body gets used to the missed estrogen," she says.

About 80 percent of all women have hot flashes. A typical hot flash lasts about 2.7 minutes. During a hot flash, your face and upper body feels as if it's been shoved into an oven. Your face reddens and you sweat heavily as your skin temperature suddenly rises 7 or 8 degrees. It usually returns to normal in about 30 minutes.

The good news is, many women feel the flash coming just before they actually break into a sweat, so they can prepare for it. Here's how.

Look cool. A positive outlook can be an effective daily tool in combating hot flashes, says Marilyn Poland, R.N., Ph.D., an associate professor of gynecology and obstetrics at Wayne State University School of Medicine.

When you feel a hot flash coming on, remind yourself of a couple of things: that hot flashes are normal, that they don't last long, and that you are able to do something about them. Most times that positive mind-set can make the flash more bearable.

Learn to relax. Women who can relax, Dr. Poland says, will be in better control. Learn meditation or yoga or just sit quietly, eyes closed, for a while every day to relax.

Control the triggers. Determine what triggers hot flashes for you, then avoid the triggers. For some women, emotional upset is a trigger. Others may find a hot meal, spicy food, a warm room, or a warm bed will trigger a flush.

Go for the layered look. Wear sweaters and vests, then peel a layer off when a hot flash threatens, suggests Dr. Poland. Add a layer when the hot flash passes because your body temperature actually falls a little below normal and can leave you feeling chilled.

Wear natural fibers. Synthetic fibers trap heat and perspiration during a hot flash, making this symptom even more uncomfortable. Natural fibers, such as cotton or wool, will give your body more ventilation and keep it cooler by wicking moisture away from your body and cooling you naturally.

Carry a fan. Buy something pretty and keep it in your purse, says Dr. Poland. Or buy a small, battery-powered electric fan and keep it on your desk. Flip it on as the hot flash begins.

Eat small meals. Rather than load your system three times a day, five or six small meals will help your body regulate temperature more easily, says Dr. Greenwood.

Drink lots of water. Don't forget to refresh yourself with cool water or juice, especially after exercising, Dr. Greenwood says. This, too, keeps body temperature in check.

Cut the caffeine. Caffeine-containing beverages stimulate production of the stress hormones that trigger hot flashes, says Dr. Greenwood.

Limit your alcohol. Some women find alcohol is another hot flash trigger, says Dr. Greenwood.

Towel off. Buy a purse-size package of moist towels and carry them with you. They'll take the edge off a hot flash, says Dr. Poland. You may want to mop your brow when the heat is most intense or you may want to remove the perspiration after the flash is over.

Turn down the heat. Heat in any form may trigger hot flashes. Turn your thermostat down, leave a window open, and avoid hot foods and beverages.

Stay sexy. Women going through menopause who continue to have intercourse on a regular basis (once a week or more) have fewer or no hot flashes compared to women who have sporadic sex, research shows. Norma McCoy, Ph.D., a professor of psychology at San Francisco State University, and Julian M. Davidson, Ph.D., professor of physiology at Stanford University, studied 43 women who were just beginning to enter menopause. They found that frequent sex helps moderate dropping estrogen levels, which reduces the occurrence of hot flashes.

Dr. McCoy believes that the high estrogen levels help maintain a healthy interest in sex and that regular sexual activity indirectly stimulates failing ovaries, which helps moderate the hormonal system and prevents extreme swings in the estrogen level.

Don't share the sheets. You don't have to have a separate bed to keep from disturbing your husband with on-again, off-again nighttime sweats, says Dr. Poland. Use separate blankets on the bed or get an electric blanket with dual controls, then you can feel free to kick off the sheets when you need to cool down.

OVERCOMING SEXUAL PROBLEMS

Our experts gave the following advice for continuing a fulfilling love life through menopause.

Lubricate your love. Vaginal dryness from a lack of estrogen decreases interest in intercourse during menopause, says Dr. Poland. A water-soluable lubricant, such as Lubifax or K-Y Jelly, vegetable oils, and unscented cream or oil, are all good choices for lubrication, says Dr. Greenwood.

Or break open a couple of capsules of vitamin E and massage them on as a lubricant, says Simpson.

Make talk. Talk to your partner, advises Simpson. Some libido-boosting comes with heart-to-heart talks about needs and feelings.

Take high adventure to the bedroom. Couples may want to try new positions in intercourse to find the most comfortable, says Dr. Greenwood. Touching can be especially important at this time. She suggests more hugs and mutual massages for closeness and sensual pleasure.

Do the Kegel. You can strengthen your anal, vaginal, and urinary muscles with a special exercise called a Kegel, says Simpson. Stronger muscles can help you relax and use these muscles with less pain and more pleasure during intercourse. They are also good for preventing urinary incontinence, a problem for some menopausal women. Here's how to do it.

Imagine you want to stop urine in midstream. Squeeze the muscles in your vaginal area firmly. Hold to the count of three, then relax. Practice with a rapid alternation between tightening and letting go. You can practice this exercise anywhere, anytime.

PANEL OF ADVISERS

Gloria A. Bachmann, M.D., is an associate professor of medicine in the Department of Obstetrics and Gynecology at the University of Medicine and Dentistry of New Jersey Robert Wood Johnson Medical School in Piscataway.

Sadja Greenwood, M.D., is a family practice physician in San Francisco, California. She is on the faculty at the University of California Medical Center in San Francisco. She is author of *Menopause, Naturally.*

Norma McCoy, Ph.D., is a professor of psychology at San Francisco State University in California.

Marilyn Poland, R.N., Ph.D., is an associate professor of gynecology and obstetrics at Wayne State University School of Medicine in Detroit, Michigan. She is coauthor of *Surviving the Change: A Practical Guide to Menopause.*

Irene Simpson is a naturopathic practitioner in Arlington, Washington.

Menstrual Cramps

13 Easy Antidotes

"A whole lot of women are still needlessly suffering from menstrual cramps," says Penny Wise Budoff, M.D., director of the Women's Medical Center in Bethpage, New York.

Menstrual cramps—or dysmenorrhea in medical jargon—are a chemical problem, Dr. Budoff explains. Each month, the lining of a woman's uterus produces chemicals called prostaglandins, which help the uterine muscles contract and expel tissue and fluids during menstruation. High levels of prostaglandins cause uterine muscle contractions, or cramps.

Not every woman suffers from cramps, but if you do, these self-help remedies might provide some relief.

Get into balance. "Too many women tend to skip meals and consume excessive amounts of sweets and salty foods just at a time when they should be so careful in their dietary choices," says Dr. Budoff. While a healthier diet won't *cure* cramps, it can do wonders for improving your overall sense of well-being, she says. Cut out salty and sweet junk foods, which can make you feel bloated and sluggish. Instead, eat more vegetables, fruit, chicken, and fish, and try to space them out in small meals throughout the day rather than having three large meals.

Take your vitamins. Many of her patients report fewer problems with cramps when they're getting a healthy daily dose of vitamins and minerals, says Dr. Budoff. Take a multiple vitamin and mineral supplement, preferably one that contains calcium and one that comes in small doses that you can take a couple of times a day after meals, she advises.

Mind your minerals. The minerals calcium, potassium, and magnesium can also play a part in relief, says Susan Lark, M.D., director of the PMS Self-Help Center in Los Altos, California. She says she has found that women taking calcium suffer less pain from cramps than those who do not. Magnesium is important, she notes, because it helps your body absorb calcium more efficiently. She suggests increasing calcium and magnesium intake before and during your period.

Cut out caffeine. The caffeine in coffee, tea, cola, and chocolate can contribute to menstrual discomfort by making you nervous, says Dr. Budoff. Go caffeine-free. The oils in coffee also may irritate your intestines.

Abstain from alcohol. If you tend to retain water during your period, alcohol will only add to your problem, says Dr. Lark. Don't drink, she advises. Or if you must, limit yourself to a glass or two of light wine.

Don't do diuretics. Many women think diuretics are great for reducing menstrual bloating, but Dr. Lark advises against them. Diuretics have the ability to take important minerals from the body along with the water. Instead, she advises, reduce your intake of water-retentive substances like salt and alcohol.

The Alternate Route

Get a Foothold for Pain Relief

Relief from cramps might be just a therapeutic touch away, says Alexis Phillips, a medical massage instructor and supervisor of the Peter Ling Clinic of the Swedish Institute in New York City.

The foot contains acupressure or trigger points that are believed to be connected along internal energy pathways to your pelvic area, she explains. Feel for these spots—which she says will be sensitive during your period—in the depressions above either side of your heel. Gently press in with your thumb and fingertips. Do the same along the sides of your Achilles tendon, moving up toward your calf muscle.

Try this acupressure technique for a few minutes on each foot.

Warm up. Warmth will increase your blood flow and relax your muscles—especially important in your cramped and congested pelvic area, says Dr. Budoff. Drink lots of hot herbal tea or hot lemonade. Also, put a heating pad or hot-water bottle on your abdomen for a few minutes at a time.

Take a mineral bath. Create your own relaxing "health spa" bath to relax your muscles and relieve cramps, suggests Dr. Lark. Add 1 cup of sea salt and 1 cup of baking soda to a warm bath. Soak for 20 minutes.

Take a brisk walk. Walk or engage in some form of moderate exercise at all times, but especially before your period. You'll feel better when it arrives, says Dr. Budoff.

Do a yoga stretch. Yoga stretches during your period can also help, says Dr. Lark. Here's one example. Kneel on the floor and sit on your heels. Bring your forehead to the floor and place your arms along the floor against your body. Close your eyes. Hold the position for as long as it is comfortable.

Make love. Having sex with orgasm is great for relieving cramps, says Dr. Lark. The vigorous muscle action moves blood and other fluids away from congested organs, relieving pain.

Take a pill. Aspirin and acetaminophen are fine for relieving cramps. Even more effective, however, are over-the-counter medications like Advil, Haltran, Medipren, and Nuprin, says Dr. Budoff. These contain a chemical called ibuprofen, which has the ability to inhibit the actions of prostaglandins. Take one of these medications—along with some milk or food to avoid stomach irritation—when your cramps start and continue taking them until the cramps go away.

PANEL OF ADVISERS

Penny Wise Budoff, M.D., is director of the Women's Medical Center in Bethpage, New York, and author of *No More Menstrual Cramps and Other Good News, No More Hot Flashes and Other Good News,* and other related books.

Susan Lark, M.D., is director of the PMS Self-Help Center in Los Altos, California, and author of *Dr. Susan Lark's Premenstrual Syndrome Self-Help Book.*

Alexis Phillips is a medical massage instructor and supervisor of the Peter Ling Clinic of the Swedish Institute in New York City.

Morning Sickness

13 Ways to Counteract Queasiness

You had planned to be a radiant madonna, one of those pregnant women who grow more beautiful with each passing month. Morning sickness just wasn't in the game plan.

Yvonne Thornton, M.D., remembers. An assistant professor of obstetrics and gynecology at Cornell University Medical College and mother of two, she used to make light of her patients' complaints—until she knew better. "What's a little nausea, I thought. And then I became pregnant. I was camped out by the toilet every 5 minutes!"

Of course, your experience with morning sickness is probably a lot different from Dr. Thornton's. Or from anybody else's, for that matter. That's because morning sickness is different from person to person. In fact, you may not even get it in the morning. It can hit at any time during the day. Maybe you'll feel worse in the evening, after a long day at work. Maybe certain smells will trigger it.

Typically, morning sickness begins around week 6 of pregnancy, about the same time that the placenta begins serious production of human chorionic gonadotropin (HCG), a special pregnancy hormone. In most women, symptoms peak during week 8 or 9 and wane after week 13.

The good news is that morning sickness seems to be a sign that the pregnancy is going well. A National Institute of Child Health and Human Development study of 9,098 pregnant women found that women who vomited during their first trimester were less likely to miscarry or deliver prematurely.

That cheers you some. But what can you do to get through it? Here's what our experts advise.

Experiment. What worked for your sister, your best friend, and the woman down the street may not do it for you. "There are as many remedies as there are women," says Deborah Gowen, a certified nurse-midwife with Women-Care in Cambridge, Massachusetts. You may have to try a couple of strategies before you find one right for you.

Eat the way your baby eats. The child growing inside you nourishes itself by raiding your bloodstream for glucose 24 hours a day. If you don't take care how you replenish the supply, your blood sugar levels can drop sharply.

Your best tactic, says Tekoa King, a San Francisco nurse-midwife, is to "switch the way you eat to the way the baby eats, a little bit at a time. Put glucose into your system quickly and easily by eating simple sugars, like fruit sugars. You want sugars already half broken down." Grapes and orange juice are excellent.

Avoid fried, fatty foods. That grilled cheeseburger with onion rings may have looked great to you last week, but you might not want to chance it now.

"Anything fried often seems to make pregnant women more nauseated," says King. The body takes longer to digest such foods, she says, which means that they sit in the stomach longer.

Carry raw almonds with you. Gowen is a big fan of raw almonds for pregnant women. Snacking on them "fulfills the requirement of small, frequent meals. They contain some fat, some protein, and are high in B vitamins. They're portable, too, and tastier than crackers."

Keep a night table nibble supply. If almonds don't appeal to you, keep soda crackers by your bed. Moving around on an empty stomach can make you feel worse, says King. So eat something to bring your blood sugar up before you get out of bed in the morning, or in the middle of the night.

Nibble to keep away heartburn, too. "You should always have something in your stomach, even if it's just a cracker or a little candy bar," advises Gregory Radio, M.D., an obstetrician/gynecologist in Allentown, Pennsylvania, and chairman of reproductive endocrinology at Allentown Hospital. "The stomach naturally makes more acids during pregnancy. Those acids need something to work against."

Drink lots of clear fluids. Dr. Radio also recommends drinking small amounts of clear fluids frequently. Clear broth, water, fruit juice, and certain herbal teas fill the bill. "I don't mean to endorse a product," he says, "but Gatorade is usually superb because it can help maintain your electrolytes [substances that regulate the body's electrochemical balance]."

MEDICAL ALERT

When Morning Sickness Should Concern You

Consult your physician about your morning sickness if:

- You notice you've lost a pound or two. Normally, weight gain during pregnancy continues even if you aren't keeping all of your meals down.
- You feel dehydrated or you are not urinating.
- You find you can't keep anything down—no water, no juice, nothing over a period of 4 to 6 hours.

At its most severe, morning sickness degenerates into a condition doctors call hyperemesis gravidarum. Left untreated, it can disturb the essential electrolyte balance in your body, cause pulse irregularities, and, in its severest form, can lead to damage of the kidneys and liver. It also endangers your unborn child. The ketones that result when your body breaks down fat already stored in the body can damage neurological development in the baby.

Women with hyperemesis gravidarum are usually hospitalized overnight and treated with an intravenous solution of glucose, water, and vitamins.

Find respite with raspberry leaf tea. If you feel queasy, try a cup of herbal tea. Raspberry leaf, chamomile, and lemon balm are among the teas that Dr. Radio recommends to his patients.

Gowen believes that herbs work best in combination. Chamomile added to peppermint is more effective than peppermint on its own, she says.

Sip ginger ale. Remember how your mom used to give you ginger ale to "settle" an upset stomach? Dr. Thornton is a ginger ale fan, too.

If you're taking prenatal vitamins, check with your doctor. In some instances, they can make you sick to your stomach, says Gowen.

The Alternate Route

Acupressure to the Rescue

The next time your mate expresses sympathy about your morning sickness, tell him he can do something to help.

That something is acupressure massage.

Daily allover massage is ideal as a preventive strategy, says Wataru Ohashi, an ohashiatsu teacher and founder of the Ohashi Institute in New York City.

But if your husband won't go for that, show him the instructions for this quickie technique. It can help in a pinch.

Have your wife lie on her right side and sit behind her, supporting her back with your left leg. Slip your left arm under hers and grasp her left shoulder.

With your right hand, massage her entire neck three times. Then place your palm against the base of her skull and stretch her head away from her shoulders.

Next, use your thumb to press down her back in the grooves between the left shoulder blade and spine and then around the perimeter of her shoulder blade out toward her side. Keep the pressure on for 5 to 7 seconds per point. If you find a sore spot, gently give it extra attention. Slip your thumb as far under her shoulder blade as is comfortable for her.

Begin with gentle pressure and let your wife tell you if she wants more pressure. Always use your body weight, not your arm muscle power. "The feeling is totally different," says Ohashi.

"If you stimulate the external, you can eliminate the internal discomfort," says Ohashi. The trigger points you use in this exercise affect the stomach and the hormonal system, he adds.

Trust your body's wisdom. "Eat whatever appeals to you, as long as you're not eating junk," says Gowen. "Avoid caffeine, artificial sweeteners, all drugs. But if all you crave is pasta, then eat it. It really does work when women listen to their bodies."

Keep calm. If you continue to put on weight, and dehydration isn't a problem for you, you're probably doing just fine.

"Women don't tend to lose beyond what their body stores can handle," says King, who has been delivering babies for ten years. "I think we just don't know the magic of what goes on inside the mother. My belief is that you can really be fairly ill with morning sickness, yet you can continue nourishing your baby very well."

PANEL OF ADVISERS

Deborah Gowen, a certified nurse-midwife, works for Women-Care in Cambridge, Massachusetts.

Tekoa King, a nurse-midwife, has been delivering babies for ten years and has taught nurse practitioners at the University of California, San Francisco. She is affiliated with the Bay Area Midwifery Service.

Wataru Ohashi is an internationally known teacher of ohashiatsu and founder of the Ohashi Institute, a nonprofit education organization in New York City.

Gregory Radio, M.D., is a practicing obstetrician/gynecologist in Allentown, Pennsylvania, and chairman of reproductive endocrinology at Allentown Hospital.

Yvonne Thornton, M.D., is a maternal fetal medicine specialist and assistant professor of obstetrics and gynecology at Cornell University Medical College in New York City. She is also director of prenatal diagnosis and an attending physician at the New York Hospital–Cornell University Medical Center.

Motion Sickness

25 Quick-Action Cures

The sky is blue, the sea is green, and you are bright-eyed and rosy-cheeked, out on the deck of a sun-dappled sailboat bobbing along in the waves. Bobbing and dipping. Dipping and lobbing. Lobbing and listing. Listing and rolling. Rolling and rising. Rising and sinking. Sinking and splashing. Splashing and crashing. Crashing and churning.

This Doctor Sets Sights on Cure

Motion sickness stems from imbalances in the inner ear, most doctors will tell you. But Roderic W. Gillilan, O.D., who for more than 24 years has focused much of his work on patients suffering from the problem, sees things differently. "Motion sickness—at least on land—is primarily visual," he says.

Dr. Gillilan's patients have ranged from people who can't read in a car without getting sick (about a third of the population can't, he says), to extreme cases who get nausea, dizziness, or headaches watching the quick action of a basketball game or walking down the aisle in a grocery store.

The problem "generally has nothing to do with the need for glasses or a person's sight," Dr. Gillilan says, but is more a matter of sensitivity to rapid eye movements and seeing motion.

To clear up the problem, his patients undergo several sessions of what he calls Dynamic Adaptive Vision Therapy, which is a process of desensitization. "It's not muscle building, but learning how to use your eyes, like learning to ski or ride a bike," he says. Once they master it, people don't usually forget it—most of his patients remain symptom-free for years.

Dr. Gillilan has given seminars in vision therapy and published a manual describing the technique for colleagues. If you're interested in receiving the training, ask your optometrist.

Listing and bobbing and dipping and rippling. Crashing and churning and stomach turning. And before you know it, you're launching your lunch into glistening green waters, quaking and quickening. It's altogether sickening.

The French call it *mal de mer,* and even the most seasoned sailors can suffer from it. In the air, it's airsickness. On land, it's car sickness. And then there's amusement park ride sickness—at least one visitor a day turns green on Disney World's Space Mountain or Big Thunder Mountain roller coaster. But it's all the same thing— that queasy, uneasy feeling collectively known as motion sickness.

"Motion sickness results when the brain receives wrong information about the environment," explains Rafael Tarnopolsky, M.D., a professor of otolaryngology at the University of Osteopathic Medicine and Health Sciences. To help keep our bodies in balance, our sensory systems continually collect information about our surroundings and send it to our inner ears, and like computers, they organize the information and send it on to the brain.

A Space-Age Cure That Goes to Extremes

". . . four, three, two, one—lift-off!" With an earth-shaking roar, white-hot jets propel Spacelab 3 and its four-member crew into the stratosphere, where it turns its back on a world still tremulously shivering. But the folks in ground control aren't the only ones shaken up by the blast. A mere 7 minutes into the flight, one of the crew members has his first "vomiting episode," an incident that is rerun numerous times during the mission.

Being motion sick in space is a serious problem for astronauts. "At any one time, the whole crew could be incapacitated," says Patricia Cowings, Ph.D., director of the Psychophysiological Research Laboratory at NASA's Ames Research Center in Moffett Field, California. "Potentially, it could be disastrous. Throwing up while wearing a helmet could be fatal." And there's no easy solution, since motion sickness medications can have dangerous side effects.

But new horizons are opening up, thanks to a biofeedback training program. For the past 15 years, Dr. Cowings and her colleagues have been making members of the American public sick in order to help astronauts feel better.

"Essentially, our routine involves bringing a person to our lab and making him throw up," says Dr. Cowings, known to her colleagues as the "Baroness of Barf." A devious device aids this process: a chair that rotates at the same time the volunteer moves his head at various angles, a process that throws off his inner ear's sense of balance in a few minutes. "It works on virtually everyone," Dr. Cowings says. "If a rock had an inner ear, it would make a rock sick."

While rotating, the subject is monitored for physiological responses such as heart rate, breathing rate, sweating, and muscle contractions. "No two people have exactly the same response," Dr. Cowings explains. "Motion sickness is actually a kind of fingerprint that's unique to each person." The fingerprint clearly drawn, each person can then be taught to control his unique responses through a combination of deep relaxation and exercise of muscles—muscles we don't realize we can exercise, like those in blood vessels.

If a person can successfully control his early responses, he may prevent more violent ones from coming up. "We've trained more than 250 people, and our track record is pretty good," says Dr. Cowings. "About 60 percent can completely eliminate their symptoms when we retest them in the chair. Another 25 percent can significantly decrease their responses. And the training remains effective for up to three years."

The results are promising enough, says Dr. Cowings, that an actual cure for motion sickness is on the horizon.

It is when our balance system notes a discrepancy between what our inner ears sense and our eyes sense that motion sickness can take hold, says Horst Konrad, M.D., chairman of the Committee on Equilibrium of the American Academy of Otolaryngology/Head and Neck Surgery. Not everyone gets it, but the signals are pretty clear when we do. We get dizzy. We sweat. Our skin turns pale. We feel nauseated. And if things don't get any better, we throw up.

Once you feel the symptoms coming on, motion sickness can be very difficult to stop, especially if you've reached your particular point of no return—usually when nausea sets in. But the following remedies can help nurse the symptoms and might be able to cut them short. Better yet, they might keep the symptoms from starting in the first place—next time you're bobbing and dipping, dipping and bobbing along on a pretty afternoon's wave.

Think about motion wellness. "Motion sickness is partly psychological," says Dr. Konrad. "If you think you're going to throw up, you're probably going to." Instead, turn your thoughts to something wonderful.

Leave nursing the sick to someone else. It's a common occurrence. You're on a fishing boat. Everything's going along fine until someone gets sick. You watch in sympathy, maybe even offer a comforting shoulder. Before long, you're the next body down. Then there goes another. It's the domino theory in action. As cruel as it may sound, do your best to ignore others who are sick, says Dr. Konrad. Otherwise you're liable to end up in the same boat.

Get your nose out of the joint. Bad odors such as engine fumes, the dead fish on ice in the back of the boat, or the sardine sandwich being made in the galley can contribute to nausea, says Dr. Konrad. Aim your nose elsewhere.

Butt out. If you're a smoker, you may think that lighting up can calm you, deterring motion sickness. Wrong. Cigarette smoke can only contribute to impending nausea, says Dr. Konrad. If you're a nonsmoker, hightail it to the nonsmoking section of the plane, train, or bus if you feel queasiness coming on.

Travel at night. Your chances of getting sick diminish when you travel at night because you can't see the motion as well as you can in daylight hours, says Roderic W. Gillilan, O.D., an optometrist in private practice in Eugene, Oregon, who has helped hundreds of patients overcome the problem.

Don't get friendly with unfriendly food. If certain foods don't like you when you're standing still, they're going to like you even less if you're moving. As tempting as plentiful meals may be during your travels, don't overindulge, advises Robert Salada, M.D., director of the Travelers Health Care Center at the University Hospitals of Cleveland, Ohio, and assistant professor of medicine at Case Western Reserve University School of Medicine.

Go ahead, get fresh. Deter nausea with a breath of fresh air, suggests Dr. Salada. In a car, open a window. On a boat, stand out on deck and take in the sea breeze. On an airplane, turn on the overhead vent.

Think before you drink. "Too much alcohol can interfere with the way the brain handles information about the environment and can set off motion sickness symptoms," says Dr. Konrad. What's more, alcohol can dissolve into the fluids of your inner ear, which can send your head spinning. Drink in moderation during plane and ship travel.

Get enough sleep. "Your chance of getting motion sickness increases with fatigue," says Dr. Gillilan. So be sure to get your usual quota of sleep before taking off on a trip. If you're a passenger in a car or plane, catching a few zzzzs while en route can help, too, if only to temporarily ward off potentially sickening stimuli.

Sit still! Your brain is already confused enough without your creating extra motion. Keep your head especially still.

Get up front and out ahead. In a car, move up to the front seat and focus on the road ahead or the horizon, says Dr. Tarnopolsky. This will bring signals from your body and your eyes into balance.

Better yet, get into the driver's seat. When you're behind the wheel, you're sensibly looking straight ahead, says Dr. Gillilan, and you have the added advantage of anticipating any quick changes in motion.

Get caught up on your reading some other time. Don't read while you're riding in a car or on a rough plane or boat trip, says Dr. Tarnapolsky. The movement of the vehicle you're in makes the printed matter on the page move, which can make you awfully dizzy.

The Alternate Route

Age-Old Cures Still in Use

They may not work for all and may not work *every* time, but folk remedies for motion sickness have probably been around since man first decided to seriously check out the scenery beyond his own backyard. Some of these remedies are still popular today and are certainly worth a try.

Gingerroot. The first settlers to the New World might have taken it to ease their transatlantic voyage. Although the tradition dates back hundreds of years, eating a bit of ginger recently passed scientific scrutiny when an experiment showed that two powdered gingerroot capsules were more effective than a dose of Dramamine in preventing motion sickness. Ginger works, researchers theorize, by absorbing acids and blocking nausea in your gastrointestinal tract.

Olives and lemons. The early stages of motion sickness cause you to produce excess saliva, which dribbles down to your stomach and makes you nauseous, some doctors say. Olives, on the other hand, produce chemicals called tannins, which make your mouth dry. Hence, the theory goes, eating a couple of olives at the first hint of nausea can help diminish it, as may sucking on a mouth-puckering lemon.

Soda crackers. They won't stop salivation, but dry soda crackers might help absorb the excess fluid when it reaches your stomach. Their "secret ingredients" are bicarbonate of soda and cream of tartar.

Coke syrup. Prescribed as an antinauseant for children, Coke syrup added to seltzer water may help. The same may be true for any carbonated cola beverage. See for yourself.

Acupressure wristbands. Sold in many marine and travel shops, these lightweight wristbands have a plastic button that is supposed to be worn over what the doctors in the Orient call the Nei-Kuan acupressure point inside each wrist. The wearer is protected against nausea, the theory goes, by exerting pressure on the button for a few minutes.

But if you must read, there are ways to do it without getting sick, says Dr. Gillilan. Among them:

- Slouch down in the seat and hold the reading material close to eye level. "It's not the reading itself that makes you sick," he says, "but the angle at which you're doing it. When you look down while traveling in a car, the visible motion from the side windows strikes the eyes at an unusual angle, and that is what triggers symptoms. This method brings your eyes into the same position as if you were looking down the road."

- Hold your hands next to your temples to block out the action or turn your back to the window nearest you.

Find the center of most resistance. On a ship, get a cabin amidships, where the least amount of rolling and bouncing occurs, advises Dr. Tarnapolsky. On a little boat you may find no such escape, although a forward cabin may be smoother than aft.

Come out from under. Staying cooped up below deck in a boat or ship, especially in a poorly ventilated area, is just asking for trouble, says Dr. Salada. Come out, come out, wherever you are.

Set your sights on something stationary. It'll help get your sensory system back in balance. Standing in a bobbing boat and watching the horizon, however, may make you sick because the horizon will bob along with you. Instead, turn your sights to a stationary point in the sky or the land in the distance.

Take a preventive pill. If motion sickness is as inevitable for you as snow in January, you might want to consider taking an over-the-counter medication like Dramamine or Bonine. Taken a few hours in advance, it can prevent symptoms from occurring in the first place, says Dr. Salada. One or two tablets last for up to 24 hours. But be sure to take it in advance, because it won't be effective if taken once the symptoms start.

Remember, time heals all wounds. And this includes motion sickness. You may feel like you're going to die—in fact, it may sound like a blessing—but motion sickness doesn't kill. Your body will eventually adjust to the environment in a ship or boat—although it might take a few days—and will stop reacting.

So be patient. Things will get better.

PANEL OF ADVISERS

Patricia Cowings, Ph.D., is director of the Psychophysiological Research Laboratory at NASA's Ames Research Center in Moffett Field, California.

Roderic W. Gillilan, O.D., is an optometrist in private practice in Eugene, Oregon, where he specializes in the treatment of motion sickness.

Horst Konrad, M.D., is chairman of the Committee on Equilibrium of the American Academy of Otolaryngology, Head and Neck Surgery, and professor and chairman of the Division of Otolaryngology at Southern Illinois University School of Medicine in Springfield.

Robert Salada, M.D., is director of the Travelers Health Care Center of the University Hospitals of Cleveland, Ohio, a first-of-its-kind service that provides health information and immunizations to travelers and immigrants. He is also assistant professor of medicine at Case Western Reserve University School of Medicine in Cleveland.

Rafael Tarnopolsky, M.D., is a professor of otolaryngology at the University of Osteopathic Medicine and Health Sciences in Des Moines, Iowa.

Muscle Pain

41 Ways to Relief

MAN: I don't understand (as he rubs his cramped calf, then his sore hamstrings, and then his strained shoulder). I exercise *almost* every Saturday. Softball, basketball, touch football. My muscles should be used to that stuff.

ALMOST EVERY MUSCLE IN HIS BODY: Give us a break. You've never met an elevator you didn't like. The only thing we're used to is pain. We should have you arrested for muscle neglect.

Enter Ted Percy, M.D., associate professor of orthopedic surgery and head of the Sports Medicine Section at the University of Arizona College of Medicine, Arizona Health Sciences Center. "Overuse—that's the key word. Doing too much *too soon.*"

WOMAN: I'm supposed to be in great shape. I walk 6 miles every single day. But my legs are killing me!

HER ANGRY LEG MUSCLES: You're killing *us!* You never take a day off. We should have you arrested for muscle abuse.

Enter Dr. Percy. "Overuse—that's the key word. Doing too much *too often.*"

So there you have the most common reasons that you hurt— the terrible trio of too much, too soon, and too often.

Now here are the treatment tips you need to know for those times when your muscles have sentenced you to pain—whether it's a cramp, a strain, or general soreness.

Take it easy. "Every time you exercise, your muscles are injured," says Gabe Mirkin, M.D., sports medicine practitioner at the Sportsmedicine Institute in Silver Spring, Maryland. "It takes 48 hours for muscles to heal from exercise. Soreness means damage, and you should stop exercising when you feel sore."

Of course, you don't have to be running a race or playing a hard tennis match to injure your muscles. Working in the yard, walking around the zoo all day, or simply sitting in an unfamiliar or awkward position, or in the same position for a long time, can cause muscle problems.

How much rest you should give your muscles depends on the severity of the injury and the situation, says Allan Levy, M.D., director of the Department of Sports Medicine at Pascack Valley Hospital in New Jersey.

A cramp may require only minutes of rest, a severe strain may need days or weeks. But sometimes you might not have the luxury of resting the muscle as long as needed. "If you're out hiking, for example, and strain a muscle [which is the same as pulling a muscle], at least rest for a couple of hours, then carefully stretch the muscle" before trying to continue, Dr. Levy advises.

Overall, don't underestimate the value of rest.

Put yourself on ice. It's still the first line of defense against swelling and should be used immediately after injury, says Carol Folkerts, orthopedic coordinator of physical therapy at the University of Maryland Hospital in Baltimore. She recommends using an ice pack or wrapping ice in a towel or plastic bag and applying it for 20 minutes at a time throughout the day.

Keep the ice off the affected area for at least as long as you keep it on. "The ice constricts your blood vessels, and it's not good to constrict your blood vessels too long," Folkerts says. "You could kill the viable tissue in that area." People with heart disease, diabetes, and vascular diseases are especially vulnerable, and "they should use ice with caution and only with the consent of their doctors."

MEDICAL ALERT

When Pain Is a Sign of Disease

A sudden muscle cramp, strain, or even extreme soreness can launch you into the pain galaxy. Sometimes it hurts so badly, you think you'll never come back to earth.

Most of the time, the pain is a lot more serious than the injury. But not always.

Cramping, for example, could be the result of a nerve injury, says Allan Levy, M.D. Or in rare cases, it could be the result of phlebitis—inflammation of a vein. Phlebitis can become serious if a deep vein is involved, but is typically not serious when the inflammation is located in a superficial vein.

A strain may not even be what it seems. "This is very rare," Dr. Levy says, "but I had a patient who thought he had badly strained a thigh muscle on a stationary bike. It didn't ever get better and we finally did surgery. He had a huge malignant tumor in the muscle."

The point here isn't to scare you but to remind you that muscle problems that take on abnormal characteristics and linger *may* be more serious. Consult your doctor.

Get wrapped up in yourself. Don't make a mummy out of that sore calf or strained ankle, but wrap it in an Ace bandage to keep the swelling down. Just be careful, Dr. Levy cautions, not to wrap too tightly, or you could cause swelling below the injured area. Compression may stop cramping, too, but Dr. Levy warns that it's a rather painful approach.

Put your feet up. This is the advice if you've injured your foot or lower leg. Specifically, raise the injured body part higher than your heart to prevent blood from pooling and causing swelling, says Bob Reese, head trainer for the New York Jets and president of the Professional Football Athletic Trainers Society.

Fire up. "After starting the ice, you may switch to heat for acute soreness or strain," Folkerts says. "Typically people like heat better; it's more relaxing. The heat will dilate the blood vessels and promote healing."

Warm baths, whirlpools, and heating pads are all effective temporary pain relievers for soreness, strains, and cramps, but use discretion with heat treatments.

Just remember not to switch from ice to heat too soon, or the injured area may swell. "And you don't have to switch over to heat at all unless you want to," Folkerts says. "You can stay with ice."

Stretch to Strengthen

Give muscles the attention they need, and they tend to do their jobs quietly. Ignore them, and they'll grab your attention—or your leg, or your arm.

When that happens, you may be able to quiet them again with some simple stretching. But if you want them to remain quiet, you probably will have to make stretching a regular part of your life.

Here are a few suggestions from doctors, athletic trainers, and physical therapists to help you keep your attention on work and play, not on muscle pain.

Toe the towel. To stretch and strengthen ankle muscles, sit on the floor and loop a towel around the ball of your foot while holding the ends of the towel in your hands. Alternately point your toes up and down while stretching the towel toward your face and keeping your legs straight. Repeat several times with both feet.

Toe the towel again. Only this time don't move your toes. Lean back with the towel looped around your foot until you feel the stretch in the calf muscle. Hold 15 seconds and repeat several times.

Stand tall. To strengthen calves, stand and slowly raise yourself on your toes, then gradually lower yourself. Do this at least ten times.

Get into bed. Actually, sit with one leg stretched out on the bed and hang the other leg over the side. Then lean forward until you feel the stretch in your hamstring (the back of the thigh) and hold 10 to 15 seconds. Repeat several times, then switch positions and stretch the other hamstring.

Use heat-penetrating rubs carefully. There isn't complete agreement here. "All the heat penetrating rubs are valuable," Dr. Levy says, "because they keep the temperature of the affected area up."

But athletic trainers, for the most part, are less enthusiastic about these popular over-the-counter analgesics. "They can irritate the skin," says Mike McCormick, director of sports medicine at DePaul University. "These rubs give a false sense of security—they warm, but it's surface warmth. They don't get the muscles warm."

Lay on some aspirin-based creams. Also sold over-the-counter, they're an alternative to the heat rubs. "They're greaseless and less likely to irritate your skin, and you won't feel the heat sensation as you would with a lot of other rubs," says McCormick. They work like aspirin, reducing pain and inflammation.

Do the flamingo. To stretch your quadricep (the front of the thigh) muscles, stand on one leg and bend the knee of the opposite leg so that the ankle is touching your buttocks. Hold 10 seconds. Repeat five times with each leg.

Reverse the conventional sit-up. For a safer way to strengthen abdominal muscles, lie back with your arms at your sides or your fingers on your stomach. Then bend your knees and raise them above your chest. Lower your legs slowly while concentrating on your abdominal muscles. Repeat five to ten times.

Reach back. For a good shoulder stretch, place one arm, with elbow bent, behind your head, and using the opposite hand, gently pull your elbow behind your head.

Reach around. Another good shoulder stretch is to hold one arm, with elbow bent, across your midriff and use the opposite hand to gently pull the arm across the front of your body.

Do the keyboard lift. It is important to strengthen those muscles that get a workout on a keyboard all day. Sit at a table and hold a light weight, say 3 to 5 pounds, in your hand with your palm up, your forearm supported on the table, and your wrist over the edge. Lift the weight up slowly, flexing the wrist. Repeat with each wrist 10 to 20 times.

Go palm down. This is another good wrist exercise that's done while sitting down. Do the previous wrist exercise as instructed above, except turn your palm toward the floor. Again, use light weights and repeat 10 to 20 times.

Bring on the A-I team. This is the anti-inflammatory team— "aspirin, ibuprofen—any of the over-the-counter nonsteroidal drugs," says Dr. Percy. "They'll help reduce pain."

S-t-r-e-t-c-h. For cramps and spasms, "gradually stretch the muscle out and you'll get the muscle to relax," says Dr. Levy.

"And stretching exercises can take care of your soreness as it exists now, as well as prevent soreness in the future," McCormick adds. Stretching is important because muscles injured during exercise shorten during the healing process, Dr. Mirkin explains. And unless the muscles are then lengthened, they will remain tight and more likely to be injured or torn. (For instructions on stretching exercises, see "Stretch to Strengthen" above.)

A Nocturnal Cramp in Your Style

You're sleeping soundly, dreaming happily.

"Ouch!! *&%*!" you shout, grabbing your calf, now obviously wide awake in a real-life nightmare of nocturnal leg cramps.

So what happened? Basically, your calf muscle got stuck. Leg muscles contract when you turn or stretch during sleep. When a muscle stays contracted, a sudden cramp can result.

Here's how to stop night cramps and, hopefully, head off a recurrence later in the night.

Grab some wall. Stand 3 to 5 feet away from a wall, keeping your heels flat and your legs straight. Lean into the wall in front of you as you support yourself with your hands. Hold for 10 seconds and repeat several times.

Pet that calf. Massage the calf by "rubbing upward from the ankle toward your heart," advises Carol Folkerts, orthopedic coordinator of physical therapy. If night cramps are a constant problem, you may want to do this before you even try to sleep, she adds.

Loosen the covers. The pressure of heavy blankets on your legs could be partly to blame, says Folkerts.

Wear roomy PJs. Pajamas that fit as snugly as straight-leg blue jeans are the last thing you want to wear to bed.

Electrify your bed. The electric blanket on your bed can do more than keep you warm all over on cold winter nights; it can also keep your calf muscles warm and pain-free, says Folkerts.

Sleep like a baby. Sleeping on your stomach with your legs straight out and your calves flexed invites cramping, says Scott Donkin, D.C. "Try sleeping on your side with your knees bent upward and a pillow between them."

Consider more calcium. "A calcium deficiency can make the muscles trigger-happy; the contractions in the muscles are stronger," Dr. Donkin says. Of course, check with your doctor before making a substantial change in your diet or adding a supplement.

Give your muscles a massage. It would be nice to have a personal masseuse or masseur at your side at all times, and in a way, you do have one—yourself. Just rub gently, and as with exercise, stop if it hurts, Dr. Levy says. You also might want to warm the sore area before massaging it.

Add warm clothing. If you're exercising in cold weather and feel yourself getting stiff and a little sore, warm up by adding more clothes. You may be able to halt muscle problems right there.

"In cold weather we use running tights under players' uniforms to retain the heat," Reese says. "They like the compressive feeling it gives them, and the tights support the muscles a little bit."

Loosen your clothing. But if it's a leg cramp you feel approaching, you may want to shed tights or any other snug clothing to give your muscles a little more room.

Change positions. Whether you're bent over a keyboard typing or bent over a bicycle pedaling, your wrists and forearms are vulnerable to cramping and soreness, says Scott Donkin, D.C., a partner in the Rohrs Chiropractic Center in Lincoln, Nebraska.

But there's one important difference between the cyclist and the office worker—the cyclist always has the opportunity to select the bike that best fits him or her. Yet office workers, who have fingers and hands of all different sizes, typically use the same office equipment.

"The wrist and hands should be used in what is known as the neutral position," according to Dr. Donkin. "In this position, the wrist is bent neither forward, backward, inward, nor outward.

If you have long hands and fingers, you can reduce the strain by adjusting the keyboard to a more horizontal position (flat with the work surface) as long as it does not put your arms or shoulders in a strained position.

For those who have short hands and fingers, a higher incline on the keyboard, typewriter, or calculator will make the keys easier to reach.

Stand up. It's simple, and perhaps that is all it will take to stop a cramp in the leg or foot, Dr. Levy says.

Repeat the activity that made you sore the very next day. Say what? "Do the activity again the very next day," Reese says, "but with much less intensity. It will help work out some of the soreness."

Then continue to follow a hard-easy/hard-easy work-out pattern. This is advisable because of the 48 hours needed for muscles to recover, says Dr. Mirkin. "All serious athletes train that way."

Branch out. This is perhaps an even better idea than the hard-easy routine, Dr. Mirkin says. If you're a walker suffering sore lower leg muscles, he suggests mixing in some swimming or bicycling (which works the upper legs) so you can continue exercising while healing.

Lose weight. If sore muscles and muscle strains have become a chronic problem, the extra weight you're asking them to move may be at least partially to blame.

Accept the truth. If running always makes you hurt, for example, then you may have to find another exercise. "Running is one of the most dangerous sports for injuries," Dr. Mirkin says.

Slow down instead of stopping suddenly. After hard exercise or physical work, the bloodstream is loaded with lactic acid, which collects in the bloodstream when there is a lack of oxygen, explains Dr. Mirkin. When the acid reaches high levels, it disrupts normal chemical reactions of the muscles and can make your muscles hurt.

"The most effective way to clear the bloodstream is to continue exercising at a slow, relaxed pace," Dr. Mirkin advises, adding that this may lessen immediate soreness but that it won't protect you from soreness the next day. That soreness, he says, is caused by torn muscle fiber.

Change your shoes. If you're wearing the wrong kind of shoes or wearing shoes that don't fit well, that could explain the foot, leg, and even back pains you're feeling while exercising, says McCormick.

Strengthen yourself. Weak muscles could be as much to blame for chronic strains as inflexibility. While men are more likely than women to be inflexible, "We tend to stress that women often need to gain strength. We stress to both men and women the need to develop strength and flexibility," McCormick says. (See "Stretch to Strengthen" on page 436 for suggested strengthening exercises.)

Be patient. The more serious the injury—a severely pulled hamstring, for example—the more of this virtue you will need to ensure a relapse-free recovery.

Drink up. Dehydration is often a big contributor to cramping, says McCormick. "We overstress the need to force liquids, especially before, during, and after physical activity. And for good reason."

PANEL OF ADVISERS

Scott Donkin, D.C., is a partner in the Rohrs Chiropractic Center in Lincoln, Nebraska. He is also an industrial consultant, providing tips on exercise to reduce stress for workstation users, and author of *Sitting on the Job.*

Carol Folkerts is orthopedic coordinator of physical therapy at the University of Maryland Hospital in Baltimore.

Allan Levy, M.D., is director of the Department of Sports Medicine at Pascack Valley Hospital in New Jersey. He also is team physician for the New York Giants football team and the New Jersey Nets basketball team.

Mike McCormick is director of sports medicine at DePaul University in Chicago, Illinois, and a certified athletic trainer.

Gabe Mirkin, M.D., is in private practice at the Sportsmedicine Institute in Silver Spring, Maryland. He is also associate clinical professor of pediatrics at the Georgetown University School of Medicine in Washington, D.C. He is the author of several sports medicine books, including *Dr. Gabe Mirkin's Fitness Clinic,* and is a syndicated newspaper columnist and radio broadcaster.

Ted Percy, M.D., is associate professor of orthopedic surgery and head of the Sports Medicine Section at the University of Arizona College of Medicine, Arizona Health Sciences Center in Tucson.

Bob Reese is head trainer for the New York Jets and president of the Professional Football Athletic Trainers Society.

Nausea

10 Stomach-Soothing Solutions

We took a survey of things that make tummies quiver and quake. In just half an hour we coughed up eggs, egg salad, eggs sunny-side up, needles, giving blood, seeing blood, hospital smells, hair in your food, bus exhaust, credit card bills, day-old grits, cooked carrots, Christmas morning anxiety, road kill, a graphic description of plastic surgery, greasy hamburger smells, "tee many martoonies," cigarette butts floating in a

---

MEDICAL ALERT

It Could Be Almost Anything

"There are at least 25 different diseases that could cause chronic nausea," says gastroenterologist Kenneth Koch, M.D. If your nausea just doesn't go away in a day or two, it's a good idea to see your doctor.

---

coffee cup, frying bacon, muck at the bottom of an old leaf pile, the smell of roasting chestnuts on the streets of New York City, a well-filled diaper, cat hairballs, bad fish, and other people being nauseous.

So, how's your tummy, *hmmmm?* Are you a little queasy? What's that lump in your throat? Do you wish the world would end—and quickly? Well, don't worry. We've got some home remedies that will denauseate your tummy before you can say "tapeworm sandwich."

As beauty is in the eye of the beholder, so nausea is in the tummy of the nauseated. So, too, are the remedies. Keep trying until you find the one that works for you.

Let's get syrupy about it. If you're not *that* nauseated, "Coke syrup is something we use that seems to work real well," says pharmacist Robert Warren, Pharm.D., who heads Pharmacy Services at Valley Children's Hospital in Fresno, California. The noncarbonated syrup has concentrated carbohydrates that may help settle the stomach. In fact, Dr. Warren says, any soft drink liquid concentrate or even plain sugar syrup may help. The dose is 1 to 2 tablespoons for adults, at room temperature, as needed, and 1 to 2 teaspoons for children.

Or go for the uncola. Emetrol is "an over-the-counter product that works the same way as Coke syrup," Dr. Warren says, but is more expensive and without caffeine. It's a phosphorated carbohydrate solution containing the sugars glucose and fructose, and phosphoric acid.

Go for Bonine. These high-sugar syrups, however, are not for diabetics or for anyone who wants to avoid the calories. Instead, Dr. Warren says, an alternative is Bonine, a chewable antihistamine tablet with no sugar. Bonine is a motion sickness drug that works on your stomach. (Dramamine, another motion sickness medication, isn't effective against other kinds of nausea because it works on your inner ear.) As with any drug, be sure to read the precautions on the label first.

Keep it all clear down below. If you want food, stick to clear liquids like tea and juices, says nausea researcher Kenneth Koch, M.D., a gastroenterologist at Pennsylvania State University's Hershey Medical Center. These liquids should be warm or room temperature, not cold, to avoid further shock to your stomach. Drink no more than 1 or 2 ounces at a time.

Make it flat. "My mom used to give me 7-Up," Dr. Warren says. Other moms gave cola or ginger ale. Since our experts advise against cold beverages and carbonated ones, do as Stephen Bezruchka, M.D., an emergency physician at Providence Medical Center in Seattle, Washington, suggests. Let carbonated drinks stand until flat and lukewarm.

Eat carbos first. If you need something to eat, and your nausea isn't too bad, eat light carbohydrates in small amounts—toast or crackers, for instance, Dr. Koch says. As your tummy de-nauseates, graduate to light protein, like chicken breast or fish. Fatty foods are the last thing to add to your diet.

The Alternate Route

Press Your Luck

The Chinese have known for centuries that acupuncture is an effective, painless, drugless medication. Acupressure is needle-less acupuncture. "The idea is to use it before you start vomiting," says acupuncturist Joseph M. Helms, M.D., a family practitioner in Berkeley, California. Who knows, this method might work for you.

Apply pressure to the webbing between your thumb and index finger on either hand. Use firm, deep pressure and a rapid massaging movement for several minutes, Dr. Helms says. "I don't mean caress it."

Using the same kind of motion and pressure, Dr. Helms says, rub with your thumb or thumbnail on the top of your foot between the tendons of the second and third toes.

Get out of the pink. The stomach soother Pepto-Bismol and others such as Mylanta and Maalox are for disease-provoked stomach upsets, not for a queasy stomach. However, if your nausea is caused by inflammation or irritation, and if it's not too severe, Dr. Koch says, "they're reasonable to start with." But none of our experts wholeheartedly recommend them, because, as Samuel Klein, M.D., an assistant professor of gastroenterology at the University of Texas Medical School at Galveston notes, "none of them is specifically designed for nausea." And they're far from being the clear liquids doctors favor.

Try the ginger cure. Daniel B. Mowrey, Ph.D., a psychologist and psychopharmacologist in Lehi, Utah, who has been researching herbal medicine for 15 years, swears by gingerroot. "It will definitely take care of nausea," he says. Take capsules of the powdered root; the amount depends on how nauseated you are. "You know you've had enough when you burp and taste ginger," he says.

Make sure it's capsulized. Fresh ginger is too strong for most people in the amounts you have to take to get the same effect as with powder, Dr. Mowrey says. Ginger ale or ginger snaps may work if your symptoms are very mild.

End it all. One of the most effective ways to stop nausea is to allow yourself to vomit, Dr. Koch says. The nausea leaves you immediately, and maybe just one good upchuck will take care of it for good. At the very least you'll have a temporary respite from that queasy feeling. He doesn't, however, recommend *making* yourself vomit.

PANEL OF ADVISERS

Stephen Bezruchka, M.D., is an emergency physician at Providence Medical Center in Seattle, Washington, and author of *The Pocket Doctor.*

Joseph M. Helms, M.D., is a family practitioner in Berkeley, California, and is president of the American Academy of Medical Acupuncture.

Samuel Klein, M.D., is assistant professor of gastroenterology and human nutrition at the University of Texas Medical School at Galveston. He is also an editorial adviser to *Prevention* magazine.

Kenneth Koch, M.D., is a gastroenterologist at Pennsylvania State University's Hershey Medical Center and a leading researcher for NASA into the causes of nausea.

Daniel B. Mowrey, Ph.D., of Lehi, Utah, is a psychologist and psychopharmacologist who has been researching the use of herbs in medicine for 15 years. He is author of *The Scientific Validation of Herbal Medicine* and *Next Generation Herbal Medicine.*

Robert Warren, Pharm.D., is director of Pharmacy Services at Valley Children's Hospital in Fresno, California.

Neck Pain

24 Ways to Get the Kinks Out

Maybe you have a boss, or a brother-in-law, whom you describe as a pain in the neck. But when it comes to neck pain, the blame—as well as the pain—is probably resting on your shoulders.

"It's keeping your head in an awkward position—that is, pushed forward with your ears in front of your shoulders—for a long time that makes your neck hurt," says Joanne Griffin, senior physical therapist and inpatient headache treatment therapist at the New England Center for Headache at Greenwich Hospital in Connecticut. "That's what many people who have neck problems are doing."

Naturally, some people—because of their occupations—are more at risk than others. "Beauticians, for example, work in a bent-over position all day long," says Robert Kunkel, M.D., head of the Section of Headache in the Department of Internal Medicine at the Cleveland Clinic in Ohio.

Regardless of your job or lifestyle, you can rid yourself of blame —and more importantly, pain—by applying a few time-tested methods, replacing bad habits with good ones, and giving your neck regular exercise. So keep your head up and your eyes open. Help is on the way.

Ice down. An ice pack or ice wrapped in a towel is a good choice when stiffness is just settling in, Griffin says. If your neck has been slightly injured, ice can help hold down swelling.

Heat up. After ice has reduced any inflammation, heat is a wonderful soother—be it from a heating pad or a hot shower.

Use a heat rub. These over-the-counter ointments are soothing but have no real healing effect because they don't really penetrate the skin's surface, says Steve Antonopulos, head athletic trainer for the Denver Broncos football team. Never use them with heating pads, he adds. At best they provide "psychological benefit."

Exercise Away Neck Pain

Yes, even your neck muscles need to be stretched and strengthened. Here are some exercises to combat stiffness and prevent problems in the future. Do each five times twice a day. Do the first three exercises for two weeks before starting the rest.

- Slowly tilt your head forward as far as possible. Then move your head backward as far as possible.
- Tilt your head toward your shoulder, while keeping your shoulder stationary. Straighten, then lean toward the other shoulder.
- Slowly turn your head from side to side as far as possible.
- Place your hand on one side of your head while you push toward it with your head. Hold for 5 seconds, then relax. Repeat three times. Then do the same exercise on the other side.
- Do basically the same exercise as above, only provide slight resistance to the front of your head while you push your head forward. Then provide slight resistance to the back of your head while you push your head backward.
- Hold light weights—say 3 to 5 pounds—in your hands while shrugging your shoulders. Keep your arms straight.

Take the old standby. Over-the-counter anti-inflammatories such as aspirin or ibuprofen will help reduce pain and inflammation. Take two pills three or four times a day.

Sit in a firm chair. Like the song says, the backbone is connected to the neck bone. And if you sit in a chair that doesn't give you good back support, you increase your chances of worsening existing neck problems and causing new ones, says Mitchell A. Price, D.C., a chiropractor in Temple, Pennsylvania.

Throw in the towel. Actually, roll a towel up and place it against the small of your back when sitting—it will better align your spine and give you additional support, says Griffin.

Take a break. Just as the feet need rest from constant standing, the neck needs a rest from constant sitting. Your head weighs approximately 8 pounds, Griffin says, and that's a lot of weight for the neck to support without much help from the rest of your body. So periodically stand up and walk around.

Keep your chin up. Keep your head level but pull your chin in, as if you were making a double chin, says Griffin. Also avoid having your head lowered all the time when working at a desk or reading, she advises. This will prevent stressing the muscles in the back of the neck.

See eye to screen. If you work with a video display terminal all day, it's important to have it positioned at eye level. If you force yourself to look up or down hour after hour, you may cause your neck to spasm, says Price.

Reach out. And consider putting down the telephone. If you talk on the phone a lot, especially while trying to write, you've got your neck in an awkward position—an invitation to stiffness and pain.

Lift carefully. It's all too easy to forget there's a right way and a wrong way to lift heavy objects. The right way, says Price, is to bend your knees and hold your spine erect while positioning the object between your feet, which should be shoulder-width apart. When you lift the object, keep it as close to your body as possible.

Sleep on a firm mattress. A lot of neck problems begin, and worsen, with poor sleeping habits. Having a firm mattress is important, Price says.

Don't fight with your pillow. Just toss it aside. "A lot of people with neck pain feel better sleeping flat—without a pillow," Dr. Kunkel says.

MEDICAL ALERT

Whiplash Needs a Doctor's Care

If you have been in an auto accident and have severe neck pain afterward, you may have whiplash and should see a doctor, advises Mitchell A. Price, D.C. In the meantime, he suggests treating with ice instead of heat because heat could inflame the injured area.

As a general rule, persistent neck pain warrants professional medical evaluation. "It's extremely remote, but it's possible that neck pain could be a signal that there's a tumor on the spine," says physical therapist Joanne Griffin.

Or get a cervical pillow. These pillows, which can be bought for as little as $20 in discount stores, give the neck proper support, Price says.

Don't sleep on your stomach. This is not only bad for your back, but your neck, too, says Price.

Sleep like a baby. In other words, sleep in the fetal position — on your side with your knees up toward your chest, Price advises.

Wrap up. When it's cold and damp outside, you probably wear a hat. But you should cover your neck as well. The weather can aggravate neck stiffness and pain, Dr. Kunkel says.

Relax. Just being tense can tighten the muscles in your neck and put you in pain. If you're under a lot of pressure or feel tense a lot, learning relaxation techniques, such as meditation or progressive relaxation, can help. Also, audiotapes are available to teach you how to relax.

PANEL OF ADVISERS

Steve Antonopulos is head athletic trainer for the Denver Broncos football team.

Joanne Griffin is senior physical therapist and inpatient heachache treatment therapist in the New England Center for Headache at Greenwich Hospital in Connecticut.

Robert Kunkel, M.D., is head of the Section of Headache in the Department of Internal Medicine at the Cleveland Clinic in Ohio. He also is vice president of the National Headache Foundation.

Mitchell A. Price, D.C., is a chiropractor in private practice in Temple, Pennsylvania.

Night Blindness

11 Ways to Deal with the Dark

Walk out of bright sunlight and into a dark movie theater and suddenly you can hardly recognize the person who walked in with you. "Everybody is night-blind momentarily in such a situation. That is, it takes a moment for the retina to adjust to the difference in light," explains Alan Laties, M.D., a professor of ophthalmology at the Scheie Eye Institute of the University of Pennsylvania Medical School.

But for some people night blindness is more than momentary. "Some people are quicker to adapt to light changes and darkness," Dr. Laties says. "Nearsighted people can at times be slower to adapt to the dark. And other people simply can't see in the dark. I can name several different reasons for this." For example, some people—though this is rather uncommon—have what is known as congenital stationary night blindness; they're born with the problem. "That's just the way the person was made," Dr. Laties says. "There's no danger to the eye."

Unfortunately, doctors don't have a bag of ready-to-issue cures for night blindness. But if you don't see well at night and your doctor has ruled out an eye disorder as the reason, here are a couple of ideas to consider, as well as good, practical advice for driving safely at night.

Do a self-evaluation. "Many people have enormous concern about their eyes," Dr. Laties says. "They are afraid of going blind." He says most people can reassure themselves that their night vision is all right. "After 5 minutes in a movie theater you should be able to see the person next to you."

Make sure you're getting vitamin A. This nutrient is important to night vision. In fact, large doses of vitamin A given to a person who is vitamin A deficient can bring improvement in night vision within hours, says Creig Hoyt, M.D., vice chairman of the Department of Ophthalmology at the University of California, San Francisco Medical Center.

449

MEDICAL ALERT

Leave Diagnosis to Your Doctor

Occasionally, night blindness can be an early symptom of a progressive eye disease. One example is retinitis pigmentosa (RP), which affects an estimated 100,000 people in the United States, according to Jill C. Hennessey, M.S., assistant to the director of science at the RP Foundation Fighting Blindness in Baltimore, Maryland.

"At this point," Hennessey says, "there's no known effective treatment." RP tends to run in families and the cause of the disease is also a mystery. It can eventually lead to blindness.

If you're having problems with night vision, you should have your eyes examined by an ophthalmologist, advises Alan Laties, M.D. It's the best way to protect your vision.

However, vitamin A deficiency is rare in the United States, Dr. Hoyt says, adding that high-level vitamin A supplementation should first be approved by a doctor.

When driving at night, do everything you can to increase visibility. On a clear day, from the driver's seat, you're usually looking about 1,200 to 1,500 feet down a straight road, says Quinn Brackett, Ph.D., a research scientist at the Texas Transportation Institute, Texas A&M University.

But at night, under good conditions and with only your headlights as your guide, you can only see 300 to 400 feet. So it's important to give yourself every advantage. "Make sure your headlights are cleaned off," says Charles Zegeer, senior staff associate at the University of North Carolina at Chapel Hill, Highway Safety Research Center. "Dirty headlights really reduce visibility" and will only make an already bad problem worse.

Don't wear sunglasses at dusk, either—no matter how stylish they may be—because they will further reduce light coming into your eyes, says Dr. Brackett.

Slow down. That way, you give yourself more time to react to any unexpected hazards.

Get a Pair of Night Glasses

Owls, famous for their nocturnal nature, have very good night vision. People, even the "night owls" of the human species, aren't so blessed. But that doesn't make improving night vision impossible. Millions of people take advantage of glasses to improve their vision, and there's no reason why glasses can't improve night myopia (defective night vision, especially of distant objects), says Creig Hoyt, M.D.

"Pilots will tell you they have more trouble seeing runways at night, and they will wear a different prescription at night," Dr. Hoyt says. So what works for a pilot trying to land a plane on a narrow strip of pavement ought to help you keep your car in the driveway and out of the front yard.

Consider, Dr. Hoyt says, wearing a stronger prescription at night or getting glasses for night driving even if you currently don't wear glasses during the day.

Expect the unexpected. These days the roads don't belong just to cars, but to walkers, runners, and cyclists as well. "And wearing white at night isn't enough to be visible," Zegeer says. So it's your responsibility to watch for pedestrians.

Respect rain and fog. These two conditions make night driving especially dangerous, Zegeer says. He recommends keeping your headlights on low beam in fog for better visibility.

Plan ahead. Careful route planning can make night driving easier. "When possible," says Brackett, "select roads that are divided or have very little traffic."

Don't take chances. If fog or travel conditions become too bad, says Zegeer, pull off at a rest area, service station, or parking lot. Stay off the shoulder of the road.

Look to the right. "Look at the roadway's edge to the right to help you avoid the glare of oncoming headlights," Brackett suggests.

Leave the driving till tomorrow. Drive only during the day. Even good lighting conditions at night, such as found in a big city, can be troublesome to someone with night blindness.

Nosebleed

17 Hints to Stop the Flow

There's nothing like a nosebleed to give you some idea about the sheer quantity of blood you routinely carry around in your head. Vast amounts circulate through capillaries in the nose alone.

Even Holden Caulfield, the memorable cynic of *The Catcher in the Rye,* knew enough to be impressed. The knockout punch his roommate delivered to his nose didn't dazzle him half as much as the sight of blood streaming down his face.

"You never saw such gore in your life," said the mouthy young hero. "I had blood all over my mouth and chin and even on my pajamas and bathrobe. It partly scared me and it partly fascinated me. All that blood and all sort of made me look tough."

Tough guy that he was, Caulfield picked an unusual home remedy: a game of canasta with Ackley next door. Our experts have more practical ideas.

The tips they give can help almost any nosebleed—whether it's from a nose made brittle by winter dryness, a side effect of high blood pressure or atherosclerosis, or a curious child putting a finger where it doesn't belong.

MEDICAL ALERT

When Your Nosebleed Needs a Doctor

You've packed your nose with cotton, applied pressure, and waited the allotted time. But you're still bleeding.

What do you do next? Go to an emergency room or head straight to your doctor's office. Nosebleeds can kill you if they go on long enough. In rare instances, continuous bleeding indicates the presence of a tumor.

If you're a senior citizen and you've got hardening of the arteries, you won't want to wait more than 10 minutes before you seek a physician's help.

Also head to the emergency room if you find yourself bleeding from the back of the nose. That's probably the case if you pack your nose and find the blood running down the back of your throat. Posterior nosebleeds often have to be packed through the mouth and require professional skill to do it right.

Blow the clot out. Before you try to stop your nosebleed, give your nose "one good, vigorous blow," says Alvin Katz, M.D., an otolaryngologist in private practice in New York City and surgeon director at the Manhattan Eye, Ear, Nose, and Throat Hospital. That removes any clots that are keeping the blood vessel open. A clot acts like a "wedge in the door," explains Dr. Katz. "Blood vessels have elastic fibers. If you can get the clot out, you can get the elastic fibers to contract around that tiny opening."

This "really, really helps," adds John A. Henderson, M.D., a San Diego otolaryngologist and allergist and assistant clinical professor of surgery at the University of California, San Diego, School of Medicine. "It saves you a lot of nonsense."

Sometimes, blowing the nose and applying a little pressure is enough to stop the bleeding pronto.

Plug the bleeding side with wet cotton. What do you wet the cotton with? Several of our experts mentioned over-the-counter decongestants like Neo-Synephrine and Afrin Nasal Spray.

But Jerold Principato, M.D., an otolaryngologist in private practice in Bethesda, Maryland, and associate clinical professor of otolaryngology at George Washington University School of Medicine and Health Sciences, favors white vinegar. The acid in the vinegar cauterizes gently, he says. Decongestants give only temporary control; if you abuse them, you can hurt the nasal lining.

Plain gauze works, too. If you don't have cotton handy, use plain sterile gauze, says Christine Haycock, M.D., a private practitioner in Newark, New Jersey, and professor of clinical surgery at the University of Medicine and Dentistry of New Jersey/New Jersey Medical School. Wet the gauze before putting it in your nose. (When it's time to take it out, cup your hands together, fill them with water, and wet the gauze. This should loosen it enough to take it out.)

Pinch the fleshy part of your nose. As soon as you've blown your nose and packed it with cotton or gauze, use your thumb and forefinger to squeeze shut the soft part of the nose. Apply continuous pressure for 5 to 7 minutes. If the bleeding doesn't stop, apply fresh packing and pinch again for another 5 to 7 minutes. The bleeding should stop by the time you're through.

"Leave the cotton in another 20 minutes before you take it out," advises Mark Baldree, M.D., a Phoenix, Arizona, otolaryngologist and staff member in the Division of Otolaryngology, Department of Surgery, at St. Joseph's Hospital there.

Sit up straight. If you lie down or put your head back, you'll just swallow blood, says Dr. Katz.

Try an ice pack. "Sometimes an ice pack can help quite a bit," says Dr. Haycock. The cold encourages the blood vessels to narrow and reduces bleeding.

Don't pick. It takes seven to ten days to completely heal the rupture in the blood vessel that caused your nose to bleed. Bleeding stops after the clot forms, but the clot becomes a scab as healing continues. If you pick your nose during the next week and knock the scab off, you'll give yourself another nosebleed, says Dr. Principato.

Apply an antibiotic/steroid ointment. "If you apply a little bit inside your nose two or three times a day, it will destroy any staph bacteria," says Gilbert Levitt, M.D., a Puget Sound, Washington, otolaryngologist and clinical instructor of otolaryngology at the University of Washington School of Medicine. This will stop the itching and prevent the crusting of mucus that might tempt you to pick.

The Ringside Remedy

In a professional boxing match, you've got exactly 1 minute between rounds to stop a nosebleed.

Angelo Dundee, a Miami Beach, Florida, trainer to 11 world champion boxers, including Muhammad Ali and Sugar Ray Leonard, has his technique down pat.

What does he do?

"You don't ever put a Q-Tip up there," says Dundee. "I take a piece of cotton and make a wick out of it. I dip it into Adrenaline 1:1000 and screw it into the nasal passage. Then I put pressure on that side of the nose.

"If you've got bleeding on both sides, I screw a cotton wick into each nostril and tell the kid, 'Breathe from your mouth and give the blood a shot to congeal.' Then I'll take a gauze pad and squeeze hard on the dead meat right in the middle of the nose. You know, the place where the nostrils meet down at the bottom of the nose? You can press as hard as you want. It won't hurt. That seems to stop it."

Adrenaline 1:1000 is available by prescription only. Its primary ingredient is epinephrine, which is also a component of several OTC nasal products.

Take iron. If you're prone to nosebleeds, consider iron supplements to help your body rapidly replace the blood supply, says Dr. Levitt. Iron is a vital component of hemoglobin, a key substance in red blood cells.

Watch your aspirin intake. Aspirin can interfere with clotting. If you're prone to nosebleeds, experts advise that you not take unnecessary aspirin.

Watch your salicylate intake, too. Dr. Henderson advises his patients to avoid foods high in salicylates, an aspirinlike substance found in coffee, tea, most fruits, and some vegetables. Foods on that list include almonds, apples, apricots, all berries, mint, cloves, cherries, currants, grapes, raisins, oil of wintergreen, bell peppers, peaches, plums, tangelos, tomatoes, cucumbers, and pickles.

Control your blood pressure. Folks with hypertension are nosebleed prone. So follow a low-fat, low-cholesterol diet, says Dr. Levitt. "If you have hypertension and a blood vessel breaks, better that it should break outside the cranial cavity than inside. That would cause a stroke. It's like God gave us a pop-off valve."

Humidify the air. When you breathe, your nose has to work to make sure that the air that reaches your lungs is well humidified. So it follows that when your surroundings are dry, your nose has to work harder. A good room humidifier, particularly one that takes several gallons to fill, can help.

Dr. Katz recommends that you fill the humidifier with distilled water to protect yourself from impurities in tap water. Also, be sure to clean the unit properly, according to the manufacturer's instructions, at least once a week. Fill it with equal parts of water and vinegar and run it for 20 minutes.

Get your fair share of vitamin C. Vitamin C is necessary for the formation of collagen, a substance essential to the health of your body tissue, says Dr. Henderson. The collagen in the tissue of your upper respiratory tract helps mucus stick where it's supposed to, creating a moist, protective lining for your sinuses and nose.

Be careful in choosing oral contraceptives. Estrogen influences mucus production. Anything that changes the estrogen balance in your body—including menstruation, for women—can make you more prone to nosebleeds. Certain oral contraceptives also alter the balance. If nosebleeds are a problem for you, be sure to discuss this with your doctor when you choose your birth control pill.

Don't smoke. You want to keep the nasal cavity moist. Smoking really dries it out, says Dr. Baldree.

PANEL OF ADVISERS

Mark Baldree, M.D., is an otolaryngologist in private practice in Phoenix, Arizona. He is a staff member in the Division of Otolaryngology, Department of Surgery, at St. Joseph's Hospital in Phoenix.

Angelo Dundee, of Miami Beach, Florida, is a boxing trainer and has been a trainer for 11 World Heavyweight boxing champions, including Muhammad Ali and Sugar Ray Leonard.

Christine Haycock, M.D., maintains a private practice in Newark, New Jersey. She is a professor of clinical surgery at the University of Medicine and Dentistry of New Jersey/New Jersey Medical School in Newark.

John A. Henderson, M.D., is an otolaryngologist and allergist in private practice in San Diego, California. He is also assistant clinical professor of surgery at the University of California, San Diego, School of Medicine.

Alvin Katz, M.D., is an otolaryngologist in private practice in New York City and surgeon director of the Manhattan Eye, Ear, Nose, and Throat Hospital there. He is past president of the American Rhinologic Society.

Gilbert Levitt, M.D., is an otolaryngologist in practice with Group Health Cooperative in Puget Sound, Washington. He is also clinical instructor of otolaryngology at the University of Washington School of Medicine in Seattle.

Jerold Principato, M.D., is an otolaryngologist in private practice in Bethesda, Maryland. He is associate clinical professor of otolaryngology in the Department of Surgery at George Washington University School of Medicine and Health Sciences in Washington, D.C. He is also an instructor at the American Academy of Otolaryngology.

Oily Hair

16 Neutralizing Solutions

You spent a good 20 minutes in the trenches this morning, blow dryer in one hand, styling gel in the other, trying to whip those recalcitrant locks into shape.

By noon, you knew you had lost the battle. One glance in the mirror and your spirits fell as flat as your hairstyle. That oil factory you call your scalp just doesn't know when to stop.

What's going on?

It could be that you have too much hair. The finer your hair, the more hair you have per square inch of scalp. And at the base of each hair shaft are sebaceous glands, which produce sebum, the fatty "oil" in oily hair. The more hair, the more oil glands, and the more oil glands, the more oil. Those with fine hair have as many as 140,000 oil glands on their scalps, according to Philip Kingsley, a New York City and London hair care specialist.

Redheads, who average 80,000 to 90,000 hairs per head, rarely have oily hair, he says. Blondes with silky, baby-fine hair tend to have the worst problems with oiliness.

"The texture of your hair does make a difference. Oil wicks onto fine, straight hair very easily. But wiry hair doesn't seem oily. It has a lot to do with perception," says Thomas Goodman, Jr., M.D., Memphis dermatologist and assistant professor of dermatology at the University of Tennessee Center for Health Sciences.

Intense heat and humidity can also accelerate oil production.

So can hormonal changes. Androgen, a male hormone, can activate the sebaceous glands. Stress boosts bloodstream levels of androgen in women as well as in men.

But androgen isn't the only factor that makes oily hair more of a problem for men. Men tend to have finer hair than women, says Kingsley. They average 311 hairs per square centimeter of scalp, as opposed to 278 for the average woman. "That's a significant 10 to 15 percent difference," says Kingsley.

What can you do about the oil factory in your scalp? Here's what our experts advise.

Shampoo frequently. Our experts agree that the most important thing you can do to combat an excessively oily scalp is to shampoo once a day, particularly if you live in a city environment. When summer heat and humidity stimulate your scalp's oil glands, shampooing twice a day may be advisable, says Lowell Goldsmith, M.D., a professor of dermatology and chairman of the Department of Dermatology at the University of Rochester School of Medicine and Dentistry who specializes in hair disorders.

"The sebaceous glands are producing oil continuously," he says. "What you're essentially trying to do is keep up with the secretion and remove it."

Choose a see-through shampoo. "Clear, see-through shampoos tend to have less goo in them," says Dr. Goodman. "They clean away oil better, without leaving a residue behind."

Give yourself a scalp massage. This should be done during the shampoo, never between shampoos, says Kingsley. "Massaging the scalp between shampoos may squeeze a little bit of extra oil out."

Bubble double. Excessively oily hair may need to be shampooed twice, says Dr. Goldsmith. "The most common mistake I see is that people don't leave the shampoo on long enough," he says. "For people with especially oily hair or scalp, I suggest a double shampoo, leaving the shampoo on the scalp for 5 minutes each time. This won't harm the hair or scalp."

Get out of condition. If you have oily hair that tends to flatten out as the day goes on, the last thing you want to do is coat it with more oil. Try going without a conditioner, suggests Dr. Goodman.

Just aim for the ends. If you find you do need a conditioner, look for a product that contains the least amount of oil or one that is largely oil-free. Condition the ends instead of the roots.

Test for oil after shampooing. "Each amount of shampoo can only take away so much oil," says Dr. Goldsmith. "So don't skimp on the shampoo. Test yourself. After you shampoo and dry your hair, does it still feel oily? If it does, you haven't cleaned it well enough."

Apply astringent to the scalp. You can help slow down oil secretion by applying a homemade astringent directly to your scalp. Kingsley suggests applying a mixture of equal parts witch hazel and mouthwash, with cotton pads, to the scalp only. The witch hazel acts as an astringent and the mouthwash has antiseptic properties, he says. If your scalp is very oily you can do this each time you shampoo.

Don't overbrush. "People with oily hair have to be extra careful not to be overly vigorous with brushing," says Dr. Goldsmith. Be aware that brushing from the roots carries oil from your scalp to the ends of your hair.

Ask your stylist to cut body into your hair. Beat the straight, matted-down hair blues by asking your stylist to cut body into your hair. "I cut from underneath, to help make the style stand up," says David Daines, owner of the David Daines Salon in New York City. "Make sure there are different lengths on top of the head. Don't wear your hair long and one length unless you don't mind having it lie flat on your head."

Dry hair in the opposite direction from which it grows. Left on its own, oily hair tends to be limp and lank. To coax more fullness into it, be creative with your blow-drying technique, says Kingsley. Use a brush to lift the hair up at the roots, or bend forward at the waist and gently brush your hair up over the top of your head.

Learn to relax. Hormones have a little-understood effect on oil production. What is known is this: When you're under stress, your body produces more androgens. And androgens help boost oil production, says Kingsley. His advice? Relaxation techniques can help.

Consider your birth control pill. Birth control pills have a decided effect on a woman's hormone balance. That in turn affects oil production. Dr. Goodman suggests that you discuss excessively oily hair with your gynecologist when you choose your oral contraceptive.

Switch to beer. "Mousse dries the hair too much and clogs the pores," says Daines. He favors fresh beer as a setting lotion for oily hair. Store it in a closed plastic container in your shower, otherwise it will only keep for a couple of days.

Freshen up with lemon. Squeeze the juice of two lemons into a quart of the best water you can find, says Daines. Distilled water is a great choice. "This is a great rinse" to help cut oiliness.

Try an apple cider vinegar rinse. Try a teaspoon of vinegar in a pint of water and use as a finishing rinse. This solution acts as a tonic for the scalp and removes soap residue that can weigh down oily hair.

PANEL OF ADVISERS

David Daines is owner of the David Daines Salon in New York City.

Lowell Goldsmith, M.D., is professor of dermatology and chairman of the Department of Dermatology at the University of Rochester School of Medicine and Dentistry in New York. He specializes in hair disorders.

Thomas Goodman, Jr., M.D., is a dermatologist in private practice and assistant professor of dermatology at the University of Tennessee Center for Health Sciences in Memphis. He is author of *Smart Face* and *The Skin Doctor's Skin Doctoring Book*.

Philip Kingsley is a trained trichologist (hair care specialist) who maintains salons in New York City and London. He is author of *The Complete Hair Book*.

Oily Skin

7 Restoratives for a Happier Face

It's not your fault, really. If you've got to blame someone, blame your ancestors. Chances are they came from someplace where oily skin served a useful purpose, such as combating the effects of excessive Mediterranean sunlight or monsoon rains. Now you're stuck with oily skin in the middle of Minnesota, where the embarrassment of a shiny forehead outweighs any possible protection your skin might afford you from scorching rays or tropical torrents.

Heredity does play a big part in oily skin, but so do hormones. Pregnant women sometimes notice an increase in skin oil as hormonal activity changes. So do women taking certain types of birth control pills. Stress can also cause the oil glands to kick into overdrive. The wrong cosmetics can easily aggravate an otherwise mild case of oily skin. Some of these causes are within your ability to control, but others you'll have to learn to live with.

There is no magic cure for oily skin. State-of-the-art advice from the experts calls for keeping it clean, and keeping at it all the time. Our tips will help you do that as well as it can be done.

On the up side, skin experts believe there are some advantages to having an oily hide, not the least of which becomes apparent with the steady passing of time. That is, oily skin tends to age better and wrinkle less than dry or normal skin. Today's curse; tomorrow's blessing.

Make mine mud. "Clay masks or mud masks are worthwhile," says Howard Donsky, M.D., an associate professor of medicine at the University of Toronto and staff dermatologist at Toronto General Hospital. But Dr. Donsky cautions that masks will make skin feel good and look better only temporarily, so don't count on the effects lasting for any length of time.

Generally, the darker brown the clay (mud), the more oil it can absorb. White or rose-colored clays, though, are gentler and work best on sensitive skin.

Masks can cleanse the skin of surface greasiness, but don't expect them to "deep-clean" the pores (the term is meaningless, some experts say) or do anything more than temporarily tone the skin.

Splash on the hot suds. "Hot water is a good solvent," says Hillard H. Pearlstein, M.D., a private practitioner and assistant clinical professor of dermatology at the Mount Sinai School of Medicine of the City University of New York. For that reason, he recommends that oily skin be washed in very warm water, with plenty of soap. "Hot water plus soap will dissolve skin oil better than cold water and soap," he says, "because more things dissolve in hot than cold, and that includes soap and the grit and grime you're trying to get rid of on your skin."

Seek out drying soaps. "Given the state of the art in oily skin treatment, all you can really do is degrease the skin," Dr. Pearlstein says, "and that has to be done repeatedly, with astringents and with drying soaps."

Finding a drying soap is not a problem (finding one that *won't* dry the skin can be, however). Many dermatologists seem to favor good old

---

Forget the Food Connection

Although some magazines and skin care books recommend special diets for reducing oily skin problems (usually by cutting out fried and fatty foods), our experts dismiss such things as pure fantasy and wasted effort.

"There's no relationship between diet and oily skin," says Hillard H. Pearlstein, M.D. "The condition is genetically determined, and you either have it or you don't. You can't turn off the oil glands with diet—all you can do is mop up."

Kenneth Neldner, M.D., agrees. "I don't think diet has any effect. If it does, there's nothing about it that's known to the medical community. I mean, if you have dry skin, there's nothing you can eat that will make your skin oily, so there's no reason to think it would work the opposite way for oily skin."

Ivory for oily skin, along with more specialized degreasing soaps such as Cuticura Mildly Medicated Soap, Clearasil soap, and Neutrogena Oily Skin Formula, to name a few.

But there's really no reason to spend lots of money, says Kenneth Neldner, M.D., a professor and chairman of the Department of Dermatology at the Texas Tech University Health Sciences Center School of Medicine. "Some people feel that soaps like Safeguard and Dial are fairly drying, and these should do the trick. The thing is to make sure you use lots of it—go heavy on the soap and scrub that skin."

Follow with astringents. Astringents with acetone are your best bet, according to Dr. Neldner. "Acetone is a great fat and grease solvent, and most astringents have a bit of acetone in them. If you use it regularly, you can surely remove oil from the skin."

Although most astringents contain alcohol, look for a brand that also contains acetones, such as Seba-Nil, says Dr. Neldner. Ordinary rubbing alcohol, however, can be used as an effective, inexpensive astringent. Those looking for something milder can try witch hazel, which contains some alcohol and also works well.

Nonalcohol astringents contain mostly water and are not as effective as those with alcohol and acetone, but they may be of help for those with sensitive skin. Worth noting: Dermatologists say that rather than washing the face several times a day, which can leave it too dry and irritated, you're better off to carry astringent pads with you and use them to cleanse the face.

Select cosmetics with care. "Cosmetics come in two major categories," says Dr. Neldner, "oil-based and water-based. If you've got oily skin, use only a water-based product."

There are many cosmetics formulated for oily skin. They are made to soak up and cover oiliness so the skin doesn't look as greasy. But no cosmetic has any magical ingredient that will slow down or stop oil production, so don't be lured into buying products that make such claims.

Take a powder. Baby powder, that is. For additional shine-free protection, some women find that simple products such as Johnson's Baby Powder make a superb face powder when fluffed lightly over makeup.

PANEL OF ADVISERS

Howard Donsky, M.D., is an associate professor of medicine at the University of Toronto and staff dermatologist at Toronto General Hospital. He is author of the book *Beauty Is Skin Deep.*

Kenneth Neldner, M.D., is a professor and chairman of the Department of Dermatology at the Texas Tech University Health Sciences Center School of Medicine in Lubbock.

Hillard H. Pearlstein, M.D., is a private practitioner and assistant clinical professor of dermatology at the Mount Sinai School of Medicine of the City University of New York in New York City.

Osteoporosis

24 Ways to Stronger Bones

An estimated 24 million Americans have osteoporosis. Many do not even know it. They are not all old. They are not all women.

Anyone can get osteoporosis, but women are much more likely to get it than men. Women develop less bone mass than men. Then, for several years after menopause, women also lose bone at an increased pace because their bodies are producing less estrogen.

But this doesn't have to happen. Anyone can take major steps to prevent osteoporosis without ever going to a doctor. And anyone who already has this bone-weakening disease can do a lot to halt its progress.

Measure Your Risk

"You can take steps to eliminate risk (in some areas) and reduce your chance of getting osteoporosis," notes Kenneth Cooper, M.D. "But, as with all aspects of health, there are some things you *can't* control."

They include:

- You have a family history of osteoporosis or some other bone disease.
- You're white and your ancestors come from Europe or from the Far East.
- You have a fair complexion.
- You have a small-boned frame.
- You have a low percentage of body fat.
- You are over 40 years old.
- You have had your ovaries removed.
- You've never had children.
- You have gone through an early menopause.
- You are allergic to dairy products.

Remember, these risk factors don't mean that you will get osteoporosis. They do serve as a warning that you should do all that you can to put the odds more in your favor.

Unfortunately, the weakening of bones can be taking place very quietly for years, even decades. In his book *Preventing Osteoporosis,* researcher Kenneth Cooper, M.D., refers to osteoporosis as the "silent destroyer."

"Most people reach their peak bone mass in the spine between the ages of 25 and 30 and reach their peak bone mass in the long bones — such as the hip — from age 35 to 40," says Dr. Cooper. "After we pass this peak bone mass age, and especially after about age 45, all the bones in the body begin to lose density."

Because official diagnosis of osteoporosis often comes too late — after a fracture — the strategy is to start fighting bone loss early and to never let up.

As you are about to see, you have many weapons in your arsenal.

Exercise to build bone. "If you don't exercise, you lose bone," says Robert Heaney, M.D., John A. Creighton University Professor at Creighton University.

But there is even more reason to exercise. "A number of studies support the theory that weight-bearing exercise can actually *increase* bone mass," says Paul Miller, M.D., an associate clinical professor of medicine at the University of Colorado Health Sciences Center School of Medicine.

One of those studies, a Stanford University project, examined male and female long-distance runners and compared them with a nonrunning group. The researchers found that both the male and female runners had about 40 percent more bone mineral content than the nonrunners.

Even walking helps your bones, doctors say. Walking is an excellent, not to mention safe, way to get your bones the exercise they need. They suggest walking at least 20 minutes a day, three or four days a week.

Of course you can't always immediately see the difference exercise can make. So if you're someone who lives by a "seeing is believing" motto, take notice of a right-handed tennis player's right forearm. Chances are good it will be considerably larger than his "passive" forearm. This is visible proof that if you use your muscles and put your bones under stress, the density and size of those bones will increase.

And you're never too old to start exercising, says Dr. Cooper. Research shows that menopausal women taking up exercise can increase their bone density.

Get enough calcium in your diet. Some scientists believe that a chronic shortage of dietary calcium is a contributing factor in developing osteoporosis.

A Yugoslavian study offers strong evidence to support calcium's importance. In one region of Yugoslavia, where dairy products were not consumed, women had half the daily calcium intake of women who lived in an area where dairy products were regularly consumed. The researchers discovered that the women who took in more calcium had substantially greater bone mass and fewer fractures after the age of 65 than did the women who had low-calcium diets.

Studies of American women with osteoporosis have supported the earlier Yugoslavian study, notes Morris Notelovitz, M.D., author of *Stand Tall! The Informed Woman's Guide to Preventing Osteoporosis*. Today the U.S. Recommended Daily Allowance (USRDA) is 1,000 milligrams of calcium. That's not enough, says Dr. Cooper and many others. He advises up to 1,500 milligrams daily. "Calcium phosphate in milk is an excellent source," he adds.

But hardly the only source. Low-fat cheeses and yogurts are also high in calcium. And skim milk offers the same calcium as regular milk without the fat, says Lila A. Wallis, M.D., a clinical professor of medicine at Cornell University Medical College. Other high-calcium foods include red salmon, sardines, nuts, and tofu. Also, some citrus juices are now being sold as calcium fortified.

Fortify your meals. Add powdered nonfat dry milk to soups, casseroles, and beverages, suggests Dr. Notelovitz in his book. Every teaspoon is worth about 50 milligrams of calcium. And no fat!

Make soup. According to Dr. Notelovitz, if you use a little vinegar when preparing stock from bones, the vinegar will dissolve the calcium out of the bones. One pint of your soup, then, will be equal to about a quart of milk in calcium content.

Pinch-hit for butter. For both good taste and calcium content, Parmesan cheese is a fine substitute.

Living with Osteoporosis

Maybe someone you know has had a hip fracture. If so, and they've managed to recover, they've been very fortunate.

Each year there are about 250,000 osteoporosis-related hip fractures in this country. Of those persons 65 and older who sustain a hip fracture, 12 to 20 percent will die within a year.

So osteoporosis can be a matter of life and death.

To help make it a matter of life, Kenneth Cooper, M.D., with the aid of the Spine Education Center in Dallas, Texas, offers several tips for preventing falls and fractures. Here are some of them.

When you stand:

- Use furniture, such as the edge of a table, to help you support your body.
- Use cushioned footwear for extra protection.

When you sit:

- Keep your knees higher than your hips. If that's not possible, lean forward and support your back by resting your arms on a desk or table.
- Don't twist. If you drop something, get up from the chair to pick the item up.

In addition, here are some suggestions for making your home safe.

- Avoid using unstable floor coverings, such as throw rugs—they could literally throw you.
- Use a night-light so unexpected night trips to the bathroom don't have to be made in the dark.
- Don't position furniture too close together—you need room to maneuver.
- Use a walker or a cane if you feel unsteady.

If you can't get enough calcium in your diet, take a supplement. Calcium supplements can work small wonders—especially for people who have trouble absorbing natural sources of calcium. There are a host of calcium supplements on the market, but what works for cousin Bessie may not work for you.

"However, calcium carbonate is well absorbed in the stomach by most people if taken in divided doses and with meals," Dr. Miller says.

There are other supplements, but most doctors recommend you try calcium carbonate first because it is typically the least expensive and offers the highest amount of calcium per tablet. Ask your doctor if a supplement program would be of benefit to you.

Test your calcium supplement at home. "Many of the generic brand supplements are so badly formulated, they don't disintegrate adequately," says Dr. Heaney.

To test your supplement, Dr. Miller suggests dropping two of the tablets in 6 ounces of vinegar and waiting for 30 minutes, while stirring every 2 or 3 minutes.

"If the tablets break up into small fragments, it's probably dissolving well in the stomach," he says. "If it stays in tablet form, take it back and get a new supplement."

Get enough vitamin D. "It's essential to calcium absorption," says Robert M. Levin, M.D., an associate professor of medicine at Boston University School of Medicine and chief of the endocrinology clinic at Boston City Hospital in Massachusetts.

Vitamin D is important to calcium in two ways. First, it increases absorption of calcium in the intestines, notes Dr. Notelovitz. And second, it increases reabsorption of calcium through the kidneys.

If you spend a lot of time in the sun, you may think you're getting more than enough vitamin D. "But because we wear clothes," says Dr. Miller, "maybe 10 percent of our needed vitamin D comes from the sun."

How much do we need? A minimum of 400 international units per day. "People above age 65," Dr. Miller says, "may need 800 international units daily if they don't get outdoors frequently and they don't eat dairy products."

You can get vitamin D in some of the same places you get calcium. An 8-ounce glass of milk contains about 125 international units. Salmon, sardines, and tuna, however, are our best natural sources of vitamin D. Four ounces of canned salmon, for example, typically contains about 565 international units.

Also be sure to read the labels of calcium supplements. Some of them contain vitamin D, too. Doctors generally do not recommend vitamin D supplements, as high levels can be toxic.

Restrict alcohol consumption. "Alcohol reduces bone formation," Dr. Cooper says, adding that research has shown that alcoholics are especially prone to losing bone density. Drink only in moderation—no more than one or two drinks per day for men, and no more than one drink per day for women, Dr. Wallis advises.

Don't smoke. As if you needed another reason. Still, here it is—cigarette smoking lowers estrogen levels, Dr. Cooper says, and women with lower estrogen levels are at increased risk for developing osteoporosis.

Put a limit on caffeine. "We've done a lot of the caffeine research, and there appears to be a slight effect on calcium being lost in the urine," Dr. Heaney says. "But two or three cups of coffee a day is no problem."

Don't eat too much meat. This doesn't mean you have to eliminate meat from your diet. But don't overdo. "We now know that protein increases calcium excretion more than it increases calcium absorption, thus leading to an overall loss of calcium from the body," writes Dr. Notelovitz.

Watch your fiber intake. A high-fiber diet may bind calcium in the stomach, thus restricting the amount of calcium that is absorbed, Dr. Cooper says.

"Certain kinds of fiber may bind calcium, but how much and what kinds is unknown," adds Conrad Johnston, Jr., M.D., a professor of medicine at the Indiana University School of Medicine.

So unless your diet is abnormally high in fiber—few Americans have this problem—don't go to the other extreme and drastically reduce fiber intake; just consider reducing it a little. After all, "There are a lot of good things about fiber," says Dr. Levin. "It's good for gut motility and it helps lower cholesterol."

Put down the salt shaker. "The more sodium in your diet, the more sodium you excrete—and the more sodium you excrete, the more calcium you excrete," writes Dr. Notelovitz.

"What probably happens is that as calcium is being excreted in the urine, the blood levels of calcium drop, causing the release of parathyroid hormone, which breaks down bone to restore calcium levels."

Watch your phosphate intake. "There is general belief, but not proof, that phosphate, such as in soft drinks, will bind calcium to the gut and prevent absorption," Dr. Miller says.

In animal studies, high doses of phosphate appeared to contribute to bone loss, Dr. Johnston adds. "But the big problem with soft drinks," he emphasizes, "is that if people are drinking them all day, they are not drinking milk and not getting enough calcium."

Ideally, "calcium to phosphorus intake should be a one-to-one ratio," says Dr. Levin. To achieve that ratio, you need much more calcium in your diet than phosphorus because calcium isn't as easily absorbed.

PANEL OF ADVISERS

Kenneth Cooper, M.D., a medical researcher, is president and founder of the Aerobics Center in Dallas, Texas, and author of *Controlling Cholesterol, Preventing Osteoporosis,* and other books.

Robert Heaney, M.D., is John A. Creighton University Professor at Creighton University in Omaha, Nebraska.

Conrad Johnston, Jr., M.D., is a professor of medicine at the Indiana University School of Medicine in Indianapolis.

Robert M. Levin, M.D., is an associate professor of medicine at Boston University School of Medicine in Massachusetts. He also is chief of the endocrinology clinic at Boston City Hospital.

Paul Miller, M.D., is an associate clinical professor of medicine at the University of Colorado Health Sciences Center School of Medicine in Denver.

Lila A. Wallis, M.D., is a clinical professor of medicine at Cornell University Medical College in New York City. She also is president of the American Medical Women's Association and founder and first president of the National Council on Women in Medicine.

Perfect Posture

20 Ways to Stand Tall

Posture is body language, a pose that tells the rest of the world how you feel—about others, about your life, about yourself.

"Posture is personality," says Suki Jay Rappaport, Ph.D., a movement educator and director of the Transformations Institute in Corte Madera, California. "And it's no coincidence we use the word 'posture' interchangeably with the word 'attitude.'"

So what does your posture say? Are you slouching, facedown on the world? Do you walk with a resigned, round-shouldered look on life? Is your back so straight that people think you are unbending? Or do you strut, head up, back straight, like a peacock—adventurous, outgoing, ready to meet all challenges?

Maybe your posture isn't an intentional stance, but simply the result of a bad habit. Even so, it can give people the wrong message.

"Try to slouch and tell someone you are excited about something," says Dr. Rappaport. "You can't do it. You have to straighten up to be excited. Good posture makes full breathing, full inspiration, possible."

Good posture is practical for other reasons, too. It's the perfect way to prevent backaches. Your backbone—the 33 bony segments called vertebrae—is your body's foundation. The vertebral column is what enables you to stand upright. It surrounds and protects your spinal cord, and it is where muscles and ligaments attach to your back. It works as a weight bearer, yet allows flexibility in movement, so you don't walk stiffly, like a zombie.

Muscles are the key to good posture. Back muscles in proper working order support the spine from the rear. Stomach muscles help to support the spine from the front.

Ever wonder why your neck and shoulders hurt at the end of the workday? Chances are you spent most of your day hunched over your desk with the muscles at the base of your neck fighting to keep your body upright.

Poor posture wears against the discs—the shock absorbers—in your spine. Poor posture strains and loosens ligaments. And it pushes and pulls unevenly on all your muscles.

A lifetime of slouching can cause chronic fatigue, headaches, and sometimes body disfigurement. Don't let it happen to you. Here's how to make your posture perfect.

Start each day in balance. Begin each day by putting your skeleton in alignment, says Dr. Rappaport. These are basic stretches she teaches in movement classes to help people find proper balance, she says. Follow this routine.

- Full extension of the spine: Stand with your knees bent slightly. Clasp your hands in front. As you breathe in, stretch your hands up, palms toward the ceiling, lifting your shoulders off your rib cage. Breath out as you bring your shoulders down, setting your shoulders squarely onto your body. Let your rib cage settle on the inside of your spine, shoulders relaxed, as you lower your arms slowly.
- Side flexion: Stand and lean to the right to touch your ear to your shoulder. Follow that through, bending as best you can toward your hip. Stand again and repeat this in the other direction.
- Repeat full extension of the spine exercise.
- Rotation of spine: Turn your head slowly to look over your right shoulder. Turn as far back as possible. Turn your head back to the center. Turn your head slowly to look over your left shoulder. Turn back to the center.
- Repeat full extension of the spine exercise.
- Forward flexion of the spine: Stand and curl your back forward, dropping your head and arms toward the floor, curving and elongating your spine.
- Repeat full extension of the spine exercise.
- Hyperextension of the spine: Sit or stand, place your hands on your hips, and lean backward very gently. Your pelvis should be tucked under.
- Finish with full extension of the spine exercise.

Look in the mirror. Relax and practice standing up straight. A stiff military posture isn't what you are looking for, says Michael Spezzano, a fitness specialist and national director of the YMCA Healthy Back Program. That's too rigid, and the small of your back would be too arched.

Stand in front of a full-length mirror to check your posture. Distribute your weight evenly on both feet and keep your shoulders back and level. Hold your chest high. Your stomach will pull in naturally as you tilt your lower pelvis slightly back. Notice that your buttocks will tuck under and the small of your back will have a very slight arch.

You'll know you are on track when you can draw an imaginary straight line from just behind your ear, through your shoulder, behind the hip and knee, and through the ankle.

Release tension. Because a round-shouldered hunch tips your head slightly forward, it tightens your shoulder and neck muscles. Release that tension with shoulder rolls and head circles, suggests Dr. Rappaport.

Start with your shoulders level and square. Roll them forward 10 to 15 times, as if you were trying to paddle a boat with your shoulders. Then roll them back. Next, hold your head high and rotate it clockwise. Repeat six to eight times, then circle in the other direction.

Test your curve. A perfect back is a curved back. Test your curve by standing with your back and buttocks against a wall. You should be able to slide your hand between your waist and the wall, says Spezzano. If you can't get your hand in there or it feels tight, you are standing too straight and have the problem called flat back. Too much curve—if you can put more than a hand behind your back—and you have a condition called lordosis.

Tilt your pelvis. You can adjust and strengthen the curve in your back with an easy exercise known as the pelvic tilt. There are three ways to do this exercise. You can do one or all three.

- Lie on your back with your knees at a 45-degree angle, feet flat on the floor. Place your hand in the small of your back. Then, flatten your back against your hand by contracting your abdominal muscles and pushing your hips downward. Do this exercise a few times twice a day.
- Sit with your thighs parallel to the floor. Place one hand on your lower back, the other in front of your abdomen just above the pubic bones. Breathe in. Then, as you breathe out, pull in your abdominal muscles, roll your lower back down so your hips roll backward and your pubic bone lifts up toward the ceiling. Breathe out. Repeat occasionally during the day if you spend a lot of time sitting.
- While you are testing the curve in your back as described earlier, place one foot on a chair seat in front of you. Your pelvis will naturally tilt up and your back will straighten and be closer to the wall than it was when both feet were on the ground.

Slouch no more. When your shoulders hunch forward, breathing is cut off, and this can make you drowsy and uninspired, says Dr. Rappaport. Here's how to correct that slouch: Stand with your arms loosely at your sides. Clasp your hands behind you, dropping them onto your buttocks. Tilt your palms under for support. Lift your shoulders toward your ears and then down, bringing your elbows toward each other. This will pinch your shoulder blades together. You will be stretching your muscles across your chest and contracting those in your back. Do this several times and repeat frequently during the day.

Keep one leg up. If you stand for long periods of time, place a box on the floor in front of you and put one foot on it, says Dr. Rappoport. This position will release back tension.

Sit with your knees level. Adjust your desk chair to make sitting straight easier. Here's how: Adjust the height of your chair so your thighs are parallel to the floor and your knees are level or slightly higher than your hips. If they aren't, your body pulls forward and your back slumps as your muscles work overtime to keep your back upright, says Spezzano.

Grab a pillow. Promote good posture by sitting in a chair molded so that your back is forced into a healthy arch. Or, if that kind of chair isn't available, put a cushion in the small of your back, between you and the chair.

Stay on the level. Advice on sitting works in a car, too, says Spezzano. Pull your seat forward, toward the pedals, until your knees are bent and slightly higher than your hips and your thighs are parallel to the floor. Use a small cushion behind the small of your back or use the seat adjustment available in some cars to support the curve in your back.

Uncross your legs. Crossed legs throw your body out of alignment. Barbers and hairstylists have known it for years, which is why a good one will tell you to uncross your legs before they cut your hair—they don't want their work to come out lopsided. Keep your feet flat on the floor, says Spezzano.

Make like Dan Rather. Want to be sure your posture is perfect for your next interview? Sit at the edge of your chair, says Jeff Puffer, television talent coach in Cedar Rapids, Iowa. That's the advice he gives news anchors who want their backs to look straight while they are on camera. Sitting at the edge encourages you to balance instead of allowing you to relax round-shouldered into the back of the chair.

Sit squarely. Sit up straight and wiggle around until you can feel the bones in your bottom against the chair. If you can feel the bones, you're on your way to sitting straight. When you can't feel those bones, you've probably rolled down in your seat and are slumping.

Keep your distance. Don't be tempted to lean your arms and elbows on your desk or table. Sit 6 to 8 inches away from it when you aren't working—too far to succumb to round-shouldered posture, says Puffer. You should be far enough away so when you try to put your arms down, only your wrists are on the edge of the surface in front of you. If you slump in this position, you'll feel how out of balance your body really is.

Keep this distance to perfect your posture if you work at a computer terminal or a typewriter most of the day.

Put your right foot forward. Here's another trick television news announcers use to keep their backs straight while they talk and gesture to the audience. Try it. While sitting at the edge of your chair, curl one foot under the chair and stretch the other out in front for balance. Your back will stay straight.

Get good sleep. Good posture throughout the night can do a lot to aid good posture throughout the day. Sleeping in the wrong position can cause backache, which can throw off your natural alignment, says Dr. Robert Bowden in his book *Self-Help Osteopathy*. Sleeping on your stomach is the worst thing you can do because it accentuates the curve in your back.

Instead, he advises, sleep on your side with knees bent and a pillow fat enough to keep your head level with your shoulders. This level maintains the alignment of your neck with the rest of your body.

Or, sleep on your back with a thin pillow under your head and a small pillow under your knees.

Choose a mattress firm enough to keep you from sinking into it when you lie down. Lying on your side, your hips and shoulders should sink just a little, allowing your spine to remain straight. Your mattress should be firm enough that you and your partner do not roll together in the middle.

Keep in tone. Walk, run, swim, bicycle, do aerobics. Stretch your muscles daily. Posture is only as good as the muscles that keep you in line. Find some kind of regular physical activity, says Spezzano, to keep your muscles strong.

Get maximum relief. At the end of the day or maybe during a break period, rest your back and improve your posture at the same time, says Dr. Rappaport. Lie on the floor with your legs on a low chair or stool. Hold for 15 minutes.

Keep your feet planted. Keep both feet flat on the floor when you stand, says Spezzano. The habit of resting weight on one leg while standing can begin an undesirable back curvature.

Arch your back. Before you begin your day and again when it is over, arch your back to counteract slumping. Here's one way: On all fours, stretch upward, as if you were an angry cat arching its back. Then lower your back to level it.

PANEL OF ADVISERS

Jeff Puffer is a television talent coach for Frank N. Magid Associates in Cedar Rapids, Iowa.

Suki Jay Rappaport, Ph.D., is director of the Transformations Institute in Corte Madera, California. A fitness consultant, her doctorate is in movement education and body transformations.

Michael Spezzano is a fitness specialist and the national director of the YMCA Healthy Back Program.

Pet Problems

33 Treatments for Cats and Dogs

Debbie's lovely, mischievous, black-and-white Old English sheepdog, Tobi, has been out chasing bunnies from the lettuce patch again. Those funny bunnies led her into Foxtail Field, through Tick Towne, and right to the doorstep of their dear friend, Sally Skunk, the local cosmetics rep. "Dingdong!" Sally chimes over her shoulder. "Try this new fragrance, Tobi. It's called Gotcha! Like it?" Tobi doesn't, but she takes a sample home to Debbie—just in case.

Meanwhile, Debbie, home from a hard day's work at the butcher shop, has collapsed on the couch. That's the signal for the Charge of the Flea Brigade, which gained access to Debbie's castle on that Trojan Cat named Marmalade. As Debbie scratches her ankles, a reeking, sticker-covered, matted Tobi bursts in and bounds into her lap. Marmalade flees. Debbie faints.

THE SKUNK WORKS

With a dog like Tobi, it's hard to know where to start, so let's begin with the most obvious.

Do the doggy douche. A commercial vinegar-and-water douche comes in handy at the oddest moments. The vinegar is helpful for covering up skunk odor, says veterinary technician Mary Ann Scalaro of Hollis Veterinary Hospital in Hollis, New Hampshire. Be sure to apply it *externally*, though. Pour it over your pet and rub it in. Sponge it on the face. Use rubber gloves to protect yourself from the skunk odor. Don't let the animal get wet again, because water will wash out the vinegar and the smell will return.

You will probably need several bottles, Scalaro says, and you'll have to repeat the treatment at least once.

476

MEDICAL ALERT

Problems That Need Help FAST!

The trouble with dogs and cats is that they can't speak a language, other than the body type. They can't tell you, "I'm throwing up today, but I'll be okay tomorrow. It must have been the garbage I ate." Many symptoms are common to both serious diseases as well as innocuous passing ailments.

This medical alert guide, with advice from Amy Marder, V.M.D., a clinical assistant professor of medicine at Tufts University School of Veterinary Medicine, tells you when a symptom is serious enough to warrant a doctor's emergency care. *These symptoms could mean your pet's life is literally on the line. Call your veterinarian immediately for advice.*

- Blood in the stool, bleeding from mouth and rectum, or vomiting and bloody diarrhea can be signs of many things, including internal hemorrhage from poisoning.
- Copious diarrhea that comes on every half hour or hour, with no eating or drinking in between, can cause shock.
- Difficulty in breathing, especially with blue gums, can be a sign of heart failure.
- Abdominal swelling with attempts to vomit, especially in the deep-chested dog breeds, is a symptom of bloat, "a serious emergency," Dr. Marder says, often requiring immediate surgery.
- Frequent drinking and urination, accompanied by depression, vomiting, diarrhea, and discharge of reddish mucus, six to eight weeks after heat in an unspayed, intact (virgin) female dog or cat are signs of pyometra, which is very common and very deadly. It comes on slowly over months or years, and is also marked by irregular heat periods.
- Difficulty in giving birth is an emergency. Some strain is involved in a normal birth, but if there's continuous labor without results, it could be life threatening.
- Seizures should be reported to a vet immediately. The cause could be poisoning. Don't try to restrain the animal during convulsions.

Get your pet juiced. Tomato juice works about the same as vinegar because of its high acidity, Scalaro says. Use it the same way you would vinegar. Its drawbacks are that it's red (meaning Tobi would be black and white and red all over). And it's messy and sticky. Also, you will need a lot of it. Still, it's better than skunk odor.

Use "made-to-odor" products. Capitalism comes to your rescue again. There are at least two enzyme odor-eaters on the market: Skunk-Off and Odor Mute. Each has its own odor. They work by combining with pure skunk to create a whole new smell that's not nearly as wretched. "Skunk-Off works surprisingly well," says Deborah Patt, V.M.D., who practices in the town of Gilbertsville, Pennsylvania, "and it won't hurt clothing or furniture."

A nonenzyme product is Skunk-Kleen. It has no odor of its own, doesn't create one when it meets up with skunk smell, and it is safe to use, say its manufacturers. Still another product is Elimin-Odor. These products should work immediately, although they often require repeat applications. They are available at pet stores.

FREEDOM FROM FLEAS

We challenge you to come up with one really good reason for fleas to exist in a just world. In nine months, two fleas can generate 222 *trillion* descendants. They can live two years, they're built to survive the most frigid winters, and they can go months without eating. They can cause anemia and transmit disease and parasites. To defeat the Charge of the Flea Brigade, Debbie has to create a flea-cological disaster area.

Go for a dip. In Texas, the fleas are so big they have dogs. Marvin Samuelson, D.V.M., director of the Veterinary Teaching Hospital at Texas A&M University, says traditional insecticide dips are the most powerful weapons against fleas. "They have better penetration than sprays or powders," he says. "And they dry as a powder to keep working."

These dips, however, can be toxic, he warns, and "misuse is common. Follow the instructions carefully. And don't use a dog dip on cats." What's good for Tobi can kill Marmalade.

Proceed prudently with powders. "Powders can be helpful but are frequently misused," Dr. Samuelson says. "The problem is in the labeling, which says to sprinkle or dust the animal. Well, 'sprinkle' means a pinch to one person and half the can to another."

Spook 'em with sprays. "It's pretty hard to overdo sprays because they're the least toxic, but that's why they're not good for heavy infestations," Dr. Samuelson says. "But they can help prevent new infestations."

Use caution with collars. Collars also can't handle heavy infestations, he says, "and they can be toxic to the pet because the exposure accumulates over a long period of time." But they work like sprays against new invasions. They can also help keep a flea-free dog free of future fleas.

Cool 'em with linalool. It's understandable if you're leery of heavy-duty chemicals. You can thank Ohio State University professor of entomology Fred Hink, Ph.D., for finding deadly (to fleas) poisons in orange peels. He discovered the newest proven flea killers on the market, D-limonene and linalool. They are probably the only insecticides available that will kill adults, larvae, and eggs, he says. Linalool is more deadly to adults and eggs than it is to larvae, but it's more deadly to larvae than D-limonene.

Linalool, however, has its limits. Neither linalool nor D-limonene works as well against adults as traditional insecticides, and neither has a residual effect—they only work when the animal's wet. "That makes coverage of large areas difficult," Dr. Hink says. You may feel the positives —low toxicity to pets and high toxicity to eggs and larvae—outweigh the negatives, though.

Linalool is available as a pump spray and a dip called Demize, and D-limonene comes as a shampoo and dip.

Catch them in bed. Sprays, dips, powders. It doesn't matter what you use. Treating the animal isn't enough. "You also have to treat the pet's bedding," Dr. Hink says, "and the immediate area where the pet hangs out—including *your* bed and furniture. It's best used in a small space where you can get thorough coverage."

"It's important to treat the environment and vehicles as well as the animal," Dr. Samuelson agrees.

Forget electronic warfare. Those high-tech, expensive flea collars that house an ultrasound monitor and look like a goiter around your pet's neck are getting a lot of attention, but "they don't work." Dr. Hink says. "They have no effect on adult fleas. Fleas and other insects, as far as we know, simply have no receptors for those wavelengths."

Protect your home against invasion. The least toxic ecological method is to use an insect growth regulator. It contains methaprene, which has the brand name Precor. "This inhibits development of the flea larvae by blocking the pupa stage," Dr. Samuelson says. "It doesn't kill existing fleas, but it stops their reproduction. It's not toxic to warm-blooded animals." Methaprene is deactivated by sunlight, so it's only good in the house, where most fleas live anyway, and in the car, where you and your pet have surely deposited them. Treat your home, especially your pet's bedding, twice a year.

Get them while they're young. Many products with methaprene also contain a pesticide to kill existing fleas, Dr. Samuelson says. These products are marked with a II—like Precor II. They are more toxic but also act more quickly. They can be used inside a doghouse or kennel not exposed to sunlight. But remember that if your animal comes indoors, indoors is where most fleas will live and breed.

Treat cats differently. Because cats groom themselves, they eat fleas and are more subject to tapeworms, which fleas carry. Because cats hate water and are not fond of hissing sounds, you can guess that cats don't like dips or sprays. Dr. Samuelson recommends you use a flea-killing dry bath foam made especially for cats. A dog preparation is too potent.

Call on Avon. Avon's bath oil, Skin-So-Soft, has been shown to be an effective flea repellent. University of Florida researchers sponge-dipped flea-ridden dogs with a solution of 1.5 ounces of Skin-So-Soft to 1 gallon of water. A day later, flea counts had dropped 40 percent. "Fleas have a keen sense of smell," the researchers reported, speculating they don't like Skin-So-Soft's woodland fragrance. Although it clearly isn't as effective as standard flea dip, they said, adding the bath oil to an insecticide dip helps mask the insecticide odor and gives the animal's coat a glossy sheen.

GETTING OUT OF A HOT SPOT

You might call them hot spots, or summer eczema, but when your pet is literally mutilating himself trying to relieve itching, you want to do something about it.

"There is no such disease as summer eczema in dogs," says Donna Angarano, D.V.M., an associate professor of dermatology at the College of Veterinary Medicine, Auburn University. Most of the time in dogs, you're seeing flea allergy at work. It's not the flea bite but the flea saliva that's driving your pet mad, and just one flea is enough. This should be diagnosed by a vet because other allergies, parasites, and illnesses can also cause "summer eczema."

Kill the fleas. If you know it's flea allergy, you know what to do, having read this far. You have to go after the fleas. The allergy often worsens with age, Dr. Angarano says. "You can't cure the allergy," adds Dr. Samuelson, "but you can remove the cause. Some studies link flea allergy to a boom-or-bust cycle. Owners let fleas get out of control, then kill them all, then lose control again." So don't let fleas run rampant in the first place.

The Alternate Route

Natural Flea Control

If chemical warfare is not for you, there are natural methods to control fleas. They may take some extra time and effort, but to many animal lovers it's the only way to go. Here are natural remedies for flea control, recommended by Richard Pitcairn, D.V.M., Ph.D.

Groom daily. This may be a big task if you have a big dog, but it's important if you want to control the flea population, says Dr. Pitcairn. Use a fine-toothed flea comb, if the coat is short enough for this technique.

Give an herb bath. At the first sign of a flea, bathe your pet with a natural pet shampoo that contains flea-repellent herbs. Pennyroyal or eucalyptus oil boost the bathwater's flea-killing power. A badly flea-infested dog needs a bath about every two weeks; a cat, about once a month.

Be clean, clean, clean. "In summer, wash the pet's bedding in hot, soapy water once a week, and dry it in a hot dryer," Dr. Pitcairn says, "Also, vacuum your rugs every two to three days. Ninety percent of fleas are found where the animal sleeps."

Use natural powders. They contain such herbs as rosemary, rue, wormwood, pennyroyal, eucalyptus, or citronella, and sometimes tobacco powder. You can also dust the powder, or just diatomaceous earth, in all the nooks and crannies you can't reach by vacuuming.

Diatomaceous earth removes the fleas' waxy coating and dries them out, which kills them. Cautions: Wear a dust mask to avoid the easily inhaled, finely ground diatomaceous earth used in swimming pool filters; and pennyroyal and tobacco powder in large quantities can be toxic to you and pets.

Attack internally. Finally, add garlic and brewer's yeast to your pet's daily diet. Even try rubbing the yeast into your pet's fur. Both ingredients are said to make a flea's taste buds curl in disgust. There's no scientific proof, but some pet owners swear by it.

Treat the wound. Clip the hair off around the hot spot, clean it with warm water, and apply an astringent to dry it out. Dr. Angarano recommends Domeboro powder available over-the-counter. Alcohol works, too, but it stings, so it should be diluted. Sulfadene is also effective, but it contains alcohol.

Ease the sting. A product containing aloe vera may help soothe and dry. "Powders and ointments often make it worse," Dr. Angarano says.

Keep it clean. An open wound like a hot spot is a natural for a bacterial infection, so the wound must be monitored and kept clean.

IT'S A MAT, MAT, MAT, MAT WORLD

Laura Martin knows mats. She raises Old English sheepdogs just like Tobi at her Jen-Kris Kennels in North Barrington, Illinois. She's got some tips for Debbie.

Cut vertically. "Most people cut mats horizontally, parallel to the skin," Martin says. "Of course, that leaves a big hole. You should cut a mat vertically, moving out away from the skin from the base of the mat. That way you cut the matted hair lying horizontally, but leave the hair that's still vertical. You'll be breaking big mats into smaller and smaller ones, and you'll have nowhere near as big a hole when you're done." Use sharp-edged but blunt-tipped scissors.

Let your fingers do dematting. When you get down to the smaller mats, pull them apart with your fingers, Martin says, and then comb or brush them out with a metal-toothed comb or a wire pin brush.

Spray 'em away. Well, not exactly. But if you use a protein-lanolin spray, let it sit 10 minutes, and then cut, Martin says, "It will cut the procedure in half time-wise."

Toe the line. "Cut them horizontally and remove the whole clump," Martin says of mats between the toes.

TICK TALK

Ticks are another form of life for which it's hard to discover a truly useful purpose. They suck blood, spread Rocky Mountain spotted fever and Lyme disease, and are ugly to boot. But at least they're easier to control than fleas.

Groom them away. After your dog comes in from the fields or woods, go over him with a fine-toothed flea comb, says Richard Pitcairn, D.V.M., Ph.D., of the Animal Natural Health Center in Eugene, Oregon. This will help to catch ticks that haven't attached themselves yet. Concentrate around the neck and head and under the ears.

Pull them out. Use your fingers. Get a good grimace on your face, grab the tick as close to your pet's skin as possible, then twist and pull gradually. Then say, "ooh yecch! Grrrosss!" and wash your hands immediately. If you pull slowly, you will get the head out, too. But if you don't, it's not a major concern. Leaving the head embedded may cause a minor inflammation, but it clears up rapidly, Dr. Pitcairn says.

Do a double dip. Most flea dips will also kill ticks, he says. Be sure, also, to treat tick infestation as you would flea infestation—ecologically.

STICKER STRATEGY

Tobi picks up stickers like Velcro. Most of the time, stickers are just a hassle to remove, and if you leave them in, they can mat fur. But sometimes they're more dangerous. Foxtails, for instance, can literally burrow their way into ears and through skin and body openings, causing severe infections, Dr. Pitcairn says. Removal of stickers is essential.

Comb or brush them out. Use a stainless steel comb with wide teeth to pull stickers out of fur before matting begins, Dr. Pitcairn advises. Hold the comb against the skin to make the grooming easier.

Use your fingers. If there are only a few stickers, or if they're in the ears or between the toes, use your fingers to pull them out (at least they're not ticks). If the sticker is too deep in the ear for you to see, however, don't try to remove it. You may push it right through the eardrum, Dr. Pitcairn warns. Instead, put some vegetable or mineral oil in the ear to soften the sticker and take your pet to the doctor as soon as possible.

MASSACRE EAR MITES

Ear mites are pesky little critters that can drive your cat or dog nuts. Once cursed, pets seem to have the problem for life. Ears that seem very itchy and have dark debris, like coffee grounds, down in the ear, are the telltale signs that your pet's ears have visitors.

Although prescription medication is the normal method of attack, Dr. Pitcairn recommends this natural remedy.

The herb mite helper. Mix ½ ounce of almond oil and 400 international units of vitamin E in a dropper bottle, Dr. Pitcairn says. Once a day for three days put a dropperful or two in each ear and massage the ear well. Let your pet shake its head and then clean out the opening with cotton swabs. The oily mixture smothers the mites and helps healing. Between uses refrigerate the mixture, and warm it up before each use.

Let the pet's ears rest for three days while you brew up a new medicine. Add 1 pint of boiling water to 1 slightly rounded teaspoon of yellow dock. Cover tightly and steep 30 minutes. Strain and let cool. Put the mixture in a clear bottle and keep it in the refrigerator.

Begin another three-day treatment as outlined above, stop for ten days, and repeat for another three days. Warm the yellow dock solution before putting it in your pet's ears; he will be more accepting of the treatment if the solution is not ice cold. Make sure it is warm and not hot.

"If your pet's ears seem irritated, either from mite infection or the herbs, use only the almond oil and vitamin E until the irritation fades," Dr. Pitcairn says. "If the ears are inflamed or very sensitive, use bottled aloe vera gel instead of the oil until the inflammation subsides."

PANEL OF ADVISERS

Donna Angarano, D.V.M., is an associate professor of dermatology at the College of Veterinary Medicine, Auburn University in Alabama.

Fred Hink, Ph.D., is a professor of entomology at Ohio State University in Columbus.

Amy Marder, V.M.D., is a clinical assistant professor of medicine at Tufts University School of Veterinary Medicine in Medford, Massachusetts. She is also president of the American Veterinary Society of Animal Behavior and a columnist for *Prevention* magazine.

Laura Martin is a breeder of Old English sheepdogs in North Barrington, Illinois. She has been breeding and showing dogs for 20 years.

Deborah Patt, V.M.D., helps run a small animal clinic, the Patt Veterinary Hospital, with her father in Gilbertsville, Pennsylvania.

Richard Pitcairn, D.V.M., Ph.D., of the Animal Natural Health Center in Eugene, Oregon, is the author of *Dr. Pitcairn's Complete Guide to Natural Health for Dogs and Cats.*

Marvin Samuelson, D.V.M., is director of the Veterinary Teaching Hospital at Texas A&M University in College Station.

Mary Ann Scalaro is a veterinary technician at the Hollis Veterinary Hospital in Hollis, New Hampshire.

Phlebitis

10 Remedies to Keep It at Bay

Phlebitis. If most people know anything at all about this disease, they know only that former President Richard Nixon had it and that it has something to do with the blood vessels in the legs.

Though correct on both counts, those who have suffered with phlebitis know it as much more—as a painful, frightening affliction that can claim a victim's life without warning via a blood clot lodged in the pulmonary veins of the lungs.

Phlebitis is more correctly known as thrombophlebitis. "Thrombo-" is for the blood clot that is its trademark and primary danger. Two basic types of phlebitis exist: deep vein thrombophlebitis, or DVT for short, the more dangerous condition, and superficial phlebitis, the type of affliction we will deal with here.

Michael D. Dake, M.D., a vascular specialist at the Miami Vascular Institute in Florida, explains the difference. "Phlebitis just means inflammation of the veins," he says, "and that can be the superficial veins near the skin or the deep veins of the legs.

"Deep vein thrombophlebitis is something we're always on guard against," he continues, "because those people can develop a moving blood clot that would have direct access to the lungs if it broke loose and traveled through the system. DVT usually requires hospitalization and treatment with anticoagulants. The blockage that occurs in superficial phlebitis, however, tends not to break loose."

For that reason, the tips we offer here are intended for use only by persons who have been diagnosed with superficial phlebitis and are under a doctor's care. These tips are designed to help relieve pain without prescription medication and help reduce the chances of a recurrence.

Get off the Pill. "If you've had a history of phlebitis or blood clots, you definitely shouldn't use oral contraceptives," says Jess R. Young, M.D., chairman of the Department of Vascular Medicine at the Cleveland

Clinic Foundation in Ohio. The incidence of deep vein thrombophlebitis in oral contraceptive users is estimated at three to four times higher than in nonusers. Such a relatively high rate of deep vein clotting also puts the superficial phlebitis sufferer at an unacceptably high risk for recurrence.

Give it rest and warmth. "Superficial phlebitis can be treated by elevating the leg and applying warm, moist heat," says Dr. Dake. While it is not necessary to remain in bed, rest, with the leg elevated 6 to 12 inches above the heart, seems to help speed healing. The inflammation of superficial phlebitis usually disappears in a week to ten days, though it may take three to six weeks to completely subside.

Know your risks. Once you've had phlebitis, you're at increased risk of getting it again. How much risk may depend largely on things you may or may not be able to control. "In general," says Dr. Young, "you have to be put in a situation where you're at increased risk for it, such as surgery or prolonged bed rest."

While you might not be able to prevent prolonged bed rest following an injury or serious illness, certain types of risks, such as elective surgery, can be avoided if you're an older individual prone to clotting disorders. Consult your doctor for specific risk factors, but keep in mind that getting up and around can help reduce the risks of developing phlebitis after surgery.

Investigate aspirin. Some studies have suggested that the blood-thinning properties of aspirin may help reduce phlebitis by preventing rapid clot formation in persons prone to the disease. These studies advise that you take aspirin before prolonged periods of bed rest, travel, or surgery, all of which tend to make circulation sluggish and increase the possibility of clotting. While such a simple recommendation sounds enticing, some doctors hedge on its effectiveness. "I'm not sure aspirin will be that protective against clotting," says Dr. Dake. Even if you do opt for aspirin, this is a *medical* treatment—see your doctor first.

Walk when you have to ride. Planning a long trip by car? If you've had phlebitis in the past, then make sure your wheels aren't the only thing in motion. "The main thing is to stop frequently and exercise when you stop," says Dr. Dake. "And don't just stop one time during the day and walk a mile, but rather, stop four or five times and walk shorter distances."

What you're trying to do, he says, is prevent the circulation from becoming sluggish as a result of sitting motionless for long periods of time. "Your circulation enters a low-flow state under those conditions and that can lead to a clot," says Dr. Dake.

Add another reason to quit. "If you get recurring cases of phlebitis and your doctor can't find any reason for it," says Dr. Young, "then you should quit smoking. You could have a case of Buerger's disease that just hasn't moved to the arteries yet." Buerger's disease is characterized by severe pain and blood clots, usually in the legs. It is directly related to smoking, and the only cure is to give up all forms of tobacco. "Occasionally, Buerger's will start out as phlebitis," Dr. Young explains. It's possible that Buerger's could be misdiagnosed as phlebitis, in which case continued smoking would be *very* hazardous to your health.

That's a long shot, Dr. Young admits, but worth considering if your doctor hasn't been able to explain recurring bouts of phlebitis. "Otherwise, there doesn't seem to be any connection between smoking and phlebitis," he says.

Get some exercise. "Exercise—primarily walking—tends to keep the veins emptied," says Robert Ginsburg, M.D., director of the Center for Interventional Vascular Therapy at Stanford University Hospital in California.

Keeping the veins emptied as much as possible is a good way to prevent a recurrence of phlebitis, he says. "The veins are a low-pressure system, and if the valves that keep blood from flowing backward in the legs aren't working properly, such as in varicose veins, the only way you're going to prevent blood from pooling is by walking."

Put your feet up when you're laid up. "If you've had phlebitis and you're going to be bedridden for any length of time," says Dr. Young, "elevate the foot of the bed several inches to increase blood flow through the veins."

He also suggests you exercise your legs as much as you can while in bed. "You can take aspirin if you want," he adds, "though there have been no good studies that show it prevents a recurrence."

Wear support stockings for relief. Some physicians advise the wearing of support stockings to prevent a recurrence of phlebitis, while others don't. While there's no documented evidence showing that support stockings do any good in *preventing* phlebitis, they do seem to

---

MEDICAL ALERT

A Sign of Infection

People often become quite worried when told they have phlebitis, believing that clots may break loose and cause death. This is rarely the case, although phlebitis can develop into life-threatening infection if left untreated.

If the symptoms of plebitis—pain, redness, tenderness, itching, and swelling—are accompanied by a fever and they do not clear up in a week or so, see your doctor. It could be a sign of infection. Your physician can clear it up with antibiotics.

---

relieve pain and make some people feel better. The best advice? Wear support stockings if they make you feel better. If they make you feel worse, though, don't think you must continue wearing them in order to prevent a recurrence.

Beware the friendly skies. The scientific literature is filled with reports of people being stricken with deep vein thrombosis following a long airplane flight. While nobody seems to be quite sure why this happens (cabin pressure, lack of motion, alcohol intake, etc.), the condition is so common that it is now known as "Economy Class Syndrome," because it rarely seems to strike those passengers seated in roomy, first-class seats.

"Long plane rides or car trips, or really any long period of inactivity, can increase the risk of thrombosis," says Dr. Young. "But on airplanes you tend to be confined to your seat a lot more than when traveling by car. So if you have phlebitis, this is a case where you ought to put on your elastic stockings before boarding, then get out of your seat and walk up and down the aisle every 30 minutes or so after taking off."

To help maintain good relations with your neighbors, he says, "It might be good to request an aisle seat."

PANEL OF ADVISERS

Michael D. Dake, M.D., is a vascular specialist at the Miami Vascular Institute in Florida.

Robert Ginsburg, M.D., is director of the Center for Interventional Vascular Therapy at Stanford University Hospital in California.

Jess R. Young, M.D., is chairman of the Department of Vascular Medicine at the Cleveland Clinic Foundation in Ohio.

Phobias and Fears

12 Coping Measures

Phobias go back a long way. Take this account of one phobia, written by a famous physician. "The girl flute player would frighten him; as soon as he heard the first note of the flute at a banquet, he would be beset by terror." Fear of the flute is called aulophobia, and the doctor describing the condition was Hippocrates.

One person's wind section can make another person writhe in fear. Nobody likes rust, except maybe automobile body shop owners, but people with a fear of rust (iophobia) probably carry a can of Rust-Oleum with them wherever they go.

Agoraphobics, of course, rarely go anywhere. They suffer from a fear of being separated from safe persons and places, and some won't even leave their houses. Claustrophobics, on the other hand, hate being confined, while panophobics fear everything.

"Just name it," says Jerilyn Ross, M.A., a psychologist who specializes in phobias and is president of the Phobia Society of America. "There are as many different kinds of phobias as there are different kinds of people."

Phobias are classified into three types — simple phobias, social phobias, and agoraphobia. People with simple phobias experience a dread of a certain object, place, or situation. Social phobics are people who avoid public situations, like a party, because they are afraid of doing something to embarrass themselves. And agoraphobics are victims of a complex phenomenon based on a fear of strange places.

"You don't go from fear to lots of fear to a full-blown phobia," says Ross. "It's not something that progresses. Usually people who develop phobias do so in areas where they had no previous fear."

But what exactly is a phobia? In the classic sense, a phobia is "an irrational, involuntary, inappropriate fear reaction that generally leads to an avoidance of common everyday places, objects, or situations," says Ross.

Blame It on Your Ears

Just when you think that your phobia may be all in your mind, along comes Harold Levinson, M.D., who says it's not in your mind, it's actually located in your inner ear.

Dr. Levinson, a Great Neck, New York, psychiatrist and neurologist who is coauthor of the book *Phobia Free,* specializes in inner ear disorders. While treating his patients for inner ear problems, he began to notice other changes. "Not only did their inner ear problems improve, but so did their phobia problems," he says.

It was his unique background as both a psychiatrist and a neurologist that led him to this conclusion. "A significant number of my patients with inner ear problems also had phobias identical to the patients I was treating in my psychiatric practice."

After 20 years of research on more than 20,000 patients, Dr. Levinson believes that 90 percent of all phobic behavior is a result of an underlying malfunction within the inner ear system.

"The mechanisms in the inner ear are not functioning correctly," he explains. For example, balance is controlled in the inner ear. If it is not working correctly and your balance is off, you might be afraid of heights or falling or tripping."

Dr. Levinson acknowledges that his is the minority point of view. But thousands of success stories are nothing to snicker at. Dr. Levinson is convinced that a trip to an ear specialist is at least worth a try for those suffering from phobias.

In the real sense, though, a phobia is a fear of fear itself. "A phobia is a fear of one's own impulses," says Ross. "It's a fear of having a panic attack and losing control. Basically it's a fear of one's own self and loss of control."

Phobics know who they are. "They always recognize that their fear is inappropriate to the situation," says Ross. "For example, if you're flying on an airplane during a thunderstorm, feeling fearful is a normal reaction. However, if your boss tells you that you'll have to take a business trip in a couple of weeks and immediately you start worrying about having a panic attack on the plane," she says, "that's inappropriate to the situation. A phobia is always irrational."

Sound like something you've experienced? If so, here's some rational advice for irrational behavior from those who deal daily with the problem.

Reverse negative thinking. In a phobic situation, the person experiences negative thoughts and scary images, which in turn trigger the physical symptoms, explains Manuel D. Zane, M.D., founder and

---

MEDICAL ALERT

When It's Time to See a Specialist

No one is certain what causes a phobia. Some experts believe it is all psychological; some believe it is biologically based. But more and more evidence indicates it is a combination of both.

What is known is that it tends to run in families. If one of your parents had a phobia, you may be predisposed to one, but not necessarily the same one. More often than not, phobias strike people who have a history of separation anxiety and perfectionism.

Some phobias are more serious than others. If your phobia is interfering with your life, you should seek professional help. Whom you seek out is as crucial as seeking help itself. "It's important that a person get help from a person who understands phobias," says Jerilyn Ross, M.A., "Many phobics end up going from doctor to doctor and hospital to hospital, so it's important to find a professional who specializes in phobias and anxiety-related disorders."

There are several hundred professionals who treat phobics in the United States and Canada. You can get a list of them and more information on phobias by sending a postcard with your name and address to The Phobia Society of America, 133 Rollins Avenue, Suite 4B, Rockville, MD 20852-4004.

One other note. People suffering from agoraphobia should not feel left out because they can't venture outside their homes. The Phobia Clinic at the White Plains Medical Center in New York has what they call phobia aides, trained people who will come to your house to help you. Many other clinics and professionals will also make house calls.

---

director of the Phobia Clinic at White Plains Hospital Medical Center in New York and associate clinical professor of psychiatry at New York Medical College. You should allow the fear to come but try to shift from the negative thoughts—"That dog will bite me"—to something realistically positive like—"The dog is tightly leashed and can't get away."

Come face-to-face with fear. Avoiding your fear will prevent you from overcoming it, says Dr. Zane. Instead, desired control can be achieved through a process called exposure treatment, in which you expose yourself to the object of your fears little by little and learn that what you imagine and expect to happen does not actually occur. Such graduated exposure can help you get used to it, he says. For example, let's say your phobia is spiders. In exposure treatment training you may start

How to Fight a Panic Attack

"I felt like I was standing in the middle of a six-lane highway with cars coming at me from either side." That's how 26-year-old Tanis felt whenever she tried to leave her home. Tanis suffers from the most common of all phobias, agoraphobia, a fear of being away from a safe person or place.

Just the thought of venturing outside of her Virginia home would bring on a paralyzing panic attack. "One moment you feel fine, then the next moment you feel like you are about to die," she says. "Physically, my heart started beating faster, I got nauseous, and I felt shaky and like I was about to faint." For Tanis, these were the signs of a full-blown phobia. Tanis did manage to leave her house for therapy, though, and that did the trick. Now she ventures out all the time, trying to help those still stuck inside. Here are some of the tactics she learned in therapy that helped set her free.

Recognize the attack. "If a panic attack comes on, recognize it for what it is," she says. "You've had them before, so you know you're not going to die. You've gotten through it before and you can do it again. Acceptance is the key."

Be sensitive to yourself. "Phobics are usually perfectionists and are usually hard on themselves, but you shouldn't be," says Tanis. "When you are going through the exposure treatment [facing your fear in stages], be easy on yourself. Give yourself credit because you did it—even if it brought on an attack."

Go slowly. "Start out slowly, but do some exposure treatment every day. Set goals for yourself; set an 8-week goal and a 16-week goal. Once you start dealing with your phobia over and over again, it really does become conditioned. As impossible as that may sound to a phobic, you can do things like a normal person again."

Believe her. When we called her house the first time to do an interview, we were told that Tanis "wasn't home."

to face your fear—usually in the presence of another person—by looking at pictures of spiders. When you learn to handle this, you may move on to looking at a dead spider, then a live spider—and you may even progress to holding one in your hand. Each time you may still feel some fear, but you learn by such exposure that the awful things you dread do not actually occur.

Play mind games. "When you feel your fear taking hold, do manageable things like counting backward by 3s from 1,000, reading a book, talking aloud, or taking deep, measured breaths," says Dr. Zane.

"When you are involved with doing something manageable in the present, you reduce your involvement with fear-generating thoughts and images. Your body quiets down and you maintain control."

Measure your fear. Label your fear on a scale of zero to ten, suggests Dr. Zane. You'll find that the severity of your fear is not constant, that it goes up and down. Write down thoughts or activities that make it increase and decrease. Knowing what triggers, increases, and decreases the fear may help you learn to control it.

Look over the rainbow. Use thoughts, fantasies, and activities that make you feel good to shift yourself away from frightening thoughts, suggests Dr. Zane. For example, think more about the high probabilities of a safe flight and the pleasures of lying on the beach in Hawaii instead of focusing on and reacting to only the unlikely dangers of the flight.

Pat yourself on the back. Functioning successfully with a level of fear is a big achievement, says Dr. Zane. Dealing with it successfully in this way is much more plausible and realistic than trying to completely erase your fear. Each encounter that you overcome in your exposure treatment training should be considered a personal victory and can build your self-confidence in being able to control the situation.

Avoid caffeine. "People who have repeated panic attacks may be very sensitive to caffeine," says David H. Barlow, Ph.D., director of the Phobia and Anxiety Disorders Clinic and a professor of psychology at State University of New York at Albany. "Caffeine re-creates some of the symptoms they have during panic attacks. People prone to panic attacks may want to omit caffeine from their diets."

As the stewardess comes walking down the aisle with the drink cart, remember that caffeine isn't limited to coffee. It's also in tea and certain soft drinks, such as colas, and chocolate.

Burn that adrenaline. "With panic attacks you have an excess of adrenaline in the body, and when you move, you burn it up," says Christopher McCullough, Ph.D., director of the San Francisco Phobia Recovery Center in California. Trying to sit still and relax is a mistake. You need to move to burn up the adrenaline, so walk around or exercise during the attack.

Play muscle games. "If you can't move around, the next best thing to do is to start tightening and untightening various muscles in your body. "Tighten the large muscles of your thigh, then do a quick release," suggests Dr. McCullough. "This kind of rhythmic tensing and releasing will also burn up the adrenaline."

PANEL OF ADVISERS

David H. Barlow, Ph.D., is director of the Phobia and Anxiety Disorders Clinic and professor of psychology at the State University of New York at Albany.

Harold Levinson, M.D., is a psychiatrist and neurologist in Great Neck, New York. He specializes in inner ear disorders. He is coauthor of *Phobia Free.*

Christopher McCullough, Ph.D., is director of the San Francisco Phobia Recovery Center in California. He is coauthor of *Managing Your Anxiety* and author of the how-to audiotape *How to Manage Your Fears and Phobias.* He has also developed a home study program, "Outgrowing Agoraphobia."

Jerilyn Ross, M.A., is president of the Phobia Society of America and associate director of the Roundhouse Square Psychiatric Center in Alexandria, Virginia.

Manuel D. Zane, M.D., is founder and director of the Phobia Clinic, White Plains Hospital Medical Center in New York and associate clinical professor of psychiatry at New York Medical College in Valhalla.

Poison Ivy and Oak

19 Skin-Soothing Remedies

If you're like most people allergic to poison ivy and poison oak (it's the most common allergy in the country, claiming at least half the population), you may not even know you've picked it up until the next day, when you are scratching like a hound at a rash of exquisite itchability.

The nagging itch and telltale red rash are caused by the toxin urushiol oil, which is found in both poison ivy and poison oak. Some people are more sensitive to it than others. And some are not sensitive to it at all—they can literally roll in the stuff and not get a reaction. But our experts don't advise those of you lucky enough to be immune to give it a try. A sensitivity to urushiol can develop at any time. The solutions to

Urushiol Oil: Evil and Persistent

Urushiol oil, the active ingredient in poison ivy and poison oak, is "one of the most potent external toxins we know," says William L. Epstein, M.D. "The amount needed to cause a rash in very sensitive people is measured in nanograms, and it could take as little as 1 nanogram. But most sensitive people will react in the 100-nanogram range." Consider that a nanogram is a mere *billionth* of a gram; that means it would take less than ¼ *ounce* of urushiol to cause a rash in every person on earth. Five hundred people could itch from the amount covering the head of a pin.

"I'm surprised it hasn't been used as a nonlethal chemical warfare weapon," says James A. Duke, Ph.D., whose interest in "this evil plant" was sparked by "an early ethnobotanical application of poison oak as a substitute for toilet paper."

Its itch torments you; its long life can fool you. Dr. Duke says "specimens of poison ivy several centuries old" have caused dermatitis in sensitive people.

"When the Japanese restored the gold leaf on the golden Temple in Kyoto, they painted urushiol lacquer on it to preserve and maintain the gold," Dr. Epstein says. "The main message for American tourists there is, 'Don't try to steal the gold.'" You'll be caught red-handed. Literally.

poison ivy or poison oak are substances that annihilate urushiol. But remember—what works for someone else may not work for you, and in severe cases may not work at all.

KILLING THE ITCH

If you've been messing around in a poison patch, you'll soon know whether you're immune or not. And as ugly as the rash looks, it's the itch that'll do you in. Here's what you can do about it, starting with the universal remedy.

Get cozy with darlin' calamine. The time-honored mainstay in poison treatment is calamine lotion, a popular skin protectant with a soothing action "that produces cooling and distracts your skin from the itching sensation," says Robert Rietschel, M.D., chairman of the Department of Dermatology at New Orleans' Ochsner Clinic in Louisiana, and clinical professor of dermatology at Louisiana State University School of Medicine. "In poison ivy and poison oak, the blood vessels develop gaps that leak fluid through the skin, causing blisters and oozing," he explains. "When you cool the skin, the vessels constrict and don't leak as much."

MEDICAL ALERT

Signs of an Emergency

About 15 percent of the 120 million Americans who are allergic to poison oak and poison ivy are so highly sensitive they break out in a rash and begin to swell in 4 to 12 hours instead of the normal 24 to 48. Their eyes may swell shut and blisters may erupt on their skin.

"This is one of the few true emergencies in dermatology," says William L. Epstein, M.D. "Get to a hospital as soon as possible. A shot of corticosteroids will bring the swelling down."

Calamine lotion also leaves a powdery residue that absorbs the oozing, develops a crust, and keeps it from sticking to your clothes, Dr. Rietschel notes. He suggests applying calamine lotion three or four times a day. To keep your rash from getting too dry and making the itch even worse, stop using calamine when the oozing stops, he says.

Subtract the additives. Antihistamines like Benadryl and painkillers like benzocaine and lidocaine are often added to certain calamine lotion products. "They may work for some people," says William L. Epstein, M.D., a professor of dermatology at the University of California, San Francisco, School of Medicine, "but they don't add much relief vis-à-vis the cost, and you run the risk of developing an allergic rash from the additives."

Pop a pill. Oral antihistamines, however, are a different story. In fact, they're high up on Dr. Rietschel's list. There are two over-the-counter brands to choose from: Chlor-Trimeton, which contains the active ingredient chlorpheniramine maleate, and Benadryl, which contains the active ingredient diphenhydramine hydrochloride. "You could take your hay fever medicine if it happens to be an antihistamine," Dr. Rietschel says.

Try other drying agents. "Although not as popular and soothing as calamine, there are other skin soothers that can be just as effective. Some of them, however, often have a lot of alcohol and tend to sting," Dr. Rietschel warns. Use them as you would calamine—until the oozing stops. Otherwise you can get the rash too dry, and it will crack and cause more itching. Zinc oxide, witch hazel, Burow's solution (aluminum acetate), and baking soda are common topical drying agents.

Cover with a compress. Put a cotton cloth soaked in cool water over the rash and let a fan blow over it, Dr. Rietschel advises. The cooling/evaporating effect works the same as calamine lotion, although there's no residue to soak up the oozing.

Irritate it to distraction. "Counterirritants like menthol and phenol confuse the nerve endings in the skin and give a cooling sensation," Dr. Rietschel says. "But they can sting and sometimes aren't sufficient to give you the relief you need." Menthol and phenol are available in anti-itch creams.

Counterattack early with cortisone. The OTC cortisone creams are too weak and "are absolutely worthless in knocking out a significant rash," Dr. Rietschel says. "But they can relieve minimal itching." Dr. Epstein recommends them as "pretty good about two weeks into the rash, when it's healing and scaling and itching."

Try an oatmeal onslaught. Colloidal oatmeal dries up oozing blisters. Aveeno is the most popular commercial preparation for skin care and comes with easy-to-follow instructions. Apply it with a cloth to the blisters, or use it in the bath if you don't mind the mess and a very slippery tub.

Get folksy with herbs. The most popular herbal treatment is jewelweed, also known as impatiens or touch-me-not, says Purdue University professor of pharmacognosy and author of *The Honest Herbal,* Varro E. Tyler, Ph.D. "There's little solid research, but in one clinical trial it worked just as well as prescription cortisone creams," he says. You can slit the stem and put the juice on the rash. U.S. Department of Agriculture economic botanist James A. Duke, Ph.D., says he uses impatiens to stop the rash from developing. "I ball up the whole plant and make sort of a washrag out of it and wipe the poison sap off," he says.

Apply plant potions. Another natural remedy is said to be the leaf of the black nightshade plant (not to be confused with the deadly nightshade). "Chop, grind, or crush it up, mix it with milk or cream, and apply it to the rash," Dr. Tyler says. He says other people have found success using the juice of the milkweed plant. "Just drip the milky latex on the rash."

Polish it off. Maybe not so natural is white shoe polish, which Dr. Tyler reports, contains pipe clay that has effects similar to calamine. Apply it as you would calamine. He says pipe clay can be found in "the old-fashioned shake-it-up kind" of polish. Another ingredient in shoe polish that has the same effect is zinc oxide.

NEVER, NEVER AGAIN!

You can try to avoid poison ivy or poison oak simply by steering clear of it—if you know what it looks like. Generally, the plants have clusters of three shiny leaves, the source of the couplet "Leaves of three, let it be." Different regions of the country, however, have different varieties. And in the winter there are no leaves to let be, but the poison lurks in roots and stems, waiting to pounce. Then there are your dog and cat, Simon and Garfunkel, who can bring the stuff on their coats right into your living room.

Thankfully, Mother Nature, the drug industry, and the cosmetics industry each provide substances that may stop the poisonous substance, urushiol, from causing a rash even after exposure to the plant.

Rub out the bad guy. Washing your exposed skin in *lots* of rubbing alcohol after you're finished playing in poison ivy for the day takes the urushiol oil out of your skin, Dr. Epstein says. But don't use a washcloth to apply alcohol—"it just picks it up [the urushiol oil] and spreads it around," Dr. Epstein says.

Wait till you're finished being exposed. Never dab alcohol on *during* your hike or picnic, because it removes your protective skin oils and the exposure you get to the poison around the next bend will be worse.

Rinse well. "Water inactivates urushiol," Dr. Epstein says. Soap is unnecessary. But after being exposed, you must douse yourself *immediately* with water from your hose or canteen or the next stream. "The best possible treatment is alcohol followed by water," he says. Again, don't use a washcloth.

Wash everything. That means everything that might have come in contact with the poisonous plant: your clothes, your dog, your backpack. Dr. Epstein says one patient who drove home after handling poison oak "kept picking it up for weeks from the steering wheel of his car."

Spray before you play. Most deodorants contain an organically activated clay known as organoclay to hold the other ingredients in suspension; almost all antiperspirants have the clay plus aluminum

---

Anything Goes in a Pinch

Horse urine. Paint thinner. Acetone. Ammonia. Clear nail polish. Meat tenderizer. Sound appetizing? Don't worry, you don't have to drink them. They've all been used successfully to treat skin exposed to poison ivy or poison oak because that's all people had handy at the time.

"Organic solvents like ammonia, paint thinner, and acetone are very good for getting the urushiol oil out of your skin before the rash occurs," says William L. Epstein, M.D. Other solvents that work are hypo sulfite, used in photographic darkrooms, and bleach, Dr. Epstein says. He warns, however, that they should be used only as a last resort. "Putting solvents on your skin isn't recommended for normal use. Still, if that's all you have, it's better than nothing. Just don't use them every day, or you can get a worse rash than poison oak. Solvents also extract all your natural protective skin oils."

But for getting the urushiol off your tools, car upholstery, and other places you suspect are contaminated, nothing beats solvents.

---

chlorohydrate. Both of these have been found by Dr. Epstein to be highly effective at neutralizing urushiol.

Since products designed to prevent poison ivy and poison oak are under the scrutiny of the Food and Drug Administration, Dr. Epstein suggests that in the meantime you may want to spray your favorite deodorant or antiperspirant on your arms, legs, clothes, and pets before rolling in poison. He says antipersirants are best because they contain both ingredients. "The aluminum salts work better than the organoclays, but they're irritating, so don't spray antiperspirants on your face or body folds," he cautions.

Hold up a shield. Multi-Shield is a barrier skin cream that's been used in industries as a defense against oils and solvents handled by employees in their work. And now it's being tested to prevent poison ivy and poison oak. Dr. Epstein did "very limited tests" and gave it a passing grade. It works for mild cases of poison. It can be purchased through Interpro, Inc., P.O. Box 1823, Haverhill, MA 01831.

Don't get burned. Don't try to rid your yard of urushiol by burning plants—urushiol takes to the air in a fire. You can inhale droplets of the oil and come down with serious lung infections, fever, and a body-wide rash. That's why you also don't want to hang around forest fires.

Postnasal Drip

13 Tips to Turn It Off

As far as you're concerned, whoever put the word "drip" after post-nasal has some wry sense of humor. "Rampant waterfall" seems more fitting to you.

Just where does all this fluid come from anyway? Well let's begin at the beginning. In the course of a single day, 2,500 gallons of air pass through an adult nose. No matter how cold and dry that air is, your nose has to make sure the air is heated to 98.6 degrees and is 100 percent humidified by the time it completes the 8-inch journey to your lungs. If the air isn't properly moist and warm, it will injure lung tissue.

Proper humidification depends mostly on glands in the lining of your nasal and sinus cavities. Each day, those glands crank out about 2 quarts of fluid to lubricate the mucous membranes in your sinuses, nose, mouth, and throat.

"Normally, those secretions flow down the back of the nose and throat, swept by the cilia," explains Gilbert Levitt, M.D., a Puget Sound,

Washington, otolaryngologist and clinical instructor of otolaryngology at the University of Washington School of Medicine. Cilia are threadlike cells that wave back and forth over some of the surface tissue. They help keep the nasal passageways clear of particulate matter.

From time to time, and especially in the winter, the mucus dries out. It begins to get "gloppy" or gluelike. That slows down the cilia. A virus can stop the cilia altogether. When the cilia stop waving, secretions pool in the back of the nose. The consistency thickens and suddenly you're aware of postnasal drip.

How can you get the mucus back to its ordinary, watery self without completely drying your upper respiratory tract?

Here's what our experts advise.

Blow your nose regularly. This may be so obvious that you overlook it, says Jerald Principato, M.D., an otolaryngologist in private practice in Bethesda, Maryland, and associate clinical professor of oto-laryngology at George Washington University School of Medicine. The simple act of blowing eliminates some excessive postnasal drainage from the front of the nose.

But don't be overzealous. Cotton swabs and even tissues should never be placed inside the nose, he says.

Flush with saltwater. Salt, water, and an infant-sized aspirator are all you need to wash away that mucus-clogged feeling—and the bad breath that often accompanies it.

Here's Dr. Principato's recipe. Dissolve ½ teaspoon of salt in 8 ounces of warm water. (Make that ⅓ teaspoon if you have high blood pressure.) Draw the water into the aspirator and put the tip of it in your nostril. Hold your nose straight back and the aspirator at a right angle to your face, parallel to the roof of your mouth. And then breathe in to "suck" the water into your nostril.

It may feel uncomfortable at first, but you'll find it gets easier with practice. Do the other nostril and spit the water back into the sink. You may need to do this a few times before you feel relief. When you're finished, blow your nose to remove the watery discharge.

Dr. Principato suggests that you irrigate the nostrils three times a day for five days when needed.

Gargle with saltwater. Use the same solution: ½ teaspoon of salt (or ⅓ teaspoon for hypertensives) in 8 ounces of warm water. This, says Dr. Principato, will help clear the throat and voice box problems created by excessive postnasal drainage.

Curb that curry craving. Maybe you're crazy for the taste of lamb curry, or a red-hot Mexican chili. But if you have a postnasal drip problem, you might want to pass for now. "Irritants in foods such as hot peppers and spices like curries can cause chronic nasal problems," says Dr. Principato.

Forgo the milk. You might want to try this to see if it helps, suggests John A. Henderson, M.D., an otolaryngologist and allergist in private practice in San Diego, California, and assistant clinical professor of surgery at the University of California, San Diego, School of Medicine. Some food experts believe that dairy products like milk and ice cream stimulate excess mucus production. Others aren't sure.

"Cow's milk is a totally different substance than human milk," says Dr. Henderson. "The problem is that it's full of sugar, and this sugar, called lactose, feeds the bacteria and molds in our throats and intestinal tracts." Overgrowth of these organisms can adversely affect the immune system.

Relax. Stress is a major cause of chronic nasal disease, says Dr. Principato. Why? The job of warming and maintaining a proper lining for the nose falls to the parasympathetic nervous system, "which is heavily influenced by stress," he says. Stress can drive the process too hard, causing the nasal lining to produce more mucus than it needs.

If you find that your postnasal drip is worse when you're under stress, relaxation techniques like progressive muscle relaxation or meditation can help you feel better all around.

Drink lots of fluids. Keeping the mucous lining moist is essential if the cilia are to do their job. Drinking lots of fluids helps to get at the mucus that's stuck in the upper part of the pharynx, says Alvin Katz, M.D., an otolaryngologist in private practice in New York City and surgeon director of the Manhattan Eye, Ear, Nose, and Throat Hospital.

"Herb tea with lemon and honey, or just warm water with lemon is excellent," adds Dr. Levitt. "Help the postnasal drainage to go down instead of fighting it by clearing the throat. Anything in the secretion is destroyed by hydrochloric acid in the stomach, so there's nothing to worry about."

Turn on the humidifier. A good humidifier, one that takes several gallons of water to fill, can help keep your nasal passages moist during the dry winter months. And this can help keep mucus from drying out and getting so thick you notice it.

Get Your Neti Ready

If you hanker after absolute purity in that schnozzola of yours, do what the yogis do. Use a neti pot daily to flush your nasal passages with saltwater. A neti pot resembles a small teapot with an extended spout. It typically holds several ounces of water.

Students of yoga believe that keeping the body's air passageways clean of dried mucus can help increase vitality throughout the system. Proponents also claim that consistent use can keep you free of all sinus problems that arise from nasal obstructions.

How do you use a neti pot? Here's the word from a spokesman for the Himalayan International Institute.

Fill the pot with warm water and a pinch of salt. Use just enough salt to approximate the salt-to-water ratio you find in your own tears. If the solution stings, you're using too much salt.

Tip your head sideways over a sink, put the spout in one nostril, and keep pouring until you've used all the fluid in the pot. The fluid should run out the other nostril.

Refill the pot, tilt your head to the other side, and irrigate the other nostril. It may require some practice to do this just right.

When you're finished, blow your nose freely through both nostrils.

You can repeat the process a second time each day if you want.

"It really is fun and easy," says the spokesman. "I use it twice a day now, which I've done for over a decade. This takes care of the mucus blockages in the most important portal in your body—the place where you get your air. When that's clogged with mucus, it affects your system dramatically."

"Use distilled water to fill the humidifiers and you won't have impurities," says Dr. Katz. Be sure to clean the unit weekly with water mixed with a little bit of white vinegar, he advises. That keeps mold and mildew away.

Don't overuse decongestants. "If nose drops are being used to control postnasal drainage, they're being used inappropriately," says Dr. Principato. They're best used when you have a documented sinus infection, he says. And he echoes other experts when he warns that you should never use nose drops or sprays for more than a few days in a row.

Consider your stomach. What you think is excessive postnasal drip could actually be esophageal reflux, more commonly known as heartburn. "This gives the symptoms of a postnasal drip," says Mark Baldree, M.D., an otolaryngologist in private practice in Phoenix, Arizona, and staff member in the Division of Otolaryngology at St. Joseph's Hospital in Phoenix. "Some of the new antihypertensive medications can cause people to have symptoms of postnasal drip when they actually have heartburn.

Consider your estrogen level. The hormone estrogen affects the mucous lining of the nasal cavity. Some oral contraceptives are high in estrogen. Increasing the amount of estrogen circulating in the body can cause the nasal lining to get more puffy and produce excess mucus.

If you have a postnasal drip problem and take the Pill, discuss this with your gynecologist. He may be able to give you a low-dose prescription.

Skip the antihistamines. "They usually aren't that helpful," says Dr. Baldree. "They don't work that well, and they do make you drowsy. A plain decongestant is better."

PANEL OF ADVISERS

Mark Baldree, M.D., is an otolaryngologist in private practice in Phoenix, Arizona. He is a staff member in the Division of Otolaryngology, Department of Surgery, at St. Joseph's Hospital in Phoenix.

John A. Henderson, M.D., is an otolaryngologist and allergist in private practice in San Diego, California. He is also assistant clinical professor of surgery at the University of California, San Diego, School of Medicine.

Alvin Katz, M.D., is an otolaryngologist in private practice in New York City and surgeon director of the Manhattan Eye, Ear, Nose, and Throat Hospital there. He is past president of the American Rhinologic Society.

Gilbert Levitt, M.D., is an otolaryngologist in practice with Group Health Cooperative in Puget Sound, Washington. He is also clinical instructor of otolaryngology at the University of Washington School of Medicine in Seattle.

Jerold Principato, M.D., is an otolaryngologist in private practice in Bethesda, Maryland. He is an associate clinical professor of otolaryngology in the Department of Surgery at George Washington University School of Medicine in Washington, D.C. He is also an instructor at the American Academy of Otolaryngology.

Premenstrual Syndrome

28 Ways to Treat the Symptoms

Think of it as biological warfare, its battles played out on the fields of a woman's body and mind. Once a month, about two weeks before her menstrual period, the opposing armies—estrogen and progesterone—begin to amass. These female hormones, which regulate her menstrual cycle and affect her central nervous system, normally work in tandem. It's only when one tries to outdo the other that trouble looms.

Some women escape the conflict altogether; their hormones strike a peaceful balance before a single sword is drawn. Others are less fortunate. For one woman, estrogen levels may soar, leaving her feeling anxious and irritable. Or her progesterone predominates, dragging her into depression and fatigue.

The battles can rage on for days. Maybe you've been there. You might feel bloated and gain weight, have a headache, backache, acne, allergies, or terrible tenderness in your breasts. You may experience all of these symptoms or just a few. You may crave ice cream and potato chips. Your mood may shift without reason, swinging from euphoria to depression. And then, suddenly, the troops clear out and peace of mind returns—you finally get your period.

Premenstrual syndrome, or PMS, is believed to affect to varying degrees between one-third and one-half of all American women between the ages of 20 and 50, says Susan Lark, M.D., director of the PMS Self-Help Center in Los Altos, California. Certain factors, such as bearing several children or being married, seem to increase the risk of having PMS, says Guy Abraham, M.D., a former professor of obstetrics and gynecologic endocrinology at the University of California, Los Angeles, UCLA School of Medicine and researcher who has conducted extensive investigation into the disorder. (PMS is a major cause of divorce, he notes.) The problem may be inherited genetically, says Edward Portman, M.D., a PMS consultant, researcher, and director of the Portman Clinic in Madison, Wisconsin, who is also doing research into PMS.

Not all PMS sufferers have the same symptoms and the same intensity of discomfort, says Dr. Abraham. Nor do all PMS sufferers respond to the same treatments. Finding the best way to handle your PMS may require some trial and error. We talked to physicians who have worked extensively with PMS. They recommend the following coping measures.

Don't worry, be happy. A positive, confident attitude can help you cope and maybe even prevent future episodes of PMS, says Dr. Lark. If you feel PMS getting the best of you, she suggests reciting some positive affirmations. Sit in a comfortable position and repeat the following two or three times: "My body is strong and healthy. My estrogen and progesterone levels are perfectly regulated. I handle stress easily and competently."

Eat a little a lot. Poor nutrition doesn't cause PMS, says Dr. Portman, but certain dietary factors can accentuate the problem. Dr. Abraham agrees. "Poor eating habits can worsen PMS." A number of other physicians recommend a hypoglycemic diet—small meals low in sugar several times a day—to help keep your body and psyche in better balance.

Avoid empty calories. Stay away from low-nutrient foods like soft drinks and sweets containing refined sugar, says Dr. Abraham. Giving in to a craving for sweets will only make you feel worse, contributing to anxiety and mood swings. Try fresh fruit as a substitute, suggests Dr. Lark.

Decrease dairy. Eat no more than one or two portions per day of skimmed or low-fat milk, cottage cheese, or yogurt, Dr. Abraham says. Reason: The lactose in dairy products can block your body's absorption of the mineral magnesium, which helps regulate estrogen levels and increases its excretion.

Ferret out fats. Replace animal fats like butter and shortening with polyunsaturated oils like corn and safflower oils, says Dr. Abraham. Animal fats contribute to the high estrogen levels that may contribute to PMS, he says.

The Supplement Solution

A number of vitamins, minerals, and even amino acids may help relieve PMS symptoms, some doctors say. Here's the lowdown on nutritional solutions.

Vitamin B₆. Research into vitamin B_6 and PMS has shown that increasing your intake of the nutrient can help alleviate symptoms such as mood swings, fluid retention, breast tenderness, bloating, sugar craving, and fatigue, says Susan Lark, M.D. But, she cautions, don't experiment with the vitamin on your own. B_6 is toxic in high doses. Any vitamin therapy, including those mentioned below, should be supervised by your doctor.

Vitamins A and D. These two vitamins work in tandem to improve the health of your skin. Because of their importance to the skin, they may play a part in suppressing premenstrual acne and oily skin, according to Dr. Lark.

Vitamin C. An antioxidant, vitamin C is believed to play a role in reducing stress. It may help relieve the stress felt during PMS, says Dr. Lark. And there's more. Vitamin C is also known as a natural antihistamine, says Dr. Lark, and can be helpful for women whose allergies worsen before a period.

Vitamin E. Another antioxidant, vitamin E may have a powerful effect on the hormonal system, helping to relieve painful breast symptoms, anxiety, and depression, says Guy Abraham, M.D.

Calcium and magnesium. These two minerals work together to fight PMS, says Dr. Lark. Calcium helps prevent premenstrual cramps and pain, while magnesium helps the body absorb the calcium. Dr. Lark also believes that magnesium helps control premenstrual food cravings and stabilizes moods.

L-tyrosine. This amino acid is required for your brain's production of the chemical dopamine, your own natural antidepressant. Edward Portman, M.D., has found that it helps some of his patients relieve the anxiety and depression associated with PMS.

The PMS pill. Your best bet for treating PMS with nutritional supplements is to take a balanced supplement every day, says Dr. Lark. Your drugstore may even sell products specially formulated for PMS symptoms.

Restrict salt. "Go on a low-sodium diet for seven to ten days before the onset of your period to offset water retention," suggests Penny Wise Budoff, M.D., director of the Women's Medical Center in Bethpage, New York. "This means no restaurants, processed foods, Chinese food, commercial soup, or bottled salad dressing."

Fill up with fiber. Fiber helps the body clear out excess estrogens, says Dr. Abraham. Eat plenty of vegetables, beans, and whole grains. Millet, buckwheat, and barley are high not only in fiber but also in magnesium, adds Dr. Lark.

Those Crazy Cravings

Did you top off dinner tonight with a giant-size chocolate bar or a quart of ice cream? Don't put yourself down, especially if your menstrual period is around the corner. Chances are, your body made you do it.

"A woman doesn't overeat at this time of the month because of a weakness of character. Research shows that she's almost driven to it by the reaction of progesterone on her brain," says Peter Vash, M.D., an endocrinologist and internist on the clinical faculty of UCLA Medical Center in California who also specializes in eating disorders in private practice. What happens, researchers theorize, is that the high levels of progesterone released by the ovaries around the midpoint of a woman's menstrual cycle seem to affect those areas of the brain responsible for carbohydrate cravings.

As disturbing as the tendency is, it may actually be a primitive protective mechanism built into a woman's biology, Dr. Vash says. "When a woman is about to have her period, she's going to lose a lot of fluid. Eating high-carbohydrate foods like potato chips and ice cream will cause her to retain fluid and will also give her additional energy." Cravings for chocolate—a common preperiod occurrence—may result because of the brain's need for amino acids contained in that substance, he says.

Try to manage your cravings, says Dr. Vash, because giving in to them will only make you feel worse. Here's how he suggests you can help yourself.

Be prepared. "Know the cravings will occur for seven to ten days a month and mark your calendar," says Dr. Vash. "And know that they will stop, too. There's a limit. You can rise above them."

Put up a fight. Get adequate sleep, drink lots of fluids, and eat fruit and vegetables when your body asks for sweets and starches.

Cut the caffeine habit. Consume very limited quantities of coffee, tea, chocolate, and other caffeine-containing substances, says Dr. Abraham. Caffeine has been shown to contribute to painful breast tenderness, anxiety, and irritability.

Abstain from alcohol. The depression that often accompanies PMS will be accentuated by alcohol, says Dr. Portman. Alcohol can also worsen PMS headaches and fatigue and cause sugar cravings, says Dr. Lark.

Say no to diuretics. As a temporary antibloating measure, diuretics are commonly used by many PMS sufferers, says Dr. Lark. But some over-the-counter diuretics draw valuable minerals out of your system along with water, she says. A better approach would be to stay away from substances like salt and alcohol that cause you to retain water in the first place.

Get more active. Moderate exercise increases your blood flow, relaxes your muscles, and fights fluid retention, says Dr. Lark. What's more, says Dr. Portman, exercise increases your brain's production of endorphins, natural opiates that make you feel better all over.

Walk at a fast pace in fresh air, swim, jog, take up ballet or karate — do something you enjoy on a daily basis, Dr. Portman suggests. For best results, increase your level of activity for the week or two before PMS symptoms set in, says Dr. Lark.

De-stress your environment. Women with PMS seem to be particularly sensitive to environmental stress, says Dr. Lark. Surrounding yourself with soothing colors and soft music can contribute to greater calm at this and other times of the month.

Breathe deeply. Shallow breathing, which many of us do unconsciously, decreases your energy level and leaves you feeling tense, making PMS feel even worse, says Dr. Lark. Practice inhaling and exhaling slowly and deeply.

Sink into a tub. Indulge yourself in a mineral bath to relax muscles from head to toe, Dr. Lark suggests. Add 1 cup of sea salt and 1 cup of baking soda to warm bathwater. Soak for 20 minutes.

Try a little romance. The aching muscles and sluggish circulation that often accompany PMS can be relieved by having sex with orgasm, says Dr. Lark. The stimulation will help move blood and other fluids away from congested organs.

Get an advance from your sleep bank. If insomnia is part of your PMS, prepare for it by going to bed a few hours earlier for a few days before the problem generally sets in, says Dr. Lark. It may help alleviate the tiredness and irritability that go hand in hand with insomnia.

Stick to a schedule. Set reasonable goals and schedules for each day to avoid feeling overwhelmed, even if this means cutting back in your routine, Dr. Lark suggests.

Save social obligations for another time. Postpone big plans like holding a dinner party until a time when you feel you can handle it better. It'll only frazzle an already frazzled situation, says Dr. Lark.

Don't hide the truth. Talking about your PMS problems with your spouse, friends, or coworkers helps, says Dr. Lark. And it can be especially beneficial. You may even find a PMS self-help group in which to share your experiences with fellow sufferers. To see if one exists in your area, ask your doctor or call a local women's center.

PANEL OF ADVISERS

Guy Abraham, M.D., is a former professor of obstetrics and gynecologic endocrinology at the University of California, Los Angeles, UCLA School of Medicine and has conducted extensive research on PMS.

Penny Wise Budoff, M.D., is director of the Women's Medical Center in Bethpage, New York, and author of *No More Menstrual Cramps and Other Good News, No More Hot Flashes and Other Good News,* and other related books.

Susan Lark, M.D., is director of the PMS Self-Help Center in Los Altos, California, and author of *Dr. Susan Lark's Premenstrual Syndrome Self-Help Book.*

Edward Portman, M.D., is a PMS consultant, a researcher, and director of the Portman Clinic in Madison, Wisconsin.

Peter Vash, M.D., is an endocrinologist and internist on the clinical faculty of the UCLA Medical Center in California and a specialist in eating disorders. He also holds a master's degree in public health.

Psoriasis

19 Helpful Healers

Georgia Mossman has five things in common with millions of others who have psoriasis.

1. Her psoriasis is like theirs because it's different, uniquely her own.

2. What works for some might not work for her.

3. What works for her might not work for some.

4. A treatment will work well once, not as well the second time, and then not at all.

5. She doesn't know why she has it.

Add unknown cause and stir in unknown cure, and you have a recipe for frustration. It's easy to see why doctors like Laurence Miller, M.D., an adviser to the National Psoriasis Foundation and the National Institutes of Health, say, "When it comes to psoriasis, modern medicine is absolutely inadequate."

Psoriasis is a disease in which the skin cells run amok. Normally, skin renews itself in about 30 days—that's the time it takes for a new skin cell to work its way from the innermost layer of skin to the surface. In psoriasis, that cell reaches the top in just 3 days, as if the body had lost its brakes. The result is raised areas of skin called plaques, which are red and often itchy. After the cells reach the surface, they die like normal cells, but there are so many of them the raised patches turn white with dead cells flaking off.

Psoriasis usually goes through cycles of flare-ups and remission, with flare-ups most often occurring in winter. Sometimes it disappears for months or years. It can improve or worsen with age.

511

The Great Cover-Up

Hollywood to the rescue (Burbank, to be precise). Cosmetologist and Hollywood makeup artist Maurice Stein helps out clients referred to him by medical doctors across the country, as well as the standard must-be-picture-perfect stars. Here are some of his recommendations.

- First of all, "Never try to cover up any open lesion," Stein says, echoing medical advice.
- "There's a very good over-the-counter cream, applied with a makeup sponge, that can be applied to the scalp to cover up the flaking," Stein says. "Get your doctor's approval first. It's called Couvre, and it comes in black, dark, medium, and light brown, and gray. It works by darkening the scalp to match the color of the hair."
- For elbows and knees, Stein recommends Indian earth mixed with your favorite emollient and spread over the plaques with a makeup sponge. A rock, ground to face powder consistency, Indian earth can be bought in salons, department stores, drugstores, or health food stores. "A dime-size portion is enough to do your whole body," he says. The emollient will keep the plaques moist, and the Indian earth will disguise their appearance. "If you have to wear clothes over it, pat it dry to remove the excess," Stein advises.
- If you can't find Indian earth, "look for a cosmetic base with a lot of pigment," he says. "The best place to find and test them is at a local cosmetologist's."

Without a cause, there is no cure. But there are many things you can do for yourself. Keep in mind, however, that what works for someone else might not work for you. You have to experiment and devise your own battle plan. Here are some strategies you can try.

Get a new attitude. Philip Anderson, M.D., a professor and chairman of the Department of Dermatology at the University of Missouri–Columbia School of Medicine, says the most important thing is to accept the fact that you have psoriasis and focus your attention on learning how to manage it and prevent it from getting serious. "Don't waste energy fussing over every bump," he says. "That's not a good idea."

Dr. Miller agrees. "I see some of my psoriasis patients maybe twice a year," he says. "There is no law that says every person with psoriasis has to get rid of every flake on the body. I put my hands about a foot apart and tell them, 'It takes this much effort to get you 80 percent clear.' Then I stretch my arms out as far as I can and say, 'For the final 20 percent, this is what you have to do.' I never say, 'Learn to live with it.' When you think you've run out of treatments, you've gone from A to Z, you start over again at A. Mild psoriasis can be controlled totally by following some of these remedies."

Lubricate your chassis. Emollients top every dermatologist's list of over-the-counter treatments. Psoriatic skin is dry, and that can mean a worsening of the psoriasis and increased flaking and itching. Emollients help your skin retain water. The emollient can be your favorite nonirritating body oil or something as mundane as vegetable shortening or petroleum jelly. They're most effective applied right after bathing, when you're still dripping wet. (For safety's sake, avoid bathing in bath oil, which can make the tub as slick as ice.) Dr. Miller recommends Sarna lotion, which contains menthol and camphor, to soothe itching.

Seek the sun. With regular doses of intense sun, 95 percent of psoriasis sufferers improve. (The Dead Sea area of Israel is famous for its climatotherapy, and many people regularly travel to sunny climes.)

"The disease seems to be so much worse in wintertime or in a variable or humid climate that you should consider moving to a warm, dry area," Dr. Anderson says. It's the ultraviolet waves that fight psoriasis, and the UVB rays work the fastest. But there's a catch-22. UVB's are also the ones that give you a sunburn and run up the risks for skin cancer. They can also cause psoriasis sufferers to break out in previously unaffected areas.

There is, however, an out. Sunscreen. "The benefits of sunbathing can outweigh the risks of skin cancer and spreading psoriasis if you use sunscreens on the places where you don't have psoriasis and only expose the affected areas to the full force of the sun," says Dr. Miller.

Turn on the lamp. Get yourself a small UVB sunlamp to treat patches of psoriasis, suggests Dr. Miller. Each person's needs vary, so consult your doctor first. You may prefer the UVA light found in tanning parlors, but it's weaker and needs much more time to work.

Use tar without feathers. Over-the-counter coal tar preparations are weaker than the prescription versions but can be effective in mild psoriasis, says Dr. Miller. You can apply the tar directly to the plaques or immerse yourself in tar bath oil and treat your scalp with tar shampoo. Since even the OTC tars can stain and smell, they're usually washed off after a certain amount of time, but some kinds can be left on the skin to enhance the effect of sunlight or UVB treatments. "Tar makes you more sensitive to the sun, so be careful," Dr. Miller warns.

He notes that some new tar products "have been made a little more elegant and cosmetically acceptable in gel form. They don't smell like tar pits, and they can be used daily and wash off easily." He gives these precautions: "If any tar product causes burning or irritation, stop using it. And tar should never be used on raw, open skin."

Get wet and warm. "Baths and heated swimming pools are excellent for psoriasis," Dr. Miller says, by flattening plaques or cutting down scaling. "But hot water can actually make itching worse."

Or get wet and cold. A cold-water bath, maybe with a cup or so of apple cider vinegar added, is great for itching. "Another thing that really works is ice," Dr. Miller says. "Just dump some ice cubes into a small plastic bag and hold it against the afflicted skin."

Try cortisone for small areas. "OTC topical cortisone creams are weaker than their prescription cousins, but they're worth trying, and they're safer on the face and genital areas," Dr. Miller says. "But if you use it all the time in these areas, it will become less effective, and when you give up on it, the psoriasis can rebound. Just use it until you show some improvement, and then gradually wean yourself off."

Seal off psoriasis. Researchers have discovered that covering lesions with tape or plastic wrap for days or weeks can help clear up psoriasis, especially if cortisone cream is applied first. "I've slept in Saran Wrap and a shower cap," says Mossman ruefully, not saying how it affected her marriage.

"The cells on the surface get real soggy and damaged," Dr. Anderson explains. "It seems to slow down the proliferation." This treatment, however, is good only for small areas, "no bigger than a half dollar. You have to be careful because the skin can get gooey and infected, and then the psoriasis can get worse."

Don't risk injury. New lesions often appear on injured skin, Dr. Anderson says. Researchers believe the trauma to the skin may send the body into ungovernable overdrive. "People with psoriasis shouldn't go out picking blackberries, just like a man with a bad back shouldn't be a piano mover," Dr. Anderson says. You can injure your skin with such things as tight shoes, watchbands, dull razors, and harsh chemicals.

The Alternate Route

Zostrix: Hot Stuff for Psoriasis

Because there is no cure for psoriasis, people scour the planet for treatments and will try anything, including medications designed for other ailments. A good example is Zostrix, an over-the-counter cream used to treat shingles.

University of Chicago Pritzker School of Medicine clinical associate professor of clinical pharmacology Joel Bernstein, M.D., invented (and holds the patent for) Zostrix. It's made from the ingredient in red pepper, capsaicin, that gives real meaning to the word hot. It's been tested on psoriasis but has been approved by the Food and Drug Administration only for shingles, Dr. Bernstein says. "It's unquestionably effective," he claims. "My only concern is that it's a little tricky to use. In fact, if and when it's approved for psoriasis, it will probably be a prescription product."

The theory is that Zostrix makes the body exhaust all its supplies of substance P, a chemical that's believed to cause inflammation and is also found in psoriatic plaques. The cream then blocks the body from making more substance P, and it also may prevent proliferation of the blood vessels needed to feed the burgeoning skin cell population in a psoriatic plaque.

Zostrix can't be used haphazardly, Dr. Bernstein cautions. "It won't help unless it's used frequently and continuously for at least three weeks." And here's the tricky part: "This stuff burns, and you'd better be prepared for it," Dr. Miller says. It burns your fingers, it burns the plaque, and it will burn your face if you should happen to rub it without first washing off the Zostrix. But the burning lessens or vanishes if you keep up the treatments, Dr. Bernstein says.

Our advice: Use it only with your doctor's approval and close supervision.

Lose weight if you're overweight. While scientists can't swear obesity worsens psoriasis, Dr. Anderson says, "it's one of the most reliable connectors. Weight loss helps many people with psoriasis. If you lose weight and maintain normal weight, the psoriasis is almost always better."

De-stress yourself. "I saw a 13-year-old girl break out in psoriasis from head to toe after her father died," Dr. Miller reports. There's overwhelming evidence that stress can trigger psoriasis, agrees Eugene Farber, M.D., president of the Psoriasis Research Institute. "If you lie on the beach in Hawaii for a week, you get better. Even going into the hospital for surgery can make your psoriasis better. Although it's stressful, you're relaxing and being cared for. Any absence from your daily stresses, for any period of time, is helpful."

Go fishing. No, this isn't stress relief. It's a cute way to say try adding fish oil capsules containing the fatty acid EPA (eicosapentaenoic acid) to your diet. Dermatology and biochemistry professor Vincent Ziboh, Ph.D., of the University of California, Davis, School of Medicine, is encouraged by what he's found. "About 60 percent of the people we studied responded well," he reports. The area and thickness of the plaques decreased, as did redness and itching.

But there are important cautions to consider. "A small number of people will not improve, and a small number will get worse," Dr. Ziboh says. "There's no guarantee." His original study was small and short-term, "so the results are not conclusive. We saw no adverse effects, but over a longer period of time, there could be some." For example, fish oil can cut down on blood clotting, so it can amplify the blood-thinning effects of other medications you may be taking. "If you take it, have your doctor monitor you," he warns.

And, Dr. Ziboh notes, not all fish oil is the same. "We analyzed the fish oils we used and found the actual percentage of EPA in capsules varied from 1 percent to 10 percent" he says. "You should expect close to 17 percent."

Although the people in his study were taking 11 to 14 grams a day, he says, "I think you could do as well or better with half that dose." But make sure you check with your doctor first. While it's a good idea to eat fatty fish, such as salmon or mackerel, he adds, you'd have to eat at least 1 or 2 pounds a day to get 5 grams of EPA.

Treat infections. There's a well-documented but unexplained link between infections and the initial onset of psoriasis. Existing psoriasis is also known to worsen when an infection strikes. Mossman suffered a case of insect bites all over her lower legs. Soon afterward, she had her first outbreak of psoriasis—on her scalp, elbows, and knees.

"We see children walk in with psoriasis covering their bodies two weeks after a strep throat," Dr. Miller says. The key here, Dr. Anderson advises, is early and proper treatment of all infections, and extra attention to psoriasis when you have any type of infection.

PANEL OF ADVISERS

Philip Anderson, M.D., is professor and chairman of the Department of Dermatology, University of Missouri–Columbia School of Medicine.

Joel Bernstein, M.D., is a clinical associate professor of clinical pharmacology, University of Chicago Pritzker School of Medicine in Illinois.

Eugene Farber, M.D., is president of the Psoriasis Research Institute and former professor and chairman of the Department of Dermatology, Stanford University School of Medicine in California.

Laurence Miller, M.D., is a member of the Medical Advisory Board of National Psoriasis Foundation and a special adviser to the director of the National Institute of Arthritis and Musculoskeletal and Skin Diseases of the National Institutes of Health.

Maurice Stein is a cosmetologist and Hollywood makeup artist. He is the owner of Cinema Secrets, a theatrical makeup house in Burbank, California.

Vincent Ziboh, Ph.D., is a professor of dermatology and biochemistry at the University of California, Davis, School of Medicine.

Raynaud's Syndrome

18 Toasty Tips

You know Raynaud's syndrome all too well. You open a refrigerator door and your hands chill out in nothing flat. Or you notice changes in your fingers when you're punching away at your keyboard.

Suddenly the blood vessels to your fingers constrict. (Sometimes your toes are affected, too.) What you get at first is a spasm. Blood flow slows to the affected area, and that lack of oxygenated blood causes it to pale, maybe even take on a bluish tinge. Sometimes you experience a sensation of numbness from the lack of blood. Your fingers turn red again when the blood returns. In advanced stages of Raynaud's, poor blood supply can weaken the fingers and damage your sense of touch.

Cold isn't the only culprit. This odd but common affliction can result from injury to the blood vessels from the vibrations of powerful equipment like chain saws and pneumatic drills and from hypersensitivity to drugs that affect the blood vessels, or disorders of the connective tissue. Other causes include nerve disorders.

How can you protect yourself from Raynaud's syndrome? Here's what our experts advise.

Condition yourself to overcome chills. Train your hands to heat up in the cold by adapting this technique that U.S. Army researchers in Alaska devised.

Choose a room that's a comfortable temperature and place your hands in a container of warm water for 3 to 5 minutes. Then go into a freezing room and again dip your hands in warm water for 10 minutes. The cold environment would normally make your peripheral blood vessels constrict, but instead, the sensation of the warm water makes them open. Repeatedly training the blood vessels to open despite the cold eventually enables you to counter the constriction reflex even without the warm water.

In the army experiments, this procedure was repeated every other day for three to six times on 150 test people. After 54 treatments, the results were impressive. Their hands were 7 degrees warmer in the cold than before.

"People are training on the rooftops in New York City, in freezer lockers, in grocery stores, and in hospitals and hotels," says Murray Hamlet, director of the army's cold research program.

Twirl your arms to generate heat. You can actually force your hands to warm up through a simple exercise that Donald McIntyre, M.D., a dermatologist in Rutland, Vermont, devised. Pretend you're a softball pitcher. Swing your arm downward behind your body and then upward in front of you at about 80 twirls per minute. (This isn't as fast as it sounds; give it a try.)

The windmill effect, which Dr. McIntyre modeled after a skier's warm-up exercise, forces blood to the fingers through both gravitational and centrifugal force. This warm-up works well for chilled hands no matter what the cause is.

Eat iron-rich foods. Lack of iron may alter your thyroid metabolism, which regulates body heat. That's what researchers at the USDA Human Nutrition Research Center in Grand Forks, North Dakota, suspect. They measured the effects of dietary iron on six healthy women when they entered a cold chamber. When the women took only ⅓ of the recommended amount of iron for 80 days, they lost 29 percent more body heat than when they were on an iron-replete diet for 114 days.

Iron-rich foods include poultry, fish, lean red meat, lentils, and leafy green vegetables. Orange juice is okay, too, since it increases the body's ability to absorb iron.

Dress smart to maintain your core body temperature. To keep warm, you have to dress warmly. Common sense, yes, but many people will slap on gloves and footwear without taking equal precautions to maintain their core temperatures, which is really more important.

Choose fabrics that wick away perspiration. Perspiration is an even bigger cause of cold hands and feet than temperature. Sweat is the body's air conditioner, and your body's air conditioner can operate in cold weather if you're not careful. The hands and feet are especially susceptible because the palms and heels (along with the armpits) have the largest number of sweat glands in the body. That's why the heavy woolen socks and fleece-lined boots you bought to keep your feet warm may instead make them sweaty and chilly.

Wear cotton-blend socks rather than pure cotton socks. You want to wear socks that wick moisture away from your feet and insulate them. All-cotton socks can soak up your perspiration and chill your feet. Those made of Orlon and cotton are a better choice.

Make sure garments are loose. None of your garments should pinch. Tight-fitting clothes, whether they are nylons, garter belts, jeans, or shoes, can cut off circulation and eliminate insulating air pockets.

Dress in layers. If you're stepping out into the cold, the best warming measure you can take is to dress in layers. This helps trap heat and allows you to peel off clothes as the temperature changes. Your inner layer should consist of one of the new synthetic fabrics, like polypropylene, which wicks perspiration away from your skin. Silk or wool blends also are acceptable. The next layer should insulate you by trapping your body heat. A wool shirt is one of your best options.

Waterproof your body. Choose a breathable, waterproof jacket or windbreaker. Gore-Tex shoes and boots are the best choice for keeping your feet warm and dry.

Wear a hat. Another good piece of clothing you can wear to warm your hands and feet is a hat. Your head is the greatest site of body heat loss. The blood vessels in your head are controlled by cardiac output and won't constrict like those in your hands and feet.

If you want to keep your hands and feet warm, says John Abruzzo, M.D., director of the Division of Rheumatology and a professor of medicine at Thomas Jefferson University, it's as important to wear a hat as it is to wear gloves and socks.

Wear mittens. Mittens keep you warmer than gloves because they trap your whole hand's heat.

Try foot powder. Clothes aren't the only way to keep dry. "Absorbent foot powders are excellent for helping keep feet dry," says Marc A. Brenner, D.P.M., a private practitioner in Glendale, New York, and past president of the American Society of Podiatric Dermatology. But he cautions people with severe cold feet problems caused by diabetes and peripheral vascular disease to use a shaker can rather than an aerosol spray, since the mist from the spray can actually freeze your feet.

Don't smoke. Smokers set themselves up for cold hands and feet whenever they light up. Cigarette smoke cools you in two ways. It helps form plaque in your arteries and, more immediately, nicotine causes vasospasms that narrow the small blood vessels.

These effects can be especially hard on people with Raynaud's. "Raynaud's patients are sensitive even to other people's smoke," says Frederick A. Reichle, M.D., chief of vascular surgery at Presbyterian–University of Pennsylvania Medical Center.

Chill out to warm up. Staying cool and calm may help some people stay warm. Why? Stress creates the same reaction in the body as cold. It's the fight-or-flight phenomenon. Blood is pulled from the hands and feet to the brain and internal organs to enable you to think and react more quickly.

Calming techniques abound. Some, like progressive relaxation—in which you systematically tense, then relax the muscles from your forehead to your hands and toes—can be practiced at any time, in any place.

Eat a hot, hearty meal. The very act of eating causes a rise in core body temperature. This is called thermogenesis. So eat something before you go out to stoke your body's furnace. And eat something hot to give the stoking a boost. A bowl of hot oatmeal before your morning walk, a soup break, or hot lunch will keep your hands and feet toasty even in inclement weather.

Drink up. Dehydration can aggravate chills and frostbite by reducing your blood volume. Ward off the big chill by drinking plenty of fluids such as hot cider, herbal teas, or broth.

But pass on the coffee. Coffee and other caffeinated products constrict blood vessels. The last thing you want when you have Raynaud's syndrome is to interfere with your circulation.

Avoid alcohol. Don't be misled by the lure of a hot toddy, either. Alcohol will temporarily warm up your hands and feet but its detrimental effects outweigh its benefits as a hand and foot warmer.

Alcohol increases blood flow to the skin, giving you the immediate perception of warmth. But that heat is soon lost to the air, reducing your core body temperature. In other words, alcohol actually makes you colder. The danger comes from drinking an immodest amount and being subjected to unexpected cold for an extended period, which can lead to severe problems like frostbite.

PANEL OF ADVISERS

John Abruzzo, M.D., is director of the Division of Rheumatology and a professor of medicine at Thomas Jefferson University in Philadelphia, Pennsylvania.

Marc A. Brenner, D.P.M., has a private practice in Glendale, New York, is past president of the American Society of Podiatric Dermatology, and author of *The Management of the Diabetic Foot.*

Murray Hamlet is director of cold research at the U.S. Army Research Institute of Environmental Medicine in Natick, Massachusetts.

Donald McIntyre, M.D., is a dermatologist in Rutland, Vermont.

Frederick A. Reichle, M.D., is chief of vascular surgery at Presbyterian–University of Pennsylvania Medical Center in Philadelphia.

Restless Legs Syndrome

20 Calming Techniques

No party, no music, no Gene Kelly. But as you lie in bed, anxious to fall asleep, your legs—*just feel like dancing.*

What's going on?

Well, maybe you've been repressing your true calling—to be a Rockette. But probably you are one of the estimated 5 percent of the population with restless legs syndrome.

The condition, also known as Ekbom syndrome, is usually a chronic annoyance rather than a symptom of a serious neurological disorder. It is characterized by an irresistible urge to move the legs, "jumping" of the legs, and deep creeping or crawling sensations in the legs.

"Typically both lower legs are affected, although the thighs and even the arms can be involved," says Lawrence Z. Stern, M.D., a professor of neurology and director of the Mućio F. Delgado Clinic for Neuromuscular Disorders at the University of Arizona Health Sciences Center. "Both sides are not always symmetrical."

The origin of the sensations is unknown. Some researchers suspect an imbalance in the brain's chemistry may be the root cause of the problem.

Whatever the physiology of it, the condition certainly isn't as much fun as dancing. So here are a few steps you can take to cut in on restless legs syndrome.

Get up and walk. Restless legs syndrome tends to strike at night, when you're at rest. So the quickest way to satisfy the legs' urge to move is to comply with a stroll around the bedroom, says Ronald F. Pfeiffer, M.D., an associate professor of neurology and pharmacology and chief of the Section of Neurology at the University of Nebraska Medical Center in Omaha.

MEDICAL ALERT

Be Conscientious: See a Doctor

If you have restless legs syndrome, you probably don't have anything to worry about—except the sleep it sometimes causes you to miss.

But if you're experiencing symptoms for the first time—pronounced sensations in the legs, usually at night—see your doctor. The symptoms of restless legs syndrome can be warning signs for serious medical problems such as lung disease, kidney disease, diabetes, Parkinson's disease, and many neurological disorders.

So for safety—not to mention peace of mind—let your doctor diagnose.

Of course, some people have trouble sleeping even without restless legs syndrome. Thus, while walking is a good way to halt a sudden, severe attack, it might also be a good idea to try the following.

Walk before going to bed. In some cases this noticeably reduces bedtime bouts of restless legs syndrome, says Dr. Stern. "Exercise changes chemical balances in the brain—endorphins are released —and may promote more restful sleep," he adds.

Wriggle. Or is that wiggle? Either way, the idea is to move your feet back and forth when symptoms arise.

Change positions. "Some people seem to develop symptoms a lot more sleeping in one position than another," says Dr. Stern. "Experiment with different sleeping positions. It's harmless and may prove to be worthwhile."

Soak your feet in cool water. "It works for some," Dr. Pfeiffer says. One caution: Do not follow a "more is better" theory and immerse your feet in a bucket of ice; you could cause nerve damage.

Warm up. While cold helps some people, others find using a heating pad more soothing and effective, Dr. Pfeiffer says.

Take one multivitamin daily. "Iron deficiency may be a cause of restless legs syndrome," Dr. Pfeiffer says, noting that several studies have found an association between iron deficiency and restless legs syndrome. Folate deficiency also has been implicated in restless legs syndrome. If you suspect a deficiency, check with your doctor.

Dr. Stern says a daily multivitamin can protect you against deficiencies of both nutrients.

Take two aspirins before bedtime. Doctors can't say why aspirin helps, but apparently it does reduce symptoms in some people.

Don't eat a big meal late. Eating a lot late at night may get the legs really jumping. "It may be the activity of digesting a big meal that triggers something that causes symptoms," offers Dr. Stern.

Lower your stress level. Easier said than done but certainly worth trying. "Stress just worsens the problem," says Dr. Stern. Being organized, giving yourself quiet time, taking deep breaths, and practicing various relaxation techniques are good ways to reduce stress.

Get plenty of rest. Symptoms may be more severe if you allow yourself to become overtired.

The Alternate Route

Different Nighttime Routines

Restless legs syndrome can be chronic—it pesters some people off and on for years and years. "So a lot of people will try different rituals," says Richard K. Olney, M.D. And some of those rituals, odd as they may be, work—at least some of the time.

Why do they work? Doctors don't even want to hazard a guess. But at the same time, if these unusual methods pose no danger and could help, you may want to give them a try.

Wear cotton stockings to bed. Maybe try this one in winter—at least they're warm.

Wear silk pajamas to bed. They'll feel good on you, and if you still have to get up and walk around, you'll be classily clothed.

Rub your legs with an electric vibrator. Some people say this reduces symptoms; in a few people, however, it could make symptoms worse.

Massage your legs. "Right before bedtime, rubbing your legs might be beneficial," suggests Richard K. Olney, M.D., an assistant professor of neurology at the University of California, San Francisco. Mild stretching also might help.

Avoid sleep-inducing medications. They may provide short-term benefits, but many people build up a tolerance to them and then they have two problems—restless legs syndrome *and* dependence on the drugs, says Dr. Stern.

Don't use alcohol as a sedative. Again, you set yourself up for double trouble, Dr. Stern says.

Stop or dramatically reduce caffeine. "Some studies have shown an association between relief of restless legs syndrome and stopping caffeine," Dr. Pfeiffer says.

Quit smoking. A 70-year-old woman who was a smoker and long-time sufferer of restless legs syndrome found relief a month after she stopped smoking, according to one Canadian doctor. Another four months later, according to the doctor's report, the woman was still free of symptoms.

Come in from the cold. Several studies have implicated prolonged exposure to cold as a possible cause of restless legs syndrome.

PANEL OF ADVISERS

Richard K. Olney, M.D., is an assistant professor of neurology at the University of California, San Francisco.

Ronald F. Pfeiffer, M.D., is an associate professor of neurology and pharmacology and chief of the Section of Neurology at the University of Nebraska Medical Center in Omaha.

Lawrence Z. Stern, M.D., is a professor of neurology and director of the Mucio F. Delgado Clinic for Neuromuscular Disorders at the University of Arizona Health Sciences Center in Tucson.

Scarring

10 Ways to Decrease the Damage

Want to look mean and tough? Dress in black, smoke a fat cigar, carry a violin case, and—above all—have a big scar running down one cheek.

Of course, looking mean and tough may not be the look you're after. If that's the case, you've come to the right place. How you treat a cut can determine what kind of scar, if any, may develop. And how you care for that scar can determine how fast and to what extent it will fade (as scars do over time).

Nip scars in the bud. If you don't want dog hair on your sofa, don't own a dog. If you don't want cavities, don't eat sugar. And if you don't want scars, don't get cut. It's that simple. "Every time the skin gets cut, it scars," says Gerald Imber, M.D., an attending plastic surgeon at New York Hospital–Cornell University Medical Center in New York City. But some people, he says, tend to scar more than others. "It's a very personal thing." However your body reacts, consider protecting your skin with gloves, long pants, and long sleeves whenever working around thorny, sharp, or jagged objects.

Help wounds heal properly. A wound that heals quickly and neatly is less likely to develop a scar than a wound that festers. Make sure all your cuts and scrapes are properly cleaned (hydrogen peroxide is a good cleanser), and try to keep the wound slightly moist with an antibiotic ointment while it is healing, says Jeffrey H. Binstock, M.D., a dermatologist in private practice and an assistant clinical professor of dermatologic surgery at the University of California, San Francisco, School of Medicine. (For proper treatment of cuts and scrapes, see page 171.)

526

The Alternate Route

Rub Oil in the Wound

Pick up a vitamin E capsule, break it open, and let the oil ooze out over a cut or a scar. Sounds simple. Sounds effective. Lots of people do it. Some swear it helps prevent scars or even makes new scars disappear.

But what it probably does is make *old* scars disappear. "Vitamin E helps a new wound heal faster than if you put nothing on at all," possibly helping to *reduce* scarring, says Stephen Kurtin, M.D.

What is it about vitamin E that helps wounds heal? It's actually the oil in the capsule that's beneficial, says Dr. Kurtin. "You're helping to keep the area moist— there's nothing magical about it. Apply the same oil with the vitamin E removed, and you'll probably get the same benefit," he says.

Don't pick at scabs. Mama was right. Picking scabs off a healing wound could increase your chances of leaving behind a visible scar, says John F. Romano, M.D., a dermatologist and an attending physician at St. Vincent's Hospital and Medical Center of New York.

Close gaps with a butterfly bandage. If you do get cut, and the cut is large enough, you should go to a doctor for stitches, particularly if the cut is on the face (where a scar would be most visible). But if a cut is small, and you are concerned about scarring, consider the use of a butterfly bandage, says Dr. Romano. These bandages, available at most pharmacies, can help to keep the wound closed for better healing and minimal scarring. They should be used only after the wound has been thoroughly cleaned.

Eat a well-balanced diet. Wounds won't heal right unless your body has what it takes to make them heal right. What does it take? Protein and vitamins—obtained by eating a good, well-balanced diet— are essential. And of particular importance to wound healing is the mineral zinc. Good sources of zinc include roasted pumpkin and sunflower seeds, Brazil nuts, Swiss and cheddar cheeses, peanuts, dark meat turkey, and lean beef.

Treat scars with tenderness. Sweat glands, oil glands, and hair glands are all destroyed by a scar, leaving it much more at the mercy of the elements than the rest of your skin, says Paul Lazar, M.D., a professor of clinical dermatology at Northwestern University Medical School. He advises keeping large scars, such as those from a third-degree burn, lubricated with a good skin cream to protect them from abrasions.

Take it easy in the shower. One common source of abrasions to tender scars is a washcloth in the hands of an overzealous washer. Dr. Lazar recommends cleaning scars very gently.

Cover your scars with sunblock. Scars have less pigment than the rest of your skin. They therefore lack the ability to develop a protective tan, and they are especially vulnerable to sunburn. You should make certain to cover all scars with a strong sunscreen whenever you head outside on a sunny day, says Stephen Kurtin, M.D., a dermatologist in New York City and an assistant professor of dermatology at Mount Sinai School of Medicine of the City University of New York.

Don't be overly alarmed. Fresh scars are often quite noticeable, but don't be too concerned. Remember that the color of a scar typically fades over time all by itself, says Dr. Lazar.

PANEL OF ADVISERS

Jeffrey H. Binstock, M.D., is a dermatologist in private practice in San Francisco and Mill Valley, California, and an assistant clinical professor of dermatologic surgery at the University of California, San Francisco, School of Medicine.

Gerald Imber, M.D., is an attending plastic surgeon at New York Hospital–Cornell University Medical Center in New York City.

Stephen Kurtin, M.D., is a practicing dermatologist in New York City and an assistant professor of dermatology at the Mount Sinai School of Medicine of the City University of New York.

Paul Lazar, M.D., is a professor of clinical dermatology at Northwestern University Medical School in Chicago, Illinois. He is a former board member of the American Academy of Dermatology.

John F. Romano, M.D., is a dermatologist and an attending physician at St. Vincent's Hospital and Medical Center of New York. He is also clinical instructor in medicine at New York Hospital–Cornell University Medical Center in New York City.

Shingles

14 Tips to Combat the Pain

Sharp, burning pain crackles like static along a nerve route in your body. Angry red blisters rise from the pain site several days later. When the bumps blister and then turn cloudy, you realize this is no ordinary rash.

You've got shingles, a viral infection of a nerve.

Blame it on the chickenpox you had as a child. The varicella zoster (VZ) virus, the same invader that caused you such misery before, never really left your system. Until now, your immune system has done great rendering the VZ virus completely inactive. And even now, that mighty immune system of yours is keeping the virus from wreaking havoc throughout your system. But that's small comfort when you're in pain. Depending upon how severe your case of shingles is, the pain can continue even after your blisters heal.

This VZ virus, also known as herpes zoster, is a member of the notorious herpes clan. The word "zoster" means belt in Greek, and until you suffer from shingles, you probably won't appreciate just how appropriately named it is.

What can you do to make yourself as comfortable as possible while your body heals?

AT THE OUTSET

Here is what the experts recommend for the beginning stages of shingles.

Reach for pain relief. Jules Altman, M.D., a private practitioner in Warren, Michigan, and clinical professor of dermatology at Wayne State University, favors extra-strength Tylenol, an aspirin substitute.

Give yourself a boost. Both your immune system and your nerves will benefit from extra doses of vitamin C and vitamin B-complex, says dermatologist John G. McConahy, M.D., of New Castle, Pennsylvania.

529

He advises his shingles patients to take 200 milligrams of vitamin C five or six times a day to build immune power and a vitamin B-complex supplement to regenerate and rebuild nerve cells. (Of course, don't take this or any vitamin therapy without your doctor's okay and supervision.)

Dr. McConahy also tells his patients to take a multivitamin tablet that contains zinc.

Try lysine. A number of studies show that the amino acid lysine can help inhibit the spread of the herpes virus. Not all studies on lysine point to that conclusion, however.

Taking lysine supplements at the onset of shingles can't hurt and might help, says Leon Robb, M.D., director of the Robb Pain Management Group in Los Angeles, California.

FOR SHINGLES BLISTERS
Once blisters appear, there are several ways you can get relief.

Do nothing. Leave the blisters alone unless your rash is really bad, says Dr. Robb. "You can retard healing if you irritate the skin by applying too many skin creams and ointments."

Make a calamine liniment. This recipe comes from James J. Nordlund, M.D., a professor and chairman of the Department of Dermatology at the University of Cincinnati College of Medicine. You might be able to get your local pharmacist to make it for you.

Add to calamine lotion, 20 percent isopropyl alcohol and 1 percent each of phenol and menthol. If the phenol is too strong or the menthol too cool, dilute the liniment with equal parts of water.

"Use this as often as you want in the course of a day until the blisters are dried and scabbed over, says Dr. Nordlund. Then don't use it anymore." Instead, switch to a lotion that contains phenol and menthol, such as Nutriderm.

Try a chloroform/aspirin paste. Dr. Robb favors this remedy, which comes from Robert King, M.D., of Syracuse, New York.

Mash two aspirin tablets (not aspirin substitutes) into a powder. Add 2 tablespoons of chloroform and mix. Pat the paste onto the affected area with a clean cotton ball. You can apply the paste several times a day. You can also ask your pharmacist to make this mixture for you.

How does it work? The chloroform is said to dissolve soap residue, oil, and dead cells in the skin. That leaves the aspirin to soak into the skin folds and desensitize the affected nerve endings. You should begin to feel better in 5 minutes. The relief can last for hours, and often days.

MEDICAL ALERT

Prevent Irreversible Nerve Damage

If your shingles pain is more than you can stand, see your doctor. This is no time for stoicism. Ignore your discomfort and you could end up with irreversible nerve damage and years of pain, says Leon Robb, M.D.

Remember, shingles is not a skin disease but a viral infection of a nerve.

Doctors typically treat the early stages of shingles with acyclovir or a steroid drug. Acyclovir slows reproduction of the varicella zoster virus and shortens the course of infection. What it doesn't seem to prevent is post-herpetic neuralgia, the nerve pain that lingers after the skin heals. Some physicians believe that steroid drugs like prednisone can prevent that pain; others are unconvinced.

The technique that Dr. Robb favors is injecting a nerve block in the appropriate place. "If you block the sympathetic nerves supplying the area of pain, you can provide definite and dramatic relief to over 75 to 80 percent of patients," he says.

Yet help is available for chronic sufferers of post-herpetic neuralgia. One method involves implanting a small electrical device in the spine that can deliver a pain-masking shock to the appropriate site when stimulated by an external transmitter.

Apply a wet dressing to severe eruptions. Take a washcloth or towel, dip it in cold water, squeeze it out, and apply it to the affected area, says Dr. Nordlund. "The cooler it is, the better it feels. This is similar to putting on ice when you burn yourself," he says.

Don't fan the flames. Avoid anything that will make your blistered skin hotter. Heat will just macerate the skin, says Dr. Robb.

Sink into a starch bath. If you have shingles on your forehead, skip to the next tip. But if the problem is below your neck, this can help. Just throw a handful of cornstarch or colloidal oatmeal, such as Aveeno, into your bathwater and settle in for a good soak, says Dr. Nordlund. "But be extra careful not to slip on the bottom of the tub.

"People find this helpful, although the relief may not last long," he adds. "I often have my patients do this 20 minutes before bed, then they take something for the pain to help them sleep."

Zap the infection with hydrogen peroxide. If the blisters become infected, try dabbing them with hydrogen peroxide. You don't need to dilute it. Straight out of the bottle is fine, says Dr. Robb.

Or use an antibiotic ointment. But be careful about which one you choose. Neomycin and neosporin are notorious as skin sensitizers, says Dr. Nordlund. Polysporin or erythromycin are better choices.

Hold the Zostrix until the blisters are gone. This will usually be about two months. Zostrix is an OTC remedy for shingles pain. Its active ingredient is capsaicin, a derivative of the red pepper used to make chili powder and cayenne pepper. Scientists believe it works by blocking the production of a chemical needed to transmit pain impulses between nerve cells.

Using this topical ointment on blistering skin is "like putting red peppers on active shingles," says Dr. Altman. "The idea behind Zostrix is its counterirritant effect. It is for healed skin that has a pain sensation, not for an open, oozing infection."

POST-BLISTER CARE

You may have some discomfort even when the blisters are gone. Here's what to do.

Chill out with ice. If you still have pain after the blisters have healed, put ice in a plastic bag and stroke the skin vigorously, says Dr. Robb. "What we're trying to do here is confuse the nerves. This has been found to be beneficial."

Do some detective work. Sometimes, for some sufferers, long-lasting shingles pain may point to some underlying emotional need that's not being met, says Dr. Altman. Is the pain diverting your attention away from some other problem? Or is the pain diverting much-needed attention to you? It's an issue to consider, says Dr. Altman, and one which you may want to discuss with your doctor.

PANEL OF ADVISERS

Jules Altman, M.D., is a private practitioner in Warren, Michigan, and a clinical professor of dermatology at Wayne State University in Detroit.

John G. McConahy, M.D., is a dermatologist with a private practice in New Castle, Pennsylvania.

James J. Nordlund, M.D., is a professor and chairman of the Department of Dermatology at the University of Cincinnati College of Medicine in Ohio.

Leon Robb, M.D., is director of the Robb Pain Management Group in Los Angeles, California, where he treats patients with shingles and conducts research. An anesthesiologist for 25 years, he is former chief of anesthesia at Hollywood Presbyterian Medical Center.

Shinsplints

13 Ways to Soothe Sore Legs

Funny thing about shinsplints. Most people know when they have them, but very few people—experts included—seem to know what they are. Most doctors prefer the terms *tendinitis*, or *periostitis*, though they can't say for certain which of those terms, if either, actually describes the condition.

"Shinsplints could be a variety of things," says Marjorie Albohm, a certified athletic trainer and associate director of the International Institute of Sports Science and Medicine at the Indiana University School of Medicine. "Many people say they're the beginning part of stress fractures, others say they're a muscle irritation. Still others say they're an irritation of the tendon that attaches the muscle to the bone. The problem in treating them goes back to the problem in defining exactly what they are."

That may explain why shinsplints plague so many active people of both sexes and of all ages. Shinsplints are one of the most common and disabling conditions in aerobic dance (about 22 percent of students and 29 percent of instructors have them), and long-distance runners (about 28 percent are afflicted) have probably suffered with them since the first road was paved.

This much is known—unyielding surfaces can produce shinsplints in an instant, and that goes for people who walk on concrete as well as for those who exercise on it. Other shinsplint culprits include faulty posture, poor shoes, fallen arches, insufficient warm-up, poor running mechanics, poor walking mechanics, overtraining, and so forth. Shinsplints aren't hard to get.

The symptoms are vague and often confused with those of stress fracture (see "When Shin Pain Isn't a Splint" on page 536). But shinsplints typically include pain in the shin of one or both legs, though there may or may not be a specific area of tenderness. Pain and aching will be felt in the front of the leg after activity, although it may occur during activity as the condition progresses.

The remedies here are designed to help keep that shinsplint condition from progressing to the point of stress fracture and to let you continue your active lifestyle without causing undue harm. Those remedies that call on you to stretch or exercise the calf muscles can be beneficial in preventing a recurrence. As always, let pain be your guide. If anything recommended here causes increased discomfort, don't do it!

Start with the ground. "Start by looking at the surface," advises Albohm. "If you're walking, running, dancing, playing basketball, or whatever on a hard, unyielding surface, then you need to change that."

For those involved in aerobic dance, injuries are highest on concrete floors covered with carpet, while wood floors over airspace are the least damaging. If you must dance on a nonresilient floor, make sure the instructor teaches only low-impact aerobics or that high-quality foam mats are provided. For runners, choose grass or dirt before asphalt, and choose asphalt before concrete. Concrete is very unyielding and should be avoided at all times.

Then move to the shoes. If you can't change your surface, or if you find that that's not the problem, then the experts say it's time to look at different footwear. "Look at the arch support," says Albohm, "look at the shock-absorption quality in the sole and through the arch. The support has to be there, and the shoe has to fit you right."

For those who participate in activities that cause a lot of forefoot impact, judge a shoe on its ability to absorb shock in that area. The best test is to try the shoes on in the store and jump up and down, both on the toes and flat-footed. The impact with the floor should be firm but not jarring.

For runners, the choice is a bit more difficult. For example, research has shown that about 58 percent of all runners with shinsplints also pronate excessively (meaning the foot rolls to the inside). Choosing a shoe for pronation control sometimes results in a loss of cushioning, but if you're a pronator with shinsplints, control is probably what you need.

Choose shoes often. Of course, one way to make sure your shoes retain as much cushioning ability as possible is to change them frequently. Gary M. Gordon, D.P.M., director of the running and jogging programs at the University of Pennsylvania Sports Medicine Center in Philadelphia, gives this advice for avoiding shinsplint pain: Runners who put in 25 miles a week or more need new shoes every 60 to 90 days — less mileage than that means new shoes every four to six months.

Those who participate in aerobics, tennis, or basketball twice a week need new shoes two or three times a year, while those who participate up to four times a week need them every 60 days.

Put it on RICE. As soon as you notice shinsplint pain, follow the rules of RICE: rest, ice, compression, and elevation for 20 to 30 minutes. The experts swear by it.

"Don't underestimate the power of ice," says Albohm. Keep your icing routine simple, she says. Just prop the leg up, wrap it with an Ace bandage, and place the ice pack on it for 20 to 30 minutes.

Go for contrast. A variation on the RICE treatment is the contrast bath, which seems especially effective for pain on the inner leg. With this method, alternate 1 minute of ice with 1 minute of heat. Do this before any activity that can cause shinsplint pain, and continue it for at least 12 minutes.

Stretch those calves. "We find that stretching the Achilles tendon and the calf muscles is an excellent preventive measure for shinsplints," Albohm says. "If you're a woman wearing 2-inch heels every day, you're not stretching either of those at all."

The reason stretching helps is because shortened calf muscles tend to throw more weight and stress forward to the shins. Place your hands on a wall, extend one leg behind the other, and press the back heel slowly to the floor. Do this 20 times and repeat with the other leg.

Now tend to the tendons. Dr. Gordon offers this simple technique for stretching the Achilles tendon: Keep both feet flat on the ground about 6 inches apart. Then bend your ankles and knees forward while keeping your back straight. Go to the point of tightness and hold for 30 seconds. "You should feel it really stretching down in the lower part of the calf," he says. Repeat the exercise ten times.

Learn to master massage. "For shinsplints in the front of the leg, you want to massage the area right near the edge of the shin—not directly on it," says Rich Phaigh, co-director of the American Institute of Sports Massage in New York City and the Institute of Clinical Biomechanics in Eugene, Oregon, and author of the book *Athletic Massage*. "If you work right on the bone, it just seems to make the inflammation worse."

To massage away shinsplint pain, sit on the floor with one knee bent and the foot flat on the ground. Start by lightly stroking both sides of the bone using the palms of your hands, gliding them back and forth from knee to ankle. Repeat this stroking motion several times. Then wrap your hands around the calf and, using the tips of your fingers, stroke deeply on each side of the bone from ankle to knee. Cover the area, using as much pressure as possible.

"What you want to do is restore length and relieve tightness in the tendons at the top and bottom of the shins," Phaigh says, noting that a good massage helps improve circulation in the area, too.

Correct faulty feet. Flat feet or very high arches can sometimes cause shinsplints, Dr. Gordon says. "If you have flat feet, the muscle on the inside of your calf has to work harder and gets fatigued quicker," he says, "making the bone take more of a pounding."

If you're flat-footed, you may need additional shock-absorbing material or arch support in your shoes. Inserts are available at sporting goods stores, but it might be best to see a podiatrist before adding inserts on your own.

Pain on the outside of the lower leg is sometimes associated with very high arches, Dr. Gordon says. "That requires a lot of stretching exercises, as well as strengthening the muscles and maybe adding orthotics."

Build muscle, reduce pain. Shinsplint pain can sometimes be prevented by strengthening the muscles surrounding the shin. These muscles help decelerate the foot and reduce shock whenever you walk or run. Help strengthen them with the following.

When Shin Pain Isn't a Splint

Because some experts believe shinsplints may actually be stress fractures in an early stage, telling the difference between the two is sometimes tricky. Even so, shinsplints can become full-blown stress fractures with continued abuse. How do you know if you've stepped over the line? We asked athletic trainer Marjorie Albohm.

"With a stress fracture, you're going to have pinpoint pain, about the size of a dime or quarter," she says. "If somebody asks you where it hurts, you'll be able to go right to it, put one or two fingers on it, and tell them exactly where it is. It'll be right on or around a bony area, and it's point specific. A shinsplint will be an aching discomfort up and down the whole lower leg."

- Try riding a bike with toe clips attached. Concentrate on pulling up with the muscles in front of the shin every time you pedal. (Bicycling also gives you a good aerobic workout without aggravating shinsplints.)
- For those who don't have access to a bike, walking around on your heels does much the same thing, forcing you to tighten and pull up with the muscles around the shin each time you take a step.
- If you're seeking a conditioner that's a bit more strenuous, try this. Sit on the edge of a table that's high enough to keep your feet from touching the ground. Place a sock filled with coins over the foot, or make a 5-pound weight from an old paint can by filling it with gravel (place this over the foot with a shoe on so the wire doesn't hurt). Flex the foot upward at the ankle, then relax, then flex the foot upward again. Repeat this as many times as you can, tightening the shin muscles as you pull the foot up.

PANEL OF ADVISERS

Marjorie Albohm is a certified athletic trainer and associate director of the International Institute of Sports Science and Medicine at the Indiana University School of Medicine in Mooresville. She served on the medical staff for the 1980 Winter Olympics and the 1987 Pan American Games.

Gary M. Gordon, D.P.M., is director of the running and jogging programs at the University of Pennsylvania Sports Medicine Center in Philadelphia. He specializes in podiatric medicine, foot surgery, and sports medicine.

Rich Phaigh is co-director of the American Institute of Sports Massage in New York City and the Institute of Clinical Biomechanics in Eugene, Oregon. He is also a massage instructor at East-West College of the Healing Arts in Portland. Phaigh is the author of *Athletic Massage* and has worked on the likes of running stars Alberto Salazar and Joan Samuelson.

Side Stitches

9 Ways to Avoid the Nuisance

A stitch or catch in the side—a sharp, temporary pain—is caused by a spasm of the diaphragm. It happens when your diaphragm, a muscle between your chest and your abdomen, can't get the oxygen it needs.

"Sometimes running can block the flow of blood to the diaphragm," explains Gabe Mirkin, M.D., a private practitioner at the Sportsmedicine Institute in Silver Spring, Maryland. "Every time you raise your knee, you contract your belly muscles, which increases the pressure inside your belly. When you breathe deeply, your lungs expand to a much larger size than during normal shallow breathing. The dual pressure from the contracted belly muscles below and the expanded lungs above can shut off the flow of blood to the diaphragm." Unable to get all the oxygen it needs, your diaphragm will go into a cramp and hurt.

If you don't breathe evenly, you can get side stitches when you're running or walking or even laughing.

Here's how to handle them.

Stop. When the pain hits, stop whatever you are doing. You need to relax to calm your twitching muscle.

Press there. Using three fingers, press on the area where the pain is the worst until the hurt stops. Or, use those three fingers to gently massage the painful area. Often this is enough to release the pain, says David Balboa, a sports psychotherapist and co-director of The Walking Center in New York City.

Exhale deeply. As you begin to knead the cramp out of your diaphragm, take a breath, then purse your lips and blow it out as hard as you can. Take another breath and exhale again. The inhaling followed by a deep exhalation works like yoga, says Balboa, giving you an internal massage for your pinched muscle.

Breathe in, breathe out. Continue to massage your aching side and work to slow your breathing to a regular pace. Getting your breathing back to a steady rhythm will help stop the ache.

Slow down and walk. If you are running when you get a stitch, sometimes just slowing to a walk is enough to calm that jerking muscle, says Suki Jay Rappaport, Ph.D., director of the Transformations Institute in Corte Madera, California, and a movement educator. When the twinge fades, speed up again.

Belly breathe. Before you go out to walk or run again, you need to know how to breathe to prevent stitches from taking sides.

Balboa suggests you try this test: Look down at your chest. Watch closely as you suck in a giant breath. What moved? If only your chest moved, you're breathing with your chest cavity and that's not enough. To fight side stitches, you want your diaphragm involved in the breathing exercise. One way to tell if you are using that muscle is to get your chest and belly to move when you breathe. Keep an eye on your belly. Inhale. Exhale. It should move in and out. People need to get out of their military-style postures to exercise comfortably, says Balboa. Besides, who is going to watch you puff your stomach while you walk or run?

As you practice your belly breathing, take deep breaths. Exhale deeply. Become superaware of your breathing while you exercise and within a couple of weeks, diaphragmatic breathing will become habit.

Massage your diaphragm. Like any muscle, the diaphragm needs to be warmed up before it exercises. So, before you stretch your legs, give your diaphragm a breath massage and get it in working order. Sit on the floor and place one hand on your chest, the other on your belly. As you breathe, you want both hands to move up and down, indicating you are using your full breathing capacity, including your diaphragm. A warmed diaphragm is less likely to stitch.

Breathe all the time. People naturally hold their breath when they are frightened, when they are cold, or when they want to avoid pain, says Balboa. If you allow yourself to feel your emotions and not try to avoid them by holding your breath, you're more likely to breathe naturally when exercise demands a constant flow of air, he suggests.

Stop to go. Even though side stitches are caused by a pinched diaphragm, some walkers and runners will get a similar feeling from trapped gas, says Dr. Rappaport.

Any aerobic activity will slow or stop the digestive process while the blood rushes to help the muscles, says Balboa. That's why runners are told not to eat at least 2 hours before a race. And that's why runners sometimes get diarrhea if they drink a lot of water during a race.

Their advice? Be careful what and when you eat before you exercise. Eat plenty of fiber. Try to have a bowel movement before you begin any exercise if you are prone to side stitches.

PANEL OF ADVISERS

David Balboa is a sports psychotherapist and co-director of The Walking Center in New York City. He is an expert on fitness walking and body/mind relationships.

Gabe Mirkin, M.D., is in private practice at the Sportsmedicine Institute in Silver Spring, Maryland. He is also associate clinical professor of pediatrics at Georgetown University School of Medicine in Washington, D.C. He is the author of several sports medicine books, including *Dr. Gabe Mirkin's Fitness Clinic,* and is a syndicated newspaper columnist and radio broadcaster.

Suki Jay Rappaport, Ph.D., is director of the Transformations Institute in Corte Madera, California. A fitness consultant, her doctorate is in movement education and body transformations.

Sinusitis

16 Infection Fighters

During the day, your head is so pumped with pressure that you feel like the Snoopy balloon in the Macy's Thanksgiving Day Parade. Later, when you try to sleep, it's as if you've sprung a slow leak. All night long, the drip, drip of nasal fluid trickles down your throat and sends you into coughing spasms. Your spouse is not amused.

Welcome to the nightmare of sinusitis, a condition in which the sinus cavities around your eyes and nose are infected, producing pressure, pain, and gobs of yellow or green mucus. How did you and 30 to 50 million other people get this stuffiness?

Change Your Habits, Not Your Address

If your sinus symptoms kick up when the blossoms start to bud, you may feel like packing up for the Sahara desert or some other dry climate. Such a move, however, won't cure your sinusitis.

"If you are allergy prone," says Stanley N. Farb, M.D., "your sensitivities will follow you wherever you go and sinusitis will reappear." In other words, you may eventually develop an allergy to desert dust. Or, if you move to a humid climate like Miami, you may develop a sensitivity to mold.

The solution? Control your exposure to allergens where you now live. (For some ideas on how to do it, see Allergies on page 7.)

To understand that, you first have to understand what your sinuses do when they're working right. Scientists believe the sinuses around your nose act like small air-quality control centers. It's their job to warm, moisten, purify, and generally condition the air you breathe before it hits your lungs. Entering bacteria gets trapped and filtered out by mucus and minute nasal hairs called cilia.

This little air-flow system may gum up, however, if something impedes the cilia, if a cold clogs the sinus openings, or if an allergen swells the sinus linings. Then air gets trapped, pressure builds, the mucus stagnates, and bacteria breed. Infection sets in and you have a whopping case of sinusitis. If you get clogged up too many times, you may wind up with a permanent thickening of the sinus membranes and a chronic "stuffy doze."

Before you get to that point, here's what the doctors say you can do to unstuff your sinuses, reduce pain and pressure, and get the air flowing freely.

Get all steamed up. "Humidity is the key to keeping the cilia working, the mucus flowing, and the sinuses drained," says Stanley N. Farb, M.D., chief of otolaryngology at Montgomery and Sacred Heart hospitals in Norristown, Pennsylvania. Twice a day, stand in a shower hot enough to fog up the mirror. Or lean over a pan full of steaming water with a towel draped over your head, creating a steam tent. Inhale the vapors as they waft up toward your nostrils.

Get a snootful at work. If stuffiness hits during the day when you're at work or on the run, get a cup of hot coffee, tea, or soup, cup your hands over the top of the mug, and sniff, suggests Howard M. Druce,

---

MEDICAL ALERT

When Self-Treatment Isn't Enough

If you've tried self-treatment for three or four days and still have sinus pain, pressure, and stuffiness, you need to see a doctor to help clear up the infection and drain your sinuses, advises Terence M. Davidson, M.D. "Otherwise, your sinuses could abscess into your eye, or worse, into your brain."

You may need to take antibiotics or, if your symptoms persist, undergo surgery to break up the blockage. A sinus specialist can also perform x-rays and help you discover what's causing your congestion, be it a virus, an obstruction like polyps, allergies, or a sensitivity to medications such as birth control pills or aspirin.

M.D., assistant professor of internal medicine and director of the Nasal and Paranasal Sinus Physiology Lab at St. Louis University School of Medicine. It won't work as well as a steam bath, but it will provide some relief.

Humidify your home. Running a cold-mist machine in your bedroom will keep your nasal and sinus passages from drying out, says Bruce Jafek, M.D., a professor and chairman of Otolaryngology/Head and Neck Surgery at the University of Colorado Health Sciences Center School of Medicine. Just make sure you clean it once a week so fungus can't set up shop.

Bathe your nostrils daily. To flush out stale nasal secretions, Dr. Jafek suggests using a commercial saline product or mixing 1 teaspoon of table salt with 2 cups of warm water and a pinch of baking soda. Pour it into a shot glass, tilt your head back, close one nostril with your thumb, and sniff the solution with the open nostril. Then blow your nose gently. Repeat on the other side.

Drink to your heart's content. Drinking extra liquids—both hot and cold—throughout the day, Dr. Farb says, thins out the mucus and keeps it flowing. Sipping hot teas made with herbs such as fenugreek, fennel, anise, or sage may help move mucus even more.

Blow one nostril at a time. This will help prevent pressure buildup in the ears, which can send bacteria further back into the sinus passages, Dr. Farb says.

Forget your manners. Go ahead and sniffle. It turns out, says Dr. Farb, that sniffling is also a good way to drain the sinuses and escort stale secretions down the throat.

Unstuff yourself with decongestant tablets. The best over-the-counter medication to dry up sinuses is single-action tablets that contain only decongestants, such as Sudafed, says Dr. Farb. Decongestants constrict the blood vessels, put air through the nose, and alleviate pressure. You should avoid products containing antihistamines if you are stuffed up from an infection, says Dr. Farb. "They work by drying nasal secretions and may plug you up more."

The Alternate Route

Order It Spicy

The way to find sinus relief may be through your stomach—by eating foods containing certain spices and condiments, says Howard M. Druce, M.D. Here's what he recommends.

Garlic. This pungent herb contains the same chemical found in a drug given to make mucus less sticky, says Dr. Druce.

Horseradish. This pungent root is another good mucus mover because it contains a chemical similar to one found in decongestants, he says. The bottled variety will work fine.

Cajun spice. You probably can't go wrong if you order Cajun food. These spicy dishes are made with cayenne peppers, little red tongue torches that contain capsaicin, a substance that can stimulate the nerve fibers and may act as a natural nasal decongestant.

But not every fiery food that makes your eyes water or nose run will burst through your sinus blockage. "Not every spice contains chemicals that work directly on the sinuses," explains Dr. Druce. In other words, eating them may make your nose drip and do nothing to drain your sinuses. And that could only compound your problem.

Use nasal sprays sparingly. Nose drops are fine to use in a pinch, but frequent use could actually prolong the condition or even make it worse, warns Terence M. Davidson, M.D., an assistant professor of head and neck surgery and director of the Nasal Dysfunction Clinic at the University of California Medical Center in San Diego. It's what the specialists call the rebound effect.

"What happens is that, initially, the sprays shrink your nasal linings," explains Dr. Davidson. "But then the mucosa reacts by swelling even more than before, creating a vicious cycle of use. It can take weeks for the swelling to finally subside after you stop using the sprays."

Walk to clear your head. Exercise, says Dr. Farb, may bring blessed relief because it releases adrenaline, which constricts the blood vessels, thereby possibly reducing swelling in the sinuses.

Press here for pain relief. Rubbing your sore sinuses brings a fresh blood supply to the area and soothing relief, suggests Dr. Jafek. Press your thumbs firmly on both sides of your nose and hold for 15 to 30 seconds. Repeat.

Wash your pain away. Applying moist heat over tender sinuses, Dr. Druce says, is an easy way to wash away sinus pain. Apply a warm washcloth over your eyes and cheekbones and leave it there until you feel the pain subside. It may take only a few minutes.

PANEL OF ADVISERS

Terence M. Davidson, M.D., is an assistant professor of head and neck surgery and director of the Nasal Dysfunction Clinic at the University of California Medical Center in San Diego.

Howard M. Druce, M.D., is an assistant professor of internal medicine and director of the Nasal and Paranasal Sinus Physiology Lab at St. Louis University School of Medicine in Missouri.

Stanley N. Farb, M.D., is chief of otolaryngology at Montgomery and Sacred Heart hospitals in Norristown, Pennsylvania. Dr. Farb is also author of *The Ear, Nose, and Throat Book: A Doctor's Guide to Better Health.*

Bruce Jafek, M.D., is a professor and chairman of the Department of Otolaryngology/Head and Neck Surgery at the University of Colorado Health Sciences Center School of Medicine in Denver. He is also chairman of the Paranasal Sinus Disease Committee of the American Academy of Otolaryngology/Head and Neck Surgery.

Snoring

10 Tips for a Silent Night

There are different levels of snoring. "If your wife moves out of the bedroom, then you snore at a moderate level," says Philip Westbrook, M.D., director of the Mayo Clinic Sleep Disorders Center in Rochester, Minnesota. "But if your neighbors move, then you're a heavy snorer."

Men are much more likely to snore than women. In a study of more than 2,000 people in Toronto, sleep researchers Earl V. Dunn, M.D., and Peter Norton, M.D., found that 71 percent of men snored, while only 51 percent of women did. In an Italian study the difference was almost two to one in favor of men—or should we say, *not* in favor of women.

Clinically, says Dr. Westbrook, moderate snorers are those "who snore every night but perhaps only when on their backs or only part of the night."

Snoring may not be music to your ears, but the sound is orchestrated by a wind ensemble located in the back of the throat. "The tissue in the upper airway in the back of the throat relaxes during sleep," says Philip Smith, M.D., director of the Johns Hopkins University Sleep Disorders Center in Baltimore, Maryland. "When you breathe in, it causes this tissue to vibrate, and that effect is very similar to a wind instrument."

For those of you with sleeping mates who are talking not about separate beds but separate bedrooms, there are ways to help stop the music.

Go on a diet. Most snorers tend to be middle-aged, overweight men. Most women snorers are past menopause. Slimming stops snoring. "Snoring is frequently related to being overweight," says Dr. Dunn of the University of Toronto Sunnybrook Medical Centre Sleep Laboratory. "We've found that if a moderate snorer loses weight, the snoring becomes less loud, and in some people it actually disappears."

"You don't have to be a 2-ton Tony to develop snoring. Just being a little overweight can bring on a problem," says Dr. Smith. "Men about 20 percent over ideal body weight can develop snoring. Women have to be much heavier, usually 30 to 40 percent over ideal body weight. But the more overweight you are, the more likely it is that your airway will collapse."

Ignore the midnight spirits. "Alcohol before bed makes snoring worse," says Dr. Dunn. Don't drink and sleep.

Stay away from sedatives. Sleeping pills may make you sleep, but they will keep your partner awake. "Anything that relaxes the tissues around the head and neck will tend to make snoring worse. Even antihistamines will do it," says Dr. Dunn.

MEDICAL ALERT

The Louder the Snore, The Bigger the Problem

"Thou dost snore distinctly. There's meaning in thy snores."

Modern science is now proving what Shakespeare knew more than 100 years ago when he wrote those lines in *The Tempest*. "In general," says Philip Smith, M.D., "the louder your snore, the more likely it is to lead to a medical problem."

One of the worst problems associated with snoring is a condition called sleep apnea. "The person literally stops breathing," explains Earl V. Dunn, M.D. "People who are heavy snorers who stop snoring at night, can have episodes where they are not breathing."

Those most prone to sleep apnea are "overweight, middle-aged men," adds Dr. Smith. "If you fall into that category, and you snore pretty loudly—that is, loud enough to be heard outside the room—the chances of your having sleep apnea are pretty high. Go see your doctor."

Sleep apnea can be controlled by wearing a device at night that forces air under pressure into the nose and the back of the throat, which keeps the airway from collapsing. Surgery is sometimes required for severe cases.

If you are a heavy snorer and/or suspect you may have sleep apnea, you might find relief by going to a local sleep clinic. For the address of a sleep clinic near you, write to the American Sleep Disorders Association, 604 Second Street SW, Rochester, MN 55902.

Put the cigarette light out. Snuff snoring by snuffing cigarettes. "Smokers tend to be snorers," says Dr. Dunn, "So stop smoking."

Back off. When you sleep, sleep on your side. "Heavy snorers snore in virtually any position," says Dr. Dunn. "But moderate snorers only snore when they are on their backs."

Get on the ball. A tennis ball, that is. "Sew a tennis ball onto the back of your pajamas," suggests Dr. Dunn. "That way, when you roll over on your back, you hit this hard object and unconsciously you roll off your back."

Have a fight with your pillow. Then get rid of it. Pillows only help elevate your snoring level. "Anything that puts a kink in your neck," reports Dr. Dunn, "like a large pillow, will make you snore more."

The Search Goes on for a Sure Cure

"There ain't no way to find out why a snorer can't hear himself snore," wrote Mark Twain in *Tom Sawyer Abroad*. But there are several hundred ways designed to get that snorer to stop. Since 1874, the U.S. Patent and Trademark Office has issued more than 300 patents for so-called antisnoring devices.

Take patent number 4644330, for instance. It's a self-contained electronic device that's worn in the outer ear. It comprises a miniature microphone for detecting snoring sounds and the means for generating an aversive audio signal. What that means is that when you snore, an alarm blasts off in your ear, waking you up. (Its basis is the theory that people who are awake seldom snore.)

Then there's patent number 4669459. This device clamps onto one molar on each side of your mouth with a connecting button that "applies pressure to the soft palate to prevent vibration thereof." Or number 4748702, which is a two-channel "antisnoring pillow." The inventor has placed "a relatively hard object" in the channel that holds the back of your head, and an object that is "not being relatively uncomfortable" in the area where the side of your face would go. Seems you get your choice. If you sleep on your back, you sleep on a rock; if you sleep on your side, it's something a bit softer. You choose.

While sleep experts say that some of the inventions may be based on sound snoring advice, they add that many of the inventions are untested and unproven. "There is very little scientific evidence supporting them," says Philip Westbrook, M.D.

Consider Yourself Lucky!

Pity Mrs. Switzer. It seems her husband, Melvin, a 250-pound British dockworker, is the sovereign of snore.

Melvin trumpeted his way into the *Guinness Book of World Records* with a snore registered at 88 decibels, about the same intensity as a motorcycle engine being revved at full throttle.

And Mrs. Switzer? She's now forced to sleep with her good ear to the pillow. Her good ear? Unfortunately, the nightly motorcycle race on the other side of the bed caused her to go deaf in one ear.

So, in the middle of the night when *you're* jolted awake by a nasal blast, remember poor Mrs. Switzer—and be glad your hubby is not a Harley.

Raise your bed to new heights. Elevating the bed can help minimize snoring. "Elevate the upper torso, not just the head," says Dr. Westbrook. "Put a couple of bricks under the legs at the head of your bed."

Blame it on your allergies. Sneezing and snoring go together. "Snoring can develop due to allergies or colds," says Dr. Westbrook. "Use a nasal decongestant, especially if your snoring is intermittent and comes during hay fever season."

Put a plug in it. When all else fails, Dr. Westbrook says, the one on the receiving end of the nasal abuse can wear earplugs to bed. They're inexpensive and can be purchased at any pharmacy.

PANEL OF ADVISERS

Earl V. Dunn, M.D., is a professor of family medicine and a researcher at the University of Toronto, Sunnybrook Medical Centre Sleep Laboratory.

Philip Smith, M.D., is director of the Johns Hopkins University Sleep Disorders Center in Baltimore, Maryland.

Philip Westbrook, M.D., is director of the Mayo Clinic Sleep Disorders Center in Rochester, Minnesota, and associate professor of medicine at the Mayo Clinic. He is also president of the American Sleep Disorders Association.

Sore Throat

27 Ways to Put Out the Fire

Swallowing your pride can be pretty painful. But when just plain *swallowing* hurts, you have a real problem. After all, it's hard to go even 15 seconds without swallowing at least once. And the more you try *not* to, the more you find yourself doing it. Combine a sore throat with a rasping cough and you know the meaning of torture.

Sore throats are often the early warning signs of colds or the flu. But they can exist independently as the result of some other viral or bacterial infection. Sometimes they're just minor irritations caused by winter's low humidity or too much cheering at a football game. Whatever the cause, here's how doctors say to make the most of a sore situation.

Suck on lozenges. If your sore throat is caused by a viral infection, antibiotics won't help it. But medicated lozenges containing phenol may do some good, says Venice, Florida, ear, nose, and throat specialist Hueston King, M.D. The phenol can kill surface germs, thereby keeping the invaders in check until your body has a chance to build up its resistance. And its mild anesthetic action numbs raw nerve endings so your throat doesn't feel as scratchy. These lozenges come in various strengths, so follow package directions.

Spray away pain. By the same token, phenol-containing throat sprays can also give topical relief. But as Ohio Northern University pharmacology professor Thomas Gossel, Ph.D., R.Ph., points out, the duration of contact between the spray and the irritated tissues is relatively brief. Lozenges simply last longer.

Give zinc a chance. Zinc lozenges can help the kind of sore throat that's associated with a cold, says Donald Davis, Ph.D., a research scientist at the Clayton Foundation Biochemical Institute at the University of Texas at Austin "We gave people one 23-milligram tablet of zinc gluconate every 2 hours—but we instructed them to let it dissolve slowly in their mouths rather than just swallowing it. The zinc relieved their sore throats as well as several other cold symptoms."

But Dr. Davis cautions against taking such large amounts of zinc for more than seven days, because it can interfere with other minerals in the body. If you don't like the taste of zinc, look for zinc-containing lozenges.

Gargle! If it hurts when you swallow, the sore area may be high enough in your throat for gargling to bathe and soothe it, says Dr. King. So gargle frequently with one of the solutions below. But be aware that if you're hoarse or have a cough, the sore spot is further down, and gargling won't help.

Stage-Door Remedies

Actors can't afford to be upstaged by sore throats. So we asked some professionals how they perform comebacks when their throats are acting up.

- Several mentioned the time-honored salvo of lemon juice and honey in hot tea or water, sipped throughout the day.
- All had their favorite lozenges. Actor, director, and writer George Wolf Reily likes Ricola herbal mints from Switzerland. "They're great when you have to do two shows a day and your throat is hurting."
- Singer Geoffrey Moore prefers Halls Mentho-Lyptus drops. "They don't contain any anesthetics to dull the feeling in my throat."
- Actor Norman Marshall favors Vocalzone lozenges for immediate relief. "These strong-tasting black lozenges were developed for Caruso many years ago and actors have been relying on them ever since."
- Another of Marshall's favorite remedies is a tablespoon of baking soda in a large glass of water. "I sip this throughout the day whenever my throat's irritated or I feel a cold coming on."
- Actress Elf Fairservis humidifies her sore throat with a facial sauna. "I just inhale the steam for about 10 minutes. If I can spare the time, I do it three times a day until I feel better."
- From a preventive standpoint, actor and singer William Perley protects his throat by "staying as healthy as I can and eating lots of carrots for their vitamin A. Also, I've been told by vocal teachers not to irritate my throat by clearing it too much."

Saltwater. Mix 1 teaspoon of table salt in 1 pint of warm or room-temperature water, says Dr. Gossel. That's just enough salt to mimic the body's natural saline content, so you'll find it very soothing. Use every hour or so, but don't swallow the liquid if you're concerned about your sodium intake.

Chamomile tea. Colorado nutrition counselor Eleonore Blaurock-Busch, Ph.D., president and director of Trace Minerals International, a clinical chemistry laboratory in Boulder, favors warm chamomile tea to relieve irritated membranes. Steep 1 teaspoon dried chamomile in 1 cup of hot water. Strain. Let it cool to lukewarm and gargle as needed.

Diluted lemon juice. Dr. Blaurock-Busch also suggests a little lemon juice squeezed into a large glass of lukewarm water.

Spirits. "Sometimes I add a spoonful of bourbon or whiskey to a large glass of warm water and use that to gargle," says Dr. Gossel. "It's just enough alcohol to help numb a sore throat."

Humidify the room.
Sometimes a sore throat upon awakening is caused by sleeping with your mouth open. Ordinarily, your nose moistens air headed for your throat and lungs. But breathing through your mouth bypasses that step, leaving your throat parched and irritated.

New Jersey otolaryngologist Jason Surow, M.D., recommends a bedroom humidifier to get the environment nice and humid. "Use a bedside model even if your heating system has its own humidifier," he says. "The built-in units just don't do a good enough job, especially if you have a forced-air heating system, which is very drying in itself."

Get up a head of steam.
In the face of a worse-than-normal dry or sore throat, supplement your bedroom humidifier with steam inhalations, says Dr. Surow. Run very hot water in the bathroom basin to build up steam. With the water running, lean over the sink, drape a towel over your head to capture some of the steam, and inhale deeply through the mouth and nose for 5 to 10 minutes. Repeat several times a day if necessary.

Open your nose.
If part of the reason you're breathing through your mouth is that your nose is clogged, says Dr. Surow, open it with an over-the-counter decongestant nasal spray, such as Afrin. But limit its use to a day or two. And follow directions carefully, he cautions, because these sprays can become addictive.

MEDICAL ALERT

Strep Throat and Other Problems

A strep throat can start suddenly and hurt like the dickens. If untreated, it can lead to more serious problems like rheumatic fever and rheumatic heart disease. Because so many different viruses and bacteria can cause sore throats, a throat culture is needed to identify strep. Fortunately, says Hueston King, M.D., strep is a bacterial infection and responds quite well to appropriate antibiotics.

Other reasons to see a doctor, says Jerome C. Goldstein, M.D., include:

- Severe, prolonged, or recurrent sore throats.
- Difficulty breathing, swallowing, or opening the mouth.
- Joint pains, earache, or a lump in the neck.
- Rash or a fever above 101°F.
- Hoarseness lasting two weeks or longer.
- Blood in saliva or phlegm.

Inhale sea breezes. If you can't actually go someplace humid like the ocean, get the same sort of salty atmosphere from a saline nasal spray, available at any pharmacy. When you inhale the mist, says Dr. Surow, the salt-based spray moistens your nose and drips down the back of your throat to help increase humidity there. Among the brands available are Ocean Mist, NaSal, and Ayr. Unlike decongestant nasal sprays, the saline formulas are not addictive.

Down some aspirin. It doesn't occur to most people that a sore throat is a pain like any other physical discomfort, says Dr. Gossel. Aspirin, acetaminophen, or ibuprofen will effectively deaden the discomfort. (No one under age 21 should be given aspirin because of the risk of Reye's syndrome, a life-threatening neurological disease.)

Increase your fluid intake. Taking in as much fluid as you can will help hydrate your parched throat tissues, says Dr. Surow. Although it doesn't really matter *what* you drink, he says, here are a few things you might want to avoid. Thick, milky drinks coat your throat and may produce mucus, making you cough and further irritating tissues; orange juice may burn an already inflamed throat; caffeine-containing beverages have a counterproductive diuretic effect.

Wrap your throat. Dr. Blaurock-Busch finds that a warm chamomile poultice, applied directly to the throat, relieves discomfort. To make the poultice, add 1 tablespoon of dried chamomile flowers to 1 or 2 cups of boiling water. Allow it to steep for 5 minutes before straining. Soak a clean cloth or towel in this tea, wring out the excess, and apply to the affected area. Leave it on until the cloth is cold. Repeat if necessary with more warm liquid.

Load up on garlic. "Garlic is one of the best natural antibiotics and antiseptics," says Dr. Blaurock-Busch. She recommends taking garlic-oil capsules (15 grains) six times a day. But if it causes you any adverse reaction, try another remedy.

Do as the Russians do. This hot idea comes from Irwin Ziment, Ph.D., director of respiratory therapy and chief of medicine at Olive View Medical Center in Sylmar, California. Mix 1 tablespoon pure horseradish, 1 teaspoon honey, and 1 teaspoon ground cloves in a glass of warm water and stir. "Sip it slowly, keep stirring—as the horseradish tends to settle—and think happy thoughts," he says. Or use it as a gargle. Dr. Ziment says it's his favorite Russian remedy."

Reach for vitamin C. Vitamin C may help build up your tissues to fight the germs that are making your throat sore. "I usually tell people to double the recommended daily requirement of 60 milligrams," says Dr. King.

Toss your toothbrush. Believe it or not, says Richard T. Glass, D.D.S., Ph.D., chairman of the Department of Oral Pathology at the University of Oklahoma College of Medicine and College of Dentistry, your toothbrush may be perpetuating—or even causing—your sore throat. Bacteria collect on the bristles, and any injury to the gums during brushing injects these germs into your system.

"As soon as you start feeling ill, throw away your toothbrush. Often that's enough to stop the illness in its tracks," he says. "If you do get sick, replace your brush *again* when you start to feel better. That keeps you from reinfecting yourself."

From a preventive standpoint, he recommends replacing your toothbrush every month and also storing it outside the moist, bacteria-prone bathroom. If you think it's expensive to buy so many brushes, he says, consider the cost of just one trip to the doctor's office. You'll do better in the long run to stay well.

Rise to the occasion. Another cause of sore throat in the morning—besides sleeping with your mouth open—is a backup of stomach acids into your throat during the night. These acids are extremely irritating to sensitive throat tissues, says Jerome C. Goldstein, M.D., executive vice president of the American Academy of Otolaryngology and a visiting professor of otolaryngology/head and neck surgery at Johns Hopkins University School of Medicine. Avoid the problem by tilting your bed frame so the head is 4 to 6 inches higher than the foot. (Try using bricks.) But don't simply pile more pillows under your head; they can cause you to bend in the middle, increasing pressure on your esophagus and making the problem worse. As an extra precaution, don't eat or drink for an hour or two before retiring.

PANEL OF ADVISERS

Eleonore Blaurock-Busch, Ph.D., is president and director of Trace Minerals International, Inc., a clinical chemistry laboratory in Boulder, Colorado. She is also a nutrition counselor specializing in the treatment of allergy and chronic diseases at the Alpine Chiropractic Center there, and is the author of *The No-Drugs Guide to Better Health.*

Donald Davis, Ph.D., is a research scientist at the Clayton Foundation Biochemical Institute at the University of Texas at Austin. He is the editor of the *Journal of Applied Nutrition.*

Elf Fairservis is a New York City actress who's done Off-Broadway productions and commercials.

Richard T. Glass, D.D.S., Ph.D., is chairman of the Department of Oral Pathology at the University of Oklahoma College of Medicine and College of Dentistry in Oklahoma City.

Jerome C. Goldstein, M.D., is executive vice president of the American Academy of Otolaryngology in Washington, D.C. He is also visiting professor of otolaryngology/head and neck surgery at Johns Hopkins University School of Medicine in Baltimore, Maryland.

Thomas Gossel, Ph.D., R.Ph., is a professor of pharmacology and toxicology at Ohio Northern University in Ada and chairman of the university's Department of Pharmacology and Biomedical Sciences. He is an expert on over-the-counter products.

Hueston King, M.D., is an ear, nose, and throat specialist in private practice in Venice, Florida. He is also a clinical associate professor of otolaryngology at the University of Texas Southwest Medical Center in Dallas.

Norman Marshall is an actor who has worked in soap operas, movies, and children's theater. He formed the No Smoking Playhouse in New York City and directed it for 11 years.

Geoffrey Moore is a semiretired professional singer living in Ridgewood, New Jersey. He has a one-man program that he performs at nursing homes.

William Perley is an actor and singer. For the past several summers he has starred in the play *The Mark Twain Drama* in Elmira, New York, which has been aired on PBS.

George Wolf Reily is an actor, director, and writer who's done Off-Broadway and regional theater.

Jason Surow, M.D., is an ear, nose, and throat specialist in private practice in both Teaneck and Midland Park, New Jersey. He's an attending otolaryngologist at both Valley Hospital in Ridgewood, New Jersey, and Holy Name Hospital in Teaneck.

Irwin Ziment, Ph.D., is director of respiratory therapy and chief of medicine at Olive View Medical Center in Sylmar, California.

Stained Teeth

7 Bright Ideas

Think of a fine porcelain cup. Fill it daily with coffee and colas, subject it to heat and cold, smoke, and alcohol. Fill it with brightly colored food. Then wash the cup in a harsh detergent. Eventually, tiny craze marks will dot the ceramic surface, and before you know it, the once-white cup looks dirty and dingy.

Your teeth are like that pretty porcelain cup. They start out shiny and white. But cola, tea, smoke, acidic juices, and highly pigmented foods slosh past them three (or more) times daily. And your teeth tell the tale in the form of stains.

Not that teeth were ever meant to be totally white. The natural color of teeth is actually light yellow to light yellow-red, says Roger P. Levin, D.D.S., president of the Baltimore Academy of General Dentistry. But as you age, your teeth tend to darken even more.

Surface enamel cracks and erodes, exposing dentin, the less dense inside of the tooth, which absorbs food color. Stains also latch onto the plaque and tartar buildup on teeth, finding anchorage among the nooks and crannies.

"There are many different kinds of stains," says Ronald I. Maitland, D.M.D., who specializes in cosmetic dentistry in his New York City practice. Stains can be caused by antibiotics, by quirks in individual metabolism, and sometimes by high fever. All these have to be fixed by a professional.

But common stains—the coffee and cigarette variety—can be washed away between professional cleanings. Here's how.

Clean after every meal. If you clean your teeth regularly and conscientiously, you have less chance of keeping stains on your teeth, says Dr. Levin.

Polish with baking soda. Mix baking soda with enough hydrogen peroxide to make a toothpaste, says Dr. Levin. Then brush those stains away.

Check your plaque quotient. Rinse with a disclosing solution that will show where plaque still remains on your teeth after brushing. Those are the spots where your teeth will stain first if you don't improve your brushing technique, says John D. B. Featherstone, Ph.D., chairman of the Department of Oral Biology at the Eastman Dental Center in Rochester, New York.

Rinse, rinse, rinse. After every meal, rinse the food from your teeth, says Dr. Maitland. If you can't get to a restroom, pick up your water glass, take a swig, then rinse and swallow at the table.

Electrify your smile. An electric toothbrush, says Dr. Maitland, will push more of the stain-collecting plaque off your teeth. Studies show an electric toothbrush can remove 98.2 percent of plaque.

Try a plaque dissolver. Mouthwashes that have an antibacterial action will reduce stain-catching plaque, says Dr. Featherstone.

Don't scrub away your smile. If you're tempted to turn to one of those super-whitening tooth polishes, don't, says Dr. Maitland. "It's a quick fix, but it's like using an abrasive on a countertop. It takes off the stain, but it wears off the enamel, too. And as your enamel gets thinner and thinner, more of the dentin shows through. And dentin is darker, so it looks like your tooth is stained."

Watch out for excessive scrubbing, too. Harder doesn't mean better, Dr. Maitland warns. A heavy-duty brush with a lot of muscle behind it can be as wearing on tooth enamel as an abrasive toothpaste.

PANEL OF ADVISERS

John D. B. Featherstone, Ph.D., is chairman of the Department of Oral Biology at Eastman Dental Center in Rochester, New York, and deputy director of the Rochester Cariology Center.

Roger P. Levin, D.D.S., is president of the Baltimore Academy of General Dentistry and a guest lecturer at the University of Maryland in Baltimore.

Ronald I. Maitland, D.M.D., is a New York City dentist who specializes in cosmetic dentistry. He is chairman of the Greater New York Dental Meeting and an expert on dental stains.

Stings

38 Hints to Relieve the Pain

When Hamlet bemoaned the slings and arrows of outrageous fortune and the thousand natural shocks the flesh is heir to, he wasn't complaining about bumblebees. Or even jellyfish. He had more pressing matters on his mind and some heavy decisions to make. But if you've just taken nasty jabs from a stinging creature, you have a decision of your own: to be or not to be in pain. Choose not to suffer by following the advice below.

BEES, WASPS, AND THEIR KIN
These insects inject venom into the skin tissue when they sting. That leads to pain, redness, and swelling at the site of the sting. Discomfort can last from several hours to a day, depending on what and how many of them sting you.

Identify your attacker. Knowing which insect did the damage can provide a clue to treatment—and help you avoid more stings. A honeybee, which has a fuzzy golden brown body, can sting only once. That's because its barbed stinger remains embedded in your skin, causing the bee to die.

Bumblebees, wasps, hornets, and yellow jackets, on the other hand, have smooth stingers that can zap you repeatedly. So be prepared to flee.

Yellow jackets pose an additional problem. Smashing one of them can lead to a full-scale attack by its nest mates. Breaking its venom sac releases a chemical that incites other yellow jackets to attack.

Act fast. The key to effective treatment is quick action. The faster you can apply some sort of first-aid treatment, the better your chances are of controlling pain and swelling.

Remove the stinger. If it was a honeybee that got you, remove the stinger as soon as possible. Otherwise, the venom sac attached to it will continue to pump for 2 to 3 minutes, driving the stinger and its poison deeper into your skin. But be careful not to squeeze the stinger or the sac—doing so will release more poison into your system.

"Scraping the stinger out is the best approach," says Edgar Raffensperger, Ph.D., a professor of entomology in the Department of Entomology at Cornell University. Use your fingernail, a nail file, or even the edge of a credit card to gently scrape under the stinger and flip it out.

Cleanse the area. Bees and their brethren are scavengers, so they often have undesirable bacteria in their venom, says Jeff Rusteen, a firefighter-paramedic with the Piedmont Fire Department in Piedmont, California. Wash the sting well with soap and water or an antiseptic.

Relieve the pain. At this point, your wound is still throbbing so you want to deaden the pain *fast*. The following substances have proven themselves effective—but you must act quickly after being stung for them to work.

Cold. An ice pack, or even just an ice cube, placed over the sting can cut down on swelling and keep the venom from spreading, says Philadelphia dermatologist Herbert Luscombe, M.D., professor emeritus of dermatology at Jefferson Medical College of Thomas Jefferson University.

Heat. Ironically, says Dr. Luscombe, heat can also make you feel better by neutralizing one of the chemicals that causes inflammation. Just take a hair dryer and aim it at your sting.

Aspirin. One of the simplest, most effective things you can do, he says, is to apply aspirin. Moisten the sting, then rub an aspirin tablet into it. The aspirin neutralizes certain inflammatory agents in the venom.

Ammonia. Sometimes household ammonia does the trick, says Dr. Luscombe. "If it's going to work, it will relieve the pain very promptly. Dab it on the sting." For outings you might want to take along a commercial product called After Bite, which contains ammonia and comes in convenient towelettes.

Baking soda. North Carolina allergist Claude Frazier, M.D., recommends applying a paste of baking soda and water.

Meat tenderizer. "An enzyme-based meat tenderizer, such as Adolph's or McCormick's, breaks down the proteins that make up insect venom," says David Golden, M.D., an assistant professor of medicine at Johns Hopkins University. You have to use it right away for it to be effective.

Activated charcoal. "A paste of powdered activated charcoal will draw the poison out very quickly so the sting won't swell or hurt," according to Richard Hansen, M.D., medical director of the Poland Spring Health Institute in Poland Spring, Maine. Carefully open a few charcoal capsules and remove the powder. Moisten it with water and apply to the sting. Cover with gauze or even plastic wrap; the charcoal works best if it stays moist.

Mud. If you don't have anything else handy, says Dr. Hansen, you can mix a little clay soil and water into a mud paste. Apply as you would the charcoal, cover with a bandage or handkerchief, and leave it on until the mud dries.

Take an antihistamine. An over-the-counter oral antihistamine may help relieve pain. In classes he teaches, Rusteen often advises parents to give their children an antihistamine-containing cough syrup, such as Benylin. "The antihistamine helps sedate the child a little and also lessens the swelling, throbbing, and redness caused by the insect venom. Adults can benefit from this treatment, too."

Don't get stung in the first place. The proverbial ounce of prevention can save you a lot of anguish later. Here's how to minimize your chances of getting stung.

Wear white. Stinging insects prefer dark colors, says Dr. Raffensperger. That's why beekeepers generally wear khaki, white, or other light colors.

Don't smell too good. Avoid perfume, after-shave, and any other fragrance that will lead a bee to confuse you with a nectar-bearing flower, he adds.

Increase your zinc intake. Insects are attracted to people who are deficient in zinc, says Illinois allergist George Shambaugh, Jr., M.D., professor emeritus of otolaryngology, head and neck surgery of Northwestern University Medical School. "I tell people to take at least 60 milligrams of zinc a day—year round. My sister had a terrible problem with bees until she started taking zinc. Now she never gets stung." (You should increase your zinc intake only with the approval and supervision of your doctor.)

Oil up. Certain bath oils can repel stinging insects, says Dr. Luscombe. Skin-So-Soft from Avon and Alpha-Keri have helped a lot of people. Rub the oil onto exposed skin before going out.

Run for shelter. If pursued by a buzzing horde, run indoors or jump into water. Or head for the woods. Stinging insects have trouble following their prey through a thicket of woods, say researchers at the Cornell University Cooperative Extension Service.

Take up painting. As a last resort, you might become a painter. Housepainters rarely get stung, says Dr. Luscombe, because the turpentine they use repels stinging insects.

JELLYFISH

Jellyfish and their larger cousin the Portuguese man-of-war are two of the most common stinging marine animals. Their long tentacles contain stinging cells. When they brush against you, the cells pierce your skin and release their poison. Even severed or damaged tentacles can inflict severe wounds. Here's what to do if you have a run-in with one of these sea creatures.

Rinse! Immediately rinse the wound with saltwater, says Arthur Jacknowitz, Pharm.D., a professor of clinical pharmacy and chairman of the Department of Clinical Pharmacy at West Virginia University. *Do not use fresh water* because it will activate any stinging cells that have not already ruptured. For the same reason, do not rub the skin.

Neutralize the stinging cells. Work on alleviating the pain by rinsing the area with one of the following. The sooner you can apply it, the better. Even so, relief may last only an hour or two, so reapply the liquid as necessary.

MEDICAL ALERT

Signs of a Severe Reaction

Bee stings cause more deaths than snakebites, says Herbert Luscombe, M.D. A normal bee sting produces pain for a brief time and swelling that usually lessens in a few hours. But more severe symptoms may indicate an allergy, which can lead to deadly anaphylactic shock. Be on the lookout for chest tightness, hives, nausea, vomiting, wheezing, hoarseness, dizziness, swollen tongue or face, fainting, or shock. The more rapidly symptoms appear, the more life threatening they are.

If these symptoms appear, says Claude Frazier, M.D., use an insect sting kit as directed. Then rush the victim to the nearest hospital or physician. If no kit is available, apply an ice pack if possible and rush the victim to help.

Severe jellyfish stings may be accompanied by headache, muscle cramps, coughing, shortness of breath, nausea, and vomiting, says Arthur Jacknowitz, Pharm.D. If the symptoms persist or worsen, contact a physician or the local emergency medical service immediately.

Alcohol. Splash alcohol over the affected areas, says Dr. Jacknowitz. Although rubbing alcohol is preferred, you may use wine, liquor, or any other alcohol that's available.

Vinegar. Dr. Luscombe recommends splashing on vinegar as soon as you can. (It wouldn't hurt to take along a large bottle of vinegar whenever you go to the beach.)

Ammonia. Ammonia is also effective, he says.

Meat tenderizer. Meat tenderizer contains an enzyme that deactivates venom protein and can help prevent the rupture of stinging cells, says Dr. Jacknowitz. Dissolve it in saltwater and pat it on.

Remove any attached tentacles. If there are tentacles clinging to your skin, now's the time to remove them. Do not, however, touch them with your bare hands. Instead, try one of these techniques.

- Wrap your hand in a towel or cloth and wipe away all attached tentacles, says Stephen Rosenberg, M.D., an associate professor of clinical public health at Columbia University School of Public Health.

- Use shaving cream and gentle shaving, says Dr. Jacknowitz.
- If that's not practical, he says, apply a paste of sand and seawater. Then scrape the tentacles off with a knife, plastic credit card, or other sharp instrument.
- Or apply a paste of baking soda and seawater, he says. Scrape the tentacles off as above.

Treat the symptoms. Take care of itching and inflammation with specific medications, says Dr. Jacknowitz.

- Relieve the itchy skin with antihistamines.
- Reduce the swelling with hydrocortisone cream.
- Take a pain reliever if pain persists.

Get a tetanus shot. Although saltwater will cleanse the sting site, it won't sterilize the wound, says Dr. Jacknowitz. So make sure your tetanus immunization is up-to-date.

Take panty hose to the beach. If you want to make sure jellyfish won't harm you, wear panty hose while you swim, says Dr. Luscombe. "It really helps."

PANEL OF ADVISERS

Claude Frazier, M.D., is an allergist in private practice in Asheville, North Carolina. He is the author of *Coping with Food Allergies* and *Insects and Allergy and What to Do about Them.*

David Golden, M.D., is an assistant professor of medicine at Johns Hopkins University in Baltimore, Maryland.

Richard Hansen, M.D., is medical director of the Poland Spring Health Institute in Poland Spring, Maine. He is author of *Get Well at Home..*

Arthur Jacknowitz, Pharm.D., is a professor of clinical pharmacy and chairman of the Department of Clinical Pharmacy at West Virginia University in Morgantown. He has published over 90 articles in professional journals.

Herbert Luscombe, M.D., is professor emeritus of dermatology at Jefferson Medical College of Thomas Jefferson University in Philadelphia, Pennsylvania. He is also senior attending dermatologist at Thomas Jefferson University Hospital in Philadelphia.

Edgar Raffensperger, Ph.D., is a professor of entomology in the Department of Entomology at Cornell University in Ithaca, New York.

Stephen Rosenberg, M.D., is an associate professor of clinical public health at Columbia University School of Public Health in New York City. He is author of *The Johnson & Johnson First Aid Book.*

Jeff Rusteen is a firefighter-paramedic with the Piedmont Fire Department in Piedmont, California. He teaches emergency medical technology at Chabot College in Hayward, California. He is the author of a videotape and companion booklet called *Until Help Arrives.*

George Shambaugh, Jr., M.D., is a medical otologist and allergist in private practice in Hinsdale, Illinois, a member of the staff at Hinsdale Hospital, and professor emeritus of otolaryngology, head and neck surgery of Northwestern University Medical School in Chicago. He writes a health and nutrition newsletter that he sends to his patients.

Stress

22 Tips to Ease Tension

Cooked, burned, whipped, beaten — we all know what it feels like to get emotionally mangled by the boulder weight of day-to-day struggles. Our bosses yell at us, our spouses yell at us — it feels like an endless circle where getting ahead at the office can leave us with so little energy for home that home turns into a battleground that leaves us with no energy for work.

But is stress really a catch-22? And is mere survival all you can ask of a hassle-filled world? No. Stress, in fact, is not only something you can beat but a force you can turn to your advantage. You don't have to run from it, and you *don't* have to go to a special stress-management seminar to find out how to manage it. The following doctor-tested tips show you how to combat stress — and win. For instant relief when the world has you in a headlock, read on.

Work on your attitude. "I think the single most important point you can make about stress is that in most cases it's not what's out there that's the problem, it's how you *react* to it," says Paul J. Rosch, M.D., president of the American Institute of Stress and a clinical professor of medicine and psychiatry at New York Medical College. And how you react is determined by how you *perceive* a particular stress.

"Watch people on a roller coaster ride," Dr. Rosch says. "Some sit in the back, eyes shut, jaws clenched. They can't wait for the ordeal in the torture chamber to end and to get back on solid ground. Up front are the wide-eyed thrill seekers who relish every steep plunge and can't wait to get on the very next ride. And in between are those who are seemingly quite nonchalant or even bored.

"They're all having exactly the same experience—the roller coaster ride—but they're reacting to it very differently: bad stress, good stress, and *no* stress."

Emmett Miller, M.D., medical director of the Cancer Support and Education Center in Menlo Park, California, a nationally known expert on stress, draws on Chinese wisdom to make this point. "The Chinese word for crisis is *weiji*—two characters that separately mean danger and opportunity. Every problem we encounter in life can be viewed that way—as a chance to show that we can handle it."

The message from both men: Changing the way you think— viewing a difficult assignment at work as a chance to improve your skills, for example—can change a life of stress and discomfort to a life of challenge and excitement.

Think about something else. "Anything that will help you shift your perspective instantly is useful when you're under the gun," says Dr. Miller. "You want to distract yourself— to break whatever chain of thought is producing the stress. And thinking about almost anything else will do that."

Think positive. "Thinking about a success or a past achievement is excellent when you're feeling uncertain—before a presentation, for example, or a meeting with your boss," Dr. Miller says. "You're instantly reminded that you've achieved before, and there's no reason you shouldn't achieve this time."

Take a mental vacation. "Taking a mini-vacation in your mind is a very good way to relieve or manage stress," says Ronald Nathan, Ph.D., director of educational development, coordinator of behavioral science, and associate professor in the departments of Family Practice and Psychiatry at Albany Medical College.

"Visualize yourself lying in warm sand on a beach in the Bahamas, a cool wind blowing in off the ocean, the surf rolling in quietly in the background. It's *amazing* what this can do to relax you."

Recite an antistress litany. Stress can strike anytime, not just at work—in the bathroom before work, in the deli at lunchtime, in the car on the way home. To help yourself unravel when unpleasant thoughts knot the muscles in your neck and tension mounts, recite the following litany, suggested by Dr. Miller.

- "There's no *place* I have to go at this moment in time."
- "There's no *problem* I have to solve at this moment in time."
- "There's nothing that I have to *do* at this moment in time."
- "The most important thing that I can experience at this moment in time is *relaxation.*"

It's necessary to think these thoughts consciously, Dr. Miller says, because doing so automatically changes the mind-set that's producing the stress. If you're reciting the litany, you're *not* thinking about whatever bothers you.

Use affirmations. "You should have a list of affirmations ready that you can start repeating when you feel stressed," Dr. Miller says. "They don't have to be complicated. Just chanting 'I can handle this' to yourself or 'I know more about this than anyone here' will work. It pulls you away from the animal reflex to stress — the quick breathing, the cold hands — and toward the reasoned response, the intellect — the part of you that really *can* handle it."

The result? You calm down.

MEDICAL ALERT

When Stress Threatens

Too much stress can directly threaten your health. Paul J. Rosch, M.D., says that any of the following stress-related symptoms may indicate that you should seek medical help promptly.

- Dizzy spells or blackouts
- Rectal bleeding (may indicate an ulcer)
- A racing pulse that won't stop
- Sweaty palms
- Chronic back and neck pain
- Chronic or severe headaches
- Trembling
- Hives
- Overwhelming anxiety
- Insomnia

"The basic rule is this: You should see a doctor if the symptoms you're experiencing are new and have no obvious cause, especially if they interfere with your quality of life," Dr. Rosch says.

Count to ten. Simply refusing to respond to a stress immediately can help defuse it, Dr. Nathan says. And making a *habit* of pausing and relaxing—just for a few seconds—before responding to the routine interruptions of your day can make a clear difference in the sense of stress you experience. When the phone rings, for example, breathe in deeply. Then as you breathe out, imagine you are as loose and limp as an old rag doll.

"One of the things pausing like this does is give you a feeling of control," Dr. Nathan points out. "Being in control is generally less stressful than being out of control. Make a habit of using rapid relaxation during the pause before you answer the phone. Deliberately pausing can become an instant tranquilizer."

Amazing! Counting to ten *works*.

Look away. "If you look through a window at a far-distant view for a moment—away from the problem that's producing the stress—the eyes relax, and if the eyes relax, the tendency is for you to do the same," Dr. Nathan says. "Take a pot off the burner and it quits boiling."

Get up and leave. "Leaving the scene can do the same as looking away," says Dr. Nathan.

Take several deep breaths. Belly breathing is what some people call it. It's an old and useful trick for defeating anxiety and nervousness.

"The basic idea is act calm, be calm," says Bradley W. Frederick, D.C., director of the International Institute of Sports Medicine in Los Angeles, California. "When you're experiencing stress, your pulse races and you start breathing very quickly. Forcing yourself to breathe slowly convinces the body that the stress is gone, whether it is or isn't."

The correct way to breathe? Abdominally—feeling the stomach expand as you inhale, collapse as you exhale.

Yell or cry. It's not always possible in the typical office, but in some situations—a private office or your car, for example—a purely emotional outburst is perfectly acceptable. Screaming or crying can provide a release for the emotions generating the stress you're feeling, Dr. Miller says.

Stretch. "Essentially everything we feel has a physical manifestation," says Dr. Frederick. "A lot of us respond to stress with muscle tension. Ideally, we'd prefer to eliminate the cause of the stress, but

---

The Way to Inner Peace

Transcendental meditation (TM), yoga, Zen—they *all* work by inducing something called the relaxation response, a body state first characterized and named by Herbert Benson, M.D., an associate professor of medicine at Harvard Medical School's internationally acclaimed Mind/Body Clinic.

"This phenomenon shuts off the distracting, stressful, anxiety-producing aspects of what is commonly called the fight-or-flight response," Dr. Benson writes in his book *Your Maximum Mind*.

"In primitive situations, where dangers from wild animals might have been the order of the day, this sort of response [fight-or-flight] was quite useful. In our own time, however, the fight-or-flight response tends to make us more nervous, uncomfortable, and even unhealthy."

A person experiencing the relaxation response turns off all the hormones and behaviors that are making him nervous. Basically any kind of meditation will produce it, though TM, yoga, and Zen require formal instruction and a good amount of self-discipline.

Dr. Benson suggests the following basic program for eliciting the response.

One, pick a focus word or phrase ("peace," for example) that is firmly rooted in your personal belief system. Two, sit quietly, close your eyes, and relax. And three, start repeating your focus word in time with your breathing, each time you exhale. Continue for 10 to 20 minutes.

Tips: Practice at least once a day, and don't worry about how you're doing. If you realize that you've been distracted by thoughts, just easily return attention to your word and continue your meditation.

---

stretching the muscles at least reduces the sensation of stress—the muscles relax, we feel less tense. And given that we often can't do anything about the source of stress, that's important."

And for many of us, that's all we need.

Massage your target muscles. "Most of us have particular muscles that knot up under stress," Dr. Miller says. "It's sort of a vicious circle: Stress produces adrenaline, which produces muscle tension, which produces more adrenaline, and so on. A good way to break the circle is to find out what your target muscles are—the ones that get tense under pressure, usually in the back of your neck and upper back—and massage them for a couple of minutes whenever you feel tense."

Press on your temples. This application of acupressure—the oriental system that uses pressure points to relieve pain and treat a variety of ailments—works indirectly. Massaging nerves in your temples, says Dr. Miller, relaxes muscles elsewhere—chiefly in your neck.

Drop your jaw and roll it left to right. "People under pressure have a tendency to clench their teeth," says Dr. Miller. "Dropping the jaw and rolling it helps make those muscles relax, and if you relax the muscles, you reduce the sensation of tension."

Stretch your chest for better breathing. The tense musculature of a person under stress can make breathing difficult, according to Dr. Frederick, and impaired breathing can aggravate the anxiety you already feel. To relax your breathing, roll your shoulders up and back, then relax. The first time, inhale deeply as they go back, exhale as they relax. Repeat four or five more times, then inhale deeply again. Repeat the entire sequence four times.

Relax all over. Easier said than done? Not if you know how. A simple technique called progressive relaxation can produce immediate and dramatic reductions in your sense of stress by reducing physical tension.

Starting at top or bottom, tense one set of muscles in your body at a time, hold for a few seconds, then let them relax. Work your way through all major body parts—feet, legs, chest and arms, head and neck—and then enjoy the sense of release it provides.

Take a hot soak. Hot water works by defeating the stress response, says Dr. Frederick. When we're tense and anxious, blood flow to our extremities is reduced. Hot water restores circulation, convincing the body it's safe and that it is okay to relax. Cold water is a no-no for the opposite reason. It *mimics* the stress response, driving blood away from the extremities. Result: Tension increases.

An office alternative might be running hot water over your hands until you feel tension start to drain away.

Move around. Regular exercise, of course, builds stamina that can help anyone battle stress. But even something as casual as a walk around the block can help you throw off some of the tension a rough business meeting or a family squabble leaves you carrying around.

"Exercise is what your body instinctively wants to do under stress: Run or fight," Dr. Miller says. "And it works. One, it burns off some of the stress chemicals tension produces. And two, a tired muscle is a relaxed muscle."

Listen to a relaxation tape. Relaxation, Dr. Miller says, is the opposite of tension — the antidote for stress. And the pre-recorded relaxation tapes he and others produce — Dr. Miller's have been used by such diverse organizations as Atari, Lockheed Corporation, and Levi Strauss & Company — are very effective.

"Good relaxation tapes are very valuable," says Dr. Nathan. "They facilitate your relaxation response. And they're inexpensive."

Available tapes offer voice only, voice with music, or just natural sounds — wind in the trees, surf on the sand. All you need is a tape recorder and a headset — to block out distractions and avoid disturbing others.

Tune in the music. Relaxation cassettes work, but they aren't your only option. Music soothes as perhaps nothing else does.

"Music is an enormously powerful tool for fighting stress," Dr. Miller says. "You can use it in two basic ways — to relax or to inspire. New-Age music is very relaxing."

PANEL OF ADVISERS

Herbert Benson, M.D., is an associate professor of medicine at Harvard Medical School in Cambridge, Massachusetts, and chief of the Section on Behavioral Medicine at New England Deaconess Hospital there.

Bradley W. Frederick, D.C., is a chiropractor and director of the International Institute of Sports Medicine in Los Angeles, California.

Emmett Miller, M.D., is medical director of the Cancer Support and Education Center and president of Source Cassette Learning Systems in Menlo Park, California. He is a nationally recognized expert on stress.

Ronald Nathan, Ph.D., is director of educational development, coordinator of behavioral science, and associate professor in the departments of Family Practice and Psychiatry at Albany Medical College in New York.

Paul J. Rosch, M.D., is president of the American Institute of Stress and a clinical professor of medicine and psychiatry at New York Medical College in Valhalla. He's also adjunct clinical professor of medicine in psychiatry at the University of Maryland School of Medicine in Baltimore.

Sunburn

37 Cooling Treatments

You could just kick yourself for getting a sunburn. And you probably would if you weren't in such pain. Really, you know better than to abuse your skin this way. You know all about sunscreens and how they protect against the ravages of old Sol's burning rays. But, well, you got *careless*, and now you're paying plenty in terms of discomfort and lost sleep. Hopefully, you've learned your lesson. Next time you won't be caught with your sunscreen down. But for now, heed this advice from the experts.

Reach for a pain reliever. The old standby aspirin can help relieve the pain, itching, and swelling of a mild to moderate burn. "Take two tablets every 4 hours," says University of Nebraska dermatologist and assistant professor of internal medicine Rodney Basler, M.D. "The same dosage of Tylenol would work also. Or, if your stomach can tolerate it, you might try three or four tablets of ibuprofen every 8 hours."

Anticipate a burn. If you know you've gotten too much sun, try taking aspirin *before* the redness appears. "Some doctors recommend 650 milligrams of aspirin [two tablets] soon after sun exposure. Repeat every 4 hours for up to six doses," says Thomas Gossel, Ph.D., R.Ph., a professor of pharmacology and toxicology at Ohio Northern University.

Apply soothing compresses. Following a burn, the skin is inflamed. Try cooling it down with compresses dipped in any one of the following substances. If desired, you can direct a fan on the sunburned area to heighten cooling.

Cold water. Use either plain water from the faucet or add a few ice cubes, says Arizona dermatologist Michael Schreiber, M.D., senior clinical lecturer in the Department of Internal Medicine at the University of

---

MEDICAL ALERT

Get Thee to a Doctor

A severe burn can take a lot out of you, says Rodney Basler, M.D. Consult a doctor if you experience nausea, chills, fever, faintness, extensive blistering, general weakness, patches of purple discoloration, or intense itching. And be aware that if the burn seems to be spreading, you could have an infection compounding the problem.

Arizona College of Medicine. Dip a cloth into the liquid and lay it over the burn. Repeat every few minutes as the cloth warms. Apply several times a day for a total of 10 to 15 minutes each.

Skim milk. Milk protein is very soothing, says Dr. Schreiber. Mix 1 cup skim milk with 4 cups water, then add a few ice cubes. Apply compresses for 15 to 20 minutes; repeat every 2 to 4 hours.

Aluminum acetate. If itching is intense, says Dr. Gossel, try mixing Buro-Sol antiseptic powder or Domeboro's powder (both available in pharmacies) with water. The aluminum acetate in either will keep the skin from getting too dry or itchy. Follow package directions.

Oatmeal. Dermatologist Fredric Haberman, M.D., a clinical instructor of medicine at Albert Einstein College of Medicine of Yeshiva University, recommends oatmeal water, which soothes the skin. Wrap dry oatmeal in cheesecloth or gauze. Run cool water through it. Discard the oatmeal and soak compresses in the liquid. Apply every 2 to 4 hours.

Witch hazel. Moisten a cloth with witch hazel, says Dr. Haberman. Apply often for temporary relief. For smaller areas, dip cotton balls into the liquid and gently stroke on.

Soak the pain away. An alternative to compresses—especially for larger areas—is a cool bath. Add more liquid as needed to keep the water at the proper temperature. Afterward, gently pat your skin dry with a clean towel. Do not rub your skin or you'll irritate it further. The following substances can reduce pain, itching, and inflammation.

The Alternate Route

Kitchen Cabinet Remedies

Common kitchen staples can be great sunburn soothers. Press the following into emergency action.

Cornstarch. Add enough water to cornstarch to make a paste, says Fredric Haberman, M.D. Apply directly to the sunburn.

Vegetable slices. Some people get relief from thin slices of raw cucumber or potato, he adds. They feel cool and may help reduce inflammation on small areas. Apple slices may also work.

Lettuce. A soothing homemade solution comes from New York City skin care specialist Lia Schorr. Boil lettuce leaves in water. Strain, then let the liquid cool several hours in the refrigerator. Dip cotton balls into the liquid and gently press or stroke onto irritated skin.

Yogurt. Plain yogurt is both cooling and soothing, she says. Apply to all sunburned areas. Rinse off in a cool shower, then gently pat skin dry.

Tea bags. If your eyelids are burned, apply tea bags soaked in cool water to decrease swelling and help relieve pain, says Schorr.

Vinegar. Mix 1 cup of white vinegar into a tub of cool water, says Carl Korn, M.D., an assistant clinical professor of dermatology at the University of Southern Californa.

Aveeno powder. If the sunburn involves a large area, use the premeasured packets or add ½ cup of Aveeno Bath Treatment, which is made from oatmeal, to a tub of cool water, says Dr. Schreiber. Soak for 15 to 20 minutes.

Baking soda. Generously sprinkle baking soda into tepid bathwater, suggests Dr. Haberman. Instead of toweling off, let the solution dry on your skin.

Go easy on soap. Soap can dry and irritate burned skin. If you must use soap, says Dr. Gossel, use only a mild brand and rinse it off very well. Do not soak in soapy water. Likewise, stay away from bubble baths.

Moisturize your skin. Soaks and compresses feel good and give temporary relief, says Dr. Basler. But they can make your skin feel drier than before if you don't apply moisturizer immediately afterward. Pat yourself dry, then smooth on some bath oil.

Let it soak in for a minute, then apply a moisturizing cream or lotion, such as Eucerin. Some people like a topical cream called Wibi, which contains a little bit of cooling menthol.

Chill out. For added relief, try chilling your moisturizer before applying it.

Seek hydrocortisone relief. Soothe skin irritation and inflammation with a topical lotion, spray, or ointment containing 0.05 percent hydrocortisone, such as Cortaid or Cortizone-5, says Dr. Basler.

Say good-bye with aloe. "We're starting to see evidence in medical literature that aloe vera may really help wound healing," says Dr. Basler. Simply break off a leaf and apply the juice. But test a small area first, he cautions, to make sure you're not allergic to aloe.

Guard against infection. If you have an infection or are worried that one will develop, use an over-the-counter antibacterial ointment such as Polysporin or Bacitracin Sterile, says Dr. Schreiber.

Try a local anesthetic. If your burn is mild, an over-the-counter anesthetic can relieve pain and itching, says Dr. Gossel. Look for brands that contain benzocaine, benzyl alcohol, lidocaine, or diphenhydramine hydrochloride. Aerosols are easier to apply than creams or ointments, but never spray them directly onto your face. Instead, put some on a piece of gauze or a cotton pad and rub it on your face to avoid contact with your eyes.

Try an ice pack. An ice pack can also provide relief if the burn is mild. Wrap it in a damp cloth and hold it over the sunburn. Improvise, if necessary, says Dr. Haberman. "You could even take a bag of frozen peas, for instance, and use that. But make sure to wrap it first so you're not placing the icy package directly against your skin."

Drink up. It's a good idea to drink lots of water to help counteract the drying effect of a burn, says Dr. Gossel.

Eat right. Eat lightly but wisely, he adds. A balanced diet will help provide the nutrients your skin needs to regenerate itself.

Are You Photosensitive?

We're not asking if you like to have your picture taken. The question is whether certain drugs, soaps, or cosmetics increase your sensitivity to the sun and lead to a burnlike dermatitis.

Antibiotics, tranquilizers, and antifungal medications can cause reactions, says Rodney Basler, M.D. So can oral contraceptives, diuretics, drugs for diabetes, and even PABA-containing sunscreens. Always ask your doctor about potential side effects of any oral drugs you may be taking.

Even common foods can trigger a bad reaction. "Two young women I know tried to lighten their hair with lime juice," he says. "They didn't realize what a potent photosensitizer lime juice can be until they developed terrible dermatitis every place the juice had run down their faces and arms."

Raise your legs. If your legs are burned and your feet are swollen, elevate your legs above heart level, says Dr. Basler. You'll feel better.

Get a good night's rest. Sleeping on a sunburn can be murder, but you need a lot of rest for your body to recover from the burn. So try sprinkling talcum powder on your sheets to minimize chafing and friction, says Dr. Haberman. A water bed or air mattress might also help you sleep easier.

Be careful with blisters. If you develop blisters, you have a pretty bad burn. If they bother you and they cover only a small area, you may carefully drain them, says Dr. Basler. But do not peel the top skin off—you'll have less discomfort and danger of infection if air does not come in contact with sensitive nerve endings.

To drain the fluid, first sterilize a needle by holding it over a match flame. Then puncture the edge of the blister and press gently on the top to let the fluid come out. Do this three times in the first 24 hours, says Dr. Basler. Then leave the blisters alone.

Beware ice and snow. Don't let your guard down in winter, says Butch Farabee, emergency services coordinator for the National Park Service. You can get a fierce burn from the sun's rays reflected off ice and snow. "I've even gotten the inside of my mouth sunburned when hiking up icy hills because I was breathing so hard that my mouth was open." So cover up appropriately and wear sunscreen on all exposed areas.

Don't make the same mistake twice. After you've gotten burned, it takes three to six months for your skin to return to normal, says Dr. Schreiber. "When you get a sunburn and the top layer of skin peels off, the newly exposed skin is more sensitive than ever. That means you'll burn even faster than you did before if you're not careful."

Follow the rules. While the memory of your burn is still painfully fresh, brush up on your sun sense with these tips from Norman Levine, M.D., chief of dermatology at the University of Arizona College of Medicine.

- Apply a sunscreen about 30 minutes before going out, even if it's overcast. (Harmful rays can penetrate cloud cover.) Don't forget to protect your lips, hands, ears, and the back of your neck. Reapply as necessary after swimming or perspiring heavily.
- Take extra care between the hours of 10:00 A.M. and 3:00 P.M. (11:00 A.M. and 4:00 P.M., daylight saving time), when the sun is at its hottest.
- If you insist upon getting a tan, do so very gradually. Start with 15 minutes' exposure and increase it only a few minutes at a time.
- Wear protective clothing when not swimming or sunbathing. Hats, tightly woven fabrics, and long sleeves help keep the sun off your skin.

PANEL OF ADVISERS

Rodney Basler, M.D., is a dermatologist and assistant professor of internal medicine at the University of Nebraska College of Medicine in Lincoln.

Butch Farabee is emergency services coordinator for the National Park Service in Washington, D.C. He has 22 years of field experience as a park ranger.

Thomas Gossel, Ph.D., R.Ph., is a professor of pharmacology and toxicology at Ohio Northern University in Ada and chairman of the University's Department of Pharmacology and Biomedical Sciences. He is an expert on over-the-counter products.

Fredric Haberman, M.D., is a dermatologist in Bergen County, New Jersey, and New York City. He is also a clinical instructor of medicine at the Albert Einstein College of Medicine of Yeshiva University in New York City. He is the author of the book *Your Skin: A Dermatologist's Guide to a Lifetime of Beauty and Health.* He is also president and founder of Save Our Children's Skin (SOCS), a foundation dedicated to preventing skin cancer and other childhood skin afflictions.

Carl Korn, M.D., is an assistant clinical professor of dermatology at the University of Southern California in Los Angeles.

Norman Levine, M.D., is chief of dermatology at the University of Arizona College of Medicine in Tucson.

Lia Schorr is a skin care specialist in New York City and author of *Lia Schorr's Seasonal Skin Care.*

Michael Schreiber, M.D., is a dermatologist in private practice in Tucson, Arizona. He is also senior clinical lecturer in the Department of Internal Medicine at the University of Arizona College of Medicine in Tucson.

Swimmer's Ear

15 Cures and Preventive Measures

If you could reduce yourself to the size of a flea and crawl into a swimmer's ear, you'd likely see an ear canal that's angry and red. It would look itchy, and you'd notice there's very little earwax. It would feel moist and smell clammy from bacteria burrowing and tunneling into the skin.

What you'd be seeing inside that swimmer's ear is a classic case of otitis externa, an infection better known — not surprisingly — as swimmer's ear.

All it takes to come down with a stubborn bout of swimmer's ear is a set of ears and unrelenting moisture. "It's like keeping your hands in dishwater. The skin gets macerated and leathery," says Brian W. Hands, M.D., an ear, nose, and throat specialist in private practice in Toronto. "The ears are constantly bathed in water — swimming, showering, shampooing. Then people try to dry the ear with a cotton-tipped swab. That takes the top layer of skin off, along with protective bacteria. Then the bad bacteria win."

Swimmer's ear begins as an itchy ear. Left untreated, it can turn into a full-blown infection. The pain can be excruciating. Once infection sets in, you'll need a doctor's help and a round of antibiotics to squelch it. But there are plenty of things you can do to keep the pain from getting worse, and even more to stop it before it starts.

Blow-dry your ears. Eliminate the moisture in your ears, says Dr. Hands, every time you get them wet, whether or not you suspect an infection. Pull the flap of your ear up and out to straighten the ear canal and aim your hair dryer into your ear from 18 to 20 inches away. Use either a warm or cool setting, but let the dryer blow for 30 seconds. That will dry the ear, eliminating the moist conditions bacteria and fungi find most attractive for growth.

Try an over-the-counter remedy. Most drugstores carry ear-drops that combat bacteria. If ear itchiness is still your only symptom, one of these preparations might snatch it back from the brink of infection, says Dan Drew, M.D., an avid swimmer and family physician in Jasper, Indiana. Use it each time your ears get wet.

Plug up the problem. Telling an avid swimmer that he can't go in the water is almost like telling someone to quit breathing, says John House, M.D., an associate professor of clinical otolaryngology at the University of Southern California School of Medicine and an otologist for United States Swimming, which selects Olympic competitors. Go ahead and swim, he says, but wear earplugs to keep the water out. Wax or silicone plugs that can be softened and shaped to fit your ear are available at most drugstores.

And don't forget to wear those plugs while shampooing or showering, says Dr. House. Keeping the ears dry is especially important for people who are prone to ear infection.

Swim on the surface. Even if you are battling swimmer's ear, you can keep on swimming, says Dr. Drew. Swim on the surface of the water. It allows less water in the ear than when you break the surface.

Use a painkiller as a temporary measure. If your ear hurts (indicating an infection), an over-the-counter painkiller such as aspirin or acetaminophen will tide you over until you can see the doctor, says Donald Kamerer, M.D., chief of the Division of Otology at the Ear and Eye Institute in Pittsburgh, Pennsylvania.

Soothe away pain with heat. Warmth — a towel fresh from the dryer, a covered hot-water bottle, a heating pad set on low — also will help ease the pain.

Leave your earwax alone. Earwax serves several purposes, including harboring friendly bacteria, say Dr. Kamerer and Dr. House. Cooperate with your natural defenses by *not* swabbing the wax out. Wax coats the ear canal, protecting it from moisture.

Tune Out to Turn Off Infection

If you wear a hearing aid, you can get swimmer's ear without even going near the water.

A hearing aid has an earplug effect, explains Brian W. Hands, M.D. In addition to picking up sound, it also picks up moisture that lodges in the ear canal. And trapped moisture can breed the germs that brew an infection.

The solution? Take your hearing aid out of your ear as often as possible to give your ear a chance to dry out.

Keep it dry. Since the irritation of swimmer's ear wears away earwax, you can manufacture your own version using petroleum jelly. Moisten a cotton ball with the jelly, says Dr. Hands, and tuck it gently, like a plug, just in the edge of your ear. It will absorb any moisture, keeping your ear warm and dry.

Take a drop. Several fluids are great for killing germs and drying your ears at the same time. If you're susceptible to swimmer's ear or if you spend a lot of time in the water, you should use a drying agent every time you get your head wet. Any of the following homemade solutions works well.

A squirt of rubbing alcohol. First, put your head down, with the affected ear up. Pull the ear upward and backward (to help straighten the canal) and squeeze a dropperful of alcohol into the ear canal. Wiggle your ear to get the alcohol to the bottom of the canal. Then tilt your head to the other side and let the alcohol drain out.

A kitchen solution. Eardrops of white vinegar or equal parts of alcohol and white vinegar will kill fungus and bacteria, says Dr. House. Use it the same way you would alcohol.

Mineral oil, baby oil, or lanolin. These can be preventive solutions before swimming. Apply as you would the alcohol.

Put a cap on it. Dr. Drew invented a bathing cap with goggles welded to it (called a Goggl'Cap) to keep goggles from floating away when swimmers dive into the pool. Then, he says, he noticed an added benefit:

The Latex version of his cap also covered the ears and helped keep water out of them. The ideal combination is a pair of earplugs with the cap holding them in place, he says.

Choose your swimming hole with care. You are less likely to pick up bacteria in a well-treated pool than you are in a pond, says Dr. Drew. Don't swim in dirty water.

PANEL OF ADVISERS

Dan Drew, M.D., is a family physician in Jasper, Indiana. An avid swimmer, he is the inventor of the Goggl'Cap, a swim cap-goggle combination.

Brian W. Hands, M.D., is an ear, nose, and throat specialist in private practice in Toronto.

John House, M.D., is an associate professor of clinical otolaryngology at the University of Southern California School of Medicine in Los Angeles. He serves as a national team physician for United States Swimming, the national governing association for competitive amateur swimming that selects the Olympic team.

Donald Kamerer, M.D., is chief of the Division of Otology at the Ear and Eye Institute in Pittsburgh, Pennsylvania. He also is a professor of otolaryngology at the University of Pittsburgh School of Medicine.

Tachycardia

12 Ways to Calm a Rapid Heartbeat

It comes on suddenly. You're not even aware of your heart and then—boom!—it starts pounding furiously. Seventy-two beats a minute become 120—180—200 beats in seconds flat. Maybe your breath catches, too, and a wave of nausea rises with your panic. You even start to sweat.

Your doctor says you have tachycardia, more specifically, paroxysmal atrial tachycardia. You're no dummy. The first time this happened, you had yourself thoroughly checked over. Together, you and your doctor ruled out ventricular tachycardia (the life-threatening type of rapid heartbeat) and all forms of organic heart disease, thyroid abnormalities, pulmonary malfunctions, etc. That was reassuring.

Yet, every so often, your atria—the chambers in your heart that receive blood from the veins and pump it into the ventricles—get a little out of control. The atria keep a steady rhythm but that rhythm can be three times faster than normal. (Tachycardia, by the way, refers to any heartbeat faster than 100 beats per minute.)

There are ways to put the brakes on your tachycardia. Below, you'll find techniques to help you cope with attacks, and lifestyle tips that can help prevent them.

Slow down. Think of that speeding heart as a flashing red light that says "stop what you're doing. Chill out. Rest." Rest, in fact, is your best mechanism for stopping an attack, says Dennis S. Miura, M.D., Ph.D., director of clinical arrhythmia and electrophysiology science at the Albert Einstein College of Medicine of Yeshiva University.

Try the vagal maneuver. How fast your heart beats and how strongly it contracts are regulated by sympathetic nerves and parasympathetic nerves (or vagal nerves). When your heart pounds, the sympathetic network is dominant. (That's the system that basically tells your body to speed up.) What you want to do is switch control to the mellower parasympathetic network. If you stimulate a vagal nerve, you initiate a chemical process that affects your heart the same way that slamming on the brakes affects your car.

One way to do this is to take a deep breath and bear down, as if you were having a bowel movement, says John O. Lawder, M.D., a family practitioner specializing in nutrition and preventive medicine in Torrance, California.

Reach for the right carotid artery. Gently massaging the right carotid artery is another vagal maneuver. Be sure to have your doctor show you the right point and the right degree of pressure. You want to massage the artery where it connects in the neck, as far underneath the jaw as possible, says James Frackelton, M.D., a Cleveland physician who researches and specializes in vascular disease and immunology.

Rely on the diving reflex. When sea mammals dive into the coldest regions of the water, their heart rates automatically slow. That's nature's way of preserving their brains and hearts. You can call on your own diving reflex by filling a basin with icy water and plunging your face into it for a second or two.

"Sometimes, that will interrupt the tachycardia," says Dr. Miura.

Break the coffee habit. Ditto for cola, tea, chocolate, diet pills, or stimulants in any form. Overuse of stimulants can put you at risk for paroxysmal atrial tachycardia, says Dr. Miura.

Baby your hypothalamus. What goes on in your head — your midbrain specifically — rules your heart, says Dr. Frackelton. That's why it's essential for you to give your hypothalamus the support it needs — through proper diet, exercise, a positive attitude — to maintain stability and control over your autonomic nervous system.

The autonomic nervous system has two subsystems: the sympathetic, which basically speeds up everything in the body but digestion, and the parasympathetic system.

Stress, poor diet, and pollutants can cause your hypothalamus to lose its grip on the autonomic nervous system, allowing the system to slip into high gear or what Dr. Frackelton terms sympathetic overload. "That's Barney Fife a half hour before his execution."

You can help your hypothalamus retain control.

Eat healthy, regular meals and go easy on the sweets. If you skip meals and then fill your stomach with a candy bar or soda pop, your pancreatic enzymes will speed in to take care of the increased sugar intake, says Dr. Frackelton. Then your insulin overshoots and you go into reactive hypoglycemia. Your adrenal glands bring adrenaline in to mobilize the stores of glycogen in your liver. The adrenaline stimulates a sudden increase in heart rate and the feeling of panic.

Tailor your meal schedule to your metabolism. People who have a rapid metabolism should eat more protein foods, says Dr. Lawder. Protein foods take longer to digest and help prevent your blood sugar from falling too low. When your blood sugar drops, it triggers the process discussed above.

Let loose. Dr. Lawder says he's noticed a relationship between perfectionistic, upwardly mobile, outer-success-oriented individuals and atrial paroxysmal tachycardia. "By and large, these are the same people who get migraine headaches," he says. "For people like this, the conduction mechanisms of the heart become highly exaggerated. There's chronic adrenaline overstimulation. When people are under a lot of stress, there is a breakthrough of autonomic conduction of the heart, a loss of rhythm."

How to compensate? Adopt a progressive relaxation program, practice biofeedback, or learn to visualize "serenity, tranquility, calmness, and peace," says Dr. Lawder.

MEDICAL ALERT

The Serious Side of Arrhythmia

Listen, we don't mean to alarm you unnecessarily. But if your ticker has lost its sense of timing, get to a doctor—pronto. Only a doctor can distinguish between paroxysmal atrial tachycardia and more serious forms of heart arrhythmia, says Arthur Selzer, M.D., a clinical professor of medicine at the University of California Medical School.

Ventricular tachycardia is an example of a more serious kind. That's what you have when one ventricle starts beating rapidly with a slightly irregular rhythm. (The ventricle is the heart chamber that pumps blood back into the arteries.) The amount of blood your heart returns to the arteries may drop markedly. You feel weak, sweaty; you may even faint.

Ventricular fibrillation—which sometimes occurs as a complication of ventricular tachycardia—is usually fatal. That's why we can't stress enough the importance of attending to any abnormal heart rhythms immediately. The right response to an attack depends on what the malfunction is.

Get your fair share of magnesium. Magnesium is a protector of the cells, says Dr. Frackelton. In the muscle cells of the heart, magnesium helps to balance the effects of calcium. When calcium moves into the cells, it stimulates muscular contractions within the cell itself. Magnesium is central to the enzymes in the cell that pump calcium out. It creates rhythmic contraction and relaxation. It makes the heart much less likely to get irritable, says Dr. Frackelton. Magnesium can be found in such things as soybeans, nuts, beans, and bran.

Keep potassium levels up. Potassium is another of the minerals that helps slow down heart action and the irritability of the muscle fibers, says Dr. Lawder. The mineral is found in fruit and vegetables, so getting enough shouldn't be difficult. But you can deplete it if your diet is high in sodium or if you use diuretics (water pills) or overuse laxatives.

Exercise. "You can do a lot by getting into good tone," says Dr. Frackelton. "When you do the kinds of exercise that raise the heart rate, it tends to reset at a lower level. People who don't exercise usually have a heart rate around 80. When they begin to do a little bit of jogging, their heart rates go up to 160, 170. Then, with a little conditioning, they can bring the resting heart rate down to 60 to 65."

Exercise also makes you resistant to excess adrenaline release, he says. "It gets your aggressions out in a healthy way. You're using adrenaline release as part of a normal function."

PANEL OF ADVISERS

James Frackelton, M.D., is in private practice in Cleveland, Ohio, and does research on vascular disease and immunology. He is past president of the American College of Advancement in Medicine and president of the American Institute of Medical Preventics.

John O. Lawder, M.D., is a family practitioner specializing in nutrition and preventive medicine in Torrance, California.

Dennis S. Miura, M.D., Ph.D., is director of clinical arrhythmia and electrophysiology science at the Albert Einstein College of Medicine of Yeshiva University in New York City.

Arthur Selzer, M.D., is a clinical professor of medicine at the University of California, San Francisco, School of Medicine and clinical professor emeritus at Stanford University. He is also a member of the cardiology staff of Pacific-Presbyterian Medical Center, where he served as department chief for 25 years.

Tartar and Plaque

24 Tooth-Care Tips

Take your fingernail and scrape it gently across the inside of one of your molars. Now look at your finger. See that white stuff under your fingernail? That's plaque.

Plaque is a sticky film of living and dead bacteria that grows on your teeth. When plaque isn't removed, it can harden—50 percent within 48 hours, becoming rock hard after 12 days. That rock, called calculus, is more commonly known as tartar.

There are a lot of reasons you don't want either one of these tooth coatings. Tartar and plaque make your teeth look ugly, feel ugly, and smell ugly.

Enough? There's one more: A plaque and tartar crust on your teeth and gums leads to even uglier tooth problems such as gingivitis and periodontal disease.

You can't remove tartar. "It gets like a barnacle on a ship," and requires professional help to remove, says Robert Schallhorn, D.D.S., a private practitioner in Aurora, Colorado, and past president of the American Academy of Periodontology. But you can remove plaque. And by getting the plaque off your teeth, you'll prevent a lot of tartar. Removing plaque is easy. So wipe your finger off and read on.

Brusha, brusha, brusha. Think of your toothbrush as your sword and plaque as the enemy. What you want to do in this case is rub the bad guy out.

The friction of a toothbrush disrupts the bacterial plaque growth on the teeth—as long as you do it correctly. And most people don't, says William Campoli, D.M.D., a dentist with a private practice in Charlotte, North Carolina.

The Alternate Route

Twig Therapy: Something to Chew On

Before praying, decreed the prophet Mohammed, people should clean their teeth with Miswak twigs. So, for centuries in areas of the Middle East and Asia, tooth cleaning has been done with roots or tiny branches from the Miswak tree.

Now studies in Egypt show that using these twigs not only cleans plaque from teeth, but it leaves a residue that continues to kill the bacteria even after a couple of days. A mouthwash containing essence of this tree reduced one kind of oral bacteria by 75 percent after only one rinse.

Bits of the Miswak are also included in some toothpastes. While traditional toothpastes rely on abrasives and synthetic detergents to clean, these twig-toting toothpastes use naturally occurring antiseptics and antimicrobial ingredients. In addition, the twigs contain tannin, which has been shown to reduce gingival bleeding and gingival inflammation. Both the twigs and the toothpaste are available in health food stores.

Users claim the Miswak is a powerful natural stain remover and say that people who use a twig instead of a brush will have whiter, brighter teeth.

If you'd like to try the original formula—the twig—it's easy, says Eric Shapira, D.D.S. First chew the twig gently to soften it. Then manipulate the stick around your mouth to push the plaque off your teeth. It's the oil in the wood, he says, that decreases the plaque. It takes about 5 to 10 minutes to get the stick pliable enough to use, then another 3 to 5 minutes to deplaque by rubbing the twig around and across all your teeth.

Up and down or back and forth isn't correct. What you need to do is turn your brush so the bristles are at a 45-degree angle to the area where your tooth and gum meet (the gum around the tooth). Now, very gently wiggle your brush in small circles, covering one or two teeth at a time.

Attack from the back. The back of your lower teeth is where the plaque is most likely to hide. "Too much emphasis is placed on brushing the smile surfaces, the upper teeth that are fairly accessible," says Dr. Campoli. "But the areas where the teeth come into contact with the tongue and cheek are neglected. That's where you need to concentrate your efforts."

Take two to clean. Two minutes, that is. "Most people brush the smile area and give the rest of the teeth a quick IOU," says Dr. Campoli. Studies show most of us brush about 30 seconds at a time and dentists— the experts who should be able to do it fastest of all—spend from 2 to 4 minutes brushing their teeth. Slow down!

Do it at night. Don't let a day's worth of debris sleep in your mouth. If you can brush only once a day, do it at night or you give your plaque 8 uninterrupted hours to set up housekeeping.

Buy a brush that fits. Think small when you choose your toothbrush. You want to reach all sides of your teeth, including those at the very back of your mouth, says Jerry F. Taintor, D.D.S., chairman of endodontics at the University of Tennessee College of Dentistry. A giant brush won't hurry your brushing along and it won't reach the little nooks and crannies those dirty germs like to hide in.

Choose soft, rounded bristles. Soft nylon bristles are easier on tooth enamel but just as tough on plaque, says Eric Shapira, D.D.S., an El Grenada, California, practitioner and assistant clinical professor and lecturer at the University of the Pacific School of Dentistry. Bristles should be rounded, not sculpted, adds Dr. Campoli. Sculpted bristles are often sharp and may slice into your gums.

Hold your brush like a pen. Finnish researchers have demonstrated that a pen grip, instead of the more common tennis racket grip, produces less gum abrasion and healthier gums and still gets rid of plaque.

C that you floss right. When it comes to plaque control, flossing is more important than brushing, says Richard Shepard, D.D.S., a retired dentist in Durango, Colorado. But you must floss correctly. Here's how. Break off 18 inches of floss and wind one end around the middle finger of one hand and the other end around the same finger on the other hand, leaving about an inch of floss between them. Using a gentle, back and forth motion, pass the floss between two teeth. When the floss gets to the gumline, curve it in a C against one tooth and slide the floss between the gum and tooth until you can feel some resistance. Now, curve it around the other tooth the same way. Scrape floss downward on upper teeth and upward on lower teeth.

Go gently. Whoa. Don't snap that floss up and down, in and out of your gums as if you were popping the plaque to death! You're whipping your gum tissue too. Slow down and take your time.

Remember that floss is floss. Find a floss you like and use it. Flavored, unflavored, waxed, unwaxed, string, or tape. Does it matter what you choose? Not really, says Dr. Taintor. Tape might be better for people with spaces between their teeth. Flavoring might make you feel a little fresher.

Get the seal of approval. Use a fluoride toothpaste recommended by the American Dental Association, says John D. B. Featherstone, Ph.D., chairman of the Department of Oral Biology at Eastman Dental Center in Rochester, New York. Generic toothpastes, he says, may not contain an active fluoride or may be too abrasive.

Try a baking soda scrub. Baking soda is an old standby that really works, says Dr. Shepard. Dip your brush directly into the box or mix a tablespoon of baking soda to a pinch of salt in a cup. Then wet your brush and scrub.

Use water alone. Don't let an empty tube of toothpaste prevent you from brushing. Wet your brush and go after the plaque, says Dr. Campoli.

Be resourceful. Your luggage is on its way to Hawaii and you are in Cleveland. No excuses! If you're left defenseless, you can use ordinary thread from your travel sewing kit, says Dr. Schallhorn. (Your airline or hotel should have some if you don't.) Use the thread like floss.

Go swish, swish, swish. After every meal, especially when you can't carry a toothbrush, dash to the bathroom and swish a mouthful of water around those teeth. One good swish will remove debris and may save you from spinach-in-the-teeth embarrassment.

Try Listerine. Listerine has been shown to be effective in reducing plaque when used alone or when used to supplement regular toothbrushing, according to studies at the University of Gothenburg in Sweden and at the University of Maryland at Baltimore. A study of 145 adults in Baltimore showed people who rinse with Listerine can reduce plaque by 22 percent and gingivitis by 28 percent.

Make your own mouthwash. For a homemade mouthwash, a half-and-half mixture of 3 percent hydrogen peroxide and water will do the trick, says Roger P. Levin, D.D.S., of Baltimore, Maryland, president of the Baltimore Academy of General Dentistry.

Put the pressure on. Gently hose down your teeth and gums with a dental water sprayer such as the Water-Pik. You will remove the food the plaque will eat. "But be careful," warns Dr. Campoli. "It's like a brushless car wash. If you use enough water pressure to blast the plaque off, it might hurt the gums." Remember, however, that using a water-spray device does not mean that you can forget about brushing and flossing.

Opt for full disclosure. Tally your score against plaque with a disclosing tablet, available at most drugstores. The tablets contain a dye that will stain plaque left on your teeth after brushing. Chew the tablet, then look in the mirror and inspect your teeth. The color will be darkest near the gums where plaque is the thickest. Brush again, and be sure to target the plaque-catching areas each time you brush.

Make your own plaque spotter. It's easy. First coat your lips with petroleum jelly to avoid staining. Then put a teaspoon full of food coloring into your mouth, swish it around, and spit it into a basin, advises John Beresford, a dentist in England and author of *Good Mouthkeeping*. Rinse with clear water. Then look for plaque, stained by the dye. Brush. Each time you brush, pay special attention to the areas stained by the dye.

Say cheese, please. Avoid the chips and reach for the cheese appetizers, suggest studies at the University of Iowa's Dow Institute for Dental Research. Researchers found that 5 grams of cheese — that's less than an ounce — eaten before meals eliminates the acid production of plaque. But you must choose an aged cheese, such as cheddar, says James S. Wefel, Ph.D., a researcher at Dow. Why?

"The mechanism is unknown," says Dr. Wefel. "It may act as a buffering agent." But he does know that young cheeses don't work.

"Something must happen in the aging process, but we haven't put our finger on it yet." Aged cheese, "the smellier, the better," works best.

Make sugarless gum your last bite. When you can't brush after a meal, pop a stick of gum in your mouth and chew your way to cleaner teeth, says Dr. Wefel. Spend about 20 minutes chewing sugarless gum after meals or snacks. As you chew, your saliva, a natural buffering agent in your mouth, will wash your teeth and neutralize the acid in the plaque before it attacks your teeth. Moving the gum around in your mouth may also dislodge food stuck between your teeth, Dr. Wefel says.

Try an electric brush. Forget the conventional toothbrushes that vibrate the plaque off your teeth. There's a new breed of electric toothbrush with bristles that rotate while the stem remains still. There are several brands for sale, including the Interplak, Rota-Dent, and Superbrush. They work like the brushes used by dental hygienists and they're the perfect instrument for people with arthritis or those who have a handicap that prevents them from using a regular toothbrush effectively. For someone not inclined to brush well, "it's a novelty item. So maybe he would use it more," Dr. Campoli says.

According to research, these new brushes remove as much as 98.2 percent of plaque from tooth surfaces versus as little as 48.6 percent removed by hand brushing.

PANEL OF ADVISERS

William Campoli, D.M.D., is in private practice in Charlotte, North Carolina.

John D. B. Featherstone, Ph.D., is chairman of the Department of Oral Biology at Eastman Dental Center in Rochester, New York, and deputy director of the Rochester Cariology Center.

Roger P. Levin, D.D.S., is president of the Baltimore Academy of General Dentistry and a guest lecturer at the University of Maryland in Baltimore.

Robert Schallhorn, D.D.S., has a private practice in Aurora, Colorado, and is past president of the American Academy of Periodontology.

Eric Shapira, D.D.S., is in private practice in El Grenada, California. He is an assistant clinical professor and lecturer at the University of the Pacific School of Dentistry in San Francisco, California, and has a master's degree in science and biochemistry.

Richard Shepard, D.D.S., is a retired dentist in Durango, Colorado. He edits the newsletter for the Holistic Dental Association.

Jerry F. Taintor, D.D.S., is chairman of endodontics at the University of Tennessee College of Dentistry in Memphis. He is author of *The Oral Report: The Consumer's Common Sense Guide to Better Dental Care.*

James S. Wefel, Ph.D., is a researcher at the Dow Institute at the University of Iowa in Iowa City.

Teething

4 Ways to Soothe the Pain

Though many folks don't know it, an infant's teeth actually start developing months before birth. In fact, tooth buds begin appearing in the fetus by the fifth or sixth week of pregnancy. By the time the baby is born, all 20 of the primary teeth that will be sprouting over the next 2½ years are already present and accounted for in the jawbone.

Usually those first teeth start pushing for daylight about four to eight months after birth. Baby's gums will become swollen and tender and your little bundle of joy will become irritable and restless. Teething has begun!

If you are like many parents, you are probably a bit concerned about how you and your baby will react to the steady onslaught of teeth against tissue.

"You could be in for nothing or for a little fussiness that goes along with the discomfort," says John A. Bogert, D.D.S., executive director of the American Academy of Pediatric Dentistry in Chicago, Illinois. "Most infants are a little fussy and cranky with the first two to four teeth."

Gee, that doesn't sound too bad. But just in case your baby's teething gets a little more intense than that, here are a few helpful hints to see both of you through it.

Cool those choppers. "Chewing on teething rings, particularly those you can put in the refrigerator and keep cold, works very well and feels good on the baby's gums," says Linda Jonides, a pediatric nurse practitioner in Ann Arbor, Michigan. "For a baby who's 6 months or older, even a clean, cold washcloth to chew on feels good," she adds.

Gauze those gums today. "You should probably start cleaning your baby's mouth before the teeth appear," says Dr. Bogert. A small gauze pad or even a soft baby washcloth can be wrapped around your forefinger, lightly moistened, and used to massage the gum pads, he says.

589

MEDICAL ALERT

Fever Is a Sign of Sickness

"One of the most common myths is that babies will run a fever when teething," says pediatric nurse practitioner Linda Jonides. "If there's a fever, it's not a teething fever. It means that something else is going on in your baby's body. You should see your doctor."

Doing so removes bacteria buildup and gets the youngster used to having someone poking around inside the mouth. "That way, when that first tooth does come in, you can start brushing it right away without a lot of trauma," Dr. Bogert notes. "And daily massaging makes for much healthier gum tissue."

How soon should you start? "We actually recommend you start doing this the day you get the child home from the hospital," Dr. Bogert says. "But you're probably not too late if you begin today. A couple of times a day is good—especially at bedtime."

Serve a tasty teether. "Take a piece of cold apple and wrap it in a wet, child-size washcloth," suggests Helen Neville, a pediatric advice nurse at Kaiser Permanente Hospital in Oakland, California.

"Most of the standard teething rings have no flavor," she notes, "so an apple will give the baby a little more incentive to bite down and work those teeth through the gums."

Use OTCs for pain and swelling. "I recommend trying the types of things most parents already keep handy for pediatric pain," says Dr. Bogert. "Usually, that would be Children's Tylenol. There are a number of topical anesthetics that are good for relieving teething pain and are available over-the-counter at any drugstore. Just wipe some on the gum pads and it'll bring quick relief."

PANEL OF ADVISERS

John A. Bogert, D.D.S., is executive director of the American Academy of Pediatric Dentistry in Chicago, Illinois.

Linda Jonides is a pediatric nurse practitioner in Ann Arbor, Michigan.

Helen Neville is a pediatric advice nurse at Kaiser Permanente Hospital in Oakland, California, where she is part of a 24-hour hotline for parents. She is the author of *No-Fault Parenting*.

Tendinitis

14 Soothing Remedies

Like simple muscle soreness from overuse, tendinitis—inflammation in or around, a tendon—can be painful. But where simple muscle soreness is temporary, tendinitis is tenacious—it's soreness that doesn't quit.

In fact, if chronic tendinitis had a credo, it might go like this: "Here today, here tomorrow, here to stay."

But does it really have to be so bleak, or is there hope for what, after all, sounds like a rather minor problem?

Yes, there is hope, says Bob Mangine, chairman of the American Physical Therapy Association's Sports Physical Therapy Section. "But if you continue to use the tendon in the same repetitive motion that triggered the problem in the first place, it's going to be very difficult to get better." And that applies to everyone from world-class marathoners to window washers and typists.

Still, it's possible to lessen the effects of tendinitis and prevent intense flare-ups, says Mangine, who is also administrative director of rehabilitation at the Cincinnati Sports Medicine Clinic. The key, he says, is unlocking your mind and freeing yourself to change some of your old ways.

Give it a rest. "That's a hard thing to get people to do," says Mangine. But a runner with Achilles tendinitis, for example, can't realistically expect any improvement if he doesn't take at least a couple of days away from the one-two pounding.

Of course, resting is easier said than done if you make your living washing windows and have tendinitis of the shoulder from constantly

---

MEDICAL ALERT

The Price of Ignoring Your Body's Warnings

If you only feel the pain of tendinitis during or after exercise, and if it isn't too bad, you may be thinking that you could run a race or swim laps with that same amount of pain—if you had to. Or maybe you already have.

In either case, you would be wise to realign your thinking. "You shouldn't play through pain unless your physician or physical therapist tells you otherwise," says the American Physical Therapy Association's Bob Mangine.

If pain is severe and you continue to abuse the tendon, it may rupture, says athletics trainer Bob Reese. And that could mean a long layoff, surgery, or even permanent disability.

In other words, exercising through tendon pain today could mean staying on the sidelines for the remainder of your tomorrows.

---

raising your arms over your head. But if tendinitis is a side effect of your job, it might not be a bad idea to save a day or two of vacation for those times when tendinitis is painfully persistent.

But don't give it too long a rest. "Muscles will start to atrophy," Mangine says. And for athletes, "we never recommend absolute rest," adds Ted Percy, M.D., an associate professor of orthopedic surgery and head of the Sports Medicine Section at the University of Arizona College of Medicine, Health Sciences Center.

Switch instead of fight. If your tendinitis is exercise induced, a new exercise may be just what your inflamed tendon needs. Runners with tendon problems in the lower legs, for example, can stay on the road if you're willing to hop on a bicycle, which will still give you a good upper-leg workout.

Give it a whirl. Taking a whirlpool bath or just soaking in warm bathwater is a good way to raise body temperature and increase blood flow. Warming the tendon before stressful activity decreases the soreness associated with tendinitis, says Mangine.

Use the ballerina treatment. The New York Jets football team finds using this method (inspired by a ballet dancer who had tendinitis) successful. With tendinitis of the knee, for example, treatment involves placing a warm, moist towel over the knee, then a plastic bag, then a heating pad, and last, a loose elastic wrap just to hold everything in place. Keep it on from 2 to 6 hours. To avoid burning yourself, keep the heating pad on low, advises Bob Reese, head trainer for the Jets and president of the Professional Football Athletic Trainers Society. For maximum success, your injured body part should be kept at a level higher than your heart.

Warm with stretching. The above heat treatments are only the first part of the warm-up equation. You should always stretch before exercising at full speed, says Terry Malone, Ed.D., executive director of sports medicine at Duke University. Stretching prevents the shortening of muscles and tendons that goes along with exercise.

In addition, says Mangine, some studies suggest that people who are less flexible are more prone to develop tendinitis. So stretching should be a regular part of your routine.

Brace yourself. Even a little extra support and warmth from a flexible brace or wrap can help during exercise and afterward, Mangine says. "There is no truth to the old wives' tale that wearing a brace will weaken the tendons and muscles, *provided*," he stresses, "you continue exercising."

Deep-freeze the pain. After exercising, ice is great for holding down both swelling and pain, Mangine says. However, people with heart disease, diabetes, or vascular problems should be careful about using ice because ice constricts blood vessels and could cause serious difficulties in people with such problems.

Wrap it up. Another alternative for reducing swelling is to wrap your pain in an Ace bandage, says Dr. Percy. Just be careful not to wrap the inflamed area too tightly or to leave the area wrapped for so long that it becomes uncomfortable or interferes with circulation.

Elevate. Raising the affected area is also good for controlling swelling.

Walk bowlegged. Okay, maybe you don't have to go that far. But for Achilles tendinitis, wearing cowboy boots or high heels some of the time is a fine idea, according to Dr. Percy. "It lifts the heel off the ground," he says, "and the muscles and tendons don't have to work as hard."

Go over-the-counter. Aspirin and other nonprescription, non-steroidal, anti-inflammatory drugs are effective temporary pain relievers for tendinitis, Dr. Percy says. They also reduce inflammation and swelling.

Strengthen. "When we say strengthen, we're not asking people to be an Arnold Schwarzenegger," Mangine says, "just to get better defined muscles by working out at home with light weights. You can even use pennies in a sock to work arm muscles." And that's a lot cheaper than a set of weights.

Take breaks. This is a simple way to at least temporarily relieve physical stress at work, says Scott Donkin, D.C., a chiropractor in Lincoln, Nebraska, and author of *Sitting on the Job*. "If you work in an awkward position," he says, "tendinitis can develop quite easily. Especially in the arms or wrists if you're working at a keyboard or typewriter all day."

PANEL OF ADVISERS

Scott Donkin, D.C., is a partner in the Rohrs Chiropractic Center in Lincoln, Nebraska. He is also an industrial consultant, providing tips on exercise to reduce stress for workstation users, and author of *Sitting on the Job*.

Terry Malone, Ed.D., is executive director of sports medicine at Duke University in Durham, North Carolina.

Bob Mangine is chairman of the American Physical Therapy Association's Sports Physical Therapy Section. He also is administrative director of rehabilitation at the Cincinnati Sports Medicine Clinic.

Ted Percy, M.D., is an associate professor of orthopedic surgery and head of the Sports Medicine Section at the University of Arizona College of Medicine, Arizona Health Sciences Center in Tucson.

Bob Reese is head trainer of the New York Jets and president of the Professional Football Athletic Trainers Society.

TMJ

15 Ideas to Ease the Discomfort

"Hmmmm, looks like you have a case of temporomandibular joint syndrome," says your dentist.

"Whagggr?" you say, your mouth still pried open wide and stuffed with cotton.

The temporomandibular joint is simply your jaw joint, he explains.

"But please explain, doctor, what's this about a syndrome?" you ask.

No matter what school of thought your dentist adheres to, his answer will no doubt be a very long and complicated one. Temporomandibular joint syndrome, commonly known as TMJ, is without a doubt among the most complex and controversial of all modern ailments.

But we won't get into the ongoing controversy as to whether TMJ is a muscle and ligament problem or a bone and cartilage problem. Nor will we argue whether the primary cause is stress or misaligned teeth or any other of the many suspected culprits. Your only concern at the moment is that you've been told that, yep, you have it, and you want to know what to do about it. Here's what the experts say you can do at home to complement the care you're getting from your doctor.

Go with the flow. That is, do anything you can to increase blood flow to the area. You may want to apply moist heat or ice, but don't interchange them. Apply ice or moist heat to the sides of your jaw, says Sheldon Gross, D.D.S., a lecturer at Tufts University and the University of Medicine and Dentistry of New Jersey/New Jersey Medical School and president of the American Academy of Craniomandibular Disorders. Heat works best for some, ice for others, he says. You should experiment to see what works best for you.

You can also try easy stretching and massage. If you get the blood flowing in the area, you are likely to alleviate some of your symptoms, says Dr. Gross.

MEDICAL ALERT

Some Symptoms are Serious

The most common signs of TMJ—among them headaches, toothaches, aching neck, shoulders, or back, and a clicking or popping noise when opening or closing the jaw—are usually nothing more than minor to moderate annoyances that will go away when the condition is corrected.

There are, however, some symptoms that are considered more serious and should be investigated by your doctor, warns Harold T. Perry, D.D.S., Ph.D.

"If you can't open your mouth, can't brush your teeth, and are having sharp headaches, go see a doctor," says Dr. Perry. It's a sign your TMJ is getting worse.

Support your jaw. Pick up the kind of mouth guard sold in sporting goods stores that you soften in hot water and then bite down on to form a better fit in your mouth. Wearing one will hold your jaw steady and may temporarily deal with your symptoms, says Dr. Gross.

Give up the bagels. If you've got a lot of pain in and around your mouth, consider an oral vacation. That is, limit yourself to soft and liquid food for a while and see if this helps, suggests Harold T. Perry, D.D.S., Ph.D., a professor of orthodontics at Northwestern University Dental School and editor of a dental medical journal that focuses on TMJ problems.

Take an aspirin and give yourself a rub. "Aspirin is a marvelous drug for any muscle or joint problem," says Dr. Perry. He suggests one tablet followed up several minutes later with a brisk self-massage of the jaw using a hot washcloth.

Check your body position. If you work at a desk, check your body position throughout the day. Make sure you—and especially your chin—are not leaning over the desk, says Owen J. Rogal, D.D.S., executive director of the American Academy of Head, Facial, and Neck Pain, and TMJ Orthopedics. His Philadelphia, Pennsylvania, practice specializes in TMJ problems. As a general guideline for sitting or standing, your cheekbone should be over your clavicle, and your ears should not be too far in front of your shoulders, he says.

Many people with TMJ also have back problems. The two are interrelated, Dr. Rogal says, not two separate problems.

Throw away your pillow. Instead, tuck yourself in with a thin towel rolled up under your neck (to about the thickness of your wrist). Have another towel under your back and a pillow under your knees. Sleeping in this position—on your back throughout the entire night—can be very relaxing to your jaws and "critical" to overcoming TMJ, says Dr. Rogal. But what if you generally sleep on your side? He suggests placing a beanbag on either side of your head to stop you from rolling over into that position.

Limit your jaw movement. Don't make like the MGM lion. If you feel a yawn coming, restrict it by holding a fist under your chin, says Andrew S. Kaplan, D.M.D., an assistant clinical professor of dentistry at the Mount Sinai School of Medicine of the City University of New York and author of *The TMJ Book*.

Seven Nasty Habits to Break

Overcoming TMJ is very much a matter of what you *don't* do, claims Andrew S. Kaplan, D.M.D. If any of these habits are yours—pay attention! These tips may be of help to you.

Don't:

- Lie on your stomach with your head twisted to one side.
- Lie on your back with your head propped up at a sharp angle for reading or watching television.
- Cradle the telephone between your shoulder and chin.
- Prop your chin on one or both of your hands for too long.
- Carry a heavy shoulder bag with the strap on the same shoulder for an extended period.
- Do work, such as painting a ceiling, that requires looking up for long periods of time.
- Wear high heels.

Stop grinding your teeth. There's little question that gnashing teeth, referred to by doctors as bruxism, can bring about or exacerbate TMJ troubles. (See Bruxism on page 102 for more on this subject.)

PANEL OF ADVISERS

Sheldon Gross, D.D.S., is in private practice in Bloomfield, Connecticut. He is a lecturer at Tufts University in Boston, Massachusetts, and the University of Medicine and Dentistry of New Jersey/New Jersey Medical School in Newark. He is also president of the American Academy of Craniomandibular Disorders and a member of both the American Pain Association and the American Headache Association.

Andrew S. Kaplan, D.M.D., is an assistant clinical professor of dentistry at the Mount Sinai School of Medicine of the City University of New York and author of *The TMJ Book*. He is director of the TMJ Clinic at Mount Sinai Hospital in New York City.

Harold T. Perry, D.D.S., Ph.D., practices dentistry in Elgin, Illinois. He is a professor of orthodontics at Northwestern University Dental School in Chicago, Illinois. He is also the editor of the *Journal of Craniomandibular Disorders—Oralfacial Pain* and a past president of the American Academy of Craniomandibular Disorders.

Owen J. Rogal, D.D.S., has a private practice in Philadelphia, Pennsylvania, limited to treating TMJ. He is executive director of the American Academy of Head, Facial, and Neck Pain, and TMJ Orthopedics. He is on the medical staff at Philadelphia's Metropolitan Hospital and is the author of *Mandibular Whiplash*.

Toothache

13 Tips for Pain Relief

A toothache hurts a lot. It hurts when you smile or frown or eat or drink, when you clench or unclench your jaw, when you move your head in any direction. Sometimes it even hurts when you breathe because cold air rushes into your mouth, over the tender tooth — and ouch!

A toothache, says Philip D. Corn, D.D.S., a private practitioner in Philadelphia, Pennsylvania, and director of the Pennsylvania Academy of General Dentistry, may be a symptom of several things. The pulp of your tooth or the gums around your throbbing cuspid could be infected. There could be decay in a molar. You may have a cracked bicuspid. Or you might have been smacked in the mouth. But the ache could simply be an irritation from a piece of food caught between two teeth, adds Jerry F. Taintor, D.D.S., chairman of endodontics at the University of Tennessee College of Dentistry. Or it could be a backlash from a sinus problem.

Only your dentist can say for sure. Until you can see him, though, you'll want to stop the pain now. Here's how.

Rinse your toothache away. Take a mouthful of water (at body temperature) and rinse vigorously, says Dr. Taintor. If your toothache is caused by trapped food, a thorough rinse may dislodge the problem.

Floss gently. If swishing doesn't work, you can try to pry the popcorn hulls or tiny bits of meat out from between your teeth by flossing, says Dr. Taintor. Be gentle! Your gums are likely to be sore.

Take a "shot" to numb the pain. Hold a swig of whiskey over the painful tooth, says Dr. Corn. Your gums will absorb some of the alcohol and that will numb the pain. Spit out the rest.

Rinse with salty water. After each meal and at bedtime, stir 1 teaspoon of salt into an 8-ounce glass of water (again, at body temperature), says Dr. Corn. Hold each mouthful, roll it around your mouth. Spit.

Try a hand massage. When you have an achy tooth, this can ease the pain by 50 percent. Rub an ice cube into the V-shaped area where the bones of the thumb and forefinger meet. Gently push the ice over the area for 5 to 7 minutes.

In a study, Ronald Melzack, Ph.D., a Canadian researcher and past president of the International Association for the Study of Pain, found ice massage eased toothaches in 60 to 90 percent of the people who tried it. His research shows this procedure works by sending rubbing impulses along the nerve pathways that the toothache pain would normally travel on. Since the pathways can carry only one signal at a time, rubbing outweighs the pain.

Oil up with oil of cloves. People have been using this over-the-counter remedy for many years, says Richard Shepard, D.D.S., a retired dentist in Durango, Colorado. Most drugstores carry tiny bottles of the oil. Drop a little directly onto the tooth, or dab a little on a cotton ball and pack the elixir next to the ache.

Be Sensitive to Your Teeth

"If you can't even touch the tooth, that's an ache," says Roger P. Levin, D.D.S. "But if the tooth is merely reacting to heat or cold, then it's a problem with sensitivity."

More than 40 million Americans have "dentinal hypersensitivity," and it begins when the dentin underneath the tooth enamel becomes exposed— usually at the gumline.

Age, receding gums, surgery, and overzealous brushing with harsh pastes and hard brushes can expose dentin. Sometimes plaque eats the tooth enamel and exposes the dentin.

Philip D. Corn, D.D.S., recommends an over-the-counter toothpaste made especially for people with sensitive teeth, applied with a soft nylon-bristle brush. Such toothpastes include Sensodyne, Promise, Protect, Thermodent, and Denquel.

And if you're noticing sensitivity for the first time, it makes good sense to see your dentist to make sure you have no other problem.

Don't bite. If the toothache is caused by a blow to the tooth, try not to use that area when you eat, says Dr. Corn. If nothing is damaged, rest for the tooth may restore its vitality.

Suck on some ice. Treat the problem like any good bruise. Use ice, says Dr. Corn. Put ice on the aching tooth or the nearest cheek for 15-minute intervals at least three or four times a day.

Keep your mouth shut. If cold air moving past the tooth is a problem, just shut off the flow, says Roger P. Levin, D.D.S., president of the Baltimore Academy of General Dentistry and a guest lecturer for the University of Maryland.

Or keep your mouth open. Some toothaches happen when a person's bite isn't quite right. In that case, says Dr. Levin, avoid shutting your mouth as much as possible until the dentist can take a look.

Swallow your aspirin. Don't believe that old-time remedy calling for placing an aspirin directly on the aching gum. This can cause an aspirin burn, says Dr. Taintor. For pain relief, take an aspirin every 4 to 6 hours as required.

Stay cool. Keep heat away from your aching cheek even if it makes the toothache feel better, warns Dr. Corn. "If it is an infection, the heat will draw the infection to the outside of the jaw and make the infection worse."

PANEL OF ADVISERS

Philip D. Corn, D.D.S., has a private practice in Philadelphia, Pennsylvania. He is a director of the Pennsylvania Academy of General Dentistry.

Roger P. Levin, D.D.S., is president of the Baltimore Academy of General Dentistry and a guest lecturer for the University of Maryland in Baltimore.

Richard Shepard, D.D.S., is a retired dentist in Durango, Colorado. He edits the newsletter for the Holistic Dental Association.

Jerry F. Taintor, D.D.S., is chairman of endodontics at the University of Tennessee College of Dentistry in Memphis. He is author of *The Oral Report: The Consumer's Common Sense Guide to Better Dental Care.*

Traveler's Diarrhea

24 Tips to Thwart Turista

You've heard all the names: Montezuma's revenge, Delhi belly, Hong Kong dog, Tiki trots, Casablanca crud, Katmandu quickstep. But citizens of Mexico, India, Nepal, Morocco, and other places might call it the New York nasties, because they can get it when they visit the United States. For now, "it" will have to be called turista, a nice name for traveler's diarrhea.

"If you're going to be abroad for any length of time, you'll probably have some episodes of diarrhea," says globe-trotter Stephen Bezruchka, M.D., an emergency physician at Providence Medical Center in Seattle, Washington. "Conceptually, it is totally preventable. In reality, it's rare you don't get an occasional loose movement." In fact, you have up to a 50 percent chance of getting turista, even if you take the recommended precautions.

The most common cause is the *Escherichia coli* bacteria. This widespread little organism normally resides in your intestines and performs a role in digestion. But foreign versions—and to a foreigner, the American version is foreign—of *E. coli* can give you diarrhea by producing a toxin that prevents your intestines from absorbing the water you ingest in the form of fluid and food.

So, as the toxin prevents the absorption of water, "you have all this extra water in there and it's got to come out," Dr. Bezruchka says. "The toxin doesn't get absorbed. You don't usually feel sick, but you might feel you have to pass some gas. Only it isn't gas at all."

Shigella and salmonella bacteria can also produce turista, while a smaller number of cases are caused by rotavirus and the giardia parasite. Changes in diet, fatigue, jet lag, and altitude sickness have been blamed, but without sufficient proof, and up to 50 percent of all turista cases are unexplained.

Thankfully, says Dr. Bezruchka, "diarrhea is a self-limiting disease. The human body has been around for at least 40,000 years, and it's built to take care of most problems it's going to encounter."

The way it takes care of *E. coli* is to purge the intestines. For one to five days, you'll have numerous runny stools. You may feel nauseated, or have cramps and even a slight fever, but often the only symptom will be the diarrhea itself. And there are ways to help your body fight it, to stop it in its tracks, and to lessen your chances of getting it. Here's how.

Drink water, water anywhere. When you have turista, your stools are mostly water. So why would the most important treatment be to drink plenty of the right fluids? Because dehydration—the loss of water and electrolytes—can kill. Diarrhea kills hundreds of thousands of children every year, often because their parents believe that giving them fluids only makes the diarrhea worse.

So rehydrating yourself when you have turista is not like bringing coals to Newcastle. "A lot of what you take in will be pumped right back out the other end," says Thomas Gossel, Ph.D., a professor of pharmacology and toxicology and chairman of the Department of Pharmacology and Biomedical Sciences at Ohio Northern University. "But you'll reach a point where you stabilize and begin retaining it. If you didn't replace any fluids at all, you could become dehydrated in a day."

How to Be a Nonturista

Sometimes no matter what you do, you'll still wind up being an unwilling host to a foreign turista. Yet there are ways to minimize your chances.

- Avoid uncooked vegetables, especially salads, fruits you can't peel, under-cooked meat, raw shellfish, ice cubes, and drinks made from impure water (the alcohol in drinks won't kill the turista bug).
- Try to make sure the dishes and silverware you use have been cleaned in purified water.
- Drink only water that has been carbonated and sealed in bottles or cans. Clean the part of the container that touches your mouth with purified water. Boiling water for 3 to 5 minutes purifies it, as does iodine liquid or tablets.
- Drink acidic drinks like colas and orange juice when possible. They help keep down the *E. coli* count, the bacteria most responsible for digestive distress.
- Drink acidophilus milk or eat yogurt before your trip. The bacterial colonies established in your digestive system before your trip and maintained during it, reduce the chance of a turista invasion.

The most basic way to rehydrate is to drink water, "if that's all you have around," Dr. Bezruchka says. "If you can't purify the water, drink it anyway. If you're so dehydrated that you get dizzy when you stand up, it's better to replace the fluids than worry about the purity."

Use the ORS solution. Another, even better way to rehydration is the so-called oral rehydration solution, or ORS, a 1960s advance over intravenous rehydration. An ORS is a drink basically containing sugar and salt, substances that help replace important electrolytes that are lost through diarrhea. They also help your intestines absorb water better, The ORS, in fact, is so beneficial that it is saving thousands of lives in the Third World.

Over-the-counter rehydration solutions are readily available in the United States, so you can buy and take them with you. Some of the name brands are Gastrolyte, Pedialyte, and Rehydralyte. Some are powders, some liquids. Each has a slightly different formula. "There isn't a whole lot of difference between them," Dr. Gossel says.

If you don't want to cart along the extra baggage, you can still get an ORS fix. Here's what you can reach for when you're overseas.

MEDICAL ALERT

Be Cautious of Infection

Although most cases of turista are self-limiting, some symptoms indicate the need for medical attention.

- Red or black stools can be a sign of bleeding or a parasitic infection, while white or pale stools can signify liver disease.
- Fever can suggest a serious infection. If you have blood in the stool or a fever, says Stephen Bezruchka, M.D., and can't get to a doctor quickly, it's advisable to take the antibiotic TMP/SMZ (found overseas over-the-counter) until you can get medical help.
- Abdominal bloating, vomiting, and pain can indicate colitis, an intestinal obstruction, or appendicitis. Vomiting means you won't be able to retain your rehydration solutions.

If you have any of these symptoms, do not take anything to stop the diarrhea, caution doctors.

The Alternate Route

A Survivor's Survival Guide

Okay, you're out in the boonies. Your Pepto-Bismol, Metamucil, antibiotics, yogurt tablets, and loperamide washed away in the rapids, which are running almost as fast as your bowels. Now what?

We asked SFC Thomas Squier, an instructor in survival training for the U.S. Army Special Forces at Fort Bragg, North Carolina, what he tells his survival training students. He says he's tried the following and they work—but you may only want to use them as his men do—as a last resort.

Clay. "We teach them to eat clay," Sgt. Squier says. "Many commercial antidiarrheal medications, like Kaopectate, contain kaolin, which is a type of clay often found on riverbanks."

Ash. "We also teach them to use campfire ashes or pulverized, dried, burned bone fragments. These have an astringent, drying-up effect when you brew them into a tea."

Tannic acid. But what if you're fresh out of pulverized, dried, burned bone fragments? "Anything that has tannic acid will stop the muscular contractions of the intestines," Sgt. Squier says. "Try acorns or the bark of oak trees or other hardwoods, boiled into a tea."

The USPHS cocktail. This is the U.S. Public Health Service recipe. In one glass, put 8 ounces of fruit juice; ½ teaspoon of honey, corn syrup, or sugar; and a pinch of salt. In another glass, put 8 ounces of purified water and ¼ teaspoon of baking soda. Drink a couple of swallows alternately from each glass until finished.

The WHO combo. "Most underdeveloped countries now are marketing packets with the World Health Organization formula," Dr. Bezruchka reports. The only problem is that they can be very expensive. But you can make your own if you happen to have access to a metric scale. Or you can call in the help of a pharmacist. Here's the formula: glucose, 20 grams; salt, 3.5 grams; baking soda, 2.5 grams; and potassium chloride, 20 grams. Just add to a quart or liter of purified water and drink.

"If your only alternative is buying a packet, you'll have to find out what the local name is," he says. "It's available over-the-counter in drugstores, medical halls, and pharmacies around the world."

Blackberry root. "Another real specific remedy that's easy to find in most of the temperate world is blackberry roots, again made into a tea," he says. "For any of these things, if you don't have hot water, you can soak them in cold, but it takes longer."

Plantain. "Plantain grows in everybody's lawns," Sgt. Squier says. "Both broadleaf and narrowleaf varieties are strongly astringent. And the other half of Kaopectate is pectin," he notes. "It comes from apples and is used for making jelly. Cooking down apple peels and drinking the liquid is another diarrhea remedy."

Blueberries. Finally, the blue-beary facts on turista. "It may be an old wives' tale, but one reason bears are so angry at certain times of the year is that they're gorging on blueberries, which make them constipated," says Sgt. Squier. "They get real severe cramps. One Alaskan trapper told me you can hear the bears' stomachs growling from quite a distance. I know I gorged myself on blueberries in Vermont and I couldn't go to the bathroom for three days. The old-timers say that if you take a few dried blueberries along on your trip, five or six of them will cure diarrhea."

Any questions?

The nonformula. If you can't get your hands on the solutions, drink clear fruit juices, caffeine-free carbonated beverages, or weak tea with sugar. Also use these to supplement your rehydration solution.

Put your bladder to the test. The more yellow your urine, the more fluid you need. It should be clear. "As a minimum," Dr. Bezruchka says, "you should pass two busting bladders of urine a day, preferably more."

Avoid milk products and solid foods. At least at the beginning. They're too hard to digest. And stay away from alcohol—it dehydrates you. When the diarrhea stops, eat easily digested solids, like bananas, applesauce, saltine crackers, or rice.

Get in the pink. Pepto-Bismol, the well-known over-the-counter stomach medication, can be the traveler's friend. It can cut down on evacuations by about 60 percent, makes stools bulkier and firmer, and kills bacteria.

Some experts believe, however, that the slowing of diarrhea means the bug will stay inside you longer. Antidiarrheal drugs may also adsorb your rehydration solution. But at a certain point, you may not care. And don't worry about your tongue and diarrhea turning black. It's a natural side effect of Pepto-Bismol. Other adsorbents are Donnagel, Kaopectate, Quiagel, and Rheaban.

Do a little coaxing. Natural fiber-based laxatives for relieving constipation, such as Metamucil and Citrucel, also help with diarrhea. Some can absorb up to 60 times their weight in water to form a gel in the intestine. "You're still going to expel excess water," Dr. Gossel says, "but it won't be so runny. It may cut you down from ten times a day to seven or eight." Other brands are Equalactin, FiberCon, and Mitrolan.

Try opiates for quick relief. Opium-based antidiarrheal drugs inhibit intestinal contractions, cutting down on bowel movements and allowing absorption of water and electrolytes. These highly effective drugs, which can be purchased over-the-counter in some states, come as liquids, tablets, or suspensions. Brand names include Banatol, Donnagel-PG, and Quiagel PG. Loperamide, found in the brand Imodium AD liquid, is the newest OTC opiatelike antidiarrheal in the United States. Some states allow OTC purchase of paregoric, which is found in Parepectolin. These products will slow your Katmandu quickstep to a crawl.

One caution: Like adsorbents, the opiates' ability to plug you up may keep the bug inside a bit longer.

Reach for easy-access antibiotics. Although antibiotics are prescription drugs in the United States, they are readily available over-the-counter in many foreign countries. "TMP/SMZ and doxycycline [Vibramycin] have been well studied, and they work," Dr. Bezruchka says. "When I tried these, almost always just one dose would do the job. I think all you're doing here is helping your body by killing off most of the bacteria and letting your body handle the rest." He advises one TMP/SMZ or doxycycline pill twice a day until the diarrhea stops. But before you leave home, get your doctor's okay to use these drugs.

Do the double dose. Your Hong Kong dog will stop barking quickly if you take an antibiotic with an antidiarrheal drug. Caution: Antibiotics are powerful drugs and can have severe side effects, including sun sensitivity, and may open the door to another invasion of turista. Again, check with your doctor.

Fight bacteria with bacteria. Khem Shahani, Ph.D., a professor of food science and technology at the University of Nebraska, and others have discovered that the bacteria lactobacillus may be just the bacteria your poor, runny insides need. "They favorably alter the gut's microecology," he says, "and produce substances that inhibit the growth of disease-causing bacteria."

And, Dr. Shahani says, "It's been proven very effective to follow antibiotic therapy with lactobacillus because the gastrointestinal system has lost most of its beneficial microorganisms."

The best form of lactobacillus seems to be acidophilus, found in acidophilus milk, followed by bulgaricus, the type found in yogurt. You can buy capsules containing acidophilus and bulgaricus in pharmacies and health food stores in the United States and take them with you. They are not as effective as yogurt or acidophilus milk, says Dr. Shahani.

Abroad, the local versions of yogurt will be the easiest forms of lactobacillus to find. In Japan yogurt is called *yakult;* in Korea, *yaogurt;* in India, *dahi;* in Egypt, *leben* and *lebenraid;* in Turkey, *eyran,* and in Sardinia, *gioddu.*

PANEL OF ADVISERS

Stephen Bezruchka, M.D., is an emergency physician at Providence Medical Center in Seattle, Washington, and author of *The Pocket Doctor.*

Thomas Gossel, Ph.D., R.Ph., is a professor of pharmacology and toxicology at Ohio Northern University in Ada and chairman of the university's Department of Pharmacology and Biomedical Sciences. He is an expert on over-the-counter products.

Khem Shahani, Ph.D., is a professor of food science and technology at the University of Nebraska in Lincoln.

SFC Thomas Squier, of the U.S. Army Special Forces, is an instructor at the JFK Special Warfare Center and School, Survival-Evasion-Resistance-Escape/Terrorist Counteraction Department in Fort Bragg, North Carolina. He is a Cherokee herbologist and grandson of a medicine man. He also writes a newspaper column called "Living off the Land."

Triglycerides

9 Ways to Lower Blood Fats

Triglycerides, along with cholesterol, are the major sources of fat circulating in your blood. Both are needed—cholesterol for building strong cells, triglycerides for energy—but when either remains at high levels for long periods of time, trouble results.

In the case of cholesterol, that trouble is clogged arteries. In the case of triglycerides, however, the trouble is not well-defined. "If you get very technical, it's probably safe to say that triglycerides are not independently important in heart disease," says John LaRosa, M.D., director of the Lipid Research Clinic at George Washington University School of Medicine and chairman of the American Heart Association's Nutrition Committee.

"But in practical terms," he continues, "high triglycerides are often associated with low levels of HDL cholesterol (the good cholesterol) and indicate a problem that's causing you to carry fat particles in the blood that do cause vascular disease. So they should be looked at as a danger signal."

Normal triglyceride levels can run from 40 to 250 milligrams per deciliter (mg/dl), a fairly broad range. Generally, levels of 250 mg/dl to 500 mg/dl are considered "borderline elevated," while levels over 500 mg/dl are considered "high." The safest bet is to keep your triglyceride levels below 150.

Keep in mind that triglycerides can be controlled in many of the same ways as cholesterol. To improve one is to improve the other. If your doctor has warned you to lower your triglyceride levels, fine— these tips will help. If he's told you to lower your LDL cholesterol (the bad stuff), fine—these tips can't hurt. It's one of those rare situations where you just can't lose either way, as long as you follow the tips.

Cut the fat. "Diet is the best way to reduce triglycerides," says Robert DiBianco, M.D., associate clinical professor of medicine at Georgetown University and director of cardiology research at Washington Adventist Hospital in Takoma Park, Maryland.

His recommendation for reducing triglyceride levels is to cut back on fat in the diet. "The lower the better when it comes to fat," he says. Reducing fat intake to less than 30 percent of daily calories is a good start, although "shooting for 20 percent would be an ideal range," Dr. DiBianco says. "And keep saturated fats at less than 10 percent."

The Alternate Route

When Nothing but Rice Is Nice

Even its developer called it disagreeable medicine. In fact, said Walter Kempner, M.D., there's only one excuse for ever using it. "It helps."

The year was 1944, and the disagreeable medicine Dr. Kempner was speaking of was the rice diet he'd just discovered. Some of his most critically ill patients had apparently been cured by eating a diet of almost nothing but rice and fruit.

Forms of that diet are still in use today, and some call it a forerunner of the healthy-for-your-heart Pritikin Diet, among others. In some places, the rice/fruit diet is still being recommended for its ability to reduce fats from the blood and lower body weight.

"We use the rice/fruit diet in people with really high triglyceride levels to clear them out," says Sonja Connor, M.S., R.D. "It also helps them with weight loss, because it's practically fat-free."

"People don't have much of a tolerance for it," she adds.

Yet some people can apparently tolerate a steady diet of rice and fruit long enough to have an effect. "We had a patient recently who went from blood triglyceride levels of 1,000 mg/dl down to 117 mg/dl in a couple of months," says Connor. "And she went out and did this herself using that diet—we didn't have to supervise her at all." But, Connor notes, "she wasn't the typical patient."

A diet this extreme should never be attempted without the approval of your doctor, however. And most doctors are not crazy about recommending it.

How long must you subsist on rice and fruit to see results? "Not long at all," Connor says. "You start getting results on this diet right away—two or three days. If we can motivate people to get rid of all fats from their diets on a short-term basis," she explains, "we could help eradicate the problem and they could start adding some fats back in."

Go in stages. One way to reduce fats to that low 20 percent level is to proceed in stages. For example, reduce your fat intake to 30 percent of calories for one month (current American levels are about 40 percent). Then return to your doctor to see if there's been an improvement in your triglyceride level. If so, he'll probably congratulate you and ask you to stay on this diet. If not, reduce your fat intake to 25 percent for one month and see what happens.

If you see no improvement at that level, lower your fat intake to 20 percent for two months. This fat level virtually ensures that you'll be getting a good portion of your calories from complex carbohydrates, and that should bring about a reduction.

Make carbohydrates complex. Populations who eat diets high in complex carbohydrates just don't have a triglyceride problem. "Substitute complex carbohydrates for fats whenever possible," advises Sonja Connor, M.S., R.D., a research associate professor of clinical nutrition at Oregon Health Sciences University. But beware of adding fat back in with traditional cooking habits. "The recipes most people have for [complex carbohydrates such as] pasta, rice, beans, and other grains force you to cook them in the company of large amounts of fat."

What you'll need to do, she says, is search out recipes for lasagna and pasta salads, scalloped potatoes, and other high-carbohydrate meals that are also low in fat. "That's the hardest thing to work on," Connor says. "There are relatively few recipes for high-carbohydrate, low-fat dishes that don't make you end up eating nothing more than plain spaghetti without any sauce." Is it worth the effort to find and prepare such dishes? "You bet," she says.

Cut the candy. "Simple carbohydrates—candy, sugar, and other sweets—are a major contributor to high triglyceride levels," says Dr. DiBianco. He recommends forgetting about sweets.

Dr. LaRosa agrees. "Low-fiber, simple carbohydrates are probably the biggest offenders of all," he says. "There's no question that simple carbohydrates are a problem."

Trim down. "Weight loss is very important," says Dr. DiBianco. "The amount of weight that needs to be lost depends on your ideal body weight, but you don't need to lose all your excess weight to see a change in triglycerides."

Just 10 pounds can bring about a reduction in people who are 20 to 30 percent overweight. Though you don't have to reach your perfect weight to bring down triglycerides, "you should try to maintain a weight that's not more than 5 or 10 percent above the ideal," Dr. DiBianco says.

Burn it off. "Exercise lowers triglyceride levels," says Dr. LaRosa. "Though it's hard to tell whether it's a result of weight loss or better metabolism; but it could be both."

The reason for such uncertainty about how exercise helps reduce triglyceride levels stems from studies showing that 1 hour of vigorous exercise three times a week can lower triglyceride levels even when weight doesn't change.

But regardless of how it produces results, exercise does work in reducing triglycerides and is highly recommended by all our experts. Check with your doctor before starting any exercise program, however.

Avoid alcohol. "I think alcohol intake is the biggest aggravator of high triglyceride levels going," says Dr. DiBianco. "Avoiding even small doses of alcohol is important."

Fix it with fish. "It's been pretty well documented that fish oil has its most marked effect on triglycerides," says Carl Hock, Ph.D., an assistant professor of medicine at the University of Medicine and Dentistry of New Jersey, New Jersey School of Osteopathic Medicine.

Several studies have demonstrated the triglyceride-lowering abilities of omega-3 fatty acids, the type found in fish oil. Though most studies use fish oil capsules to ensure accuracy, you can get an equivalent amount by eating fish regularly, or by combining a high-fish diet with occasional use of capsules.

Most studies have used about 15 grams of fish oil a day, equivalent to an 8-ounce serving of salmon, herring, or mackerel. Newer studies, however, have produced the same results with 10 grams per day.

"You can get enough fish in the diet to bring triglycerides down," says Dr. DiBianco. "In fact, the fish oils seem to be most beneficial in those patients who are lacking it in their diets from a regular intake of fish. If somebody's eating fish as a part of his regular diet, he should be okay."

PANEL OF ADVISERS

Sonja Connor, M.S., R.D., is a research associate professor of clinical nutrition at Oregon Health Sciences University School of Medicine in Portland and coauthor of *The New American Diet.*

Robert DiBianco, M.D., is associate clinical professor of medicine at Georgetown University in Washington, D.C., and director of the cardiac risk factor reduction program and cardiology research at Washington Adventist Hospital in Takoma Park, Maryland.

Carl Hock, Ph.D., is an assistant professor of medicine at the University of Medicine and Dentistry of New Jersey, New Jersey School of Osteopathic Medicine in Camden.

John LaRosa, M.D., is director of the Lipid Research Center at George Washington University School of Medicine in Washington, D.C., and chairman of the American Heart Association's Nutrition Committee.

Ulcer

15 Soothing Treatments

Just a few years ago, doctors might as well have told patients with ulcers to surrender their taste buds because they were already asking them to completely give up just about every food they could taste.

Chili, pizza, and tacos were out. Toast, crackers, and the rest of the bland band were in. It was anything but sweet music to the ears of people who were trying to live with recurring, raging infernos in the depths of their stomachs.

Now specific anti-ulcer diets, including those widely prescribed bland regimens, are out, says Steve Goldschmid, M.D., an assistant professor of medicine in the Division of Digestive Diseases at Emory University Hospital in Atlanta, Georgia. "There is no proof of a therapeutic benefit from altering your diet," he says.

MEDICAL ALERT

Be Wise to These Symptoms

Much of the time an ulcer is just a literal pain in the gut. But a *bleeding* ulcer can become serious, even life threatening.

A bleeding ulcer can drain you of enough blood to drastically lower blood pressure and stop vital organs from functioning, says Steve Goldschmid, M.D.

"If you have an ulcer and get really nauseated and suddenly throw up blood or what looks like old coffee grounds, see your doctor immediately," he says. Other symptoms of serious trouble include passing a stool that is black or one containing bright red blood. A person with a bleeding ulcer also may become dizzy and pass out.

What doctors currently recommend recalls that old doctor/patient conversation that, today, might go like this: "Hey Doc, whenever I eat rocky road ice cream covered with kiwi sauce, it feels like there's a blowtorch in my belly."

"Well," says the doctor, "don't eat rocky road ice cream covered with kiwi sauce."

In other words, listen to your ulcer and use common sense—whether you have a gastric ulcer (on the lining of your stomach) or a duodenal ulcer (on the duodenum, the part of the small intestine nearest the stomach).

Scientists have yet to say what, specifically, causes ulcers. But stomach acid is the prime suspect and certain bacteria and stress are viewed as possible accomplices.

Certainly ulcers are not rare—an estimated 5 million Americans have them, says John Kurata, Ph.D., an epidemiologist and associate

---

The Alternate Route

Pepto-Bismol to the Rescue

The next best thing to a cure for ulcers already may be in your medicine cabinet—Pepto-Bismol.

So claims Australian researcher Barry Marshall, M.D., who tested hundreds of patients with duodenal ulcers and found that they had one thing in common: most carried the same type of bacteria. His conclusion: Bacteria, not stomach acid, may cause ulcers.

When Dr. Marshall treated his patients with bismuth (an ingredient in Pepto-Bismol that kills the bacterial invader in the stomach), the bacteria tended to disappear, and so did the ulcers.

No one, however, is going so far as to claim that Pepto-Bismol is a cure for ulcers. And some, such as Michael Kimmey, M.D., are even skeptical about the bacteria theory. "The bacteria research is interesting," Dr. Kimmey says, "but it's not been proven that bacteria cause ulcers."

But Pepto-Bismol could be worth a try, says David Earnest, M.D. "It might be useful," he says, "in certain cases where a person continues to relapse and the bacteria are shown to be present." But ask your doctor about the side effects of taking large doses of Pepto-Bismol over a long period. Pepto-Bismol does not have the approval of the Food and Drug Administration as an ulcer medication.

The Stress Connection

Can stress *cause* ulcers?

Many doctors are skeptical. "Most of us think there is a lack of good evidence to show stress causes ulcers," says John Kurata, Ph.D. "But if you already have an ulcer, stress may worsen the disease."

Consider this, however: The incidence of duodenal ulcers in New York City is greater proportionally than it is in surrounding areas, according to Steve Goldschmid, M.D. And is there anyone who'll argue that New York City is less stressful than, say, New Rochelle?

Also worth considering: the case of Richard Maschal, art and architecture critic for the *Charlotte Observer*. He discovered he had a gastric ulcer during a period of "extreme stress on the job," he says. "I didn't see eye-to-eye—actually, detested—the person who was supervising my area." And he let it drive him crazy. He became *tense!*

It's not so much the stressful event that happens to us, but how we interpret it and react or overreact to it, explains Georgianna S. Hoffmann, coordinator of the Family Stress Clinic in the Department of Family Practice at the University of Iowa College of Medicine.

With that in mind, here are a few suggestions for handling stress—and the ulcer it may be aggravating.

Think pleasant thoughts and talk to yourself. Maschal has a new boss, and that's helped a lot, as has the medication his doctor prescribed. But he also still catches himself heading toward tension. And only he can stop it. "Now," he says, "I take time to talk myself down."

Breathe slowly and deeply. Three or four deep breaths provide the most immediate feeling of calmness anywhere, anytime.

Exercise. "Moderate physical exercise is a very good coping mechanism," Hoffmann says.

Practice relaxation techniques. "When you relax the body, you relax the mind," Hoffmann says. "And when you relax the mind, you relax the body." Meditation, yoga, imagery, or listening to relaxation tapes, done regularly, are among the relaxation techniques you might want to explore.

adjunct professor at the University of California, Los Angeles, and research director of the San Bernardino County Medical Center in California.

Unfortunately, ulcers are also stubborn. "Ulcer disease is really a chronic disease," Dr. Goldschmid says. "Ulcers come and go." So here are some tips for living with ulcers that will hopefully make them go sooner.

Avoid the arsonists. Whether it's an ice cream sundae or a pepperoni pizza, if it starts a fire in *your* stomach, don't eat it. "The foods that bother people seem to vary with each individual," says David Earnest, M.D., a professor of medicine at the University of Arizona College of Medicine Health Sciences Center and chairman of the Committee on Patient Care for the American Gastroenterological Association. "But obviously spicy foods may bother some people."

Take it easy with milk. Long thought to be a great soother for a burning ulcer, milk's rebound effect is now well established. "Although it buffers acid for a while [and thus provides brief relief]," Dr. Goldschmid says, "it actually stimulates more stomach acid secretion" and causes more pain later.

Use over-the-counter antacids. They may not cure an ulcer, "but they are a good treatment for symptoms," says Dr. Earnest.

Don't take too many pain relievers. Aspirin has the bad reputation, but nonsteroidal anti-inflammatory drugs—which have become very popular—are at least as hard on the stomach lining as aspirin is, says Thomas Brasitus, M.D., a professor of medicine and director of gastroenterology at the University of Chicago Pritzker School of Medicine.

Don't light up. Yes, smoking even gets indicted for contributing to ulcers. Although there is no evidence that smoking causes ulcers, they are less likely to heal in smokers than nonsmokers, says Dr. Brasitus.

Let it out. "Some evidence suggests that people who are frustrated and don't express their feelings very well are more likely to get ulcers," says Michael Kimmey, M.D., an assistant professor of medicine at the University of Washington School of Medicine.

Double your meals. Although many doctors are saying three normal-size meals are fine, some people may have less ulcer upset if they eat six smaller meals, says Dr. Brasitus. Food neutralizes stomach acid.

Don't pump iron. "Iron is a gastric irritant," Dr. Goldschmid says. "People who take iron supplements might have a lot of upset if they have a gastric ulcer."

Live by the moderation motto. Too much of one food or beverage could upset an ulcer. Alcohol, by the way, is not necessarily an irritant. "Moderate drinking probably does not increase the risk of developing new ulcers," says Dr. Kurata.

Give it time. Sometimes that's all you can do. "Ulcers have cycles," Dr. Brasitus says. "A lot of them will burn out within a few years."

PANEL OF ADVISERS

Thomas Brasitus, M.D., is a professor of medicine and director of gastroenterology at the University of Chicago Pritzker School of Medicine in Illinois.

David Earnest, M.D., is a professor of medicine at the University of Arizona College of Medicine Health Sciences Center in Tucson. He also is chairman of the Committee on Patient Care for the American Gastroenterological Association.

Steve Goldschmid, M.D., is an assistant professor of medicine in the Division of Digestive Diseases at Emory University Hospital in Atlanta, Georgia.

Georgianna S. Hoffmann is coordinator of the Family Stress Clinic in the Department of Family Practice at the University of Iowa College of Medicine in Iowa City.

Michael Kimmey, M.D., is an assistant professor of medicine at the University of Washington School of Medicine in Seattle.

John Kurata, Ph.D., is an epidemiologist and associate adjunct professor at the University of California, Los Angeles. He also is research director at San Bernardino County Medical Center in California.

Varicose Veins

15 Helpers and Healers

If you were to wake up tomorrow morning, rub the sleep from your eyes, and find a slew of gaping crocodiles at the foot of the bed, would your very first thought be, "Oh my, what *ugly* reptiles!" Of course not. Yet, were you to look down and notice varicose veins for the first time, your first thoughts might turn to matters of appearance.

MEDICAL ALERT

Clots: A Cause for Concern

One hundred years ago, doctors would yank out varicose veins with hooks. Rest assured the treatment today is much more humane—and helpful. Today injection therapy is used with resounding success against even the wiliest varicose veins.

But when do varicose veins warrant a trip to the doctor? Brian McDonagh, M.D., says that there are two major complications presented by varicose veins: vein clotting and rupture.

How do you recognize a clot? "It will become very painful, sore, and tender—it just hurts," says Dr. McDonagh. Clots are usually visible as red lumps in the veins that don't decrease in size even when you put your legs up.

Varicose veins around the ankle areas are more inclined to rupture and bleed. This is much more dangerous than clotting because you can lose blood very rapidly. If this happens, put pressure on it to slow the bleeding and get to your doctor.

"Most people don't even see varicose veins as a disease—they think of them only as something cosmetic. But this is far from the case. "People with varicose veins have a disease, a disease with a cosmetic aspect," says Brian McDonagh, M.D., a Chicago, Illinois, phlebologist (vein specialist) and founder and director of Vein Clinics of America.

Bluish, swollen, lumpy-looking veins—and their cousins the crimson "spider veins"—are only the most evident signs of varicose vein disease. Veteran sufferers know all too well that with these visible veins often come achy, tired, listless legs.

The condition is usually not life threatening (certainly not on a par with having a slew of crocodiles in bed with you). So there is no reason to panic nor to rush to a doctor. But if you are afflicted with varicose veins, you—and your poor legs—will be infinitely better off knowing how to manage them.

Here are some suggestions from the experts.

Don't feel guilty. By far the greatest risk factor for varicose veins is having a parent with the problem, says Dr. McDonagh. Myths abound to explain the existence of this largely hereditary disease—the largest

---

The Alternate Route

Assume a Different Pose

The ancient system of yoga has much to offer sufferers of varicose veins, says John Clarke, M.D., a cardiologist with the Himalayan International Institute.

This yogic breathing practice can be done without instruction, without danger, and with a good chance that your discomfort from varicose veins will be relieved, claims Dr. Clarke. Try this exercise right now. Lie flat on your back and prop your feet up on a chair. Breathe slowly and evenly from your diaphragm, through your nose. That's it!

While gravity is pulling excess blood out of your raised legs, your full, steady inhalations will create negative pressure in your chest, Dr. Clarke says. This negative pressure helps pull in air to the chest cavity, as well as blood from all over the body, including your blood-gorged legs, he says.

---

myth being that varicose veins are caused by crossing one's legs. "That's nonsense," says Dr. McDonagh. You are simply one of the 17 percent of all Americans who possess the culprit genes (most of you are women).

Get gravity on your side—lift your feet. Varicose veins are weakened veins that lack the strength they once had to return blood to the heart. Veins in the legs are the most susceptible, for they are farthest—and straight downhill—from the heart. You can make their job much easier by putting gravity on your side. It's easy. Using an ottoman, pillows, or an easy chair, raise your legs up above hip level whenever they're aching, and the discomfort should start to go away, says Dudley Phillips, M.D., a family practitioner in Darlington, Maryland.

Wear support hose. They help provide relief. These stockings, available in pharmacies and department stores, resist the blood's tendency to pool in the small blood vessels closest to the skin, explains Dr. Phillips. (Instead, the blood is pushed into the larger, deeper veins, where it is more easily pumped back up to the heart.)

Throw those veins a one-two punch. Dr. Phillips suggests that sufferers of varicose veins combine the powers of gravity and support hose in the following exercise: Slip on your support hose. Then lie flat on your back and raise your legs straight up in the air, resting them against a wall. Hold this position for 2 minutes. This allows the blood to flow out of the swollen leg veins back toward your heart. Repeat throughout the day, if possible, as often as needed.

Tilt your bed. You can make gravity work for you through the night by raising the foot of your bed several inches, says Paul Lazar, M.D., a professor of clinical dermatology at Northwestern University Medical School. He cautions, however, that if you have a history of heart trouble or if you have any difficulty breathing during the night, it's best to consult a doctor before adjusting your bed.

Wear sensible shoes. Varicose veins are discomforting enough to the legs. Don't give your gams any extra troubles by wearing high heels or cowboy boots, says Dr. Phillips.

Buy a pair of elastic stockings. These special stockings, generally sold in medical supply stores rather than in pharmacies, are to support hose what a 45 Magnum is to a BB gun. Specially fitted elastic stockings, worn up to knee level, can give you considerable relief, depending on the severity of the varicose veins, says Dr. McDonagh. Get measured for a good-quality stocking.

Watch your weight. Added body weight means more pressure on your legs, one reason why pregnant women often suffer from varicose veins. Keep your weight down, and chances are you'll have fewer problems with bulging veins, says Lenise Banse, M.D., a dermatologist and director of the Mole and Melanoma Clinic at Henry Ford Hospital in Detroit, Michigan.

Stay away from tight-fitting clothes. Tight garments, particularly a girdle that is too tight or panty hose that are too constricting in the groin area, can act like tourniquets and keep blood pooled in your legs, says Dr. Banse.

On the Pill? Be suspicious. Hormonal imbalances, which sometimes occur with birth control pills, can be the cause of spider veins. If your problem appeared after you started the Pill, there might well be a connection, says Dr. McDonagh.

Don't smoke. A report from the Framingham Heart Study noted a correlation between smoking and the incidence of varicose veins. The researchers conclude that smoking may be a risk factor for those with varicose veins.

Go for a walk. Prolonged sitting or standing can cause problems in your legs because the blood tends to pool. A little bit of exercise throughout the day, particularly walking, can often prevent this pooling, says Eugene Strandness, Jr., M.D., a professor of surgery at the University of Washington School of Medicine. In fact, the Framingham study found that sedentary adults were more likely to have varicose veins than those who were active.

Don't hide from your problem. Much of the discomfort and pain of varicose veins can be masked with pain pills. Don't do it, says Dr. McDonagh. "Varicose veins are a problem that should not be dealt with by hiding the pain," he says. If you've gone down the list of tips and nothing helps, seek medical attention.

PANEL OF ADVISERS

Lenise Banse, M.D., is a dermatologist in Detroit, Michigan, where she is director of the Mole and Melanoma Clinic at Henry Ford Hospital.

John Clarke, M.D., is a cardiologist with the Himalayan International Institute in Honesdale, Pennsylvania.

Paul Lazar, M.D., is a professor of clinical dermatology at Northwestern University Medical School in Chicago, Illinois. He is a former board member of the American Academy of Dermatology.

Brian McDonagh, M.D., is a phlebologist (vein specialist) based in Chicago, Illinois. He is the founder and director of Vein Clinics of America, the largest medical group in the country dedicated solely to the treatment of vein disorders.

Dudley Phillips, M.D., of Darlington, Maryland, has practiced family medicine for more than 40 years.

Eugene Strandness, Jr., M.D., is a professor of surgery at the University of Washington School of Medicine in Seattle.

Vomiting

13 Feel-Better Remedies

Vomiting is the logical conclusion of nausea. Mr. Tummy is saying, "Yecch!" as loudly as possible so that you pay attention. Mr. Tummy's goal is to get rid of whatever you did that made it sick. Your goals are to help Mr. Tummy settle down and to prevent dehydration. Here's what the experts advise.

Forget the stomach settlers. It's too late. Those familiar potions—Pepto-Bismol, Maalox, Mylanta—are not designed to stop vomiting, says Samuel Klein, M.D., an assistant professor of gastroenterology and human nutrition at the University of Texas Medical School at Galveston. "Take them only if the vomiting is related to too much stomach acid. For instance, if you have a stomach ulcer or something you ate is causing irritation," he says. Then they might work by neutralizing excess acid or soothing irritation. Otherwise, forget it.

Replace fluids. "The ultimate goals for someone who's got a lot of vomiting are to not get dehydrated and to not lose weight," says nausea researcher Kenneth Koch, M.D., a gastroenterologist at Pennsylvania State University's Hershey Medical Center. You lose a lot of fluid in vomiting, so the best thing you can do is drink fluids to replace those lost.

These fluids should be clear liquids, Dr. Klein says: water, weak tea, juices. Even fluids like milk or heavy soups may be too much to handle.

Replace important nutrients. Vomiting also flushes out minerals. Dr. Klein recommends you take electrolyte drinks to replace these nutrients: Gatorade and Pedialyte, clear soups, or juices like apple or cranberry. Water is better than nothing, but ideally you should add a couple pinches of salt and sugar to each glass. "I often have patients sipping Gatorade every half hour," Dr. Koch says.

MEDICAL ALERT

Don't Wait Too Long

Vomiting can be a sign of something serious. "If it's profuse or persistent or bloody, seek help," advises Stephen Bezruchka, M.D., an emergency physician at Providence Medical Center in Seattle, Washington. Also see a doctor "when you've gone 24 hours without being able to keep any food down, and nothing seems to help," Kenneth Koch, M.D., says.

"If your thirst is severe and you notice you're not urinating very much, and especially if you're also getting light-headed when you stand up, which are signs of dehydration, see a doctor," he says. "If you know it's the flu or you've just eaten something a little strange, you might try to go a bit longer."

Sip, not slurp. Sipping your fluids in tiny swallows lets your irritated stomach adjust, Dr. Koch says — no chug-a-lugging. Sip no more than 1 or 2 ounces at a time, Dr. Koch advises. Otherwise, it could be, *après fluid, le deluge.*

Determine your own timing. The less fluid you're sipping at a time, the more often you have to sip. How frequently you take fluids depends on how your stomach reacts. Once you know you can keep the last sip down, sip some more.

Use the color code. If your urine is deep yellow, you're not getting enough fluid. The paler it gets, the better you're doing to prevent dehydration.

Go for warmth. Our experts advise against cold drinks, which shock sensitive stomachs. Room temperature or warm drinks are best, Dr. Koch says.

Let the fizz out. Tiny bubbles — just what you don't need if you're vomiting. Let your favorite clear carbonated drinks stand until they go flat before you start sipping.

Settle down with syrup. A good stomach settler, says Robert Warren, Pharm.D., director of Pharmacy Services at Valley Children's Hospital in Fresno, California, is Coke syrup. "We don't know why it works," Dr. Warren says, "but it does." It also is a good source of easily digestible concentrated carbohydrates (and it tastes good, too!). The children's dose is 1 to 2 teaspoons, adults' dose is 1 to 2 tablespoons, as often as needed between bouts of vomiting.

Or try the drugstore alternative. If you want a more medical-sounding syrup, try Emetrol, Dr. Warren suggests. It's a phosphorated carbohydrate solution that works the same way. A caution: None of these sugar-rich syrups is recommended for diabetics without a doctor's okay, Dr. Warren says.

Start with carbohydrates. Sooner or later, vomiting will end. The experts say the best way to start eating again is with a gelatin dessert.

"Jell-O is the traditional hospital way to begin eating after a period of vomiting," Dr. Warren says. It's mostly liquid, easy on the stomach, high in carbohydrates, and tastes good. Other bland foods like nonbuttered toast or crackers are also good postvomiting treats.

Add a light protein. "When you're feeling a little better, you can move on to a light protein like chicken breast or fish," Dr. Koch says. Chicken noodle or chicken with rice soup is perfect for this, he says. Be sure to skim off as much fat from the soup as you can.

Leave fat for last. Fat stays in the stomach too long and can thus add to the bloated, full feeling, Dr. Koch says. So avoid fatty meats and cream soups.

PANEL OF ADVISERS

Stephen Bezruchka, M.D., is an emergency physician at Providence Medical Center in Seattle, Washington, and author of *The Pocket Doctor.*

Samuel Klein, M.D., is an assistant professor of gastroenterology and human nutrition at the University of Texas Medical School at Galveston. He is also an editorial adviser to *Prevention* magazine.

Kenneth Koch, M.D., is a gastroenterologist at Pennsylvania State University's Hershey Medical Center and a leading researcher for NASA into the causes of nausea.

Robert Warren, Pharm.D., is director of Pharmacy Services at Valley Children's Hospital in Fresno, California.

Warts

26 Ways to Win the War

Okay, we're only going to say this once, so listen up. Toads have nothing to do with warts. They don't cause them; they don't spread them; they don't even know what warts are. Got that?

Warts are benign skin tumors that can occur singly or in large packs on just about any part of the body. And while each type carries its own special name, all are caused by various strains of the fiendish papilloma virus. It masterfully tricks the body into providing it with free room and board in a sheltered "house" that is known medically as the wart proper.

MEDICAL ALERT

Are You Sure That's a Wart?

Remember what Davy Crockett said: "Be sure you're right and then go ahead." That advice applies to treating warts as surely as to anything else in life. The absolute first rule of thumb (and finger, foot, and elbow) is: Make sure it *is* a wart and not a corn, callus, mole, or cancerous lesion. According to Alvin Zelickson, M.D., "Normally, you'd think it would be pretty easy to identify a wart, but it's amazing how many people end up treating skin cancers or other growths as warts." So if you have the slightest doubt about what you're dealing with, see a doctor.

In general, warts are pale, skin-colored growths with a rough surface, even borders, and blackened surface capillaries. Normal skin lines do not cross a wart's surface. And contrary to popular opinion, warts are very shallow growths—they don't have "roots" or "runners" that go down to the bone.

At any one time, says Robert Garry, Ph.D., an associate professor of microbiology and immunology at Tulane University School of Medicine, about 10 percent of the population has a wart. Probably 75 percent of all people will get one sometime in their lives. No wonder we spend an estimated $125 million annually on wart treatments! After acne, warts are the most common dermatologic complaint.

Unfortunately, standard medical treatment often comes in the form of nasty-sounding destructive methods such as burning, scraping, cutting, freezing, injecting, or zapping with a laser. These techniques may or may not be effective. Many of them are painful and may leave scars. To add insult to injury, warts often reappear, no matter what treatment is used.

Knowing all this, you may want to try some home remedies before heading to the doctor's office. But, by all means, heed the advice of Memphis dermatologist Thomas Goodman, Jr., M.D., an assistant professor of dermatology at the University of Tennessee Center for Health Sciences. "Don't injure yourself with wart treatments. Start with simple measures and persist for several weeks before proceeding to stronger ones."

Unless otherwise noted, the following are effective for both common warts and plantar warts (those found on the foot).

Leave 'em alone. Like Little Bo Peep's sheep, many warts respond to a loose hand. According to one estimate, 40 to 50 percent of all warts eventually disappear on their own, typically within two years. Children in particular often lose warts spontaneously.

Marc A. Brenner, D.P.M., past president of the American Society of Podiatric Dermatology and a private practitioner in Glendale, New York, does caution that warts constantly shed infectious virus, and if left untreated they may get larger or spread to other areas. So if your warts start multiplying, take action.

Call in the A-team. Dr. Garry has had great success applying vitamin A directly to warts. "Get capsules that contain 25,000 international units of natural vitamin A from fish oil or fish-liver oil. Simply break open a capsule, squeeze some of the liquid onto the wart, and rub it in. Apply this once a day." He emphasizes that the vitamin should be applied to the skin only. Taken orally in large doses, vitamin A can be toxic.

"Different warts respond differently to this treatment. Juvenile warts can be gone in a month, although two to four months is more like it. Plantar warts might take two to five months or longer," he says.

Dr. Garry recalls one woman who had more than 200 warts on her hand. By persisting with the vitamin A therapy for seven or eight months, she was able to lose all but one stubborn wart under her fingernail.

How to Avoid a Wart

Warts are caused by a virus. It's in the air, and you pick it up the same way you do any viral infection. If you're susceptible to the virus and if you have an appropriate cut or crack in the skin for it to take hold, you'll get a wart. It's that simple. Even so, there are a few things you *can* do to lessen your chances of sprouting a wart.

Keep your shoes on. The wart virus thrives in a very moist environment, says Suzanne M. Levine, D.P.M., so always wear plastic thong sandals around swimming pools, health clubs, and locker rooms to avoid foot contact with it. By not going barefoot, you also sidestep minute cracks or cuts in your feet through which the virus could easily enter.

Change shoes frequently. Since the wart virus breeds in moist places, you should change your shoes frequently and allow shoes to dry out between wearings, says Dr. Levine.

Clean up. "At a health club or gym, you might even want to clean the shower out first with a product like Lysol," says Dr. Levine. "Even just household bleach works to kill viruses and bacteria."

Look but don't touch. "Warts spread easily," says Marc A. Brenner, D.P.M. "So if you have one on the bottom of your foot, for instance, try not to touch it with your hand. If you have even a small cut on your finger, you risk getting a wart there."

Pamper your cuticles. If the wart virus enters a cut or opening around your cuticle, it can cause a particularly nasty type of wart. Called periungual warts, they're very difficult to treat, says Dr. Levine. "If you do get a cut in the cuticle, put on a topical antibiotic cream (such as Bacitracin) and then cover it with a bandage until it heals."

Play it cool. "My own feeling is that people seem to be more susceptible to warts when they're under stress and eating poorly," says Dr. Levine. "And the warts seem to spread more then." So try to take it easy.

See what another vitamin can do. Making a paste from crushed vitamin C tablets and water has helped some people. Apply to the wart and then cover with a bandage so the paste doesn't rub off. Jeffrey Bland, Ph.D., who spent many years studying vitamin C at the Linus Pauling Institute in Menlo Park, California, says that "although no formal research has been done in this area, there is some evidence that the high acidity of ascorbic acid [vitamin C] can kill the wart-producing virus." Keep in mind, though, that vitamin C (at least in its ascorbic acid form) may irritate the skin, so you should try to cover only the wart with the paste.

Keep that wart under wraps. "I've had success applying a tape bandage to warts," says Dr. Goodman. "Use any kind of medical or first-aid tape. Apply it *snugly* over the wart and leave it there 24 hours a day, 7 days a week. Change the tape only when you need to look clean. Be patient and persist for at least three weeks. It really does work for some people if they do it properly."

Try a dose of castor oil. For a variation on the tape technique, says Dr. Goodman, apply a drop of plain castor oil to the wart twice daily and then tape it as above.

Herbal consultant and educator Jane Bothwell of Arcata, California, also believes in the usefulness of castor oil, this time mixed into a thick paste with baking soda. Apply the paste a couple of times a day. To keep it from rubbing off, either apply a bandage or put on a glove or sock.

Stay dry. Warts thrive on moisture, so keeping the feet very dry might help eliminate plantar warts. Says Dr. Brenner, "If you wanted to work on a plantar wart without using chemicals, you could try changing your socks at least three times a day. And apply a medicated foot powder such as Zeasorb frequently—ten times a day if necessary. There are other drying agents that might help. Believe it or not, I have used a Clorox solution on people who have not responded to anything else, and occasionally it has worked."

Opt for an OTC. Probably the most popular commercial wart remedies are the over-the-counter salicylic acid preparations. Salicylic acid is believed to work against warts by softening and helping dissolve them. These products come in liquid, gel, pad, and ointment form. Diabetics and those with impaired circulation should not use them.

There are three rules for dealing with an acidic OTC, says podiatrist Glenn Gastwirth, D.P.M., of Bethesda, Maryland, director of scientific affairs at the American Podiatric Medical Association. "First, be certain that it *is* a wart you're treating (see "Are You Sure That's a Wart?" on page 624). Second, follow package instructions to the letter. And third, if the wart does not respond within a reasonable amount of time—say a week or two—see a doctor."

The Alternate Route

Some Simple Folk Cures

When all is said and done, you never know just what will cure any particular wart. The remedy that so neatly dispatched one little growth might leave another completely unscathed. So perhaps your most powerful weapon in the war of the warts is an open mind. That's why you shouldn't be quick to overlook the healing potential of so-called folk cures: treatments that have never undergone formal scientific scrutiny but that have worked just fine for many people. Here are a few that some folks swear by:

• Apply vitamin E oil, clove oil, aloe vera juice, milkweed juice, the milky juice of the sow's thistle plant, or the milky juice of unripe figs directly to the wart.
• Take garlic capsules or tablets.
• Soak lemon slices in apple cider with a little salt. Let stand two weeks. Then rub the lemon slices on the wart.
• Rub with a piece of chalk or a raw potato.
• Tape the inner side of a banana skin to a plantar wart.

"A liquid product like Compound W can work if you use it on a small wart," says Christopher McEwen, M.D., chairman of the Department of Dermatology at the Ochsner Clinic in Baton Rouge, Louisiana. Adds New York City podiatrist Suzanne M. Levine, D.P.M., clinical assistant podiatrist at Mount Sinai Hospital, "One good thing about Compound W in particular, is that it contains a little oil, which makes it less irritating to the skin than some other salicylic acid products."

Dr. Brenner advises, however, that the liquid and gel products, which typically contain only about 17 percent salicylic acid, may not be strong enough to work on plantar warts that have a thick callus covering them.

Pad the wart. "If I had to pick one over-the-counter product," says Dr. McEwen, "I'd go with a 40 percent salicylic acid plaster such as Mediplast. It works fairly well for plantar warts and can also be effective on hand warts, although it's harder to keep the patch in place on the hand."

"The main drawback to pads," says Dr. Levine, "is that people often use too large a piece, which exposes the surrounding skin to serious irritation. And they put on a new pad every day. Pretty soon they have an ulcer around the wart that's far worse than the wart they started with. The best course of action is to use one little pad every four or five days."

To ensure a good fit, cut out a little cardboard template exactly the shape and dimensions of your wart. Then use that template to precut a supply of patches from the adhesive plaster. Lightly coat the perimeter of the wart with petroleum jelly to prevent any of the medication from touching the skin.

Go with an ointment. Rounding out the salicylic acid arsenal is 60 percent ointment. For best results, advises Dr. Levine, soak the area in lukewarm water for about 10 minutes to allow for greater penetration. Dry well, then apply a drop of the ointment to the wart. Cover with a bandage. If you're dealing with a plantar wart, do this at bedtime so you won't have to walk around on the wart and rub off the ointment. In the morning, soak the area again and lightly pumice off any softened skin.

Try an old-fashioned cream. "A product that has historically been used for warts is Vergo cream, which has calcium pantothenate [a B vitamin], ascorbic acid [vitamin C], and starch in it," says Nicholas G. Popovich, Ph.D., an associate professor of pharmacy practice at Purdue University. "Those particular ingredients have never been demonstrated by the Food and Drug Administration panel on wart products to be effective for wart removal. That doesn't necessarily mean the product doesn't work; it's just that its effectiveness is probably based on testimonial evidence rather than clinical studies."

Unlike the salicylic acid products, Vergo cream is not caustic and will not burn, blister, or injure surrounding tissue. Average treatment time is two to eight weeks.

Get timed-release relief. If you're ready to see a doctor but not ready for him to freeze or laser your wart off, there's a brand-new product designed for self-care use that you can ask him about. The Trans-Ver-Sal transdermal patch is "very effective in treating warts," says Dr. McEwen, who's gotten good results with it. Like other transdermal patches, it's applied directly to the skin (in this case to the wart) and delivers a continuous dose of medication for several hours. And like other transdermal patches, it's available only by prescription.

The active ingredient in the patch is salicylic acid, the same drug used in over-the-counter wart removers. The big difference, according to Alvin Zelickson, M.D., a clinical professor of dermatology at the University of Minnesota Medical School, "is that the salicylic acid *is* transferred to the wart. With standard plaster pads, for instance, very little actually

Mind Games:
Who's in Control Here?

Go into a trance. "You are getting very sleepy—soon you will be in a deep trance—soon your warts will disappear." Hogwash? No, hypnosis. And it may be a formidable weapon against warts.

According to psychiatrist Owen Surman, M.D., of Massachusetts General Hospital in Boston, "Hypnosis does seem to be a scientifically validated tool for treating warts. Why it would be is subject to guesswork. Currently, people are very interested in this area called psychoneuroimmunology. It's attractive to think that mental phenomena could affect immune function."

In one study, Dr. Surman hypnotized 17 people who had warts on both sides of their bodies for a series of five sessions and told them that their warts would disappear from one side only. Another 7 people were not hypnotized and were instructed to abstain from using any wart remedies on their own. Three months later, more than half of the hypnotized group had lost at least 75 percent of their warts. The people who hadn't been hypnotized still had their warts.

And although the warts that did go away disappeared from *both* sides of the hypnosis group's bodies, "we felt the experiment was a success," says Dr. Surman.

Imagine your warts away. The power of suggestion alone—without hypnosis—may be equally effective at wasting warts. Perhaps the most research in this area has been done by Nicholas Spanos, Ph.D., a professor of psychology, and his colleagues at Carleton University in Ottawa. "We tell patients to imagine that their warts are shrinking, that they can feel the tingling as their warts dissolve and their skins become clear. Initially, we give them about 2 minutes of this type of imagery, then we have them practice on their own at home for 5 minutes a day.

"Believe it or not, we can actually predict who will achieve results based on the very first session. People who report really vivid imagery that first day are more likely to lose warts than those who say their imagery was relatively weak."

Be a believer. Other doctors have had plenty of informal success with the power of suggestion. Says Christopher McEwen, M.D., "I've treated a couple of kids who could not tolerate freezing, which is how we usually remove warts. So I gave them a harmless substance to use and impressed upon them that it was a very strong medicine that would knock out the warts. And it worked." Strong belief in a cure may also explain the continued popularity of such offbeat, old-fashioned folk remedies as rubbing the wart with a penny and then burying the penny under the porch.

gets released into the wart. These patches are easy to use and don't require presoaking the skin. You put one on at bedtime and remove it in the morning. It's available in two sizes (and strengths), so it's appropriate for both common and plantar warts."

Dr. Zelickson, who conducted full-scale tests of the patch on about 40 patients, found that the patch removed warts about 80 percent of the time, typically in four to twelve weeks.

PANEL OF ADVISERS

Jeffrey Bland, Ph.D., was formerly a senior researcher at the Linus Pauling Institute in Menlo Park, California. He is president of HealthComm, a wellness-education consulting service in Gig Harbor, Washington.

Jane Bothwell is a practicing herbal consultant and educator in Arcata, California. She was formerly an instructor at the California School of Herbal Studies.

Marc A. Brenner, D.P.M., has a private practice in Glendale, New York, is past president of the American Society of Podiatric Dermatology, and author of *The Management of the Diabetic Foot.*

Robert Garry, Ph.D., is an associate professor of microbiology and immunology at Tulane University School of Medicine in New Orleans, Louisiana.

Glenn Gastwirth, D.P.M., a podiatrist in Bethesda, Maryland, is director of scientific affairs at the American Podiatric Medical Association.

Thomas Goodman, Jr., M.D., is a dermatologist in private practice and assistant professor of dermatology at the University of Tennessee Center for Health Sciences in Memphis. He is the author of *Smart Face* and *The Skin Doctor's Skin Doctoring Book.*

Suzanne M. Levine, D.P.M., is a podiatrist in private practice and clinical assistant podiatrist at Mount Sinai Hospital in New York City. She is author of *My Feet Are Killing Me* and *Walk It Off.*

Christopher McEwen, M.D., is chairman of the Department of Dermatology at the Ochsner Clinic in Baton Rouge, Louisiana.

Nicholas G. Popovich, Ph.D., is an associate professor of pharmacy practice at Purdue University in West Lafayette, Indiana.

Nicholas Spanos, Ph.D., is a professor of psychology at Carleton University in Ottawa.

Owen Surman, M.D., is a psychiatrist at Massachusetts General Hospital in Boston and an assistant professor of psychiatry at Harvard Medical School there.

Alvin Zelickson, M.D., is a clinical professor of dermatology at the University of Minnesota Medical School in Minneapolis.

Wrinkles

24 Tips to Slow Aging

A lot of good can come with age—things like wisdom, grandchildren, and senior citizen discounts. But there are a few not-so-terrific things, like gray hair and wrinkles.

Gray hair, of course, can be touched up with a little dye. Simple enough. Wrinkles, however, are an altogether different story. No, you can't iron them out. And you can't (like Peter Pan or Dorian Gray) simply wish them away. But experts say there are a number of strategies to keep you from looking old before your time.

Don't be a California raisin. In other words, stay out of the sun. This is the first line of wrinkle defense suggested by every one of our experts. Too much sun eventually does the same thing to your skin that it does to dried fruit: It shrivels it up. This is *especially* true today, as depletion of the earth's ozone layer allows more of the sun's harmful rays to reach your vulnerable skin, says Norman A. Brooks, M.D., a dermatologist in private practice in Encino, California, and an assistant clinical professor of dermatology at the University of California, Los Angeles, UCLA School of Medicine. (For more on avoiding sun-induced wrinkles, see "Fun—And Wrinkles—In the Sun," on the opposite page.)

Avoid tanning booths. They produce the very same wrinkling rays as the sun, says Jeffrey H. Binstock, M.D., a dermatologist in private practice and an assistant clinical professor of dermatologic surgery at the University of California, San Francisco, School of Medicine.

Scrunch not. It's okay to occasionally make a funny face, but constantly furrowing your brow, squinting, or puckering your lips will, in time, create wrinkles or make those you already have worse, says Mari-

Fun—And Wrinkles—In the Sun

Doctors say that too much sun causes wrinkles. The problem, of course, is that unless you're a vampire or a roll of film, avoiding sunlight completely isn't something you want to do. So here's what experts suggest for balancing fun in the sun with wrinkle control.

Leave the midday sun to mad dogs and Englishmen. About 95 percent of the sun's wrinkling rays hit the Earth between the hours of 10:00 A.M. and 2:00 P.M. (11:00 A.M. and 3:00 P.M., daylight saving time), according to Stephen Kurtin, M.D.

Slather on the sunblock. Whenever you're out in the sun, the use of a sunscreen—the higher the sun protection factor (SPF) number, the better—is advised, says Dr. Kurtin. To be most effective in battling wrinkles, sunscreens should be applied to the skin at least ½ hour before going out and reapplied after swimming.

Beware of reflective surfaces. It's always the same sun up there, but circumstances on Earth do change. Keep in mind that the wrinkling effects of the sun will be strongest off light-colored (and therefore reflective) surfaces, such as snow, sand, and concrete, says Jeffrey H. Binstock, M.D.

Pay attention to your locale. Be aware that the sun's skin-shriveling rays are strongest at high altitudes (where the air is thinner) and southern latitudes (closer to the equator).

Make sure you get enough vitamin D. If you're really serious about staying out of the sun, remember that sunlight normally provides us with essential vitamin D. You can, however, get all the vitamin D you need either from vitamin D–enriched milk or a multivitamin, says Marianne O'Donoghue, M.D.

anne O'Donoghue, M.D., an associate professor of dermatology at Rush-Presbyterian–St. Luke's Hospital in Chicago, Illinois.

Test your face. How do you know if you're scrunching your face? Look at yourself in a mirror as you're chatting on the telephone, suggests Dr. Binstock. Or try wearing a piece of cellophane tape over your forehead (just around the house, of course). Every time you furrow your brow, you'll feel the tape start to crinkle, says John F. Romano, M.D., a dermatologist and clinical instructor in medicine at New York Hospital–Cornell University Medical Center in New York City.

Avoid the bare-faced double whammy. A great recipe for wrinkling is to go out into the sun without sunglasses or a peaked hat. Not only do you then have to contend with the sun's damaging rays falling on your face, but your inclination will be to squint, which eventually can forge little wrinkles around your eyes, says Dr. O'Donoghue.

Keep pillows away from your face. "Watch out for sleep wrinkles," says Dr. Binstock. These are wrinkles that are caused by pressing your face into the pillow at night. If you're guilty of this habit, learn to sleep on your back instead, or experiment to find a position where your face is not pressing the pillow. You may see some of your smaller lines fade away.

Don't be a yo-yo dieter. Gaining a lot of weight can stretch your skin. Then losing weight (especially if you're older and your skin is less elastic) can result in wrinkles because the skin will not completely retract to its original size, says Stephen Kurtin, M.D., a dermatologist practicing in New York City and an assistant professor of dermatology at Mount Sinai School of Medicine of the City University of New York. The smart thing to do is to never get overweight in the first place, or, if you do, lose that excess fat and keep it off before the age of 40, says Dr. Kurtin.

Exercise regularly. People who are generally in good shape seem to have healthier, more elastic skin than those who aren't. One Finnish study found that middle-aged athletes had skin that was denser, thicker, and stronger than that of a similar group of nonexercisers. The elastic quality that allows the skin to spring back to its original shape after being stretched was also significantly better in the athletes.

Eat right. Vitamins and minerals are important to maintaining youthful skin. Among the most important are the B-complex vitamins (found in beef, chicken, eggs, whole wheat and enriched flour, and milk, among other food) and vitamins A and C (found in fresh fruit and vegetables). Dr. O'Donoghue says the best foods for healthy skin are green leafy vegetables, carrots, and fresh fruit.

Don't smoke. Smoking, in addition to being bad for your general health, can result in premature wrinkling around your mouth due to all those years of puckering lips around cigarettes. Smoking also tends to decrease blood supply to the small blood vessels under your skin, which could exacerbate wrinkling, says Gerald Imber, M.D., an attending plastic surgeon at New York Hospital–Cornell University Medical Center in New York City.

Stick with checkers (or some other sobering activity) on Saturday night. Party goers and others who hit the bottle too heavily may find that while alcohol drowns their sorrows, it also brings on wrinkles. Why? Because your face puffs up in the morning after you've had too much to drink. And that temporarily stretches the skin. This swelling and subsequent shrinking can create wrinkles much the same way that putting on a lot of weight and then going on a crash diet will, says Dr. Imber.

Use a moisturizer. No moisturizer on the market can reverse the aging process. If you have dry skin, however, the use of a moisturizing lotion can hide some of the smaller wrinkles that form on the surface, says Dr. Kurtin. He emphasizes that it is important to dampen the skin first before applying moisturizing cream.

The Alternate Route

Deal with Wrinkles the Oriental Way

Can wrinkling be stopped or minimized? "We do it here all the time," says Marshall Ho'o, a doctor of oriental medicine at the East-West Clinic in Reseda, California. The way wrinkles are dealt with in oriental medicine is "from the inside out," says Dr. Ho'o.

That is to say his patients are taught a number of exercises designed "to develop tone and symmetry" in their faces and necks. They may also be given acupressure treatments. But what can you do at home without any special training from Dr. Ho'o?

"Massage your face," he says. Using your fingertips, your thumbs, and the palms of your hands, rub every part of your face and neck. Any kind of massage, he explains, will help "to maximize stimulation and circulation. It can also round out the facial muscles, whose symmetry is often lost in fixed or rigid expressions."

Dr. Ho'o also emphasizes the importance of living a happy and stress-free life. "Chinese people who have big families, who talk and laugh a lot, seem to have less wrinkles. And when wrinkles do appear, they are not unattractive."

Don't be fooled into buying "miracle" creams. Especially since the headline-grabbing advent of Retin-A, a *strictly prescription* topical drug that can actually reduce wrinkling, false advertising about certain over-the-counter lotions has popped up everywhere. "The claims being made by some cosmetic companies for anti-aging creams have been found by the Food and Drug Administration [FDA] to be quite misleading," says Emil Corwin, an information officer with the Center for Food Safety and Applied Nutrition at the FDA.

Go easy on the suds. "If anything, people in our society tend to *over*wash," says Dr. Kurtin. Overwashing can lead to dryness, which can create temporary wrinkling. Solution? Wash less and use only extra-mild soaps. And rinse extremely well. "People should spend more time rinsing and less time washing," says Dr. Kurtin, who explains that a soapy film left on the skin will exacerbate drying.

Use a humidifier. Keeping the air in your house moist is great for your skin and may prevent the smaller, temporary wrinkles that sometimes come with dry skin, says Dr. O'Donoghue.

See a makeup artist. "The judicious use of good makeup can do a very good job of hiding wrinkles," says Paul Lazar, M.D., a professor of clinical dermatology at Northwestern University Medical School. He suggests you consider seeking out a professional. "Just as good makeup artists can make someone look old for a movie, they can also make you look younger," he says.

Buff yourself with a little powder. Jack Myers, director of the National Cosmetology Association and a professional cosmetologist for the past 30 years, says that sometimes when people try to hide wrinkles with makeup, they wind up actually *emphasizing* wrinkles. That's because they rub cream- or oil-based makeup into their skin and it tends to cake up between the wrinkles. The key to hiding wrinkles, he says, is to use only powder-based (such as cornstarch) products. Here, as with moisturizers, don't expect miracles, says Myers.

Live with less stress. Dr. Lazar says the link between wrinkles and emotions is probably a superficial one. But happy people tend to carry smiles, he says, and a smile will divert other people's attention away from any wrinkles.

Yeast Infections

26 Natural Antidotes

Candida albicans—yeast—is a fungus that grows naturally and harmlessly in women's vaginas and in the intestines in both men and women.

"They are natural flora. They live there just like bacteria live in the mouth," says Michael Spence, M.D., an obstetrician and gynecologist at

Hahnemann University School of Medicine. "If there is an upset in the balance or ecology of the area by taking antibiotics, or if you have diabetes, for instance, then you get more yeast and a vaginal infection."

Other things that can provoke a yeast infection include pregnancy, birth control pills, hormones for menopause, chemical douches, spermi-

Three Ways to Kill an Infection

News Item: *Boise, Idaho (UPI)—Firefighters went on a panty raid of sorts when a woman called the department complaining of smoke in her attic.*

When firefighters arrived at the scene, they discovered that the source of the smoke was a pair of the woman's panties in the microwave oven.

The woman, whose name was not released, told firefighters she put the nylon panties in the microwave to get rid of a yeast infection.

For the record, microwaving may be a great way to cook vegetables, but it is not a sensible way to cure a vaginal yeast infection, as this news item attests.

The microwave "cure" is the result of a study by University of Florida and Baylor College researchers who discovered that the yeast-causing organism, *Candida albicans,* can be killed by microwaving. The scientists said women leave yeast spores in their panties when they have an infection. Normal laundering won't kill the fungus. But microwaving them, they proved, does. It also starts fires.

Cooking your panties in the microwave isn't good advice, says Marjorie Crandall, Ph.D., a candida specialist who has written a booklet called *How to Prevent Yeast Infections.* What the researchers proved, she says, is that *Candida albicans* survives normal wash-and-dry cycles, once deposited in a woman's panties, meaning it can reinfect the wearer. But most women don't want to take the chance of a panty raid in the kitchen.

So what's the answer?

Give those panties an extra scrub. As a precaution, scrub the crotch of your panties with unscented detergent before dropping them into the wash, says Dr. Crandall. Avoid bleach, she adds, and fabric softener, which irritate tender skin.

Or boil the fungus away. Still another laundry and underwear study reports you can boil your underpants or soak them in bleach for 24 hours prior to reuse to kill the candida. Wash with unscented soap before wearing.

Kill it with heat. Also, candida can die when panties are touched with a hot iron.

cides, nicks in the vaginal wall from tampons, too little lubrication during intercourse, or intercourse with someone who has a yeast infection.

When you get a yeast infection, a doctor confirms the problem by examining some of the discharge under a microscope. Then he prescribes a medicine that kills the excess yeast in the vagina.

It sounds simple, but women who get yeast infections know it isn't. Yeast, which causes itching and burning and carries a yeasty smell and causes a white, cheesy discharge, has a way of coming back. Some people are prone to yeast infections.

Marjorie Crandall, Ph.D., a candida specialist and founder of Yeast Consulting Services in Torrance, California, understands why women will try almost anything to relieve the discomfort. For 20 years, she fought chronic yeast infections that made her life miserable. Today she is infection-free, and she is also one of the top authorities on ways to control the problem.

Here's what she and other experts recommend for those troubled by yeast infections.

Sleep like Eve. Yeast thrives in a warm, damp atmosphere, says Dr. Spence, so one of the best preventive measures you can take against this fungus is to keep your vaginal area ventilated—that is, cool and dry. Sleep naked or take your panties off underneath your nightgown when you go to bed and give your body 8 hours of unencumbered relief.

Wear loose clothing. During the day, avoid tight-fitting clothing or clothing made from fibers that don't allow good air circulation. Those include plastic, polyester, and leather fabrics, says Dr. Spence. Cut down on the layers of clothing you wear. Don't wear panties under panty hose under tight jeans. When you get home, peel off extra layers, such as panty hose, and let your body breathe. Wear skirts when you can.

Don't dust. Starch is the perfect medium for growing fungus cultures, says Dr. Spence. Since most after-bath powders have a starch base, you're encouraging an infection when you use a dusting powder. Keep powder out of your panties.

Use an over-the-counter vaginal medicine. There are some places you just can't scratch (at least in public) and this is one of them. While your prescription medicine works on eliminating the fungus, you can reduce the itch with an OTC such as Benadryl or Cortaid. Or dab an over-the-counter hydrocortisone cream around the vulva and vaginal

---

MEDICAL ALERT

Let Your Doctor Diagnose

Doctors often take a culture or examine vaginal discharge under a micro-scope because not all discharges are caused by relatively harmless yeast. Anything from a forgotten tampon to life-threatening pelvic inflammatory disease can cause similar symptoms: itching and an odd-smelling discharge.

Other causes include gardnerella vaginalis, a bacterial infection; trichomonas, a parasitic infection; and chlamydia, gonorrhea, and syphilis. So don't play doctor. Get a professional diagnosis.

---

opening to lessen the itch. Just be sure you don't use these creams before seeing a doctor because they may cover up an infection and prevent a proper diagnosis.

Use a natural lubricant. Mineral oil, petroleum jelly, egg whites, and plain yogurt are dandy substances for lubrication during intercourse, says Dr. Crandall, because they aren't chemically irritating unless you are allergic to them. (Do not use petroleum jelly with condoms, because it will cause holes to form in the rubber.) Do not use baby oil, because it contains perfume, which can irritate.

Say no to chemical potions. A sure way to aggravate an already delicate situation is to add chemicals to your smoldering yeast infection. Avoid douches, contraceptive jellies, foams and sprays, yeast-killing tablets, and feminine deodorants, says Dr. Crandall.

Mix yourself a healing bath. One alternative to douching is the sitz bath. Fill a shallow tub (just to the hip) with warm water, then do one of the following.

- Add salt (enough to make the water taste salty, about ½ cup) to match the body's natural saline state.
- Add vinegar (½ cup) to help rebalance the vaginal pH to 4.5.

Now, sit in the water, knees apart, until it gets cool. The bath will do the cleansing.

Put spermicides in their place. Spermicides are another chemical to keep out of your vagina, especially if you are prone to infections. If you plan to use a spermicide during intercourse, put the spermicide inside the reservoir tip of the condom, where it can do the work it was meant to do, says Dr. Crandall.

No scents is good sense. Choose plain, unscented personal products. Perfumes and deodorants on tampons and sanitary pads can irritate or trigger another episode of vaginitis.

Wash with water. Soap, shampoo, bath salts, and oils remove the natural oils that protect your skin and may leave an irritating residue. Wash your vaginal area with plain water and friction when you shower. A hand held shower head is perfect for directing the spray.

Make cotton queen. Choose cotton panties because they wick moisture away from your skin. Nylon will retain heat and moisture, which invites yeast to grow. If you prefer the feel of nylon against your skin, choose panties with a built-in cotton crotch. If your panties don't have a cotton crotch, a panty liner or mini-pad may be a good substitute.

Always wear panty hose with a cotton crotch, so air can pass through to cool and dry the vagina. And remember, you don't have to wear panties with panty hose! The fewer layers of clothing you wear, the more ventilation you get.

Use uncolored toilet paper. Dye is another chemical with chafing potential. Dr. Crandall suggests you avoid unnecessary irritation by using plain white, unscented toilet paper.

Keep germs in their place. Wipe from front to back after a bowel movement. Wash anything that comes in contact with the anus before touching the vagina.

Wash before intercourse. If you and your partner are both squeaky clean, there's less chance of transferring yeast germs into your vagina. Wash your hands and genitals before intercourse.

Rinse with water only. The vagina is naturally self-cleaning, but some women feel they need to douche. If you douche, Dr. Crandall recommends a gentle cool-water douche used on an infrequent basis because it is the least irritating thing you can use.

Do not douche during your period when your cervix is open; the upward flow might push infection into your uterus. Also, never douche during pregnancy unless your doctor recommends it.

Douche with vinegar. Vinegar has approximately the same acidity as the vagina, which is one reason a lukewarm vinegar and water mix (4 teaspoons vinegar to 1 pint of water) is sometimes suggested as a douching liquid. Some doctors suggest that a vagina with the correct pH balance is less likely to grow excess yeast.

Also, there are premixed vinegar-and-water solutions available for women who don't want to mix their own.

Avoid sex when you have vaginitis. Intercourse can further irritate the inflammation caused by a yeast infection. Also, yeast can spread to your partner who may reinfect you later, says Dr. Crandall.

Urinate before and after. Men and women should wash and urinate before and after sex to flush germs out of the urethra and avoid bladder infections, says Dr. Crandall.

Use a condom. An unribbed, unlubricated condom will be less irritating. It will also protect partners from passing yeast back and forth.

Control yeasts and molds. Women who have recurrent yeast infections may become allergic to foods containing yeasts and molds. Avoid foods and beverages such as bread, doughnuts, beer, wine, vinegar, pickles, fermented foods, cheese, mushrooms, and fruit juices.

Keep your blood sugar under control. Yeast thrives on sugar, according to a study at Mount Sinai Hospital in Hartford, Connecticut. High sugar intake contributes to yeast infections. It provides food for yeast. People with diabetes, who are more prone to yeast infections, should monitor their blood sugars. Also, excessive lactose in dairy products and artificial sweeteners increase the likelihood of yeast infections.

Raise your resistance. A healthy person fights infection more easily than someone whose body isn't up to par. Boost your immunity by exercising regularly, eating properly, getting plenty of sleep, not smoking or using drugs, drinking in moderation, and using caffeine sparingly.

Choose natural fibers first. Use cotton tampons instead of synthetic fiber tampons. Superabsorbant tampons and those left in more than 12 hours will stop natural drainage and encourage bacterial growth. Another idea: Use pads at night and tampons during the day.

PANEL OF ADVISERS

Marjorie Crandall, Ph.D., is a candida specialist and founder of Yeast Consulting Services in Torrance, California. She has written a self-help booklet, *How to Prevent Yeast Infections.*

Michael Spence, M.D., is an obstetrician and gynecologist at Hahnemann University School of Medicine in Philadelphia, Pennsylvania.

Index

Calcium *(continued)*
    magnesium and, 582
    from nonmilk sources, 408
Calcium gluconate, 56
Calcium supplements, 467, 468
Calf
    cramp in, 438
    pain in, 382–85
    stretching of, 535
Calluses, 165–70
Calories
    in diabetic diet, 199, 201
    emphysema and, 237
    fat and, 15, 17, 609–10
Camphor, 70, 149, 153
Candida albicans, 637, 638
Canker sores, 110–13
Capsaicin, 515, 532, 543
Carbamide peroxide, 111
Carbohydrates
    craving for, 508
    in diabetic diet, 198–99
    malabsorption of, 269
    nausea treated by, 442, 443
    triglycerides and, 610
Carbon dioxide, 352
Carmex, 133
Carmol (10 or 20), 166, 195
Carotid artery, right, 580
Carpal tunnel syndrome, 114–18
Carrots, 140, 214
Car seats, 43
Cascara sagrada, 164
Castor oil, 90, 109, 302, 627
Cataracts, dermatitis and, 196
Cats. *See also* Pet problems
    bites from, 58–59
    fleas and, 478, 480
Cellulite, 119–22
Cervical cancer, herpes and, 301
Cetylpridinium chloride, 306
Chafing, 122–24

Chamomile, 166, 260, 425, 551, 553
Chapped hands, 125–30
Chapped lips, 131–34
Charcoal, activated, 139, 269–70, 310, 559
Cheese, 47, 409–10, 587–88
Cherries, 310
Chest pain, from angina, 14, 15
Chicken soup, 146
Chickweed, 349
Children. *See also* Aspirin; Infants
    bed-wetting by, 50–51
    diarrhea in, 214
    ear infections in, 230–33
    fever in, 258, 259, 262
    hiccups in, 347
    insect stings in, 559
    Reye's syndrome in, 231, 262, 273, 552
    thermometer use for, 261
    Tylenol for, 590
Chlorine, 56, 158, 223
Chloroform, 530
Chlor-Trimeton, 349, 496
Chocolate, 327, 331–32, 508
Cholesterol, 135–42, 608
    angina and, 15, 17
    in diabetic diet, 199
    impotence from, 356
    intermittent claudication and, 384–85
Chromium G.T.F., 204
Cigarette smoking. *See* Smoking, conditions caused or aggravated by
Cilia, 501, 541
Circadian rhythms, 252–53, 375, 377, 391
Circulation
    bandaging and, 173–74
    phlebitis and, 486, 487

Rodale Press, Inc., publishes PREVENTION, America's leading health magazine.
For information on how to order your subscription,
write to PREVENTION, Emmaus, PA 18098.